AF778482

Mechanical Circulatory Support in End-Stage Heart Failure

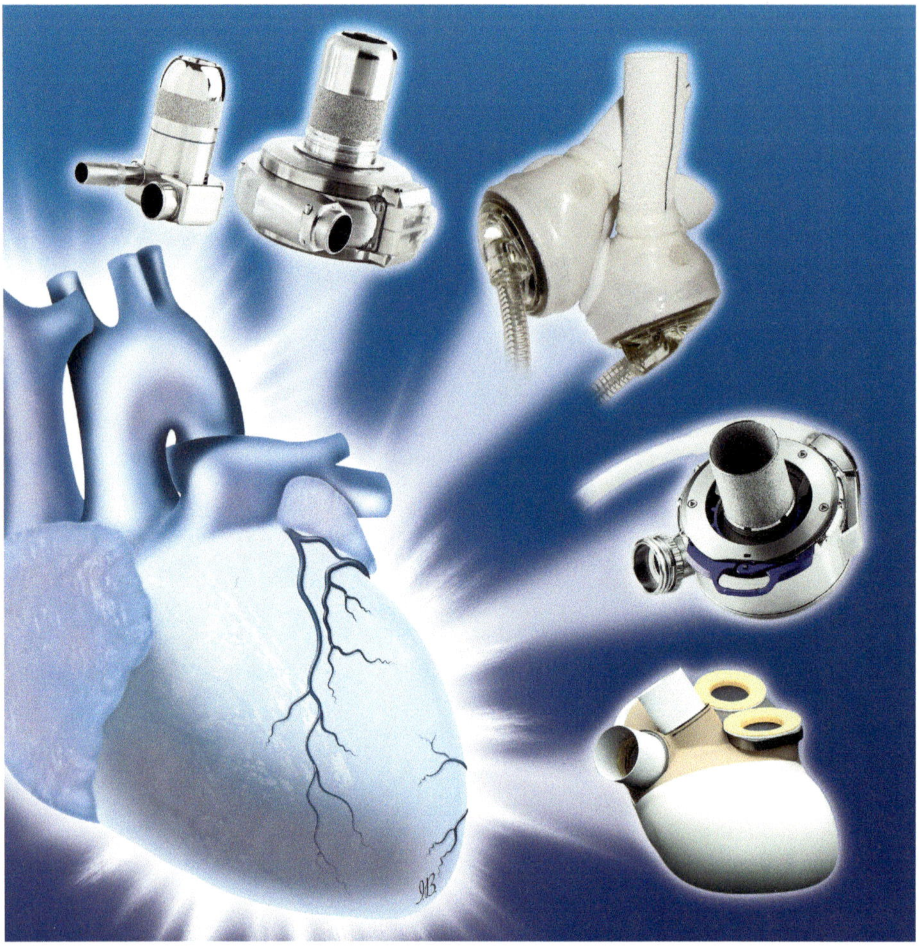

Andrea Montalto
Antonio Loforte
Francesco Musumeci
Thomas Krabatsch
Mark S. Slaughter
Editors

Mechanical Circulatory Support in End-Stage Heart Failure

A Practical Manual

In collaboration with Cristiano Amarelli

Springer

Editors
Andrea Montalto
San Camillo-Forlanini Hospital
Rome, Italy

Antonio Loforte
Cardiac Surgery
S.Orsola-Malpighi Hospital
Bologna, Italy

Francesco Musumeci
San Camillo-Forlanini Hospital
Rome, Italy

Thomas Krabatsch
Deutsches Herzzentrum Berlin
Berlin, Germany

Mark S. Slaughter
Department of Cardiovascular
and Thoracic Surgery
University of Louisville
Louisville, KY, USA

ISBN 978-3-319-43381-3 ISBN 978-3-319-43383-7 (eBook)
DOI 10.1007/978-3-319-43383-7

Library of Congress Control Number: 2017943505

© Springer International Publishing Switzerland 2017
This work is subject to copyright. All rights are reserved by the Publisher, whether the whole or part of the material is concerned, specifically the rights of translation, reprinting, reuse of illustrations, recitation, broadcasting, reproduction on microfilms or in any other physical way, and transmission or information storage and retrieval, electronic adaptation, computer software, or by similar or dissimilar methodology now known or hereafter developed.
The use of general descriptive names, registered names, trademarks, service marks, etc. in this publication does not imply, even in the absence of a specific statement, that such names are exempt from the relevant protective laws and regulations and therefore free for general use.
The publisher, the authors and the editors are safe to assume that the advice and information in this book are believed to be true and accurate at the date of publication. Neither the publisher nor the authors or the editors give a warranty, express or implied, with respect to the material contained herein or for any errors or omissions that may have been made. The publisher remains neutral with regard to jurisdictional claims in published maps and institutional affiliations.

Printed on acid-free paper

This Springer imprint is published by Springer Nature
The registered company is Springer International Publishing AG
The registered company address is: Gewerbestrasse 11, 6330 Cham, Switzerland

To all patients whose desire for a better life inspired me

Andrea Montalto

To my beloved daughter, Alessandra, and wife, Elisa

Antonio Loforte

To my relatives and friends
who cared and loved me, supporting my curiosity and perseverance after the loss of my father

Cristiano Amarelli

Preface

> *We are all God's knights and knights of life.*
> *This is my destiny, this is the message that God tells me to bring.*
> *A message of life and hope for me and for others.*
> *Whatever happens do not close my sufferings in a drawer or a sad thought.*
> *I was always smiling. Remember my smile and my will to live.*
> *Go ahead and tell it so that it can be of relief and hope for others.*
> *It should be a happy memory.*
> *So in the worst case a knight will become an angel.*
> *Mario C.*

End-stage acute and chronic heart failure refractory to maximal pharmacological therapy carries a poor chance of survival for patients unless they undergo heart transplantation. Heart transplantation is restricted by age and comorbidities to a small group of patients, and the actual donor's shortage does not meet properly the demand of patients on waiting list. Mechanical circulatory support is a valid temporary solution before heart transplantation, whose results are playing the role of a game-changer in such a challenging field. The choice and management of the right device for every patient remains tricky. Giving the equipoise of the short and even the midterm results between LVADs and heart transplantation experienced in the last decade, the use as destination therapy is gaining space, permitting to promptly treat a wider patient population. Prompt availability and cost-effectiveness as unique constraint are the mainstreams of the mechanical solution. The proper selection of candidates for VAD or TAH implantation remains a challenging clinical decision. Patients who are too compromised may have an elevated risk of mortality postoperatively while patients with an early heart dysfunction scenario may have a poor benefit, thus being more exposed to device-related complications. Preoperative hemodynamic and clinical scenarios which may occur are extremely different from those the clinicians routinely have to face up to with traditional cardiac surgery therapy. Proper management and interpretation of MCS-related complications is an additional concern to deal with particularly in the case of non-hub and well-trained centers. Moreover, the psychological aspects and views of long-term VAD/TAH recipients which may influence the overall outcome should not be underestimated.

The complexity of MCS therapy and its clinical landscape, as well as the devotion of free minds in discovering, always case by case, the adequate treatment of such a delicate patient population, stimulated all of us to develop such an ambitious project. We aimed at building a textbook that would be a practical guide in terms of correct and well-accepted management of patients undergoing implantation of VAD and TAH. Our goal was to move up from a pioneer's phase of MCS adopted in few centers in the world to a world-wide standardized and shared management of a such effective therapy. In order to accomplish all of the above, we approached all those renowned centers and physicians worldwide who, over the years, have spent interest and time mostly in studying deeply such a delicate medicine field which is heart failure mechanical treatment. We encouraged all authors to enrich their contributions with tables and algorithms in order to render each chapters adoptable as a guiding protocol, thus providing keys for the resolution of any kind of traditionally discussed issue. Our goal has been welcomed with great enthusiasm by all authors who have fully grasped the essence of this project. It is therefore with great satisfaction that we thank all those who, despite the onerous work commitments, have devoted their time to the realization of this book which we hope will be a valuable tool to improve survival and quality of life of those people who are living thanks to an artificial heart support system.

Andrea Montalto
Rome, Italy

Antonio Loforte
Bologna, Italy

Francesco Musumeci
Rome, Italy

Thomas Krabatsch
Berlin, Germany

Mark S. Slaughter
Louisville, USA

Contents

II Intraoperative Tips and Pitfalls

Editors and Contributors

About the Editors

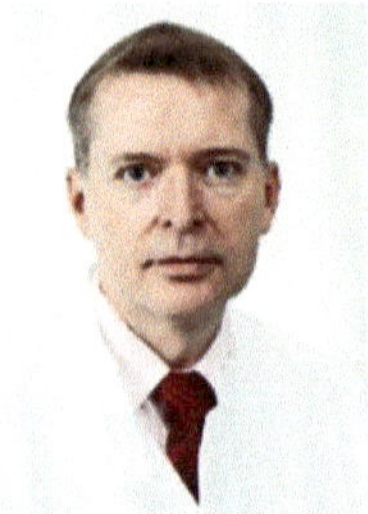

Thomas Krabatsch, MD, PhD

Dr. Krabatsch is senior cardiac surgeon at the Deutsches Herzzentrum in Berlin with expertise in the surgical treatment of a variety of cardiovascular diseases in adults including severe diffuse coronary artery disease and valvular heart diseases, in mechanical circulatory support, and in transplantation. He is the director of the Deutsches Herzzentrum Berlin's mechanical circulatory support team, which has carried out over 2800 implants. Dr. Krabatsch's basic science research interests include processes and mechanisms at the machine-human body interface, pump technology, and heart failure. He is a member of the ISHLT, EACTS, DGTHG, the German Society for Gene Therapy, and the BBGHK and author or coauthor of more than 150 scientific articles. Dr. Krabatsch also collaborates with several universities and cardiosurgical hospitals in Eastern Europe, such as Russia, Belarus, Bosnia, and Hungary. He is honorary professor in one of the Russian largest medical schools.

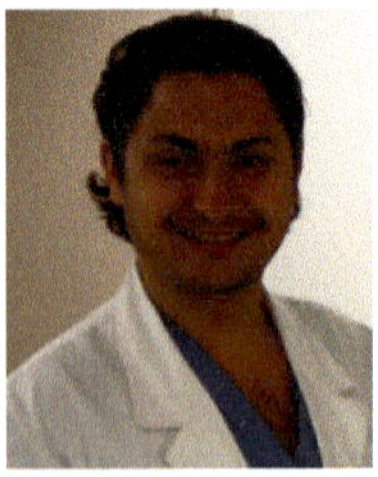

Dr. Antonio Loforte, MD, PhD

Dr. Loforte is currently staff surgeon and cochair of the mechanical circulatory support program at the Department of Cardiothoracic, Transplantation and Vascular Surgery, S. Orsola Hospital, University of Bologna, Italy. He completed his cardiothoracic surgery residency at the University of Bologna, S. Orsola Hospital (Italy); at St. Antonius Ziekenhuis, Nieuwegein (the Netherlands); and the Deutsches Herzzentrum Berlin (Germany). He additionally joined the Michael E. DeBakey Department of Surgery, Division of Transplant and Assist Devices, in Houston, Texas, USA. Dr. Loforte is member of a number of professional organizations including the prestigious STS, ISHLT, ASAIO, EACTS, RHICS, and SICCH among others. His bibliography lists over 60 peer-reviewed original articles, 180 abstracts (communications) for international meetings and 10 book chapters. He serves as a reviewer for 21 international journals and is on the editorial board in 9. He got a "European PhD label" in organ transplantation and three international awards in Europe and the USA.

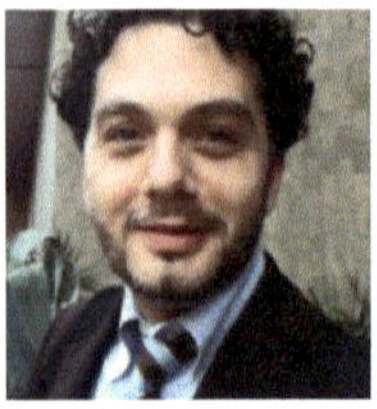

Dr. Andrea Montalto, MD

Dr. Montalto obtained his medical degree at the University of Naples "Federico II" School of Medicine in Naples, Italy. After completing the residency in cardiac surgery at the University of Naples Federico II, he completed his training at the Cardiac Surgery Center of the San Camillo Hospital in Rome, Italy. Since 2006, he is permanent staff surgeon at the Department of Cardiac Surgery and Transplantation of the San Camillo Hospital. Dr. Montalto has shown particular interest in the field of surgical treatment of advanced heart failure, becoming familiar with the management of patients implanted with mechanical devices and is head of the VAD program of the Cardiac Surgery Center at the San Camillo Hospital since 2012. He is an active member of SICCH and EUROMACS.

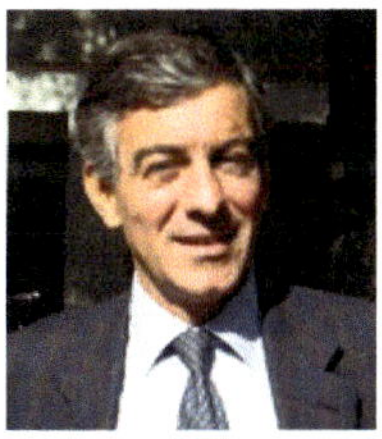

Francesco Musumeci, MD, FECTS

Dr. Musumeci is director of the Cardiac Surgery and Transplantation and director of the Department of Cardiovascular Medicine at the San Camillo Hospital in Rome, Italy. He had his cardiac surgical training in London and between 1987 and 1990 he was senior registrar at the Harefield Hospital. In 1991 he was appointed consultant cardiac surgeon at the University Hospital of Wales. In 1998 moved back to Rome as director of Cardiac Surgery at the San Camillo Hospital. His clinical interests have been focused on heart failure surgery including transplantation and mechanical circulatory support and on minimally invasive surgery which is the standard surgical approach for all valve pathologies. In November 2011 the Robot Assisted Cardiac Surgical Program was started. The department has also a large experience in TAVI. Dr. Musumeci is elected president of the SICCH (Italian Society of Cardiac Surgery) for the years 2017–2018.

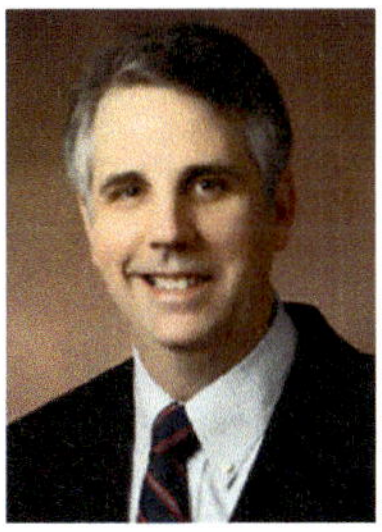

Dr. Mark S. Slaughter, MD

Dr. Slaughter is professor of surgery and chair of the Department of Cardiovascular and Thoracic Surgery at the University of Louisville, KY, USA, and is an adjunct professor in the Department of Bioengineering. Dr. Slaughter currently serves as a consultant to the FDA Medical Device Review Panel and a National Science Foundation SBIR/STTR grant reviewer and previously served two terms for the Health and Human Services Medicare Coverage Advisory Committee. In addition, he serves on the Ethics Committee and the Education Committee for the American Association for Thoracic Surgery and is a councilor for the Southern Thoracic Surgical Association. Dr. Slaughter has served as the president of the American Society for Artificial Internal Organs and president of the International Society for Rotary Blood Pumps. He currently is the editor in chief of the *American Society for Artificial Internal Organs* journal and also serves as an associate editor for the *Annals of Thoracic Surgery*.

Contributors

Robert M. Adamson
Department of Cardiothoracic Surgery
Sharp Memorial Hospital
San Diego, CA, USA

Larry A. Allen
Section of Advanced Heart Failure
Division of Cardiology
University of Colorado School of Medicine
Aurora, CO, USA

Cristiano Amarelli
Department of Cardiovascular Surgery
and Trasplantation
Monaldi Hospital
Naples, Italy

Antonio Amodeo
Department of Pediatric Cardiac Surgery
Ospedale Pediatrico Bambino Gesù
Rome, Italy

Emanuela Angeli
Department of Pediatric Cardiac Surgery and
Transplantation
S. Orsola-Malpighi Hospital, Bologna
University
Bologna, Italy

Martine Antoine
Department of Cardiac Surgery
Erasme Hospital, Free University of Brussels
Brussels, Belgium

Francisco A. Arabia
Heart Institute, Cedars-Sinai Medical Center
Los Angeles
California, USA

Matteo Attisani
Division of Cardiac Surgery
Città della Salute e della Scienza University
of Turin
Turin, Italy

Lorenzo Bagozzi
Division of Cardiac Surgery
Department of Cardiac
Thoracic and Vascular Sciences
University of Padua
Padova, Italy

Massimo Baiocchi
Anesthesia and Intensive Care Unit
Cardiovascular and thoracic Department
S. Orsola-Malpighi University Hospital Bologna
Bologna, Italy

Alessandro Barbone
Department of Cardiac Surgery
Istituto Clinico Humanitas
Rozzano, Milan, Italy

Rachel A. Beaupré
Center for Circulatory Support
Texas Heart Institute
Baylor College of Medicine
Houston, TX, USA

Jonida Bejko
Division of Cardiac Surgery
Department of Cardiac, Thoracic and Vascular
Sciences
University of Padua
Padua, Italy

Fabio Bellotto
Preventive Cardiology and Rehabilitation
Institute Codivilla-Putti
Cortina D'Ampezzo, Italy

Giovanni Benedetti
Cardiothoracic Department
University Hospital
Udine, Italy

M. Benedetto
Anesthesia and Intensive Care Unit
Campus BioMedico University Hospital
Rome, Italy

Felix Berger
Department of Pediatric Cardiology
and Congenital Heart Diseases
Deutsches Herzzentrum Berlin
Berlin, Germany

Giacomo Bortolussi
Division of Cardiac Surgery
Department of Cardiac, Thoracic and
Vascular Sciences
University of Padua
Padua, Italy

Robin Bostic
Thoratec Inc.
Pleasanton, CA, USA

Tomaso Bottio
Division of Cardiac Surgery
Department of Cardiac, Thoracic
and Vascular Sciences
University of Padua
Padua, Italy

Nicolas A. Brozzi
University of Miami
Division of Thoracic Transplant
and Mechanical Circulatory Support
Miami, FL, USA

Holger Buchholz
Integrative Health Institute (IHI)
University of Alberta
Edmonton, AB, Canada

Marianna Buonocore
AZ Sint Jan
Brugge, Belgium

Edward J Burke
Thoratec Inc.
Pleasanton, CA, USA

Alain Carpentier
Department of Cardiovascular Surgery
Hôpital Européen Georges Pompidou
Assistance Publique-Hôpitaux de Paris
Université Paris Descartes
Paris, France

Lucio Careddu
Department of Pediatric Cardiac Surgery
and Transplantation
S. Orsola-Malpighi Hospital
Bologna University
Bologna, Italy

Evaristo Castedo
Espamacs and Hospital Universitario Puerta
de Hierro Majadahonda
Madrid, Spain

Katherine Chorpenning
HeartWare Inc.
Miami, FL, USA

Dawn M. Christensen
MyLVAD, Innovative Program Solutions, LLC
Pine Grove, PA, USA

Manlio Cipriani
"A. de Gasperis" CardioCenter
Niguarda Great Metropolitan Hospital
Milan, Italy

Colleen Pietras
Division of Cardiovascular Surgery
Mayo Clinic
Rochester, MN, USA

Leonida Compostella
Preventive Cardiology and Rehabilitation
Institute Codivilla-Putti
Cortina D'Ampezzo, Italy

Jennifer Conway
Integrative Health Institute (IHI)
University of Alberta
Edmonton, AB, Canada

Jack Copeland
UCSD Cardiovascular Center
The University of Arizona Health Network
University of Arizona
Tucson, USA

Michael Dandel
Department of Cardiology
Deutsches Herzzentrum Berlin
Berlin, Germany

Theo M.M.H. de By
Euromacs e.V. c/o Deutsches Herzzentrum
Berlin
Berlin, Germany

Fabrizio De Rita
Department of Congenital Cardiothoracic
Surgery
Freeman Hospital
Newcastle Upon Tyne, UK

Ezin Deniz
Department of Cardiothoracic, Transplantation
and Vascular Surgery
Hannover Medical School
Hannover, Germany

Walter P. Dembistky
Department of Cardiothoracic Surgery
Sharp Memorial Hospital
San Diego, CA, USA

Arianna Di Molfetta
Bambino Gesù Childrens Hospital
Department of Pediatric Cardiac
Surgery
MCS Unit
Rome, Italy

S. Ersel
Berlin Heart GmbH
Berlin, Germany

David Feldman
University of Cincinnati Medical Center
Cincinnati, OH, USA

Christina Feldmann
Department of Cardiothoracic, Transplantation,
and Vascular Surgery
Hannover Medical School
Hannover, Germany

Sergio Filippelli
Department of Pediatric Cardiac
Surgery
Ospedale Pediatrico Bambino Gesù
Rome, Italy

Arnt E. Fiane
Department of Cardiothoracic Surgery
and Transplantation
Oslo University Hospital
Oslo, Norway

Rodger G. Ford
ReliantHeart Inc.
Houston, TX, USA

O.H. Frazier
Center for Cardiac Support, Cardiovascular
Surgery Research
Texas Heart Institute University of Texas Health
Science Center in Houston
Houston, TX, USA
e-mail: lschwenke@texasheart.org

Guido Frascaroli
Anesthesia and Intensive Care Unit,
Cardiovascular and Thoracic Department
S. Orsola-Malpighi University Hospital Bologna
Bologna, Italy

Maria Frigerio
"A. de Gasperis" CardioCenter
Niguarda Great Metropolitan Hospital
Milan, Italy

Gaetano Gargiulo
Department of Pediatric Cardiac Surgery
and Transplantation
S. Orsola-Malpighi Hospital
Bologna University
Bologna, Italy

Gino Gerosa
Division of Cardiac Surgery
Department of Cardiac, Thoracic
and Vascular Sciences
University of Padua
Padua, Italy

Paul W. Goetz
Division of Cardiac Surgery
Department of Surgery and Department
of Psychiatry Feinberg School of Medicine
Chicago, IL, USA

Andrew B. Goldstone
Department of Cardiothoracic Surgery
Stanford University school of Medicine
California, USA

Kathleen L. Grady
Division of Cardiac Surgery
Feinberg School of Medicine
Northwestern University
Chicago, IL, USA

Francesco Grigioni
Department of Cardiology and Transplantation
S. Orsola-Malpighi Hospital
Bologna University
Bologna, Italy
e-mail: francesco.grigioni@unibo.it

Jan Gummert
Department of Cardiothoracic Surgery
Heart and Diabetes Center
North Rhine-Westphalia
Bad Oeynhausen, Germany

Shelley A. Hall
Department of Cardiac Transplant
Baylor University Medical Center at Dallas
Dallas, TX, USA

Margaret M. Hannan
Mater Misericordiae University Hospital
University College Dublin
Dublin, Ireland

Jasmin S. Hanke
Department of Cardiothoracic, Transplantation, and Vascular Surgery
Hannover Medical School
Hannover, Germany

Asif Hasan
Department of Congenital Cardiothoracic Surgery
Freeman Hospital
Newcastle Upon Tyne, UK

Axel Haverich
Department of Cardiothoracic, Transplantation, and Vascular Surgery
Hannover Medical School
Hannover, Germany

Michael Hübler
University Children's Hospital
Department of Congenital Pediatric Surgery
Zurich, Switzerland

Piet Jansen
Carmat SA
Vélizy-Villacoublay, France

Robert Jarvik
Jarvik Heart Inc.
New York, USA

David L. Joyce
Division of Cardiovascular Surgery Mayo Clinic
Rochester, MN, USA

Friedrich Kaufmann
Department of Cardiothoracic and Vascular Surgery
Deutsches Herzzentrum Berlin
Berlin, Germany

Reiner Koerfer
Klinikum Niederrhein, Department of Thoracic and Cardiovascular Surgery
Duisburg, Germany

Andreas Koster
Department of Anesthesiology,
Heart and Diabetes Center North Rhine-Westphalia
Bad Oeynhausen, Germany

Thomas Krabatsch
Department of Cardiothoracic and Vascular surgery
Deutsches Herzzentrum Berlin
Berlin, Germany

Marian Kukucka
Department of Anesthesiology
Deutsches Herzzentrum Berlin
Berlin, Germany

Mark Lamotte
Physiotherapy and Rehabilitation Department
Erasme Hospital, Free University of Brussels
Brussels, Belgium

Jeff A. LaRose
HeartWare Inc.
Miami, FL, USA

Christian Latrémouille
Department of Cardiovascular Surgery
Hôpital Européen Georges Pompidou,
Assistance Publique-Hôpitaux de Paris
Université Paris Descartes
Paris, France

Karl K. Limmer
Department of Cardiothoracic Surgery
Sharp Memorial Hospital
San Diego, CA, USA

Ugolino Livi
Cardiothoracic Department
University Hospital
Udine, Italy

Matthias Loebe
Leonard M. Miller School of Medicine at
University of Miami
Division of Thoracic Transplant and Mechanical
Circulatory Support
Miami, FL, USA

Antonio Loforte
Department of Cardiovascular Surgery and
Transplantation
S. Orsola-Malpighi Hospital
Bologna University
Bologna, Italy

Angela Lorts
Cincinnati Children's Hospital Medical Center
Cincinnati, OH, USA

Ciro Maiello
Department of Cardiovascular Surgery and
Trasplantation
Monaldi Hospital, Az. dei Colli
Naples, Italy

Simon Maltais
Department of Cardiac Surgery Mayo Clinic
Rochester, MN, USA

Ares K. Menon
Berlin Heart GmbH
Berlin, Germany

Giuseppe Marinelli
Department of Cardiovascular Surgery
and Transplantation
S. Orsola-Malpighi Hospital
Bologna University
Bologna, Italy

Antonella Marino
Ventricular Assist Devices, Vega S.p.A
Bollate, Italy

Marco Masetti
Department of Cardiology and Transplantation
S. Orsola-Malpighi Hospital
Bologna University
Bologna, Italy

Anna L. Meyer
Department of Cardiothoracic Surgery
Heart Center Leipzig, University of Leipzig
Leipzig, Germany

Bart P. Meyns
Department of Cardiac Surgery
Katholieke Universiteit Leuven
Leuven, Belgium

Oliver Miera
Department of Pediatric Cardiology
and Congenital Heart Diseases
Deutsches Herzzentrum Berlin
Berlin, Germany

Carmelo A. Milano
Department Cardiovascular and Thoracic
Surgery Duke University Medical Center
Durham, NC, USA

Nader Moazami
Kaufman Center for Heart Transplantation and
Mechanical Circulatory Support - Department
of Thoracic and Cardiovascular Surgery,
Cleveland Clinic
Department of Biomedical Engineering
Lerner Institute of Research
Cleveland, OH, USA

Paul Mohacsi
Department of Cardiology
Swiss Cardiovascular Center
University Hospital (Inselspital)
Bern, Switzerland

Andrea Montalto
Department of Cardiac Surgery and Heart
Transplantation
San Camillo Hospital
Rome, Italy

David L.S. Morales
Department of Cardiothoracic Surgery
The Heart Institute Cincinnati Children's Hospital Medical Center
University of Cincinnati College of Medicine
Cincinnati, OH, USA

Jeffrey A. Morgan
Center for Cardiac Support, Cardiovascular Surgery Research
Texas Heart Institute
University of Texas Health Science Center in Houston
Houston, TX, USA

Francesco Moscato
Center for Medical Physics and Biomedical Engineering
Medical University of Vienna, Ludwig Boltzmann Cluster for Cardiovascular Research
Vienna, Austria

Francesco Musumeci
Director of Cardiovascular Medicine
Director of Cardiac Surgery and Transplantation
San Camillo-Forlanini Hospital
Rome, Italy

Yoshifumi Naka
Division of Cardiac, Thoracic and Vascular Surgery
Columbia University Medical Center
New York, NY, USA

Ivan Netuka
Department of Cardiac Surgery
Institute for Clinical and Experimental Medicine
Charles University in Prague
Prague, Czech Republic

Alina Nicoara
Duke University Medical Center
Durham, NC, USA

Fabrizio Oliva
"A. de Gasperis" CardioCenter
Niguarda Great Metropolitan Hospital
Milan, Italy

Helena Ortis
Cardiothoracic Department
University Hospital
Udine, Italy

Federico Pappalardo
Department of Anesthesia and Intensive Care
IRCCS San Raffaele Scientific Institute
Milan, Italy

Centofanti Paolo
Division of Cardiac Surgery
Città della Salute e della Scienza University of Turin
Turin, Italy

Christopher Parker
Thoratec Inc.
Pleasanton, CA, USA

Gianluigi Perri
Department of Pediatric Cardiac Surgery
Ospedale Pediatrico Bambino Gesù
Rome, Italy

Vito Piazza
Division of Cardiology
Department of Cardiac Surgery and Heart Transplantation
San Camillo Hospital
Rome, Italy
vitopiazza@inwind.it

Marina Pieri
Department of Anesthesia and Intensive Care
IRCCS San Raffaele Scientific Institute
Milan, Italy

Massimiliano Polastri
Physical Medicine and Rehabilitation
University Hospital S. Orsola-Malpighi
Bologna, Italy

Evgenij Potapov
Department of Cardiothoracic and Vascular Surgery
Deutsches Herzzentrum Berlin
Berlin, Germany

Luciano Potena
Department of Cardiology and Transplantation
S. Orsola-Malpighi Hospital
Bologna University
Bologna, Italy

Luca Ragni
Department of Pediatric Cardiac Surgery
and Transplantation
S. Orsola-Malpighi Hospital
Bologna University
Bologna, Italy

Mauro Rinaldi
Division of Cardiac Surgery
Città della Salute e della Scienza
University of Turin
Turin, Italy

Sebastian V. Rojas
Department of Cardiothoracic, Transplantation,
and Vascular Surgery
Hannover Medical School
Hannover, Germany

Diyar Saeed
Department of Cardiovascular Surgery
Heinrich-Heine University of Düsseldorf
Düsseldorf, Germany

Anna Mara Scandroglio
Department of Anesthesia and Intensive
Care
IRCCS San Raffaele Scientific Institute
Milan, Italy

Heinrich Schima
Center for Medical Physics and Biomedical
Engineering
Medical University of Vienna, Ludwig
Boltzmann Cluster for Cardiovascular
Research
Vienna, Austria

Thomas Schlöglhofer
Center for Medical Physics and Biomedical
Engineering
Department of Cardiac Surgery Medical
University of Vienna
Vienna, Austria

K.R. Schmitt
Department of Pediatric Cardiology and
Congenital Heart Diseases
Deutsches Herzzentrum Berlin
Berlin, Germany

Jan D. Schmitto
Department of Cardiothoracic, Transplantation,
and Vascular Surgery
Hannover Medical School
Hannover, Germany

Stephan Schueler
Department of Cardiothoracic Surgery
Newcastle Upon Tyne Freeman Hospital
Newcastle Upon Tyne, UK

Martin Schweiger
University Children's Hospital
Department of Congenital Pediatric
Surgery
Zurich, Switzerland

Melody Sherwood
Department of Cardiac Transplant
University Medical Center at Dallas
Dallas, TX, USA

Yasuhiro Shudo
Department of Cardiothoracic
Surgery
Stanford University school of Medicine
Stanford, CA, USA

Mark S. Slaughter
Professor and Chair
Department of Cardiovascular
and Thoracic Surgery
University of Louisville
Luoisville, KY, USA

Gro Sorenson
Oslo University Hospital
Oslo, Norway

Sotirios Spiliopoulos
Department for the Surgical Therapy of
End-stage Heart Failure and Mechanical
Circulatory Support
Heart and Vascular Center Duisburg
Duisburg, Germany

Alexander Stepanenko
Department of Cardiothoracic
and Vascular Surgery
Deutsches Herzzentrum Berlin
Berlin, Germany

Hiroo Takayama
Divisions of Cardiac, Thoracic
and Vascular Surgery
Columbia University Medical Center
New York, NY, USA

Koji Takeda
Divisions of Cardiac, Thoracic
and Vascular Surgery
Columbia University Medical Center
New York, NY, USA

Daniel Tamez
HeartWare Inc.
Miami, FL, USA

Paul C. Tang
University of Wisconsin Hospitals
and Clinics Madison
Madison, WI, USA

Vincenzo Tarzia
Division of Cardiac Surgery
Department of Cardiac, Thoracic
and Vascular Sciences
University of Padua
Padua, Italy

Gero Tenderich
Department for the Surgical Therapy of
End-stage Heart Failure and Mechanical
Circulatory Support
Heart and Vascular Center Duisburg
Duisburg, Germany

Steven Tsui
Department of Cardiothoracic Surgery
Papworth Hospital
Papworth Everard, CA, UK

Nir Uriel
New York Presbyterian Hospital Columbia
University Medical Center
New York, NY, USA

Christina VanderPluym
Boston Children's Hospital
Boston, MA, USA

Juliane Vierecke
Deutsches Herzzentrum Berlin
Berlin, Germany

Chet R. Villa
Department of Pediatric Cardiology
The Heart Institute Cincinnati Children's
Hospital Medical Center
University of Cincinnati College of Medicine
Cincinnati, OH, USA

Oliver Voigt
SynCardia Systems Europe GmbH
Bad Oeynhausen, Germany

Hanjay Wang
Department of Cardiothoracic Surgery
Stanford University School of Medicine
Stanford, CA, USA

Georg Wieselthaler
Cardiac Transplantation and Mechanical
Circulatory Support
University of California
San Francisco, CA, USA

Y. Joseph Woo
Department of Cardiothoracic Surgery
Stanford University School of Medicine
Stanford, CA, USA

Daisuke Yoshioka
Divisions of Cardiac, Thoracic
and Vascular Surgery
Columbia University Medical Center
New York, NY, USA

Daniel Zimpfer
Department of Cardiac Surgery Medical
University of Vienna
Vienna, Austria

Invited Lecture "Pioneering the Future: From Transplant to Device Development"

O.H. Frazier

© Springer International Publishing Switzerland 2017
A. Montalto et al. (eds.), *Mechanical Circulatory Support in End-Stage Heart Failure*,
DOI 10.1007/978-3-319-43383-7_1

One of the most important scientific breakthroughs of the modern era has been the ability to support or replace the failing heart. Heart transplantation and mechanical circulatory support (MCS) are now so widely accepted that it is easy to forget what a short history they have. However, the concept of cardiac support and replacement is not new. It may even have been foreshadowed by the biblical prophet Ezekiel, who said, "A new heart also will I give you, and a new spirit will I put within you: and I will take away the stony heart out of your flesh, and I will give you an heart of flesh" [1].

Until the twentieth century, the heart was considered off-limits to surgeons except for occasional desperate repairs of cardiac wounds. Ironically, World War II provided an important stimulus for the growth of cardiovascular surgery because of the experience gained in treating battlefield injuries. The next breakthroughs were achieved in the field of congenital heart defects, including ligation of a patent ductus arteriosus (Robert E. Gross, 1938) and the use of extracardiac shunts to correct cyanotic congenital heart defects, predominantly caused by tetralogy of Fallot (Alfred Blalock and Helen B. Taussig, 1944). A few surgeons also performed closed-heart procedures to treat valvular defects. Without stopping the heart and opening it, however, they were unable to view the intracardiac structures. Numerous researchers were working to design a heart-lung machine that could temporarily assume cardiopulmonary function. The first surgeon to perform a successful open-heart operation was John H. Gibbon, Jr. In 1953, he used a machine of his own design that allowed him to repair an atrial septal defect in an 18-year-old girl. Although the patient survived, Gibbon's three other young open-heart patients died. He was so discouraged that he gave up on "his" machine. Subsequently, other researchers continued to develop and improve it [2]. However, Gibbon deserves special credit for being the first to show that a mechanical pump could at least temporarily sustain human life.

Around the same time, an unusual open-heart technique was singularly developed by C. Walton Lillehei at the University of Minnesota. This technique, known as cross-circulation [3], was used for correcting congenital heart defects in children. One of the child's parents served as a "living heart-lung machine." After the child's circulatory system was connected to that of the parent, the child's heart could be stopped and the defect repaired. Lillehei introduced this approach to open-heart surgery in 1954 with some success, thus demonstrating that open-heart surgical repairs could be successfully performed. However, its limited application to children with parents made it imperative that the heart-lung machine be successful. Dr. Denton Cooley visited with Lillehei in 1955 and saw the bubble oxygenator being developed by Lillehei and DeWall and performed the first heart surgery in Houston using a similar device in April of 1956 [4]. By the end of that year, Dr. Cooley reported performing 94 cases [5], twice the number of the University of Minnesota and the Mayo Clinic (the only other sites performing open-heart surgery) combined. The program at the Texas Heart Institute continued to perform more heart surgery than any program in the world for the next 30 years.

In the middle of the twentieth century, the USA was the world's economic leader, with enough capital to fund many scientific and medical advances. In the early 1960s, during the charismatic presidency of John F. Kennedy, Americans were increasingly optimistic about the possibility of achieving many humanitarian and scientific goals, including halting wars, ending hunger, and curing disease. We were also determined to set foot on the moon by the end of the decade as well as developing an artificial heart. We did perform the impressive feat of landing on the moon, but the other goals remain elusive.

With regard to heart transplantation and replacement, significant advances had already been achieved in animals, most notably by Alexis Carrel, a French surgeon, and by Vladimir Demikhov, a Russian scientist. Between 1902 and 1909, Carrel performed successful transplants of the heart and other organs in dogs [6]. As a fourth-year biology student, Demikhov designed an implantable total artificial heart (TAH), which he tested in a dog that survived for 2.5 h; although this experiment was performed in 1938, Demikhov's work was largely unknown outside the Soviet Union until the 1960s [7]. These feats were highly experimental and had never been attempted in the clinical arena.

In 1964, with the support of President Lyndon Johnson, Dr. Michael DeBakey convinced the US National Institutes of Health to fund the development of a workable TAH. As chairman of the Department of Surgery at Baylor College of

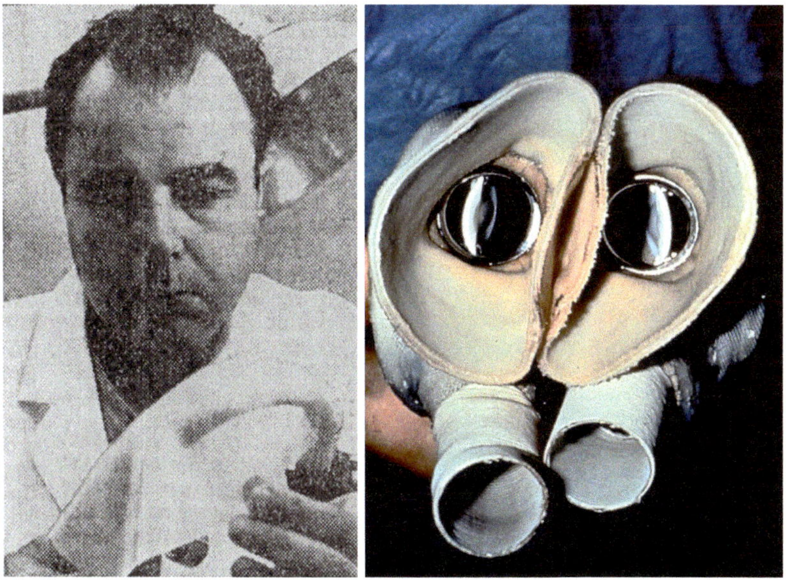

Fig. 1.1 Dr. Domingo Liotta (*left*) and his TAH (*right*)

Medicine, in Houston, DeBakey was a pioneering heart surgeon with considerable political clout. He believed that the development of a TAH, like the moon landing, could be accomplished within the decade. Accordingly, Baylor researchers began a series of calf experiments led by Domingo Liotta, an Argentinian physician with a long-standing interest in the artificial heart (Fig. 1.1).

My own involvement with MCS systems dates from 1965, when I was a medical student at Baylor. All medical students were required to have a research project, and as a result I worked under Liotta's direction on the TAH. Although the Baylor TAH worked well for short periods in calves, none of the early experiments resulted in 24-h survival. As a result, DeBakey decided that the TAH was unready for clinical use. The clinical efforts of the program shifted to the partial artificial heart or left ventricular assist device (LVAD). In 1966, DeBakey performed the first successful clinical implantation of an LVAD. The patient, a 37-year-old woman, was supported by the device for 10 days. During this period, she recovered sufficiently that the pump could be removed. By the late 1960s, DeBakey had used the LVAD in several patients, two of whom survived [8]. I was on his service at the time, and the experience further enhanced my dedication to this endeavor.

On December 9, 1967, the first human heart transplant was performed on December 9 by Christiaan Barnard, in Cape Town, South Africa. The initial results were so promising that the procedure was soon adopted by many other surgeons throughout the world. Application of this therapy was severely limited by the scarcity of donor hearts. At Baylor, Dr. Liotta envisioned that the TAH could serve as a short-term "bridge" until a donor heart was available to heart transplantation. At that time, Denton Cooley was also on the staff at Baylor. As a renowned cardiovascular pioneer, Cooley was the world's most experienced heart surgeon. He had founded the Texas Heart Institute (THI), of which he was surgeon-in-chief. In May 1968, Cooley performed the first successful heart transplant in the USA [9]. Within a few months, he had gained the world's most extensive experience with this procedure. In late 1968, Liotta approached Cooley and asked if he would consider using a TAH as a bridge to transplantation. Cooley agreed to this plan but insisted that the device be used only in an emergency and after the completion of more animal experiments. Before long, Dr. Liotta had a calf that survived for 44 h while being totally supported by the TAH.

In April 1969, Cooley implanted the artificial heart in Haskell Karp, a 47-year-old man who could not have survived without the device [10]. After the implant, the patient was alive, awake, and in stable condition. The TAH kept him alive for 64 h, until a transplant could be performed. Unfortunately, immunosuppression was poorly understood at that time. Mr. Karp began receiving immune suppressants when the TAH was implanted. By the time of the transplant, his

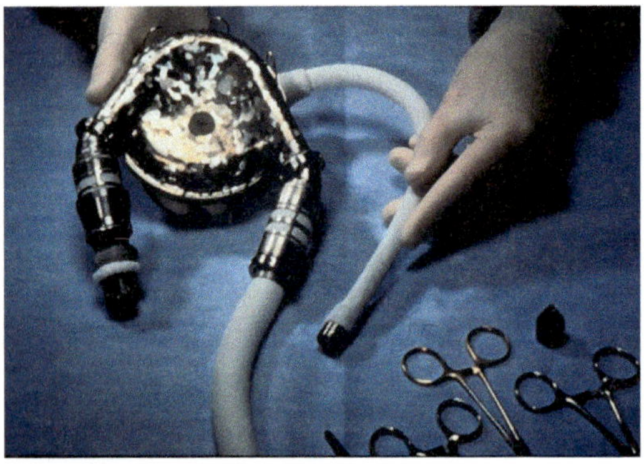

Fig. 1.2 The HeartMate I LVAD

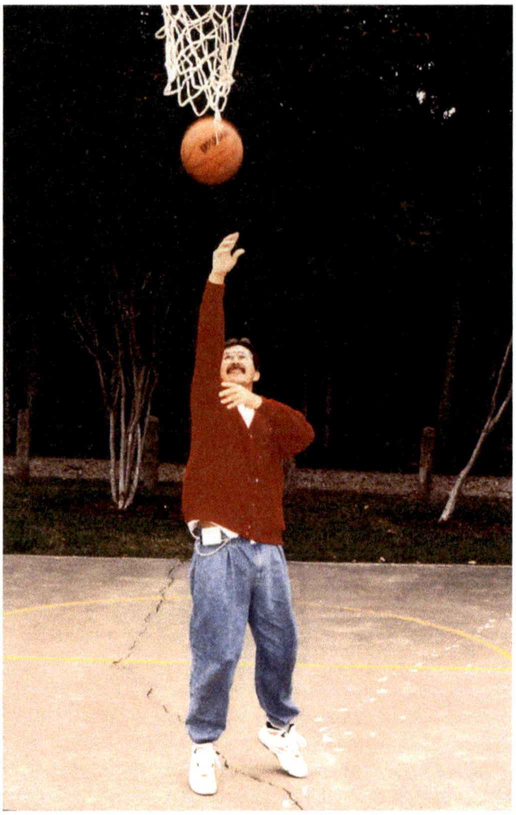

Fig. 1.3 First patient to have the HeartMate XVE implanted and the first patient to be discharged with an LVAD (Image reproduced with permission from Frazier [21]. Figure 1. Copyright Elsevier)

white blood count had fallen to below 2000 cells mc/L. He died of overwhelming sepsis 32 h after the transplant. Nevertheless, this first clinical TAH experience proved that a patient could be supported by a mechanical heart.

Despite its promise, the early era of heart transplantation soon ended in disappointment. By the early 1970s, most of the recipients had died of infection or organ rejection. For this reason, cardiac transplantation was almost universally abandoned for at least a decade. The US government redirected its research funds toward the development of an implantable LVAD, not as a bridge to transplantation but as a permanently implantable device. By that time, I was involved in heart surgery and MCS research at THI. After transplantation was renewed in the early 1980s, the pulsatile HeartMate implantable pneumatic LVAD was developed in our laboratory. In 1994, it became the first implantable pump to be approved for clinical use by the US Food and Drug Administration (FDA). The HeartMate vented electric (VE) LVAD (Fig. 1.2) was implanted in 1991, and this untethered device was the first device that allowed patients to leave the hospital (Fig. 1.3). As of early 2012, more than 10,000 HeartMate pumps had been implanted worldwide. However, they were too large to fit in smaller patients, including many women and children. Perhaps even more important, the durability of these pumps was limited.

While the human body is at rest, a healthy heart beats 70 times a minute. This is equivalent to 4200 beats an hour and more than 100,000 beats a day. Therefore, the ideal circulatory support pump must be durable enough to beat more than 36 million times a year. Because the initial LVADs could function reliably for only about 2 years, long-term LVAD support would have necessitated frequent pump replacement. As a result, these devices were impractical as destination therapy and were practical only for bridging to transplantation. Therefore, the number of patients who could benefit from LVADs long term was limited to the number of available donor hearts – about 2400 in the USA and 3500 worldwide each year. Thus, LVAD technology would have no epidemiologic effect on the approximately 100,000 patients in the USA alone who faced premature death without a replacement heart. This caused Norman Shumway, a heart transplant pioneer at Stanford University, to comment during a nationally televised debate with Dr. Jarvik that bridging to transplantation would have no statistical benefit; it would simply result in a nightmare – further prolonging the waiting list for heart transplants.

Contemporaneous with what I referred to as "Shumway's nightmare," I began to further explore the use of implantable continuous-flow (CF) blood pumps, which would function without creating a

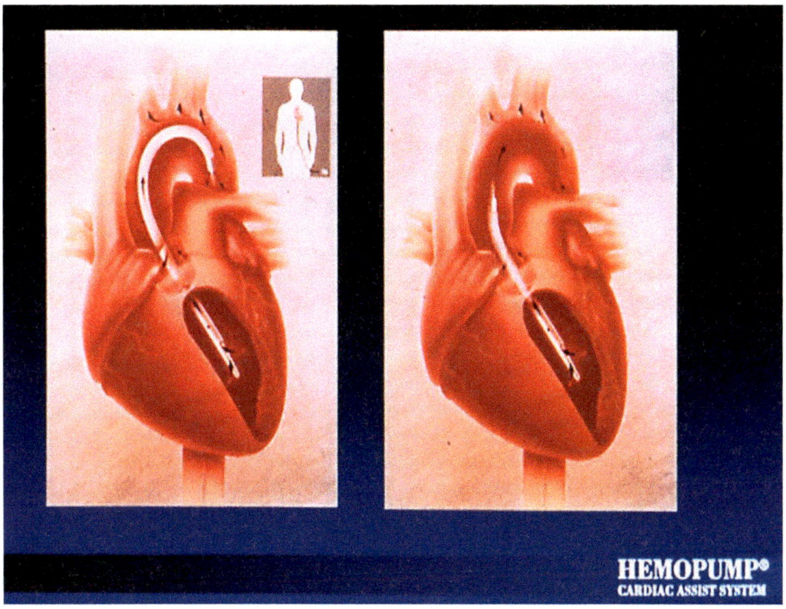

Fig. 1.4 The Hemopump

pulse. When the idea of using implantable, long-term, nonpulsatile pumps was first proposed, it incurred severe criticism from the medical community. The concept gave rise to a debate about whether or not a pulse is necessary. However, the heart is the only organ that actually needs a pulse, which is required not for systole but for the diastolic blood flow that provides an energy source. If the heart fails, however, this becomes a moot point. The heart could potentially be unloaded by a CF pump, which would perhaps restore the normal Starling response. Heart surgeons of that era knew that patients who could not be weaned from CPB but who had a heartbeat could usually be maintained by a CPB flow of about 2 L/min; however, their heart could not compensate if they were separated from this support. As a preliminary experiment, in 1984, I had implanted a small CF pump supplied by Bio-Medicus, Inc. (currently Medtronic, Minneapolis, Minnesota, USA), in two pigs. In each case, the heart was fibrillated, but an adequate cardiac output was maintained by the CF pump in the left ventricle. I believed that such devices would offer much longer durability (potentially up to 20 years) than the flexing membrane in pulsatile pumps. In addition, because CF pumps were much smaller, they would fit a wider range of patient body sizes.

From the early 1980s, I was a clinical advocate of implantable long-term CF pumps. For this reason, at a 1986 conference I was approached independently by two medical engineers, Robert Jarvik and Richard Wampler, who asked me to test their respective designs for implantable CF blood pumps. At first, I was skeptical of these devices, but I thought that we should follow Claude Bernard's advice to proceed with the experiment and let nature provide the answer [11].

The first of these cf-LVADs to be implanted clinically was the Hemopump (Fig. 1.4), designed by Wampler. It was about the size of the eraser on a number 2 lead pencil and spun at up to 25,000 rpm. I was initially concerned that it might act like a kitchen blender and destroy the blood cells, but our laboratory showed that the device was safe in short-term experiments in calves. In 1988, we successfully implanted it in a 55-year-old man with heart failure (Fig. 1.5), thereby rescuing him from certain death [12, 13]. This pump may be likened to the Wright brothers' flying machine, which also was initially regarded as impractical; the Hemopump got pulseless blood flow technology "off the ground" as a feasible approach to temporary circulatory support. Later, the Hemopump was implanted numerous times, both in the USA and abroad, but insufficient funding was available to make the device comply with FDA requirements. Fortunately, in 1994, I was at a congress in Germany, where I encountered an old friend, Dr. Helmut Reul, of Aachen. He was a pioneering biomedical engineer who had trained in Houston. I encouraged him to look at the technology represented by the Hemopump, as I felt that

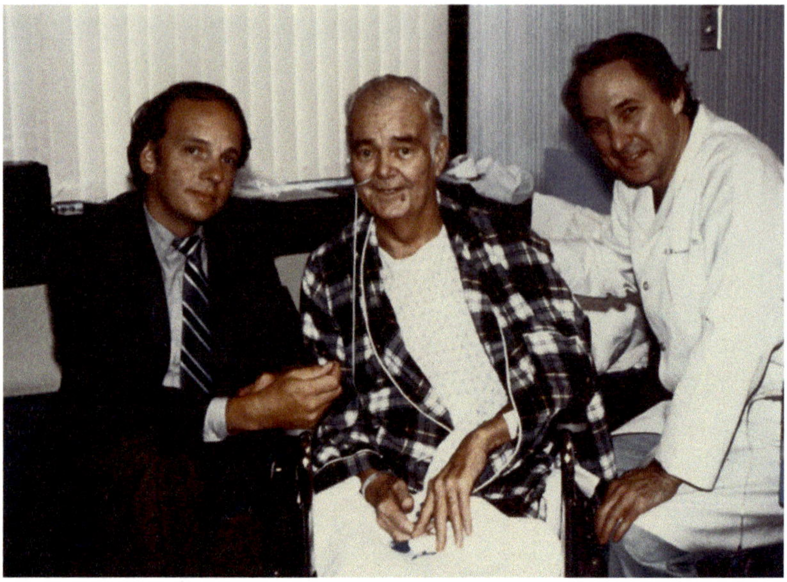

Fig. 1.5 Dr. Richard Wampler (*left*), Dr. O. H. Frazier (*right*), and the first patient to receive a Hemopump (*center*) (Image reproduced with permission from Frazier [21]. Figure 2. Copyright Elsevier)

it was an important step forward. Dr. Reul soon began developing this technology in Germany. His work resulted in the device currently known as the Impella LVAD for temporary support, which is currently approved for clinical use in both Europe and the USA.

The second CF device tested in the THI laboratory – the Jarvik pump – spun at 8000 to 12,000 rpm. For successful long-term use, an axial-flow blood pump requires blood-washed bearings that continuously spin at a high rate. In the early 1980s, it was generally believed that non-lubricated bearings would be impossible to maintain in the bloodstream for very long. Like automobile bearings, LVAD bearings require lubrication. Within the bloodstream, the only source of lubrication is the blood itself. However, use of blood as a lubricant was not deemed feasible. In 1986, Rob Jarvik and I began working on a non-lubricated, implantable long-term pump with a blood-washed bearing. After fabricating the pulseless axial-flow pumps in New York, Jarvik sent them to us in Houston for animal testing. The first pump lasted for only 3 days before its bearings became stuck; this seemed to confirm the original belief that special lubrication was needed. Nevertheless, over a 4-year period, Jarvik gradually refined the pump and its bearings, each pump lasting longer than its predecessor. Eventually, the Jarvik heart (using bearings washed only by blood) was able to support calves in our laboratory for more than 8 months. This experiment conclusively proved that the device would be safe for human implantation.

It is impossible to overstate the importance to the field of these two advances: the concept of a small, high-speed (25,000 rpm) blood pump (Wampler) and of blood-washed bearings (Jarvik) became the basis for initial clinical progress in this field, ultimately resulting in thousands of pumps implanted and lives saved. I had the privilege of performing the first clinical implantation of the Jarvik heart in 2000 (Figs. 1.6 and 1.7) [14] and of the HeartMate II LVAD (an implantable version of the Hemopump) in 2003 [15]. Both of these devices propel blood by means of axial flow, a method introduced by the ancient Greek scientist Archimedes for transporting liquids with a screw-type pump. The idea of applying this principle to blood pumps first occurred to Wampler when he was visiting Egypt and observed Archimedes screw pumps propelling water in the fields. Therefore, this 2000-year-old concept became the inspiration for today's lifesaving axial-flow LVADs.

A different type of flow, in which blood is propelled by centrifugal force, has also been a focus of our work at THI. We began studying implantable centrifugal force pumps in 1994. I felt that the inflow responsivity of centrifugal force, as demonstrated at that time by the Bio-Medicus device, made these pumps potentially superior hemodynamically to axial-flow devices, particularly with regard to safety. In addition, centrifugal force pumps offered the possibility of magnetic

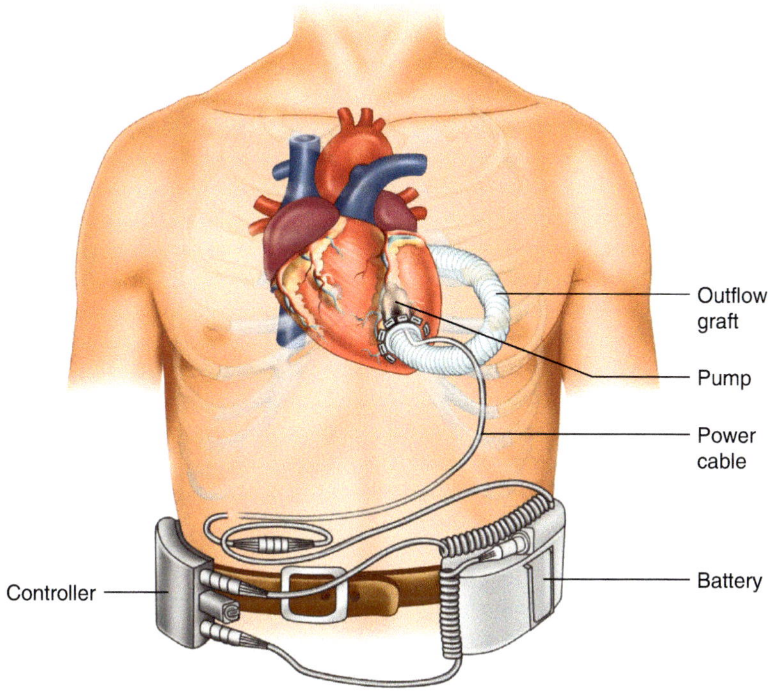

Fig. 1.6 Diagram of the Jarvik 2000 Heart (Figure reproduced with permission from Frazier et al. [16]. Figure 1. Copyright American Heart Association)

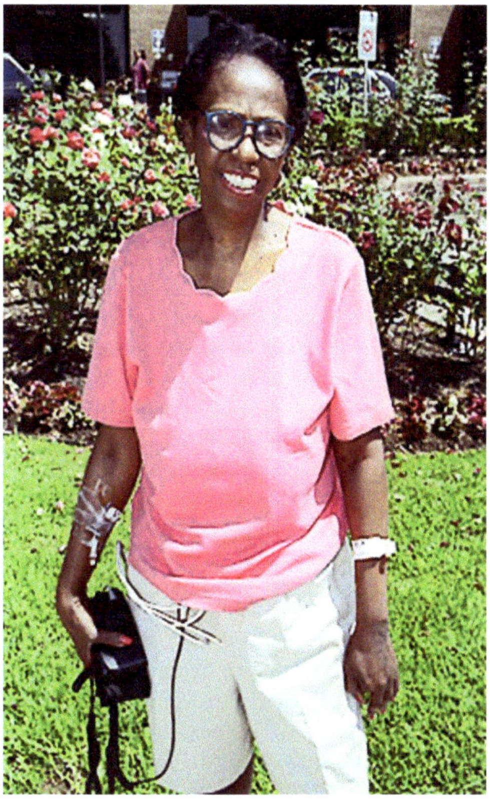

Fig. 1.7 The first patient to have the Jarvik 2000 Heart implanted (Image reproduced with permission from Frazier [21]. Figure 3. Copyright Elsevier)

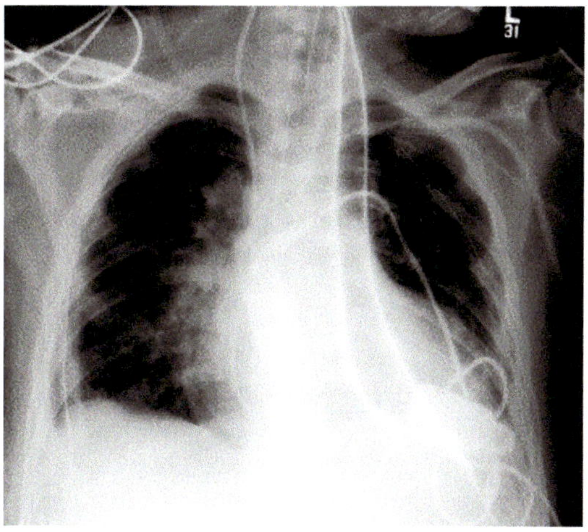

Fig. 1.8 Postoperative chest radiograph of first long-term implantable right-sided pump (Image reproduced with permission from Frazier et al. [22] Figure 1B. Copyright Elsevier)

suspension, therefore requiring no bearings at all. Another important advantage of such pumps is that they are easily adaptable for assisting the right side of the heart. I had implanted the first long-term implantable right-sided pump in 2003 (Fig. 1.8) [16]. Another potential advantage of centrifugal force technology was the ability to place the pump entirely within the pericardium, thus avoiding the

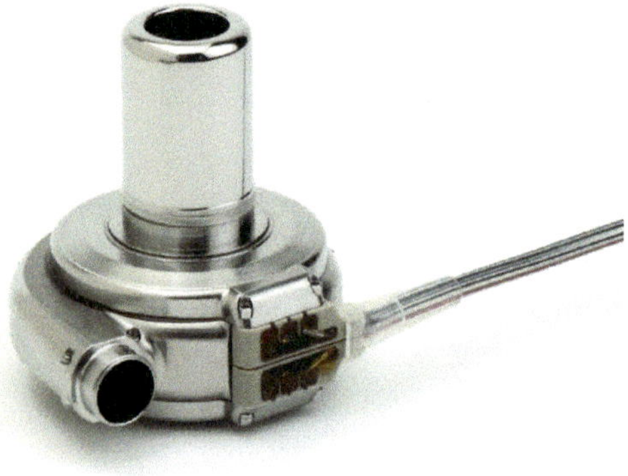

■ **Fig. 1.9** The HeartWare LVAD

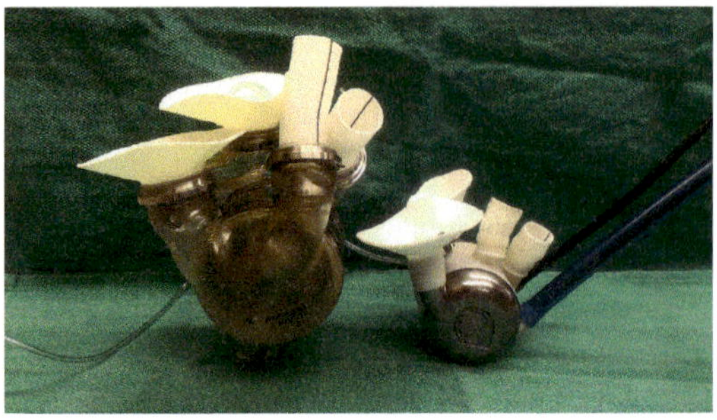

■ **Fig. 1.10** The AbioCor TAH (*left*) and the BiVACOR TAH (*right*) (Image reproduced with permission from Frazier [21]. Figure 7. Copyright Elsevier)

need to create a pump pocket, which is a potential source of infection.

At THI, we initiated our research on implantable centrifugal force pumps in collaboration with Richard Wampler and a single investor, Robert Fine. The resulting device was developed under the name of Kriton. Research progressed from 1994 until 2001, at which time the company was reformed under the name of HeartWare. Since that time, this technology has been an important contribution to advancement in this field. The HeartWare LVAD is presently the second most frequently implanted circulatory support pump (■ Fig. 1.9) [17, 18]. Another currently used centrifugal force LVAD, the HeartMate III, was developed in the 1990s by Vic Poirier and Kurt Dasse at Thermo Cardiosystems, which later merged with Thoratec (Pleasanton, California, USA).

Experience with LVAD systems has been an important factor in furthering efforts to create a usable long-term TAH, which has proved more elusive than researchers envisioned in the 1960s. The advent of CF pumps, with their smaller size and increased durability, greatly expanded the number of patients in whom such devices could be used. Since the early 2000s, when these pumps were introduced clinically, more than 30,000 of them have been implanted in a wide spectrum of patients, ranging from children to 400 lb. adults. Over 100 individuals to date with HeartMate II, Jarvik, and HeartWare pumps have survived for up to 10 years with the same pump without its showing signs of wear. Current research is aimed at improving these devices and creating even smaller ones, which could be implanted in adults without opening the chest and in children. This would increase the safety of the implant procedure and allow the devices to be used much earlier in the course of cardiac failure. As a result, the heart might have sufficient time to recover its normal function, sparing the patient the need for a transplant or a long-term LVAD.

Unfortunately, heart failure remains the foremost cause of premature death in the USA and Europe. Whereas most heart failure patients can be helped by an LVAD, others can be saved only by a total heart replacement. These include patients whose heart muscle has been destroyed by severe heart attacks and patients with refractory cardiac rhythm disturbances, malignant cardiac tumors, or other rare cardiac conditions. In all of these cases, a permanent TAH may be the only hope for survival.

Experience with CF assist devices has confirmed that humans can live without any pulse at all. Indeed, both in animal experiments (2005) [19] and in a human patient (2011) [20], THI researchers have shown that the heart can be successfully replaced by two CF pumps. In 2013, with the goal of developing a CF-TAH, we joined with an Australian engineering team led by Dr. Daniel Timms. The resulting pump, known as the BiVACOR (■ Fig. 1.10), has only a single moving part, fits into the palm of the hand, provides flows of up to 20 L/min, and offers the automaticity of a Starling response not seen in other total heart replacement devices. Early animal experiments have confirmed the feasibility of this device as a cardiac substitute, and we anticipate its use in man within 5 years [21].

Looking back, I am indebted to that young Italian boy whose death reinforced my decision to pursue MCS research. Since that time, incredible progress has been made in this field. We now have pumps that can be pulled "off the shelf" to assume the function of a failed heart, even one that requires internal massage. Many patients worldwide have been saved by this technology. Over the course of my career, I have been involved in the development or testing of many of the LVADs in clinical use today. I am gratified that these efforts – and those of my dedicated colleagues in this field – have resulted in an array of lifesaving devices that were hardly imaginable half a century ago.

References

1. Ezekiel 36:26 KJV.
2. Cohn LH (2003) Fifty years of open-heart surgery. Circulation 107(17):2168–2170
3. Meisner H (2014) Milestones in surgery: 60 years of open heart surgery. Thorac Cardiovasc Surg 62(8):645–650
4. Cooley DA (2008) A brief history of the Texas heart institute. Tex Heart Inst J 35(3):235–239
5. Cooley DA, Belmonte BA, Debakey ME, Latson JR (1957) Mechanical heart lung for temporary cardiopulmonary by-pass: report of 95 cases. Tex State J Med 53(6):397–400
6. Sade RM (2005) Transplantation at 100 years: Alexis Carrel, pioneer surgeon. Ann Thorac Surg 80(6):2415–2418
7. Glyantsev SP, Tchantchaleishvili V, Bockeria LA (2016) Demikhov's "Mechanical Heart": the circumstances surrounding creation of the world's first implantable total artificial heart in 1937. ASAIO J 62(1):106–109
8. DeBakey ME (1971) Left ventricular bypass pump for cardiac assistance. Clinical experience. Am J Cardiol 27:3–11
9. Cooley DA, Nora JJ, Trentin JJ, Hallman GL, Bloodwell RD, Leachman RD (1969) Clinical experience in transplantation of the human heart: report of ten cases. Transplant Proc 1(2):703–712
10. Cooley DA, Liotta D, Hallman GL, Bloodwell RD, Leachman RD, Milam JD (1969) Orthotopic cardiac prosthesis for two-staged cardiac replacement. Am J Cardiol 24(5):723–730
11. Bernard C, Greene HC, Henderson LJ (1927) An introduction to the study of experimental medicine. The Macmillan Company, New York
12. Wampler RK, Moise JC, Frazier OH, Olsen DB (1988) In vivo evaluation of a peripheral vascular access axial flow blood pump. ASAIO Trans 34(3):450–454
13. Frazier OH, Wampler RK, Duncan JM et al (1990) First human use of the Hemopump, a catheter-mounted ventricular assist device. Ann Thorac Surg 49(2):299–304
14. Frazier OH, Gregoric ID, Delgado RM et al (2001) Initial experience with the Jarvik 2000 left ventricular assist system as a bridge to transplantation: report of 4 cases. J Heart Lung Transplant 20(2):201
15. Frazier OH, Delgado RM 3rd, Kar B, Patel V, Gregoric ID, Myers TJ (2004) First clinical use of the redesigned HeartMate II left ventricular assist system in the United States: a case report. Tex Heart Inst J 31(2): 157–159
16. Frazier OH, Myers TJ, Gregoric ID et al (2002) Initial clinical experience with the Jarvik 2000 implantable axial-flow left ventricular assist system. Circulation 105(24):2855–2860
17. Wieselthaler GM, O Driscoll G, Jansz P, Khaghani A, Strueber M, Investigators HC (2010) Initial clinical experience with a novel left ventricular assist device with a magnetically levitated rotor in a multi-institutional trial. J Heart Lung Transplant 29(11): 1218–1225
18. Slaughter MS, Sobieski MA 2nd, Tamez D et al (2009) HeartWare miniature axial-flow ventricular assist device: design and initial feasibility test. Tex Heart Inst J 36(1):12–16
19. Cohn WE, Winkler JA, Parnis S et al (2014) Ninety-day survival of a calf implanted with a continuous-flow total artificial heart. ASAIO J 60(1):15–18
20. Frazier OH, Cohn WE (2012) Continuous-flow total heart replacement device implanted in a 55-year-old man with end-stage heart failure and severe amyloidosis. Tex Heart Inst J 39(4):542–546
21. Frazier OH (2014) Mechanical circulatory assist device development at the Texas Heart Institute: a personal perspective. Semin Thorac Cardiovasc Surg 26(1):4–13
22. Frazier OH, Myers TJ, Gregoric I (2004) Biventricular assistance with the Jarvik FlowMaker: a case report. J Thorac Cardiovasc Surg 128(4):625–626

Preoperative Evaluation

Contents

Physiopathology and Fate of End-Stage CHF in the Era of MCS

Vito Piazza, A. Montalto, C. Amarelli, A. Loforte, and Francesco Musumeci

© Springer International Publishing Switzerland 2017
A. Montalto et al. (eds.), *Mechanical Circulatory Support in End-Stage Heart Failure*,
DOI 10.1007/978-3-319-43383-7_2

2.1 Introduction

Heart failure is a clinical syndrome with different etiologies and quite variable presentation. The acute onset can be due to exacerbation of signs and symptoms of known HF (acute decompensated heart failure) or to the sudden appearance of HF in a patient with previous normal cardiac function (new-onset or de novo HF), as it happens after myocardial infarction or myocarditis. In chronic HF the symptoms of ventricular dysfunction occur in a time span of weeks or months and generally are caused by long-lasting ischemic heart disease, dilated cardiomyopathies, and hypertensive and valvular disease. With the advent of echocardiography, HF has been classified into two major subclasses: (1) heart failure with reduced ejection fraction (HFrEF), also called systolic heart failure, and (2) heart failure with preserved ejection fraction (HFpEF), also known as diastolic heart failure. The prevalence of heart failure increases rapidly with age. The Framingham Heart Study showed a prevalence of 8/1000 and up to 66/100 in 50–59 and 80–89 aged men, respectively [1]. In women, the prevalence of cardiac insufficiency was 8/1000 for the age group of 50–59 years and 7/1000 for age between 80 and 89 years. The incidence has similar trends, doubling for each subsequent decade of life. There are several reasons for this increase: the aging of the population, the improved efficacy of treatments of acute coronary syndromes with prolonged life span expectancy, and the significant increase of diabetes and obesity. As a consequence the hospitalizations are progressively raising, due not only to the occurrence of worsening symptoms but also to comorbidities such as renal failure, electrolyte abnormalities, and multiorgan dysfunction. Risk factors for heart failure include age, sex, hypertension, diabetes, obesity, coronary artery disease, insulin resistance, genetic factors, and use of cardiotoxic drugs. In the SOLVD registry, 70% of patients suffering from heart failure had coronary heart disease and 7% hypertensive disease [2].

2.2 Systolic Heart Failure

In systolic heart failure, the left ventricle dilates and becomes more spherical so that the transverse diameter increases more than the longitudinal one and the distance between the papillary muscles raises, causing a misalignment that often results in secondary or functional mitral insufficiency. The wall thickness remains unchanged or reduced, the wall stress is increased, the end-diastolic and systolic volumes are increased, but the rise of end systolic is higher than the end diastolic, so that ejection fraction is lowered [3, 4]. These alterations trigger neurohumoral responses that lead to the activation of vasoconstrictors (catecholamines, angiotensin, aldosterone, and cytokines) and of vasodilators (natriuretic peptides, nitric oxide). When the balance between vasodilator and vasoconstrictor systems is maintained, the progression of heart failure is prevented; otherwise ventricular remodeling is promoted and the ventricular failure progresses. The neurohormones, such as vasoconstrictor angiotensin II, also promote atherosclerosis, causing vascular smooth muscle proliferation, myocyte necrosis, and apoptosis. Norepinephrine levels are higher the more severe the ventricular dysfunction and are associated with enhanced systemic vascular resistance with consequent increase in ventricular afterload and further deterioration of the left ventricular function. The raised sympathetic activity also results in an increase of venous constriction leading to an increment of the preload of the left ventricle, which is useful in the early stages to preserve stroke volume, but responsible for augmented wall stress and impairment of the ejection fraction in later phases [5, 6]. By means of these mechanisms, the reduced left ventricular function leads to a vicious cycle that further causes left ventricular remodeling and dysfunction (◘ Fig. 2.1). Looking at the volume-pressure curves, we observe a downward and rightward shift of the left ventricle end-systolic pressure that reflects the reduced contractile function. Initially, stroke volume

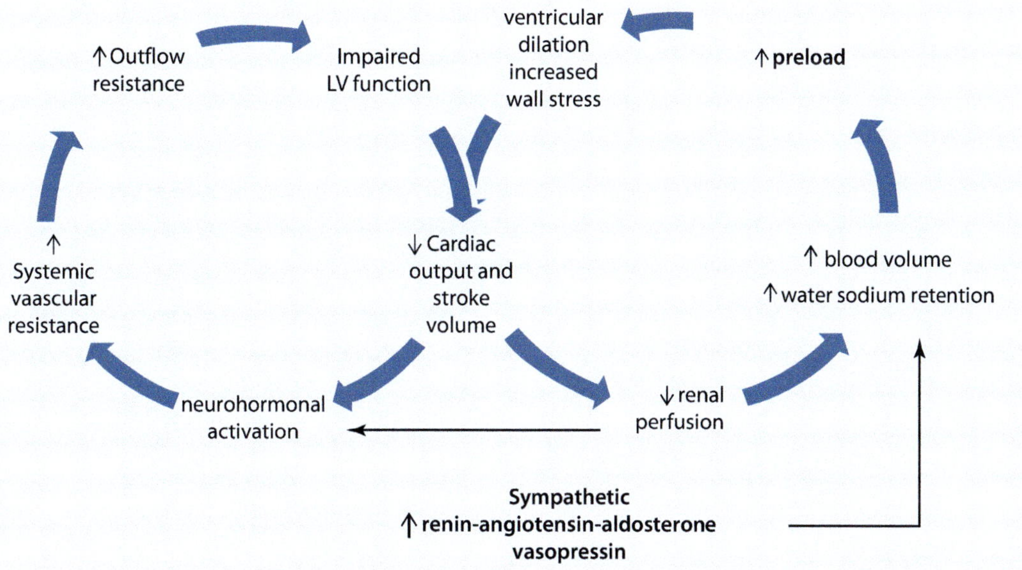

Fig. 2.1 Cycle of left ventricular remodeling triggered by systolic dysfunction

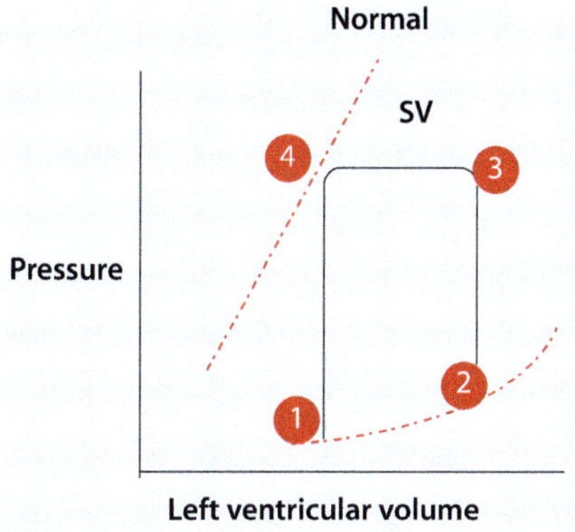

Fig. 2.2 Illustration of left ventricular pressure-volume loops in normal individuals

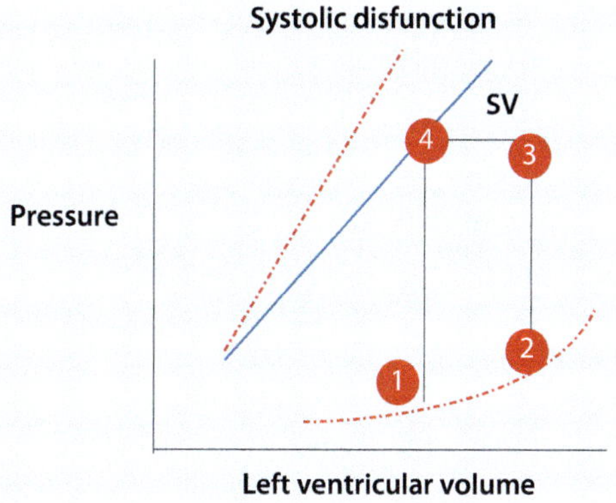

Fig. 2.3 Illustration of left ventricular pressure-volume loops in individuals with systolic dysfunction

is maintained, thanks to the Frank-Starling mechanism, but with further reduction of ventricular function, the stroke volume decreases resulting in augmentation of residual volume (Figs. 2.2 and 2.3).

2.3 Diastolic Heart Failure

Several definitions have been proposed to indicate the HF arising from diastolic dysfunction. A first one defined diastolic dysfunction as a clinical

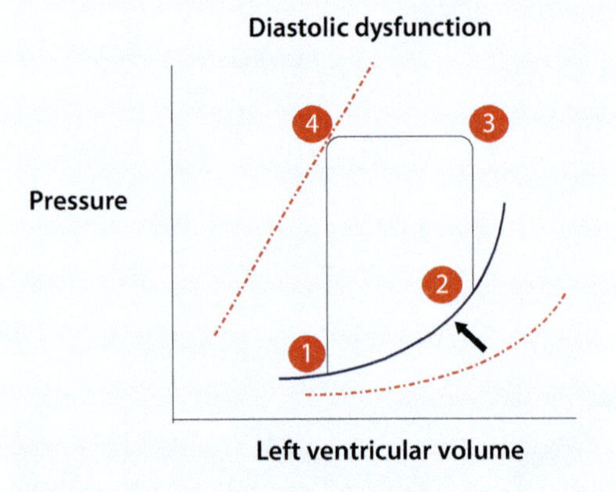

■ **Fig. 2.4** Left ventricular pressure-volume loops in individuals with diastolic dysfunction

syndrome characterized by signs and symptoms of heart failure, preserved ejection fraction, and abnormal diastolic function [7]. In clinical practice, the most widely used definition defines diastolic dysfunction as the clinical condition in which the signs and symptoms of HF are associated with EF greater than 45%. The left ventricle shows normal size, normal or increased wall thickness (concentric hypertrophy), normal or decreased end-diastolic and end-systolic volumes, and increased mass/cavity ratio. Since the wall thickness is increased without increment of ventricular volumes, wall stress is reduced and this guarantees a normal EF [8, 9]. As already seen for the systolic failure, diastolic heart failure is associated with neurohormonal abnormalities such as increased levels of norepinephrine, interleukin-6 and interleukin-8, and tumor necrosis factor-alpha (TNF) [10–12]. The main functional anomaly is the increased stiffness of the ventricular walls and the reduced compliance of the left ventricle. The diastolic relaxation curve moves upward and to the left (■ Fig. 2.4) resulting in a disproportionate increase in ventricular diastolic pressure to any increment in left ventricular end-diastolic volume. In patients with severe diastolic dysfunction, the early diastolic pressure is elevated, and the left atrial pressures rises creating the conditions for pulmonary congestion and hypertension. While the systolic dysfunction causing pulmonary hypertension in patients with HFrEF is usually easy to detect, the proper distinction between pulmonary arterial hypertension and pulmonary hypertension associated with HFpEF is much more challenging. The gold standard for the assessment of LV diastolic function is the invasive assessment of the pressure-volume relationship which usually requires an estimation of LV volume by the conductance method [12, 13]. An alternative and reliable method to diagnose HFpEF is a comprehensive echocardiographic study in combination with natriuretic peptides, as proposed by a consensus statement [14]. Echocardiographic assessment for HFpEF includes estimation of LVEDP by E/E′, assessment of left atrial size, E/A ratio, and deceleration time [15]. Since single echocardiographic parameters such as E/E′ have limitations in accurately diagnosing HFpEF, an integrative score of five echocardiographic variables (RV/LV ratio, left ventricular eccentricity index, E/E′, RV forming apex, width and inspiratory collapse of the inferior vena cava) as well as additional parameters such as the shape of the RV outflow tract Doppler envelope (“RVOT notching”) may be utilized to discriminate between pre- and postcapillary PH [16, 17].

2.4 Cardiorenal Syndrome

The term “cardiorenal syndrome” (CRS) indicates a concomitant dysfunction of the heart and kidney in which an acute or chronic impairment of the function of one of the two organs results in an acute or chronic reduction of the other organ functional capacity. Ronco et al. suggested a classification of the cardiorenal syndrome which takes account of the fact that the syndrome is due to primary or secondary alteration of the heart or kidney or if the dysfunction of these two organs is the consequence of systemic diseases affecting both organs (■ Table 2.1) [18]. Type 1 indicates the acute worsening of renal at function (AKF) that follows the rapid deterioration of cardiac function. The risk of AKF is increased by pre-existing chronic kidney disease; its severity is higher in subjects with HFrEF compared to patients with HFpEF and occurs in 70% of patients suffering from cardiogenic shock [19]. The type 2 refers to chronic renal impairment due to long-standing cardiac failure and reduced perfusion and is often exacerbated by coexisting micro- and macrovascular pathology. The type 3 (acute reno-cardiac syndrome) indicates acute worsening of renal function that can adversely affect the myocardium, inducing ischemia, arrhythmias, or

Table 2.1 Cardiorenal syndrome classification

Type	Name	Description
Type 1	Acute cardiorenal syndrome	Abrupt worsening of cardiac function leading to acute renal injury
Type 2	Chronic cardiorenal syndrome	Chronic abnormalities in cardiac function causing progressive and potentially permanent chronic kidney disease
Type 3	Acute reno-cardiac syndrome	Abrupt worsening of renal function causing acute cardiac disorders
Type 4	Chronic reno-cardiac syndrome	Chronic kidney disease contributing to decreased cardiac function.
Type 5	Secondary cardiorenal syndrome	Systemic pathologies causing both cardiac and renal dysfunction

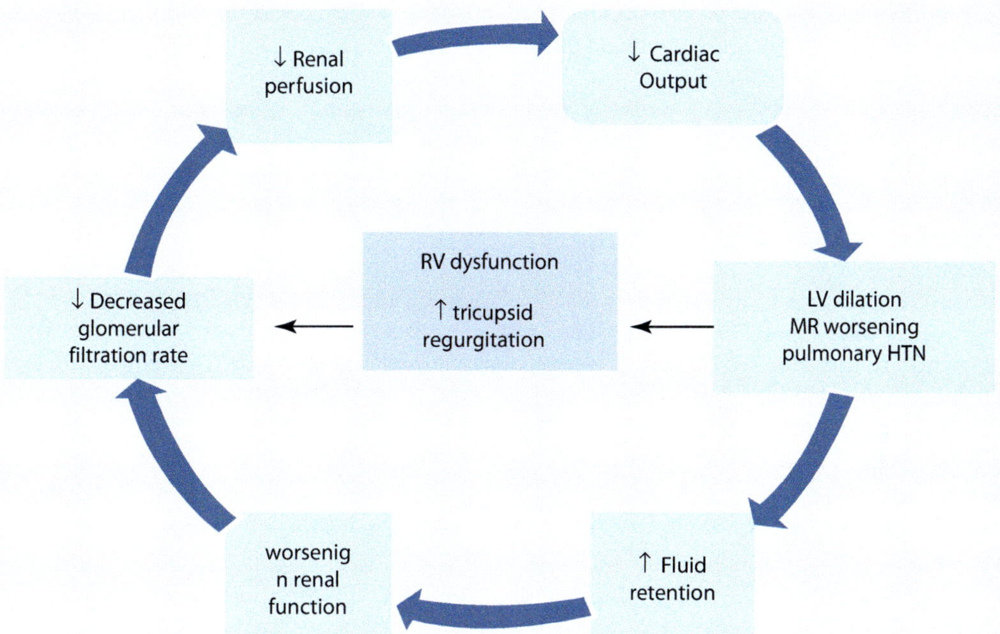

Fig. 2.5 Schematic illustration of the development of the cardiorenal syndrome

ventricular failure. In patients with acute reno-cardiac syndrome, fluid overload can result in pulmonary edema and hyperkalemia, responsible for arrhythmias and cardiac arrest. Patients with bilateral renal artery stenoses are more likely to develop diastolic heart failure due to high blood pressure by releasing vasoconstrictor neurohormones and retention of sodium and water [20]. The type 4 cardiorenal syndrome occurs when a chronic kidney disease (CKD) contributes to aggravate systolic and diastolic dysfunction and type 5 when cardiac and renal function are compromised by systemic diseases such as sepsis, hypertension, diabetes, amyloidosis, and autoimmune diseases.

The functions of the heart and of the kidney are closely linked through changes of CO and atrial volume and pressure. In normal subjects, an abrupt increment in the left atrial pressure results in increased urine output through suppression, mediated by the vagus, of the antidiuretic hormone arginine vasopressin (AVP) and reduction of renal sympathetic activity (Fig. 2.5). The reduction of CO and of systemic blood pressure removes the inhibition on the central nervous system leading to increased sympathetic stimulation and AVP release. The effect of stimulation of the adrenergic receptors and angiotensin receptors in the proximal tubule determines a sodium and water reabsorption. In patients with advanced HF, the vasoconstrictive and sodium retentive responses are accentuated, and the vasodilating and diuretic effects of increased AVP are blunted. In these patients marked cardiorenal dysfunction can develop that can be reversed after the implantation of ventricular assist device [21]. The relationship between renal function and congestion is complex and not entirely understood. Some studies have shown that baseline renal dysfunction is related to elevated central venous pressure (CVP) only when the renal blood flow is reduced [22], others found only a weak correlation [23], and others showed a biphasic correlation with renal failure being associated with low or high CVP [24]. On the other hand, the reduction of renal function during the course of hospital stay (so-called worsening renal function) has been variably related to persistently elevated CVP [25], to CVP but only when the basal value was below 10 mmHg [26], to hemoconcentration due to aggressive diuresis, and to consequent lowering of filling pressures [27]. From a pathophysiological point of view, the increase of CVP reduces the renal perfusion pressure gradient, acts directly on the glomerular filtration pressure, and is a potent activator of direct renal vasoconstrictive reflexes that further reduce renal perfusion and promote sodium reabsorption [28]. Furthermore, persistent congestion can increase the intra-abdominal pressure in approximately 60% of patients with advanced heart failure, even in the absence of ascites, and has been associated with impaired renal function independently of systemic hemodynamics, due to increase of intrarenal interstitial pressure, further reduction of renal perfusion pressure gradient, and local neuro-sympathetic activation. Small increases of the endoabdominal pressure, in the order of 8–12 mmHg (normal value 5–7 mmHg) in critically ill adults, can cause renal failure and can be easily detected with transvesical monitoring [29]. While the therapy of chronic heart failure is based on the pharmacological modulation of neurohumoral activation, the treatment of acute decompensated heart failure is based on the manipulation of hemodynamic alterations characterized by reduction of systemic perfusion pressure and relative underfilling of the arterial vessels in the face of expansion of total plasma volume and increased filling pressures. Hemodynamic monitoring studies have shown that the increase of the filling pressures precedes the onset of clinical signs of congestion and the hospital admission by days or even weeks [30] and that the management of heart failure based on hemodynamic data reduces the 30-day readmissions [31]. The increase in central venous pressure (PVC) may be due to water and sodium retention, redistribution of blood volume within the vascular tree from the large splanchnic veins, and right ventricular failure [32–34] and is related to the appearance or worsening function of many organs, mainly the kidneys.

2.5 Hepatorenal Syndrome

The characteristics of the liver circulation expose particularly this organ to the risk of hypoperfusion in heart failure owing to the combination of elevated CVP and reduced cardiac output. Approximately ¾ of liver blood flow come from the portal vein and only ¼ from the hepatic artery, and the two flows mix at the entrance of the sinusoids. The cells in the central zone of the hepatic lobule (zone 3) receive blood at a lower oxygen tension than the peripheral cells (zone 1) and therefore more readily become anoxic and necrotic [35]. The rise in the right atrial pressure increases hepatic venous pressure and causes sinusoidal distension and hemorrhage, while the reduction of the arterial blood flow causes necrosis of the zone 3 cells [36]. Since the portal vein has predominantly alpha-adrenergic receptors and the hepatic veins beta-adrenergic receptors, sympathetic stimulation combined with elevation of hepatic venous pressure can reduce significantly the liver flow. This causes necrosis of the centrilobular zone with a cholestatic enzyme profile; the local accumulation of adenosine, which activates renal vasoconstriction through synapses between hepatic and renal nerves; and the production of cAMP, which promotes sodium reabsorption (hepatorenal syndrome) [37].

2.6 Splanchnic Circulation

The circulation of the intestinal villi is arranged very similar to the renal medulla. The direction of the blood flow in the central arterioles which perfuse the villous tip is contrary to that of the capillaries returning blood to the base of the villi so that a countercurrent exchange mechanism can be established. This creates an osmotic gradient from the tip to the base of the villi that facilitates the reabsorption of water but causes shunt of oxygen from arterioles to capillaries at the base of the villi which exposes the tip to the risk of anoxia. The countercurrent exchange is more efficient when blood flow is reduced so that the reduction of cardiac output seen in patient with heart failure can cause "nonocclusive ischemia" [38]. Moreover the reduction of blood flow is associated with an increase of the intestinal lumen pressure and wall tension, and the luminal distension is correlated to the reduction of flow to the mucosa [39]. The mucosal ischemia and the hypoxic damage of the tip of the villi can increase the intestinal permeability and the concentration of endotoxin and cytokines in blood samples of patients with acute heart failure [40]. In these patients the thickness of the intestinal wall and the concentration of bacteria adherent to the mucus of the intestinal wall are increased [41] and the bowel thickening is associated with gastrointestinal symptoms, reduced intestinal absorption capacity, cachexia, and right ventricular dysfunction [42].

2.7 Pulmonary Hypertension

In patients with heart failure, moderate and severe mitral regurgitation can be detected respectively in about 50% and 10% of cases, with frequency almost doubled in patients with left ventricular ejection fraction less than 30% [43]. Mitral regurgitation is due to different mechanisms: left ventricular dilation with tethering of the leaflets, kinetic anomalies of the base of the papillary muscles in patients with ischemic heart disease, and asynchrony of contraction in patients with left bundle branch block, and is not related to ejection fraction or to global left ventricular remodeling [44]. Mitral regurgitation brings additional volume overload and left ventricular dilation that aggravates the valvular regurgitation and thus creates a vicious circle that worsens the left ventricular function. The normal response to the elevation of the left atrial pressure and pulmonary capillary pressure, consisting in reduction of the release of arginine vasopressin and of sympathetic tone and increase of natriuretic peptides, is blunted in patients with heart failure [32]. Importantly, the rise of left atrial pressure regurgitation affects the pulmonary circulation so that mitral regurgitation is the major determinant of pulmonary hypertension in patients with heart failure [45] and is associated with increased risk of heart failure and cardiac mortality [43].

Pulmonary hypertension is defined by a mean pulmonary artery pressure greater than or equal to 25 mmHg [46]. In heart failure the pulmonary hypertension is typically postcapillary, with a pulmonary capillary pressure greater than 15 mmHg, transpulmonary pressure gradient (TPG, the difference between the mean pulmonary artery pressure and pulmonary capillary wedge pressure) less than 12 mmHg, and pulmonary vascular resistance (PVR) less than 3 Wood units. When pulmonary vasoconstriction or structural abnormalities of pulmonary vessels supervene, pulmonary artery pressure increases disproportionately, and TPG and PVR are elevated (reactive or mixed pulmonary hypertension). The TPG depends on pulmonary blood flow, left atrial pressure, and pulmonary vascular distensibility [47]. If the flow is reduced (low output), the pulmonary vessels are less relaxed so that the TPG can be falsely increased, while if the left atrial pressure is elevated, retrograde distention of the pulmonary vessels can cause TPG and PVR falsely decreased [48].

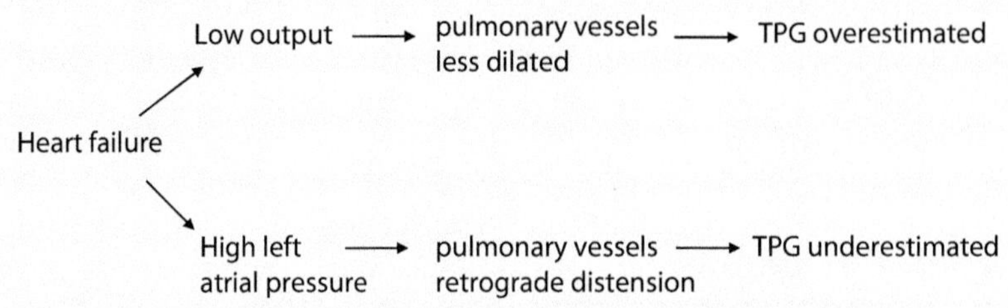

The diastolic pulmonary gradient (the difference between pulmonary artery diastolic pressure and pulmonary capillary wedge pressure, DPG) is theoretically less sensitive to variations in flow and thus could reflect better than TPG the effective pulmonary resistance [49]. It corresponds to the critical closing pressure of the pulmonary vessels. If the left ventricular pressure rises, DPG is reduced until it disappears: in this case the pulmonary artery diastolic pressure corresponds to the diastolic pressure of the left ventricle [49]. The normal value of the DPG is equal to or less than 5 mm Hg, and the presence of DPG equal to or greater than 7 in combination with PVR > 3 Wood units defines the combined pre- and postcapillary pulmonary hypertension [46]. Despite these pathophysiological advantages, recent studies have not confirmed the prognostic value of the DPG in patients with heart failure. In a retrospective study on 1236 patients with dilated cardiomyopathy, mortality was not related to DPG but to TPG and PVR. Patients with DPG < 7 mmHg had significantly worse hemodynamic profile, with lower pulmonary artery pressure and higher pulmonary capillary pressure. The study's results suggest that integrated measures which include not only mean pulmonary artery pressure but also pulmonary blood flow probably have closer relationship with the patient's hemodynamic profile and prognosis [50].

The pulmonary arterial capacitance is expressed by the ratio between the stroke volume and the pulmonary artery pulse pressure and is inversely proportional to the mean pulmonary artery pressure. While in the systemic circulation, 80% of the arterial compliance is localized at the level of the aorta, and the resistance in small peripheral arterial branches, in the pulmonary circulation compliance and resistance, are placed in the same distal branches [51, 52]. The compliance of the pulmonary circulation is four times higher than in the systemic circulation and is an important determinant of right ventricular afterload. The afterload of the right ventricle is due to:

1. Resistive or nonpulsatile component, measured from the pulmonary vascular resistance, reflects the energy expenditure to produce the mean pulmonary flow.
2. Pulsatile or oscillatory component, measured by pulmonary arterial compliance, is related to pulmonary artery pulse pressure.
3. Flow impedance is related to the inertia of blood and to the vascular properties.

The first can be considered beneficial (flow producing) and the second dissipative (does not produce primitively flow). Since in the systemic circulation, the ratio of the pulsatile to the resistive component is equal to approximately 10%, while in the pulmonary circulation reaches up to 25–30%, the pulmonary circulation is much more exposed to work "loss" [52]. Although the external work of the left ventricle is about five times larger than that of the right ventricle, the pulsatile component of the right ventricular work is increased by an amount equivalent to 23%. So the use of the PVR as a measure of right ventricular afterload underestimates the actually developed work which is on average 1.3 times higher [52]. In patients with heart failure, pulmonary arterial compliance is inversely correlated with mean pulmonary artery pressure, capillary wedge pressure, and pulmonary resistance. When the pulmonary capillary pressure increases, the pulmonary compliance decreases so that the pulsatile load to the right ventricle and the pulmonary artery pressure are increased ("reactive" pulmonary hypertension) [53]. A value less than 2–2.5 ml/mmHg shows correlation with mortality more strictly than other hemodynamic parameters [54, 55].

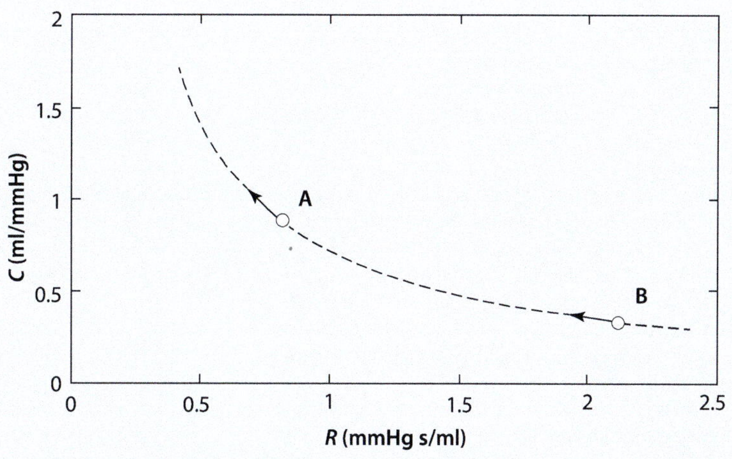

Fig. 2.6 Relationship between the decrease of PVR and the increase of pulmonary arterial compliance according to baseline PVR (With permission from: Lankhaar et al. [51])

In the pulmonary circulation, pulmonary artery compliance and resistance are inversely proportional, according to a constant (time constant of the fall of diastolic pulmonary pressure) that has the dimensions of time (seconds) [51]. In patients with heart failure, the increased pulmonary capillary wedge pressure shifts the curve upward and rightward reflecting the reduction of pulmonary arterial compliance [53]. So the same reduction of pulmonary vascular resistance in a patient with high baseline pulmonary resistance reduces the pulmonary artery compliance less than in a patient with low baseline pulmonary resistance (Fig. 2.6). The latter patient will reduce both the resistive and pulsatile component of the right ventricular afterload, the first only the resistive component [51]. In heart failure, the prevalence of pulmonary hypertension evaluated by echocardiography is 25–50%. In advanced heart failure, pulmonary hypertension measured at the right heart catheterization has been shown in at least 50% of cases, is more frequent in more compromised patients, and is an independent predictor of mortality [56–58]. Pulmonary hypertension causes right ventricle failure and dilatation, tricuspid regurgitation, and increase of right atrial pressure. The rise of right atrial pressure induces atrial enlargement and systemic and abdominal congestion, promotes the reabsorption of sodium and the onset or worsening of renal and liver failure, increases the intra-abdominal pressure, and modifies the intestinal function and permeability. The reduction of the right output and pulmonary blood flow can reduce pulmonary pressures which can be "falsely" normal or reduced. Probably for this reason in less advanced heart failure, pulmonary hypertension and right ventricular failure are associated with poor prognosis [57, 58], while in patients more severely compromised, as those evaluated for VAD implantation, low pulmonary pressure is a prognostic indicator [59]. Since the increase of the right atrial pressure and the relative reduction of the pulmonary pressure are the expression of right ventricular dysfunction, recently has been proposed the pulmonary arterial pulsatility index (PAPi), the ratio between pulmonary pulse pressure and PVC. A recent retrospective analysis of patients undergoing left VAD implantation showed that 1-point increase of PAPi is associated with lower risk of right VAD implantation and right heart failure with an optimal cutoff value of 2 [60]. Pulmonary pressure can also be falsely reduced in patients undergoing aggressive diuresis resulting in reduction of left filling pressures and can be revealed by the rapid infusion (5–10 min) of 0.5 L saline [61].

References

1. Ho KK, Pinsky JL, Kannel WB et al (1993) The epidemiology of heart failure: the Framingham Study. J Am Coll Cardiol 22:6A–13A
2. Bourassa MG, Gurne O, Bangdiwala SI et al (1993) Natural history and patterns of current practice in heart failure. The Studies of Left Ventricular Dysfunction (SOLVD) Investigators. J Am Coll Cardiol 22:14A–19A

3. Konstam MA (2003) Systolic and diastolic dysfunction in heart failure? Time for a new paradigm. J Card Fail 9:1–3
4. Aurigemma GP, Zile MR, Gaasch WH (2006) Contractile behavior of the left ventricle in diastolic heart failure with emphasis on regional systolic function. Circulation 113:296–304
5. Swedberg K, Viquerat C, Rouleau JL et al (1984) Comparison of myocardial catecholamine balance in chronic congestive heart failure and in angina pectoris without heart failure. Am J Cardiol 54:783–786
6. Hasking GL, Esler MD, Jennings GL et al (1986) Norepinephrine spillover to plasma in patients with congestive heart failure: evidence of increased overall and cardiorenal sympathetic nervous activity. Circulation 73:615–621
7. Zile MR, Brutsaert DL (2002) New concepts in diastolic dysfunction and diastolic heart failure: part I: diagnosis, prognosis and measurements of diastolic function. Circulation 105:1387–1393
8. Quinones MA, Zile MR, Massie BM et al (2006) Chronic heart failure: a report from the Dartmouth Diastolic Discourses. Congest Heart Fail 12:162–165
9. van Heerebeek L, Borbely A, Niessen HW et al (2006) Myocardial structure and function differ in systolic and diastolic heart failure. Circulation 113:1966–1975
10. Klitzmann DW, Little WC, Brubaker PH et al (2002) Pathophysiological characterization of isolated diastolic heart failure in comparison to systolic heart failure. JAMA 288:2144–2150
11. Mak GJ, Ledwidge MT, Watson CJ et al (2009) Natural history of markers of collagen turnover in patients with early diastolic dysfunction and impact of eplerenone. J Am Coll Cardiol 54:1674–1682
12. Zile MR, Baicu CF, Gaasch WH (2004) Diastolic heart failure – abnormalities in active relaxation and passive stiffness of the left ventricle. N Engl J Med 350: 1953–1959
13. Wachter R, Schmidt-Schweda S, Westermann D et al (2009) Blunted frequency-dependent upregulation of cardiac output is related to impaired relaxation in diastolic heart failure. Eur Heart J 30:3027–3036
14. Paulus WJ, Tschope C, Sanderson JE et al (2007) How to diagnose diastolic heart failure: a consensus statement on the diagnosis of heart failure with normal left ventricular ejection fraction by the Heart Failure and Echocardiography Associations of the European Society of Cardiology. Eur Heart J 28:2539–2550
15. Nagueh SF, Appleton CP, Gillebert TC et al (2009) Recommendations for the evaluation of left ventricular diastolic function by echocardiography. Eur J Echocardiogr 10:165–193
16. D'Alto M, Romeo E, Argiento P et al (2015) Echocardiographic prediction of pre- versus postcapillary pulmonary hypertension. J Am Soc Echocardiogr 28:108–115
17. Arkles JS, Opotowsky AR, Ojeda J et al (2011) Shape of the right ventricular Doppler envelope predicts hemodynamics and right heart function in pulmonary hypertension. Am J Respir Crit Care Med 183:268–276
18. Ronco C, House AA, Haapio M (2008) Cardiorenal syndrome. Refining the definition of a complex simbiosi gone wrong. Intensive Care Med 34:957–962 (Liang KV, Williams AW, Greene EL, et al. Acute decompensated heart failure and the cardiorenal syndrome. Crit Care Med. 2008;36:s75–88)
19. Mebazaa A, Gheorghiade M, Pina IL et al (2008) Practical recommendations for prehospital and early in-hospital management of patients presenting with acute heart failure syndrome. Crit Care Med 36:S129–S139
20. Bongartz LG, Cramer MJ, Doevendans PA et al (2005) The severe cardiorenal syndrome: "Guyton revisited". Eur Heart J 26:11–17
21. Khot UN, Mishra M, Yamami MH et al (2003) Severe renal dysfunction complicating cardiogenic shock is not a contraindication to mechanical support as bridge to cardiac transplantation. J Am Coll Cardiol 41:381–385
22. Damman K, Navis G, Smilde TDJ et al (2007) Decreased output, venous congestion and the association with renal impairment in patients with cardiac dysfunction. Eur J Heart Fail 9:872–878
23. Nohria J, Hasselblad V, Stebbins A et al (2008) Cardiorenal interactions. Insights from the ESCAPE trial. J Am Coll Cardiol 51:1268–1274
24. Damman K, van Deursen VM, Navis GN et al (2009) Increased central venous pressure is associated with impaired renal function and mortality in a broad spectrum of patients with cardiovascular disease. J Am Coll Cardiol 53:582–588
25. Muellens W, Abrahams Z, Francis G et al (2009) Importance of venous congestion for worsening renal function in advanced decompensated heart failure. J Am Coll Cardiol 53:589–596
26. Uthoff H, Breidthardt T, Klima T et al (2011) Central venous pressure and impaired renal function in patients with acute heart failure. Eur J Heart Fail 13:432–439
27. Testani MJ, Chen J, McCauley BD, Kimmel SE, Shannon RE (2010) Potential effects of aggressive decongestion during the treatment of decompensated heart failure on renal function and survival. Circulation 122: 265–272
28. Abildgaard U, Agerskov K, Sjontoft E et al (1987) renal vascular adjustments to partial renal venous obstruction in dog kidney. Circ Res 61:194–202
29. Muellens W, Abrahams Z, Skouri HN et al (2008) Elevated intra-abdominal pressure in acute decompensated heart failure. J Am Coll Cardiol 51:300–306
30. Bourge RC, Abraham WT, Adamson PB et al (2008) randomized controlled trial of an implantable continuous hemodynamic monitor in patients with advanced heart failure. J Am Coll Cardiol 51:1073–1079
31. Adamson PB, Abraham WT, Stevenson L et al (2016) Pulmonary artery pressure-guided heart failure management reduces 30-day readmissions. Circ Heart Fail 9:e002600
32. Gheorghiade M, Filippatos G, De Luca L et al (2006) Congestion in acute heart failure syndromes: an essential target of evaluation and treatment. Am J Med 119:S3–S10
33. Cotter G, Metra M, Milo-Cotter O et al (2008) Fluid overload in acute heart failure – Re-distribution and

other mechanisms beyond fluid accumulation. Eur J Heart Fail 10:165–169
34. Greyson CR (2008) Pathophysiology of right ventricular failure. Crit Care Med 36:S57–S65
35. Richardson PDI (1982) Physiological regulation of the hepatic circulation. Fed Proc 41:2111–2116
36. Sherlock S (1951) The liver in heart failure: relation of anatomical, functional and circulatory changes. Br Heart J 13:273–293
37. Verbrugge FH, Dupont M, Steels P et al (2013) Abdominal contributions to cardiorenal dysfunction in congestive heart failure. J Am Coll Cardiol 62:485–495
38. Mailman D (1982) Blood flow and intestinal absorption. Fed Proc 41:2096–2100
39. Chou CC, Gallavan RH (1982) Blood flow and intestinal motility. Fed Proc 41:2090–2095
40. Peschel T, Schonauer M, Thiele H et al (2003) Invasive assessment of bacterial endotoxin and inflammatory cytokines in patients with acute heart failure. Eur J Heart Fail 5:609–614
41. Sandek A, Bauditz J, Swidinski A et al (2007) Altered intestinal function in patients with chronic heart failure. J Am Coll Cardiol 50:1561–1569
42. Valentova M, von Haehling S, Bauditz J et al (2016) Intestinal congestion and right ventricular dysfunction: a link with appetite loss, inflammation, and cachexia in chronic heart failure. Eur Heart J 37:1684–1691
43. Agricola A, Ielasi A, Oppizzi M et al (2009) Long-term prognosis of medically treated patients with functional mitral regurgitation and left ventricular dysfunction. Eur J Heart Fail 11:581–587
44. Siu FY, Enriquez-Sarano TC et al (2000) Determinants of the degree of functional mitral regurgitation in patients with systolic left ventricular dysfunction. Circulation 102:1400–1406
45. Enriquez-Sarano M, Rossi A, Seward JB et al (1997) Determinants of pulmonary hypertension in left ventricular dysfunction. J Am Coll Cardiol 29:153–159
46. Rosenkranz S, Gibbs JS, Wacher R et al (2016) Left ventricular heart failure and pulmonary hypertension. Eur Heart J 37:942–954
47. Guazzi M, Borlaug BA (2012) Pulmonary hypertension due to left heart disease. Circulation 126:975–990
48. Naeje R, Vachiery JL, Yerly P et al (2013) The transpulmonary pressure gradient for the diagnosis of pulmonary vascular disease. Eur J Respir Dis 41:217–223
49. Harvey R, Enson Y, Ferrer IM (1971) A reconsideration on the origins of pulmonary hypertension. Chest 59:82–94
50. Tampakis E, Leary PJ, Van N (2015) Selby et al. The diastolic pulmonary gradient does not predict survival in patients with pulmonary hypertension due to left heart disease. JACC Heart Fail 3:9–16
51. Lankhaar JW, Westerhof N, Faes TJC et al (2006) Quantification of right ventricular afterload in patients with and without pulmonary hypertension. Am J Physiol Heart Circ Physiol 291:H1731–H1737
52. Saouti N, Westerhof N, Helderman F et al (2010) Right ventricular oscillatory power is a constant fraction of total power irrespective of pulmonary artery pressure. Am J Respir Crit Care Med 182:1315–1320
53. Tedford RJ, Hassoun PM, Mathai SC et al (2012) Pulmonary capillary wedge pressure augments right ventricular pulsatile loading. Circulation 145:289–297
54. Pellegrini P, Rossi A, Pasotti M et al (2014) Prognostic relevance of pulmonary arterial compliance in patients with chronic heart failure. Chest 145:1064–1070
55. Dupont M, Mullens W, Skouri HN et al (2012) Prognostic role of pulmonary artery capacitance in advanced heart failure. Circ Heart Fail 5:778–785
56. Georgiopoulou VV, Kalogeropoulos P, Borlaug BA et al (2013) Left ventricular dysfunction with pulmonary hypertension. Part 1: epidemiology, pathophysiology and definitions. Circ Heart Fail 6:344–354
57. Ghio S, Gavazzi A, Campana C et al (2001) Independent and additive prognostic value of right ventricular systolic function and pulmonary artery pressure in patients with chronic heart failure. J Am Coll Cardiol 37:387–388
58. Ghio S, Temporelli PL, Klersy C et al (2013) Prognostic relevance of a noninvasive evaluation of right ventricular pressure in patients with chronic heart failure. Eur J Heart Fail 15:408–414
59. Cowger Matthews J, Koelling TM, Pagani FJ et al (2008) The right ventricular risk score. J Am Coll Cardiol 51:2163–2172
60. Kang G, Ha R, Banerjee D (2016) Pulmonary artery pulsatility index predicts right ventricular assist device implantation. J Heart Lung Transplant 35:67–73
61. Robbins IM, Hemnes AR, Pugh ME et al (2014) High prevalence of occult pulmonary venous hypertension revealed by fluid challenge in pulmonary hypertension. Circ Heart Fail 7:116–122

Cardiomyopathies and Clinical Features

F. Grigioni, L. Potena, G. Marinelli, and Marco Masetti

© Springer International Publishing Switzerland 2017

A. Montalto et al. (eds.), *Mechanical Circulatory Support in End-Stage Heart Failure*,
DOI 10.1007/978-3-319-43383-7_3

Heart failure (HF) is the end-stage scenario common to all different types of cardiomyopathies. It is characterized by an imbalance between the oxygen delivered by the cardiac output and the need of peripheral organs and tissues [1]. However, the clinical picture, the time course of its occurrence, and its treatment can vary according to the different underlying diseases.

Schematically, heart failure can be classified according to:

1. Heart systolic function: reduced (HFrEF) or preserved (HFpEF)
2. Modality of presentation (acute or chronic)
3. Main symptoms: anterograde or retrograde heart failure, being the first characterized by low-output symptoms and the latter by congestion-related symptoms
4. Etiology: being ischemic heart disease and cardiomyopathies are the most frequent ones, even if other non-heart-related conditions can at least favor or worsen HF occurrence

3.1 Heart Failure with Preserved Ejection Fraction (HFpEF)

This topic will be treated briefly, as mechanical circulatory support devices (MCS) are not normally used in this scenario.

Among patients with heart failure, its prevalence is approximately 50% [2], even if it is difficult to be estimated because several different criteria have been used to define this condition. The diagnosis of HFpEF is challenging because it is normally made after having excluded other potential noncardiac causes of symptoms suggestive of HF. However, the diagnostic criteria include signs or symptoms of HF, evidence of preserved LVEF (>50%), and abnormal LV diastolic dysfunction determined by Doppler echocardiography or cardiac catheterization. Obesity, coronary artery disease (CAD), diabetes mellitus, hypertension, atrial fibrillation (AF), and hyperlipidemia are highly prevalent, even if hypertension remains the most important cause of HFpEF.

3.2 Heart Failure with Reduced Ejection Fraction (HFrEF)

In this condition, ejection fraction is reduced, leading to low cardiac output and elevated left filling pressures. This scenario, if chronically perpetuated, can lead to pulmonary hypertension and increased pulmonary vascular resistances.

The general clinical picture of heart failure is characterized by:

- Dyspnea: it is due to pulmonary venous congestion that causes an increase in hematic volume of the lungs and leads to a restrictive respiratory syndrome; other causes are dilatation of pulmonary capillaries that causes a decrease in bronchioles and reduced pulmonary muscles perfusion. In the early phases, dyspnea appears during exertion-related activities; later, it appears also at rest.
- Orthopnea: in orthostatism, the increased preload can increase pulmonary congestion. This causes dyspnea especially in the nocturnal hours, when also adrenergic tone is higher.
- Pulmonary edema: it is due to accumulation of fluid in the interstitial space than in alveolus.
- Cheyne-Stokes breathing: alternation of apnea (when pO2 decreases and pCO2 increases) and hyperventilation, causing hypocapnia, that leads again to apnea.
- Oliguria: due to reduced renal perfusion.
- Asthenia.
- Hepatalgia: it is due to hepatic congestion and increased venous pressure in splanchnic circulation (it occurs often in right heart failure).
- Neurological symptoms: due to low cerebral perfusion, hallucinations, loss of memory, and insomnia.
- Cardiogenic shock and multiorgan failure: in end-stage phases of the disease, with a low cardiac output leading to a low perfusion of all organs.

According to INTERMACS report [3], CAD and cardiomyopathies with a dilated phenotype are the most frequent etiologies leading to the need for mechanical circulatory support (MCS) and/or heart transplantation (HT). In the other cardiomyopathies, LVAD implantation needs to be evaluated only in selected cases, after a careful assessment of comorbidities and of hemodynamic situation.

In the following sections of this chapter, the main clinical and pathophysiological aspects of the most frequent cardiomyopathies will be discussed.

Schematically, as pointed out recently by the Guidelines of the European Society of Cardiology

[4], according to their morphological and functional phenotypes, cardiomyopathies can be distinguished in the following types:

1. Dilated cardiomyopathy
2. Hypertrophic cardiomyopathy
3. Restrictive cardiomyopathies
4. Arrhythmogenic right ventricular cardiomyopathy (ARVC)

Other cardiomyopathies, like tako-tsubo and non-compaction, are classified as "others."

The diagnostic process is made of the recognition of phenotype, a careful assessment of familial history that can give information about inheritance modality, and of other potential extracardiac conditions that can be associated to some specific forms.

3.3 Dilated Cardiomyopathy

Dilated cardiomyopathy (DCM) is characterized by an increased volume and a reduced systolic function of the left ventricle (LV), without any other condition leading to volume overload (i.e., severe valvulopathies or systemic hypertension) and without a significant coronary artery disease responsible of left ventricular dilatation. In the most advanced stages of the disease, also the right ventricle (RV) is dilated, leading to a biventricular involvement. In rare cases, the disease begins from the right ventricle and then spreads to all the heart.

Incidence is 0.7–6/100000 new cases/year and prevalence is 8.3–36.5/100000. In most multicenter RCTs and registries in HF, approximately 30–40% of enrolled patients have DCM.

3.3.1 Etiology

Even if several genes have been advocated to be involved in its pathogenesis, in most of the cases, a primary cause cannot be identified.

A familial history of DCM can be found in about 30% of cases, and it should be suspected when there is a family history of sudden death, especially in the younger age, or of musculoskeletal disease or of abnormalities in the heart conduction system.

The most frequent form of transmission is autosomal dominant, but there are also X-linked forms; among autosomal dominant forms, the most frequent mutations involve genes codifying for the cytoskeletal, sarcomeric protein, Z-band, nuclear membrane, and intercalated disc; X-linked forms include frequent mutations in genes codifying for dystrophin and can be therefore associated with muscular dystrophies, like Becker or Duchenne dystrophy. Also mitochondrial mutations can lead to DCM.

Beside genetic forms, there are acquired forms of DCM; they can be related to toxic effects of substances or drugs. The most frequent case is alcoholic cardiomyopathy, followed by post-chemotherapy or postradiations DCM.

Other acquired forms include peripartum DCM and the dilated evolution after a myocarditic process.

Finally, there is a group in which, even if a clear myocarditic episode is not identifiable, a possible infective-inflammatory process can be advocated in the etiology.

Beside the above considerations, however, in most of the cases, a clear etiology cannot be identified; in the common medical language, these latter forms are generally named as "idiopathic" DCM.

3.3.2 Clinical Picture

The symptoms are typical of heart failure: exertion dyspnea, orthopnea, and low-output symptoms. The disease's onset can be acute with pulmonary edema, cardiogenic shock, biventricular failure, or characterized by aspecific symptoms, leading to an occasional diagnosis.

3.3.3 Instrumental Findings

ECG

Electrocardiogram is abnormal in most of the cases and can be the exam leading to the clinical suspicion. The findings can be various; the most frequent ones are:

- Left bundle branch block (incomplete or complete)
- Left ventricular hypertrophy
- Right bundle branch block
- Ventricular repolarization abnormalities
- Normal ECG

A wide QRS complex is associated with worse prognosis; its presence after 3-6 months of optimal medical therapy is a clinical indicator of response to cardiac resynchronization therapy with a biventricular pacing (CRT). Arrhythmias are frequent in the course of DCM, especially at the onset of the disease and in advanced cases. The most frequent arrhythmia is atrial fibrillation (AF), present in 20% of cases in the acute phase. Ectopic heart beats, like premature ventricular contraction beats (PVC), are very frequent. Ventricular tachycardia can occur; it can be distinguished in non-sustained ventricular tachycardia (NSVT, duration of <30 seconds). or sustained ventricular tachycardia (>30 seconds, SVT). PVCs are asymptomatic in most cases or can be referred by the patient as chest discomfort or palpitation. NSVT can be detected at the earlier stage of the disease in asymptomatic patients at 24-h-ECG monitoring (Holter ECG); SVT instead of VT is symptomatic and can lead to worsening of heart failure symptoms, syncope or to ventricular fibrillation.

Some peculiar electrocardiographic aspects can move the clinician toward the suspicion of particular forms of DCM. For example, ECG aspects of posterolateral necrosis can orient the diagnostic suspicion toward a dystrophinopathy, whereas high-grade recurrent atrioventricular blocks can raise the suspicion of laminopathies A/C, a particular form characterized by a high arrhythmogenic risk.

▪▪ Echocardiography

Echocardiography *is* the fundamental step for the diagnosis. It allows to assess the grade of left (LV) and right ventricular dilatation and systolic function of the left ventricle, through the calculation of ejection fraction (LVEF). According to the Guidelines of American Society of Echocardiography [5], LVEF can be classified as: mildly reduced (41–50%), moderately reduced (30–40%), and severely reduced (<30%). The LV is remodeled, more spherical, and with reduced wall thickness; the degree of LV dilatation is assessed according to the diastolic volumes indexed for body surface area.

The most common finding is a global hypokinesia without regional wall abnormalities that are typical of coronary artery disease. However, some regional wall abnormalities can occur: akinesia or dyskinesia of the posterior basal portion of LV wall (without coronary artery disease) in case of dystrophinopathies or regional akinetic or dyskinetic areas not following a coronary distribution in patients with a previous myocarditis or with sarcoidosis. Left atrial size is often increased, whereas right atrial size is increased in case of severe pulmonary hypertension or of atrial fibrillation.

Diastolic function is studied by assessment of LV filling pattern, through evaluation of the different phases of diastole by pulsed-wave (PW) Doppler. In particular, filling velocities early diastolic velocity (E wave) and A wave (reflecting atrial contraction occurring during the final phase of diastole) are studied; a high (>2) E/A wave ratio, combined with a short deceleration time (reflecting a rapid slope in early diastolic velocity), is indicative of a restrictive pattern (also called grade III diastolic dysfunction), due to impaired diastolic function and to elevated left atrial pressures. According to the relationship between E and A wave peak velocities and deceleration time, different grades of diastolic dysfunction can be defined. The information derived by PW-Doppler study of LV filling pattern is usually combined with assessment of tissue Doppler imaging (TDI) of LV that adds additional information about the different phases of systole and diastole and therefore of their function.

A detailed description of this technique goes beside the aims of this Chapter, but TDI is nowadays a fundamental step in assessing both systolic and diastolic function in DCM. Moreover, it has been demonstrated that the longitudinal assessment of variations in LV filling pattern can provide useful prognostic information and can help in guiding therapy. For example, the transitioning to higher grade of diastolic dysfunction is indicative of arising left atrial and left ventricular pressure, requiring adjustments in therapy, like increased dose of diuretics. An irreversible transition to a higher grade of diastolic dysfunction is a marker of poor prognosis.

Echocardiography allows also to assess the degree of functional mitral regurgitation (MR), due to the increased size of LV and of mitral annulus. The degree of MR is an independent incremental prognostic marker in these patients [6] and can lead to or worsen pulmonary hypertension. The degree of tricuspid regurgitation (TR) is also an important parameter to be calculated, particularly when deciding if the patient is suitable or not for a LVAD; through the continuous-Doppler (CW) evaluation of the regurgitant flow and the calculation of peak regurgitant velocity, it is possible to calculate the pressure gradient through the right atrium and RV, and therefore systolic pulmonary pressure is estimated (right atrial pressure is usually estimated by studying respiratory excursions of inferior vena cava or by evaluating with physical exam central jugular pressure).

The assessment of right heart function is particularly difficult, as RV is not completely visible from transthoracic echocardiography, and it is not possible to calculate RV volumes by 2D exam. While the assessment of LV function is mainly based on calculation of one parameter (LVEF), the evaluation of overall systolic function is based on the information derived from multiple data: (1) RV shortening fraction, (2) tricuspid annular plane systolic excursion (TAPSE), (3) S (systolic) wave by TDI, and (4) myocardial performance index (MPI) or Tei index. A detailed presentation of these parameters will be treated in another Chapter of this book. RV function is impaired in about 25% of cases.

Inferior vena cava diameter and its dynamic respiratory variations are also common parameters evaluated.

▪▪ Magnetic Resonance Imaging (MRI)

In the last years, the use of MRI as diagnostic tool in patients with DCM is increased; this technique, particularly the studying of the late gadolinium enhancement (LGE), can add important information both for clarifying diagnosis and for guiding medical treatment. It can calculate the volumes of heart chambers and systolic function more accurately than echocardiography; and help in distinguishing a LV dilatation due to DCM or to coronary artery disease or to other conditions (i.e., myocarditis, dilated evolution of hypertrophic cardiomyopathy, ARVD, sarcoidosis).

3.4 Specific Cardiomyopathies with a Dilated Phenotype

3.4.1 Alcoholic Cardiomyopathy

Chronic alcoholism is one of the most important causes of DCM [7]. Clinical and phenotypic characteristics are the same of "idiopathic" DCM. The effect of alcohol on the myocardium is dose related, and it is responsive to cessation of its consumption. The mechanisms are alcohol direct toxicity, damage induced by its metabolite acetaldehyde and of other eventual substances (i.e., cobaltum), and thiamine deficit. The diagnosis is suspected when biventricular dysfunction and dilatation are observed in a heavy drinker in the absence of other known causes for myocardial disease. It most commonly occurs in men 30–55 years of age who have been heavy consumers of alcohol for >10 years [8]. Women are less frequently affected but may be more vulnerable with less lifetime alcohol consumption. The risk of asymptomatic alcoholic cardiomyopathy is increased in those consuming >90 g of alcohol per day (7–8 standard drinks per day) for >5 years. Recovery of LV function after cessation of drinking has been reported. The coexistence of hepatic cirrhosis and alcoholic DCM is rare. Arrhythmias are also frequent, especially atrial fibrillation and SVTs. Physical exam findings are similar to the "idiopathic" forms of DCM; however, in this disease, associated muscle myopathy is more common. A frequent presentation is "holiday heart syndrome": chest discomfort, syncope, and palpitations after binge drinking episodes. Complete cessation of alcohol consumption is the therapeutic cornerstone for this disease, together with heart failure therapies.

3.4.2 Cardiotoxicity Related to Cancer Therapies

Several cytotoxic antineoplastic drugs, especially the anthracyclines, are cardiotoxic and can lead to long-term cardiac morbidity. Myocardial damage is mediated by oxidative stress; histologically, it is characterized by severe lesions, up to necrosis and substitutive fibrosis.

Other antineoplastic chemotherapies with cardiac toxicity are the monoclonal antibody against HER-2 receptor of breast cancer (trastuzumab), high-dose cyclophosphamide, taxoids, mitomycin C, 5-fluorouracil, and the interferons [9]. The true incidence and reversibility of chemotherapy-related cardiotoxicity are not well documented.

3.4.3 Myocarditis

Inflammation of the heart may cause HF in about 10% of cases of initially unexplained cardiomyopathy [10]. Myocarditis can arise from viral (or other pathogens) infections, toxins, and medications or as part of other systemic diseases such as systemic lupus erythematosus and other myocardial muscle diseases such as HIV, cardiomyopathy, and possibly peripartum cardiomyopathy. Presentation may be acute, with severe hemodynamic compromise and severe LV dysfunction as seen in acute fulminant myocarditis, or it may be subacute, with an indistinct onset and better-tolerated LV dysfunction [11]. Prognosis varies, with spontaneous complete resolution (paradoxically most often seen with acute fulminant myocarditis) to the development of DCM despite immunosuppressive therapy. The role of immunosuppressive therapy is controversial. Targeting such therapy to specific individuals based on the presence or absence of viral genome in myocardial biopsy samples may improve response to immunosuppressive therapy.

Giant cell myocarditis is a rare form of myocardial inflammation characterized by fulminant HF, often associated with refractory ventricular arrhythmias and a poor prognosis. Histologic findings include diffuse myocardial necrosis with numerous multinucleated giant cells without granuloma formation.

3.4.4 Acquired Immunodeficiency Syndrome

The extent of immunodeficiency influences the incidence of HIV-associated DCM [12–13]. In long-term echocardiographic follow-up, 8% of initially asymptomatic HIV-positive patients were diagnosed with DCM during the 5-year follow-up. DCM could be related to a direct action of the virus on the myocardial tissue or to proteolytic enzymes or cytokine induced by HIV. Mortality is high, independently of CD4 count, race, and sex. Other cardiac manifestations, like pericardial effusion, infective endocarditis, and pulmonary hypertension, can coexist.

3.4.5 Chagas Disease

It is an important cause of death in Central and South America [14]; it usually develops in 10–30% of infected persons, years or even decades after the *Trypanosoma cruzi* infection. Cardiac changes may include biventricular enlargement, thinning or thickening of ventricular walls, apical aneurysms, and mural thrombi. The conduction system is often affected, typically resulting in right bundle branch block, left anterior fascicular block, or complete atrioventricular block.

3.4.6 Peripartum Cardiomyopathy

In peripartum cardiomyopathy, LV dysfunction occurs between the last trimester of pregnancy or the early puerperium and 6-month postpartum [15]. The etiology is not clear, even if inflammatory processes have been advocated. It is reported in 1:1300–1:4000 live births, and it is more common in African countries. Risk factors for peripartum cardiomyopathy include advanced maternal age and multiparity. Clinical presentation is similar to "idiopathic" DCM, but a higher frequency of venous thromboembolism is reported. The clinical onset can be in some cases severe. Regarding prognosis, there are two different scenarios: an improvement in myocardial function in the first 6 months after presentation (30–50% of cases) or a rapidly worsening disease, with poor prognosis (50% mortality rate at 6 years). Subsequent pregnancy in women with a history of peripartum cardiomyopathy may be associated with a further decrease in LV function and clinical deterioration, including death. However, if ventricular function has normalized in women with a history of peripartum cardiomyopathy, the risk may be less. The main mechanisms involved are probably viral or autoimmune myocarditis and prior existing DCM, worsened by pregnancy.

3.4.7 Hemochromatosis

It is characterized by an excessive deposition of iron in different tissues: the heart, liver, gonads, and pancreas [16]. The most frequent form is an autosomal recessive disorder, due to a mutation in HFE gene, which codes for a protein involved in regulation of iron uptake in the intestine and liver. Hemochromatosis can be due also to chronic liver disease or to lifetime transfusion requirements as seen in people with beta-thalassemia major. In this latter disease, HF is one of the most frequent causes of death. The classic clinical picture is characterized by: HF, cirrhosis, impotence, diabetes, and arthritis. Cardiac involvement leads to both systolic and diastolic dysfunction.

Echocardiogram reveals increased wall thickness and LV dilatation; hemodynamic characteristics can show a restrictive physiology. Plasma iron levels are high; serum ferritin and urinary iron are elevated. Chelation therapy and phlebotomy have dramatically improved the outcome of hemochromatosis. Mortality is higher in males, especially in the ones with clinical onset at younger age.

3.4.8 Cardiac Sarcoidosis

Systemic sarcoidosis is characterized by a diffuse granulomatous infiltration of different organs, especially the lungs, skin, and reticuloendothelial system [17]. Cardiac sarcoidosis may affect up to 25% of patients with systemic sarcoidosis. Clinical manifestations are mainly arrhythmias: PVCs, junctional tachycardias, atrioventricular blocks, VTs, and sudden cardiac death. The most frequent clinical phenotype is DCM; in some cases, a restrictive phenotype can be present. Echocardiography can show LV dilatation; in some cases, there are regional hypo- or akinetic regions or aneurisms (with or without global dilatation) in regions unusual for ischemic cardiomyopathy, like the anterobasal portion of interventricular septum. Cardiac magnetic resonance and cardiac positron emission tomographic scanning can identify cardiac involvement with patchy areas of myocardial inflammation and fibrosis. However, diagnosis is difficult and requires a high grade of suspicion; a delay in conduction delays or malignant arrhythmias in young patients with a dilated or restrictive phenotype can help in suspecting the disease.

3.5 Hypertrophic Cardiomyopathy

It is characterized by an unexplained LV hypertrophy associated with non-dilated ventricular chambers. In particular, conditions causing hemodynamic overload, like arterial hypertension and valvulopathies, need to be excluded. The disease is present in every age group, and incidence is the same between males and females [18].

Hypertrophy is typically asymmetric, and in some cases can be very represented, like leading to a severe reduction in LV volumes. Most frequently, hypertrophy is localized at interventricular septum, especially in the anterobasal portion; their frequent localizations are the apex and medioventricular portion of LV; in less frequent cases, also the free wall of the right ventricle can be interested by the disease. The typical histological feature is myocardial disarray; frequently, small vessels of the coronary arteries can have intimal thickening and lumen narrowing; this morphologic alteration can cause the myocardial ischemia and angina pectoris, especially in the end-stage form of the disease. The length of anterior leaflet of the mitral valve is usually increased; moreover, anterior papillary muscle is dislocated toward interventricular septum. These features can lead to the systolic anterior movement of the mitral valve (SAM) that can cause dynamic left ventricular obstruction.

3.5.1 Etiology

The disease has an autosomal dominant transmission, with high penetrance; in >60% of cases, genes codifying for sarcomeric proteins are involved, most frequently beta myosin heavy chain protein, myosin-binding protein C, tropomyosin alpha-1 chain, troponin, and myosin light chain.

Other genetic disorders, with mutations not involving sarcomeric proteins, can lead to morphological phenotypes similar to HCM; the most frequent ones are:

- Anderson-Fabry disease: X-linked disease, characterized by alpha galactosidase enzyme deficit (frequent renal and neurological manifestations)
- Danon disease: X-linked, often with preexcitation aspects at ECG
- Pompe disease: glycogenosis with recessive transmission; in the adults, associated with limb myopathy
- Mitochondrial diseases (like MELAS syndrome)
- LEOPARD syndrome and Noonan syndrome: autosomal dominant transmission
- Friedreich ataxia: autosomal recessive transmission

The pathophysiology of HCM is characterized by:

- Dynamic left ventricular obstruction: it is caused by the anterior systolic movement of the mitral valve. It increases when the preload

is reduced (i.e., orthostatic position, high doses of diuretics, tachycardia) and can be exacerbated by physical exercise. Up to 30% of patients have an obstruction in basal conditions and an equal proportion during physical exercise.
- Diastolic dysfunction, due to the impaired relaxation.
- Myocardial ischemia.

The clinical picture can vary from completely asymptomatic patients to sudden death. The most common symptoms are exertion dyspnea, angina, and syncope. Physical exam reveals elective murmur pro-mesosystolic, with maximal intensity on mitral and aortic auscultation foci that increases with Valsalva maneuvers or with physical exertion.

▪ ECG

In most cases, it is pathologic. Most common findings are severe left ventricular hypertrophy with overload signs, ST–T wave abnormalities, pathological Q waves in inferior and lateral leads, and high R waves in anterior leads.

▪▪ Echocardiography

It is the fundamental exam for diagnosis, and it allows to localize and assess the magnitude of hypertrophy (i.e., typically >15 mm). LV volumes are normal or reduced, LVEF is normal or highly normal, but the longitudinal function of LV is usually reduced (S wave <8 cm/s). The exam of the mitral valve can reveal SAM and quantify the degree of mitral regurgitation. One of the most important information is to measure the gradient at left ventricular outflow tract (LVOT); in obstructive HCM gradient is >30 mmHg at rest, or after exercise or Valsalva maneuvers. It becomes hemodynamically significant when it is >50 mmHg; in such cases, surgical myectomy can be considered in some cases, it can reach values >100 mmHg. In forms with mild hypertrophy, differential diagnosis must be done with other forms, like athletes' heart; in these cases, a careful physical examination and familial history can help in distinguishing the two forms.

▪▪ MRI

It allows to assess the localization and the degree of hypertrophy, and to evaluate dynamic obstruction, and the degree of myocardial fibrosis, through LGE.

Overall, differential diagnosis must be made with athletes' heart, secondary causes of hypertrophy (i.e., subvalvular aortic stenosis), and genetic disorders due to non-sarcomeric mutations and mitochondrial forms, as above specified.

The clinical course of HCM is very heterogeneous. Some patients are asymptomatic for all their life; other patients develop HF, angina, atrial fibrillation, or sudden death.

A minority (5–10%) of patients evolves toward LV dilatation (end-stage HCM), with a final clinical phenotype very similar to DCM; this group is carried by the worse prognosis among all patients. About 20% of patients develop atrial fibrillation. Sudden death is due in most cases to VTs or cardiac arrest; known risk factors for sudden death are familial history of death related to HCM or of sudden death, unexplained syncope (especially in young people), NSVTs at 24 h ECG Holter, severe LV hypertrophy (thickness >30 mm), and hypotension or absent increasing of blood pressure during exertion. Patients with a sarcomeric mutation usually have a higher rate of arrhythmias and of sudden death [19].

3.6 Restrictive Cardiomyopathies

This is a heterogeneous group of diseases characterized by an impaired ventricular filling, requiring high filling pressures, especially in the first phase of diastole. This group constitutes only rarely an indication for MCS implantation; therefore, given the scopes of this book, they will be treated very shortly.

RCMs can involve the myocardium or endocardium.

In the first case, we can distinguish three forms, based on the localization of the pathologic process:
- Infiltrative RCM: extracellular deposition of abnormal substances (i.e., amyloidosis)
- Accumulation forms: intracellular deposition (i.e., glycogenosis, hemochromatosis)
- Neither infiltration nor accumulation: desminopathies, post-actinic cardiopathy, idiopathic RCM, and sarcomeric forms with restrictive phenotype

In cases of endocardial involvement, most frequent forms are endomyocardial fibrosis and hypereosinophilic forms (Loeffler endocarditis).

Pathophysiology is common to all these forms and it is characterized by a high frequency of HF with normal ejection fraction. From an epidemiologic point of view, the most important forms are amyloidosis, idiopathic RCM and forms with endocardial involvement.

3.6.1 Amyloidosis

Cardiac amyloidosis involves the extracellular deposition of insoluble proteins as fibrils in the heart, resulting in HF. The most frequent forms are:

- AL amyloidosis (monoclonal kappa or lambda light chains)
- Familial TTR amyloidosis (mutant transthyretin), with an autosomal dominant expression
- Senile TTR amyloidosis (wild-type, non-mutant transthyretin)

Other less frequent forms are secondary amyloidosis (protein A) and dialysis-associated amyloidosis (beta-2 microglobulin) or can affect the heart, but cardiac involvement is primarily encountered in AL and TTR amyloidosis [20]. Amyloid infiltrates interstitium, leading to a physical and electrical separation of myocardial cells. The main consequence is an RCM with severe HF episodes; also atrial fibrillation and atrioventricular blocks are frequent. Often, there are extracardiac manifestations: orthostatic hypotension (AL and aTTR), carpal tunnel syndrome (TTR and SSA), and proteinuria (AL). The disease can be rapidly progressive, and in patients with ventricular septum thickness >15 mm, LVEF <40%, and symptoms of HF, median survival may be <6 months. Cardiac biomarkers (e.g., B-type natriuretic peptide [BNP], cardiac troponin) have been reported to predict response and progression of disease and survival. Three percent to four percent of African Americans carry an amyloidogenic allele of the human serum protein transthyretin (TTR V122I), which appears to increase risk for cardiac amyloid deposition after 65 years of age. Neurological involvement can be severe and progressive, especially in TTR-related forms and is characterized by an autonomic neuropathy.

ECG

It can show atrioventricular blocks or diffuse low voltages, due to infiltration of the amyloid or to pericardial effusion.

Echocardiography

The main findings are LV hypertrophy, diffuse thickening of atrioventricular valves and of interatrial septum, mild pericardial effusion, and granular sparkling; LV function is normal, but myocardial velocities at TDI and strain and strain rate are impaired. In some cases, there is a discrepancy between diffuse low voltages at ECG and hypertrophy at echocardiography.

MRI

The typical aspects for diagnosis are high avidity of the myocardium for gadolinium and late enhancement of gadolinium with diffuse subendocardial diffusion.

TTR and senile amyloidosis are detectable at 99mTcDPD scintigraphy. The histologic diagnosis is made by subcutaneous fatty tissue biopsy (for AL) and by endomyocardial biopsy (for TTR forms).

Natural history of the disease is characterized by rapid progression of heart failure. In cases of AL amyloidosis, combined autologous stem cell transplantation and heart transplantation can be considered [21]. In selected cases of TTR amyloidosis, without a severe neurological involvement, a combined heart-liver transplantation may be considered in high specialized centers [22].

3.7 ARVC

ARVC is a genetic form of cardiomyopathy characterized by a fibro-fatty infiltration of the right ventricle and is caused by mutations in genes that encode elements of the desmosome [23]. Desmosomal gene mutations explain 50% of cases, and ten genes are currently associated with the disease. In most cases, inheritance is autosomal dominant; in a minority of cases, the transmission is recessive (in Naxos island, where it is associated with cutaneous manifestations). It is responsible of 20% of cases of sudden death. In the most advanced stages of the disease, the pathological process involves also LV. Overall prevalence is between 1:1000 and 1:5000; mean age of affected individuals is between 7 and 40 years.

ECG

It can show negative T waves in right precordial leads (V1–V3) without right bundle brunch block and epsilon waves (from the end of QRS to the beginning of T wave). PVCs and VTs are frequent; VTs have a left bundle brunch morphology.

Echocardiography

In the advanced stages, it shows dilatation and hypokinesia of RV; in the initial stages, diagnosis can be challenging, and the clinician must pay attention to these signs: akinesia, dyskinesia, or aneurisms at apex or at RV outflow tract and increased trabeculation and fissuring of the RV walls.

MRI

It can identify, through LGE, areas of fibrosis; moreover, it can identify areas of adipose infiltration.

The diagnostic process is very challenging; for this reason, diagnostic score has been build, comprehensive of major and minor diagnostic criteria: morphologic, histologic, electrocardiographic, arrhythmic, and familial history.

The natural story of the disease is characterized by different phases: an asymptomatic stage with structural abnormalities, a phase characterized by electrical disturbances, and finally the progression to right ventricular failure and then biventricular failure.

A substantial proportion of patients with sudden death had previously developed a history of syncope. Risk factors for arrhythmias are previous cardiac arrest, syncope, familial history of sudden death, VTs, severe RV dysfunction, and LV involvement. In these cases, ICD implantation is recommended.

3.8 Other Cardiomyopathies

3.8.1 Stress (Tako-tsubo) Cardiomyopathy

Tako-tsubo cardiomyopathy is an acute reversible LV dysfunction in the absence of significant CAD, triggered by acute emotional or physical stress. This phenomenon is most common among middle-aged women and appears to be related to catecholamine release; it is identified by a distinctive pattern of "apical ballooning." A majority of patients have a clinical and ECG presentation similar to that of acute coronary syndrome (ACS) and may have transiently elevated cardiac enzymes.

3.8.2 Non-compaction Myocardium

This condition is characterized by a diffuse trabeculation in LV; the ventricular wall has a normal basal layer and a "spongy" internal layer. It can be diagnosed by echocardiography, but MRI has the best sensitivity. It can be associated to DCM, but even to HCM or congenital heart diseases. In the clinical practice, the association of DCM and non-compaction myocardium must orient the clinician toward the research of neuromuscular diseases.

References

1. Ponikowski P et al (2016) 2016 ESC Guidelines for the diagnosis and treatment of acute and chronic heart failure. Eur Heart J 37:2129–2200
2. Owan TE, Hodge DO, Herges RM et al (2006) Trends in prevalence and outcome of heart failure with preserved ejection fraction. N Engl J Med 355: 251–259
3. Kirklin JK et al (2015) Seventh INTERMACS annual report: 15,000 patients and counting. J Heart Lung Transplant 34(12):1495–1504
4. Elliott P, Andersson B et al (2008) Classification of the cardiomyopathies: a position statement from the european society of cardiology working group on myocardial and pericardial diseases. Eur Heart J 29:270–276
5. Lang RM et al (2015) Recommendations for cardiac chamber quantification by echocardiography in adults: an update from the American Society of Echocardiography and the European Association of Cardiovascular Imaging. J Am Soc Echocardiogr 28:1–39
6. Grigioni F et al (2005) Contribution of ischemic mitral regurgitation to congestive heart failure after myocardial infarction. J Am Coll Cardiol 45(2): 260–267
7. Piano MR (2002) Alcoholic cardiomyopathy: incidence, clinical characteristics, and pathophysiology. Chest 121:1638–1650
8. Cerqueira MD et al (1991) Rarity of preclinical alcoholic cardiomyopathy in chronic alcoholics less than 40 years of age. Am J Cardiol 67:183–187
9. Bovelli D et al (2010) Cardiotoxicity of chemotherapeutic agents and radiotherapy-related heart disease: ESMO Clinical Practice Guidelines. Ann Oncol 21:v277–v282
10. Kindermann I et al (2012) Update on myocarditis. J Am Coll Cardiol 59:779–792

11. McCarthy RE et al (2000) Long-term outcome of fulminant myocarditis as compared with acute (nonfulminant) myocarditis. N Engl J Med 342:690–695
12. Grody WW et al (1990) Infection of the heart by the human immunodeficiency virus. Am J Cardiol 66:203–206
13. Raidel SM et al (2002) Targeted myocardial transgenic expression of HIV Tat causes cardiomyopathy and mitochondrial damage. Am J Physiol Heart Circ Physiol 282:H1672–H1678
14. Kransdorf EP, Zakowski PC, Kobashigawa JA (2014) Chagas isease in solid organ and heart transplantation. Curr Opin Infect Dis 27(5):418–424
15. Elkayam U et al (2001) Maternal and fetal outcomes of subsequent pregnancies in women with peripartum cardiomyopathy. N Engl J Med 344:1567–1571
16. Gujja P et al (2010) Iron overload cardiomyopathy: better understanding of an increasing disorder. J Am Coll Cardiol 56:1001–1012
17. Srichai MB et al (2011) Cardiac sarcoidosis. J Am Coll Cardiol 58:438
18. Elliott P et al (2014) 2014 ESC guidelines on diagnosis and management of hypertrophic cardiomyopathy. Eur Heart J 35:2733–2779
19. Biagini E et al (2014) Significance of sarcomere gene mutations analysis in the end-stage phase of hypertrophic cardiomyopathy. Am J Cardiol 114(5): 769–776
20. Quarta CC et al (2014) Left ventricular structure and function in transthyretin-related versus light-chain cardiac amyloidosis. Circulation 129(18): 1840–1849
21. Potena L et al (2014) Prognostic stratification and treatment of cardiac light chain amyloidosis: a narrow path in the jungle. J Heart Lung Transplant 33(2):136–138
22. Reich HJ et al (2015) Combined heart and liver transplantation: the Cedars-Sinai experience. Transplant Proc 47(9):2722–2726
23. Basso C et al (2009) Arrhythmogenic right ventricular cardiomyopathy. Lancet 373(9671):1289–1300

MCS Candidate Selection Criteria

Cristiano Amarelli, Marianna Buonocore, Ciro Maiello, Andrea Montalto, and Georg Wieselthaler

© Springer International Publishing Switzerland 2017
A. Montalto et al. (eds.), *Mechanical Circulatory Support in End-Stage Heart Failure*,
DOI 10.1007/978-3-319-43383-7_4

4.1 General Perspective

Following the definition from the 2009 ACCF/AHA HF guidelines, a patient affected by stage D heart failure (HF) is defined as having a "truly refractory HF who might be eligible for specialized, advanced treatment strategies, such as MCS, procedures to facilitate fluid removal, continuous inotropic infusions, or cardiac transplantation or other innovative and experimental procedures or for end-of-life care, such as hospice" [1].

Among the available choices in this armamentarium for the treatment of heart failure, mechanical circulatory support (MCS) faced a considerable expansion during the last decade as witnessed by the seventh and latest annual report of the Interagency Registry for Mechanically Assisted Circulatory Support (INTERMACS) [2]. This is due to the important technological advancements across the three generations of ventricular assist devices (VADs), with the new miniaturized continuous-flow devices that have likely 10 years free from mechanical failure, thus leading to significant improvement in terms of patients' survival [3].

During the same period, we experienced a slight decline in the number of heart transplants performed, due to a reduced availability of suitable heart donors [4], and an increasing number of patients on the waiting list, without a concomitant introduction of new drugs capable to modify or even reverse the progression of the disease, especially when applied in a very late state.

Even if heart transplantation is still considered the gold standard treatment for stage D HF, early results with VAD implantation are comparable in terms of survival at 1 and 2 years (80% and 70%, respectively) particularly when implanted only as left ventricular assist device (LVAD). Biventricular assist devices (BiVAD) or TAH, whose survival is only around 50% at 1 year [5], used for patients with severe biventricular HF, indicating increased risk of the advanced disease.

Taken these facts into consideration it can be concluded that MCS represents nowadays a valid therapeutic option for end-stage HF.

Nevertheless, in order to reach a solid improvement in patient outcome and a cost-effective balance for this still considerable expensive technology, a careful patient selection and a proper timing of the implantation is needed [6–9].

LVADs have been predominantly implanted in transplant candidates who are not expected to reach transplant, deemed too sick for transplant or with potentially reversible transplant contraindications [10]. Main goals of LVAD therapy in such a population are to improve symptoms, quality of life, and prognosis. Equally important goals are to stabilize or reverse organ dysfunction and/or pulmonary vascular hypertension, thus increasing the likelihood of a successful transplant. Finally, prevent progressive right ventricular dysfunction that might contraindicate future LVAD implantation is the key strategy to expand the population of patients benefiting of the LVAD technology.

Clinical decision support tools and criteria for HTx listing are well validated and generally agreed upon: peak VO_2, its percentage of predicted VO_2, the Heart Failure Survival Score (HFSS), and the number of admission for inotropic support. In contrast, there are no validated selection criteria and indeed no consensus when it comes to candidate selection for LVAD, and selection relies instead on clinical status, inotrope dependence, and invasive hemodynamic parameters. With worsening clinical status, the need for LVAD and its clinical benefit increases but so does the perioperative risk, and optimal operative timing becomes difficult.

In this chapter, considering the different technological solutions (ECMO, LVAD, BiVAD, TAH), indications for MCS will be addressed leaving the choice of the device open but trying to support the advantages of different strategies in different clinical settings. In fact, if the indications for a short-term MCS (temporary circulatory support, TCS) and for a mid- and long-term MCS might be considered ideally the same in a system without economic constraints. The implanting centers should be committed to warrant a fair treatment to all the patients (whose number are rapidly rising) without risk to lower the general perception of the effectivity of this emerging technology [11].

To correctly define the indication for every clinical condition and to standardize the targets of MCS is important to clarify the variables that the surgeon and the cardiologist have to keep in mind when giving indication to MCS:

- INTERMACS classification
- Underlying disease/etiology and eventual reversibility
- Patient comorbidities and reversibility
- Device strategy
- Costs/benefit
- Frailty, nutritional status, and risk of infections
- Assessment of hemorrhagic and thromboembolic risk

Once the decision of an LVAD implantation has been considered as a valuable option, the subsequent evaluations should be:

- Available risk scores
- Right heart dysfunction reversibility and/or need of management of right ventricle to reduce perioperative unplanned RVAD implantation
- Management of aortic valve to avoid the approach of the aortic valve during midterm follow-up
- Surgical management and/or need of eventual concomitant procedures
- Need of pulsatility and eventual strategies to preserve from hemorrhagic complications

In case of severe right ventricular reversibility with need of biventricular support, the choice between TAH and BiVAD should be taken considering the following factors:

- Policy of implantation and quality of life
- Technical feasibility of intracorporeal implantation
- Need to explant the heart
- Possible reversibility of right ventricular dysfunction over long time
- Patient choice and informed consent

In case of indication to a TCS, the following factors have to be evaluated on:

- Which device provide the most minimal risks?
- Is there need for an oxygenator in the system and/or for how long is there needed?
- What is the final goal for this patient?

Keeping in mind two simple flow charts (◘ Figs. 4.1 and 4.2), this chapter will try to address the need to be exhaustive but simple for the reader.

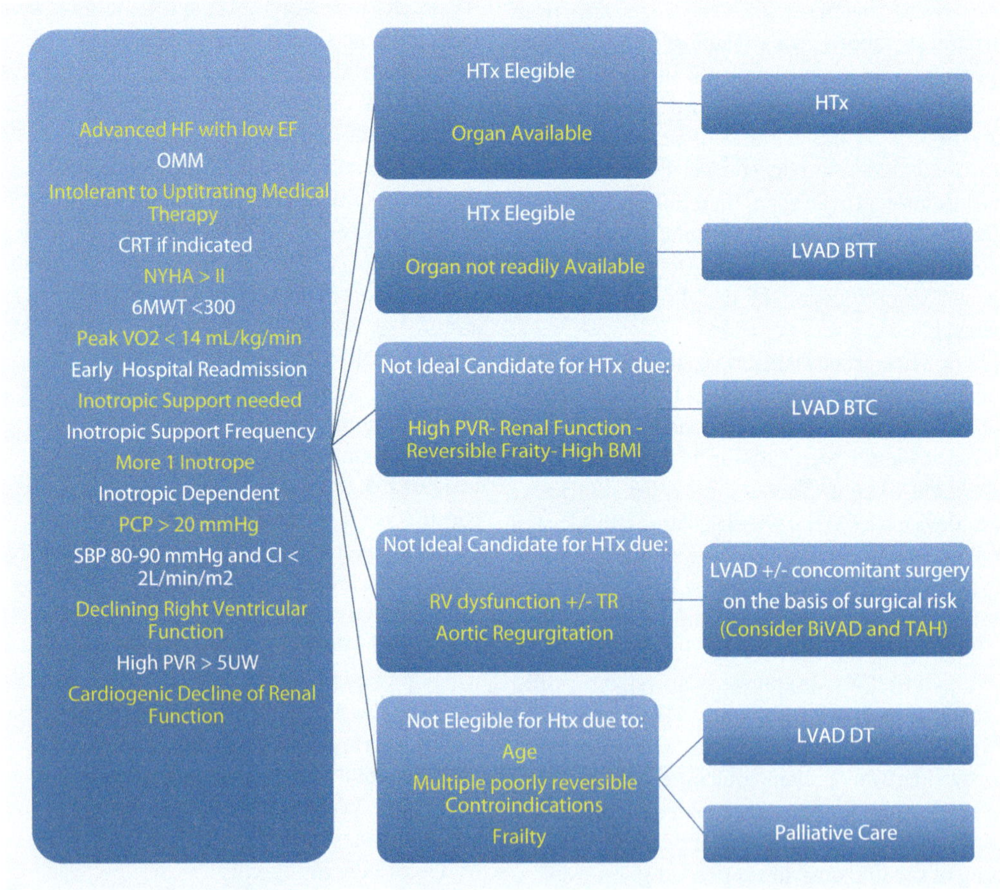

◘ **Fig. 4.1** Patient selection workflow. *HF* heart failure; *EF* ejection fraction; *OMM* optimal medical management; *CRT* continuous replacement therapy; *6MWT* 6-minutes walking test; *PCP* pulmonary capillary pressure; *SBP* systolic blood pressure; *HTx* heart transplant; *RV* right ventricle; *TR* tricuspid regurgitation; *LVAD* left ventricular assist device; *BTT* bridge to transplant; *BTC* bridge to candidacy; *BiVAD* bi-ventricular assist device; *TAH* total artificial heart; *DT* destination therapy

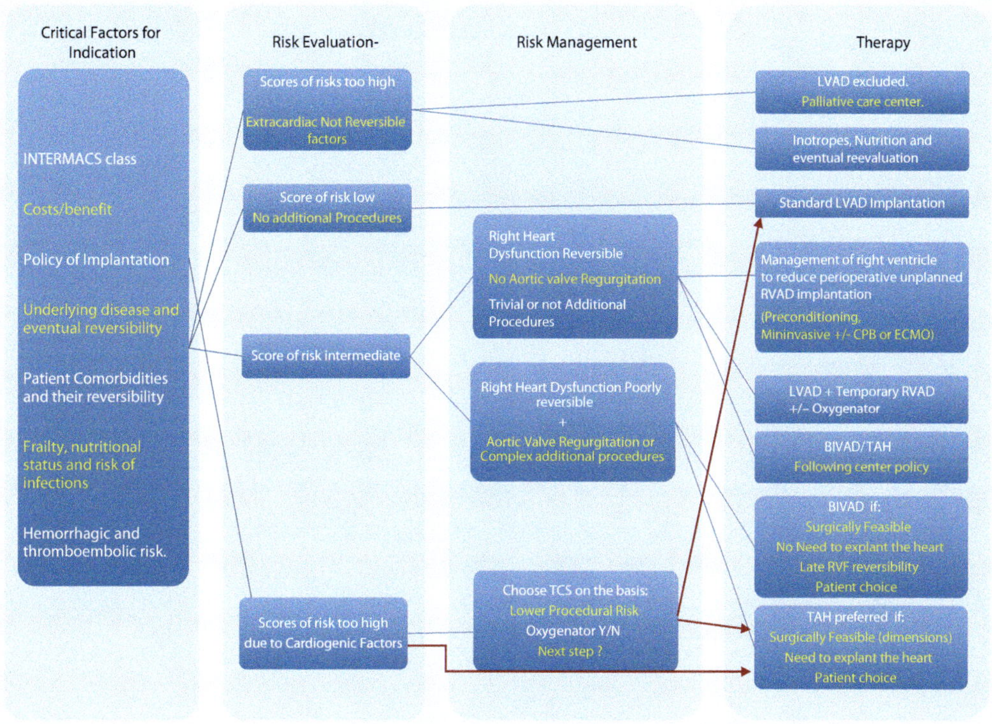

Fig. 4.2 Risk/Benefit Evaluation for patients candidate to LVAD implantation

4.2 INTERMACS Classification

One of the parameters most commonly used to guide the selection of the right treatment for every patient is the Interagency Registry for Mechanically Assisted Circulatory Support (INTERMACS) classification (Table 4.1), a risk stratification tool for durable MCS support candidates aiming to normalize the outcomes of the implanting centers in the US to the preoperative patients' clinical conditions.

The classification appears extremely easy to apply and aims to overcome the wide spectrum of the possible preoperative clinical scenarios. Meanwhile the INTERMACS classification was adopted by the whole heart failure community and is now accepted worldwide.

The classification appears extremely easy to apply and aims to overcome the great spectrum of possible preoperative clinical scenarios. Meanwhile the INTERMACS classification was adopted by the whole heart failure community and is now accepted worldwide. The classification has been shown to be effective to evaluate the short-term mortality risk of a VAD patient as well as to identify adverse events associated with different INTERMACS profiles. As a consequence of the fact that patients in INTERMACS profile 1 ("critical cardiogenic shock") experience higher mortality (from 65% up to 76% at 1 year) and morbidity, a shift was noticed from implanting durable VADs in patients with INTERMACS profile 1 [2] towards patients characterized by a lower acuity and severity of illness (30% implants in INTERMACS class I in 2008 to only 15% in 2013) [12]. Only durable VADs and TAH go into the INTERMACS registry. Unfortunately, this leaves behind the possibility of outcome analysis of TCS, mainly used for bridge-to -decision applications. In order to lower the costs and avoid futile implantations of expensive durable VADs the strategy of bridge-to-decision with TCS is becoming widely adopted within our community [10, 13].

To even better stratify the VAD population and evaluate concomitant risk factors, three modifier factors (TCS, arrhythmia, and frequent flyer (FF)) were successively added [14]. The TCS modifier is meant to be assigned to patients in profiles 1–3 who are supported with either with an intra-aortic balloon pump (IABP), an extracorporeal

Table 4.1 INTERMACS classification

Levels	Description	Time to MCS
1	"Crashing and burning" critical cardiogenic shock	Within hours
2	"Progressive decline" inotrope dependence with continuing deterioration	Within a few days
3	"Stable but inotrope dependent" describes clinical stability on mild-moderate doses of intravenous inotropes (patients stable on temporary circulatory support without inotropes are within this profile)	Within a few weeks
4	Recurrent advanced heart failure "recurrent" rather than "refractory" decompensation	Within weeks to months
5	"Exertion intolerant" describes patients who are comfortable at rest but are intolerant of exercise	Variable
6	"Exertion limited" a patient who is able to do some mild activity, but fatigue results within a few minutes or any meaningful physical exertion	Variable
7	"Advanced NYHA 3" describes patients who are clinically stable with a reasonable level of comfortable activity, despite history of previous decompensation that is not recent	Not a candidate for MCS

Modifiers:
TCS: Includes inpatients supported with IABP, ECMO, TandemHeart, Levitronix, Impella
A: Arrhythmia modifies any profile. Recurrent tachyarrhythmias should be investigated if reversible or treatable
FF: Modify outpatients in classes III–VI with frequent emergency department visits or hospitalizations (>2 emergency department or hospital visits in 3 months or three visits in 6 months) for heart failure management, including use of intravenous diuretics, inotropes, or ultrafiltration

membrane oxygenator (ECMO), or a temporary ventricular (right or left) support (TCS) prior to their durable VAD implantation. The arrhythmia modifier can be applied to any profile and classifies patients with recurrent ventricular tachyarrhythmia that evoke clinical compromise. Finally, the FF modifier applies to patients in profile 3 at home on inotropes and patients in profiles 4–7. The FF modifier denotes a patient with frequent emergency department visits or hospitalizations for heart failure symptoms (Table 4.1).

When IABP is removed from the TCS definition, the TCS modifier conferred >40% higher mortality [14]. The strategy of using TCS, might save costs in patients with otherwise durable VAD implantations, but can end up in a very complex management with multiple procedures and a predicted long ICU stay. Looking at the accuracy of prediction, the TCS modifier should probably only be applied only in patients supported with ECMO or temporary VAD support and should be always assigned to a profile 1 TCS. The real discriminant to clarify the effectiveness of such a strategy is to determine the percentage of patients receiving a TCS and being actively withdrawn from support, in order to establish the real amount of resources spared. Finally, addressing INTERMACS I those patients with a bridge-to-decision approach has the potential to reduce the higher mortality rate of this challenging patient population.

Arrhythmias as cause of decompensation should be always adequately addressed and eventually treated before or during LVAD implantation if its resolution is not deemed as a goal trough wall-stress reduction due to LVAD implantation. The clinical profile of patients with the arrhythmias was that of sicker patients, requiring more vasopressors and ventilator and dialysis support than patients without high-burden arrhythmias. However, arrhythmias may limit the impact of preoperative interventions such as IABP and inotrope support thus warping the accuracy of INTERMACS levels.

The FF modifier portended worse outcome beyond that of INTERMACS profile and other known risk factors; unfortunately, only 47% of patients with profiles 3–7 had the FF designation recorded, and this reduces the quality of prediction of such a modifier. However, these data should mandate an indication to MCS implantation when a patient does not recover an acceptable clinical stability after a first treatment with inotropes. A second episode of decompensation during the next 6 months should be a red flag indicating prompt MCS implantation.

Today, INTERMACS data fully support MCS implantation with durable devices when the patients are in classes I up to III. However, the feared increased risk of mortality and of adverse events in the lower INTERMACS classes dampened the use of implantable LVAD in such patients so that, despite the maximum clinical benefit, LVADs have been less commonly implanted in these settings.

It should be noted that the clinical results and the consequential benefit in this setting were realized in an era in which the largest amount of pumps implanted was pulsatile [2] and indeed not necessarily these data could be replied in the era of continuous-flow pumps. In the 2013 report the incidence of right ventricle failure (RVF) in INTERMACS I patients is significantly higher reaching an incidence up to 40% [2], thus mandating a careful selection of LVAD candidate versus BiVAD and TAH [15]. Weighting the clinical benefits and the costs, the adoption of a short-term easy-to-implant device in class I has become a common pathway of treatment for such complex patients especially when a complete neurological evaluation is not available and the metabolic status impedes to establish the reversibility of clinical conditions [16–19]..

On the other hand, the excellent outcome reached by LVAD implantation in the last registered trials and in the real-world practice might be comparable to midterm results of heart transplantation in the era of marginal donors [20], and this is stimulating to plan studies in order to expand LVAD implantation to the higher INTERMACS classes [8, 21]. Until now, the high cumulative risks of complications causing re-hospitalization during the first year [2] and the amelioration of the outcomes of medical treatment (ROADMAP) prevented the expansion to less sick patients. Long-term data from a trial on medical management of patients suffering of end-stage heart failure (MEDAMACS) are awaited to further define the benefit of MCS in such patients and to identify clusters of patients with more aggressive clinical course beside a high INTERMACS profile.

Preliminary data recently available from the MEDAMACS Registry of patients in INTERMACS 4–7 showed a high overall event rate in the entire study [21, 22]. Of the total study population of 144 patients, 75.7% were alive without a transplant or LVAD, 11.8% had died, 4.9% received a transplant, and 6.3% had an LVAD implantation. The high mortality rates were driven by patients that were transplant/DT-LVAD ineligible. Transplant/DT-LVAD ineligible patients had substantially higher mortality rates (23.3% versus 8.0% in DT-LVAD eligible and 5.9% in transplant eligible, $p = 0.02$), a larger number of patients were requiring inotropes, and greater number of re-hospitalizations. These data clearly suggest that there is still an important unmet clinical need (>30% of patients in INTERMACS IV–VII) among those patients with a weak evidence for a VAD implant according to the guidelines, but with an overall bad final outcome. In the registry, clinically perceived frailty, social factors, and risk of nonadherence to therapies were the principal explanation of being labeled as transplant/DT-LVAD ineligible. These patients will be probably the new frontier for MCS in the near future waiting for a less invasive and easy to manage strategy of circulatory support such as cheaper and easy to handle pumps for partial support.

4.3 Costs

The management of End-Stage-CHF with MCS carries high costs due both to device direct costs and to indirect costs mainly related to the prolonged ICU/Hospital stay. Cost-effectiveness of MCS experienced a meaningful improvement in the recent era, partially due to the reduction of implant costs and also due to the improved knowledge of care with consecutive reduction in length of stay. The hospital costs decreased by 50% with the evolution from the pulsatile devices to continuous-flow device implantation [11, 23]. On the other end, the incidence of the pathology and also the socioeconomic weight in terms of re-hospitalization, with the relative consumption of human and economic resources, still represent a serious factor limiting the expansion of this technology.

LVAD therapy represents a mainstream therapy for advanced heart failure with a relative 75% reduction in cost/QALY over the past decade. The overall high costs for MCS is outweighed by the definitive clinical benefit of CHF patients in comparison to patients with other life-threatening diseases. The anticipated reduction of adverse events should further reduce the costs of MCS [24].

The British BTT experience was the initial cost-effectiveness analysis of continuous-flow LVADs, showing a cost per QALY of £258,913 ($414,275) (depending on the choosen device) [25]. This estimate outweighed of £30,000 for cost-effectiveness of the treatment, and the two determinants of poor cost-effectiveness were improved survival of advanced heart failure patients awaiting transplant and the high cost of the LVAD. Cost-effectiveness of LVADs from BTT trials is further complicated by the additional costs due to the subsequent transplantation. The more the follow-up is long the more the difference in costs increase due to the different survival between the two cohorts.

Real-life experience showed comparable length of hospital stay, number of readmissions, and 1-year survival between patients receiving a continuous-flow LVAD as a bridge and those going straight to heart transplant.

A different scenario has to be considered for the implantation of TCS systems in the highest-risk patients in which a higher hazard of failure, the increased risk of complications, the increased costs due to prolonged ICU stay, and the hazards due to multiple procedures may lead the patients treated with a TCS both to unacceptably high costs and to a bad outcome. In this view TCS should be used as bridge to decision only for brief periods and principally as a strategy of optimization of the main treatment, upgrading to a durable device as soon as the patient reaches criteria to be implanted. Data from the Medicare population ineligible for transplant disclosed an average cost of treating advanced heart failure with optimal medical management (OMM) of approximately $180,000, spent previously during the last 6 months of life [26].

Cost-effectiveness analyses, when applied to orphan diseases or other end-of-life treatments, can be challenging, as the evaluation does not consider the innovative nature of medicine or the availability of an alternative treatment.

Finally, current data suggest that the cost-effectiveness of VAD therapy as DT is improving but has yet to achieve the goal of <$100,000 USD/QALY through a careful patient selection and management [23]. Moreover, the sicker the patient the higher are the adjunctive costs strictly dependent from the increased survival. Thus, if futile implantations encompass high costs that could be completely spared without treatment, effective implantations spare life that cannot be saved differently.

However, looking at the possible future benefits of MCS in congestive heart failure given the social impact of the increasing prevalence of this disease and the increasing length of life, when coupled with more robust data on long-term survival and quality of life, it is reasonable to anticipate that mechanically assisted circulation will ultimately achieve cost-effectiveness.

4.4 Device Strategy and VAD Selection

Nowadays the distinction between bridge to transplant policy and destination therapy may be justified principally by the strict historical relation between MCS and transplantation at the dawning of MCS. In the actual situation of organ shortage (worsened by the increased survival of patients treated with medical therapy and with MCS), MCS is increasingly used as a treatment for HF because of its prompt availability, leaving heart transplantation (HTx) as a solution for patients not amenable of MCS implantation and for patients with a failure of MCS. However, ideally, HTx should be reserved to the few recipients that could experience a follow-up long up to 20 years or a significant amelioration of quality of life and consider MCS for all the others. Moreover, the MCS has also changed the clinical course of patients affected by ES-CHF so that patients with a low likelihood of HTx before MCS may become ideal candidates after an effective mechanical support. In a paper of Uriel [27], it was well pointed out how the definition of the strategy (◘ Table 4.2) may be subject to repeated changes during the support of the patient, and this led in Europe to label a new therapeutic strategy, known as "bridge to candidacy" (BTC). Finally, today it could be more appropriate [28] to distinguish the "indication" to HTx from the

Table 4.2 Policies of implantation

Bridge to decision: Use of MCS in patients with drug-refractory acute circulatory collapse and at immediate risk of death to sustain life until a full clinical evaluation can be completed and additional therapeutic options can be evaluated
Bridge to candidacy: Use of MCS to improve end-organ function in order to make an ineligible patient eligible for transplantation
Bridge to transplant: Use of MCS to keep a patient at high risk of death before transplantation alive until a donor organ becomes available
Bridge to recovery: Use of MCS to keep patient alive until intrinsic cardiac function recovers sufficiently to remove MCS
Destination therapy: Long-term use of MCS as an alternative to transplantation in patients with end-stage heart failure ineligible for transplantation

"candidacy" to HTx, considering for the latter a timely MCS implantation in case a suitable organ is not available in a reasonable time, in order to prevent a further decline of patient's conditions and miss even the possibility for a safe LVAD implantation.

Destination therapy (DT) is the strategy for patient not eligible for HTx, either due to age or comorbidities. Destination therapy is meant to be a permanent, lifelong form of left ventricular support, and it represents a growing indication, offering the greatest potential for improvements in HF morbidity and mortality. An intriguing perspective is to provide early unloading to prevent remodeling in a cardiomyopathy with hopes for recovery (i.e., myocarditis) [29].

Implanting a patient as bridge to transplant (BTT), the effectiveness in terms of end-organ recovery should be kept in mind as first issue, trying to choose a device capable to offer full support to the patient and to perform a safe HT. An extensive work-up has to be performed [10, 30] to verify if end-organ dysfunction may be reversible keeping in mind the difference between acute (shortly reversible), chronic (often reversible over a mid-time), and acute on chronic illness (often requiring a very long period to recovery).

An intriguing perspective is the "bridge to recovery" (BTR) strategy, that aims to provide an early unloading to prevent ventricular remodleing in a cardiomiopathy considered to be reversible (i.e., myocarditis) [30]. Destination therapy (DT) is the strategy for patient not eligible for HTx, either due to age or comorbidities. Destination therapy is meant to be a permanent, lifelong form of left ventricular support, and it represents a growing indication, offering the greatest potential for improvements in HF morbidity and mortality. When implanting a patient as destination therapy, the principal target is to choose the device capable to improve clinical conditions and possibly quality of life of the patients while reducing the incidence of complications [31, 32]. The ENDURANCE trial (still unpublished data) disclosed different kinds of complications between the two most commonly implanted pumps (Heart Mate II and HeartWare) that should be balanced with preoperative features of the patients (i.e., risk of strokes after HW in patients with history of hypertension). In the effort to tailor the approach to the patient characteristics, some centers prefer to implant a device with partial [33–36] support (i.e., CircuLite Synergy) or less complete but without the abdominal driveline (i.e., Jarvik) wishing to give a better clinical perception to the patient and trying to eliminate the risk of driveline infection during the long term. In this perspective the knowledge of temporal course of complications and the capability to anticipate the kind of complications with respect to the baseline clinical characteristics may become a new horizon to offer the best results to a variegate population of patients. Indeed, the choice of a device with higher shear stresses may increase the probability of bleeding complications over the long term especially in an elderly patient, and, on the other end, early implantation with pumps capable to give a lower output may be preferred to preserve patient's right ventricular function and to keep arterial pressure pulsatility in order to protect from gastrointestinal bleedings [37, 38]. Development of aortic valve regurgitation should be avoided [39, 40]. In such elderly patients with mildly incompetent fibrotic aortic valve (or dilated aortic root), an additional care may be to choose a device capable to preserve flow pulsatility by specific softwares generating periodic flow changes [41, 42]. Recently, some interesting data regarding pulsatility emerged also from the analysis of the Evaheart cohort [43]. It has been postulated that the peculiar flow-pressure curve of the pump and its design is capable to best preserve pulsatility and its effect both on coagulative disorders (less gastrointestinal bleedings) [44, 45] and on right ventricular dysfunction [46]. Another factor to be evaluated is the width of the driveline: devices with a thinner driveline seem to account to less driveline infections [47].

In conclusion, when implanting an elective patient with the aim of destination therapy, it should be fairly discussed with the patient the choice and the risk both of the available models and of the surgical approach trying to give to the patient the best outcome with the lowest incidence of complications.

4.5 Left Heart Underlying Condition and Eventual Reversibility

The underlying disease is an important factor when planning the implantation of a system of TCS or MCS. In case of TCS the principal aims are the lower biological impact to reduce complications and the left ventricle unloading to increase the likelihood of recovery. In fact, the most common indication of TCS today is bridge to recovery. An alternative strategy is represented by the bridge-to-decision policy: this solution is increasingly used as soon as the patient recovers an optimal metabolic and end-organ function and neurologic dysfunction has been excluded. The bridge to transplant with ECMO should be carefully considered looking at the data coming from ISHLT database as the short- and midterm survival is heavily impaired. The length and the quality of TCS may represent the real discriminant factor with respect to transplant results. ECMO is the most commonly used system for TCS as documented by a recent study from Bartlett [48], and the maximum chance of recovery is reached after minimum 6 days of support [49]. A study on ECMO [18] showed that an ECMO support longer than 14 days is associated with a bad outcome with respect to a quick transition to durable MCS. Efforts should be always spent to plan the next step when the patients is bridged with a TCS and an organ is not timely available. According to the data from the ISHLT, patients coming out from ECMO have a lower survival after HTx that is similar to the survival of TAH/BiVAD [2]. Adjunct of a left ventricular drainage seems to increase the likelihood of a recovery [50].

In the case of durable MCS, the underlying disease in the light of a possible recovery [20] is becoming more and more debated looking at the possibility to heal the heart and not to replace it. Intriguingly, in the era of cf-LVAD, the incidence of recovery appears reduced. It is not clear if it depends from a lack of arterial wave pulsatility or if it depends from a different clinical profile of the candidate for LVAD implantation today compared to the era of pf-LVAD. Certainly time of implantation is important if aiming to a possible recovery both in myocarditis and in idiopathic cardiomyopathy (the most commonly recovering underlying diseases). In this setting, also if some evidence of reversal of fibrosis has been reported [51], the likelihood of a recovery appears really unpredictable when a significant grade of myocardial fibrosis has been already established.

Care must be taken when choosing patients with restrictive and hypertrophic cardiomyopathy both for surgical issues and for an increased risk of complications due to the placement of the inflow cannula [52]. However, these recipients if carefully selected may really benefit from LVAD implantation, in consideration of the increased risk of primary graft failure associated with heart transplantation [53].

Another fascinating and growing indication to LVAD implantation that should be accurately assessed in the near future is the support of congenital adult cardiomyopathies. Patients with a univentricular physiopathology have been treated with an LVAD implantation from many surgeons after the first report in 2005 from Frazier [54]. Numerous small series are showing the possible role of LVAD implantation and also of TAH in such a setting. The burden of the treatment of a failing Fontan is another big issue to approach. A number of patients with surgically corrected or palliated congenital heart disease are left with abnormal anatomy that makes VAD implantation difficult, impossible, or even unpredictable. Artificial conduits, valvular insufficiency and residual shunts may portend complications within the inflow or outflow of the device. Repair residual defects and then place a VAD or a biventricular assist device (BiVAD) is an attracting solution [55], but the morbidity/mortality profile will be then certainly higher compared to an isolated VAD placement, thus leading many authors to prefer directly a TAH solution [56].

4.6 Right Heart Dysfunction Reversibility

LVAD implantation is based on the assumption of a normal right ventricular function, capable to maintain a sufficient preload warranting an optimal filling of the left ventricle. The capability to predict postoperative right ventricular failure (RVF) is one of the trickiest evaluations in the field of MCS: careful evaluation of preoperative parameters, timely diagnosis, and perioperative management are the key. Unplanned postoperative temporary RVAD/ECMO implantation for right ventricular failure may be a catastrophic complication with a significant impact on the length of postoperative ICU stay and mortality [57].

Without entering into specific considerations that will be explained further in this book, there are several factors that have to be considered when evaluating right ventricular function in a possible candidate to LVAD implantation:

- Assessment of extracardiac factors:
- Metabolic
- Renal function
- Liver function
- Inflammatory
- Assessment of systolic and diastolic right ventricular function
- Assessment of filling state
- Assessment of load dependency of right ventricular function
- Assessment of right ventricular contractility reserve

Many scores try to predict adequately the incidence of RVF, but scores alone shouldn't contraindicate implantation of an LVAD, being more a tool to address a more careful management of right ventricle from preoperative to postoperative course.

In the era of CF-LVAD, the incidence of delayed RVF is increased [58–60], partly due to different clinical profiles of the patients implanted nowadays, partly due to the absence of pulsatile flow, with a consequent dampened pulsatility in the right sections [61]. The adoption of solutions to preserve aortic valve opening and systemic pressure pulsatility try to address such an issue [38, 39].

In case of preoperative right ventricular dysfunction, right ventricle function has to be carefully evaluated in the attempt to distinguish reversibility of right ventricular dysfunction. The different possible solutions in case of concomitant right ventricular failure are shown in ◘ Table 4.3.

The fear of the absence of a backup circulation and the dimension of the device (lately resolved by the 50 cc TAH fitting approximately to all adults and small adults) is one of the main factors limiting expansion of TAH technology nowadays.

◘ **Table 4.3** Principal solutions for patients with moderate/severe right ventricular dysfunction

LVAD Implantation + Peripheral ECMO: This may warrant a safe surgical implantation without need of CPB (less biologic impact) and without right ventricular distension that could impair right ventricular function
LVAD Implantation + Percutaneous RVAD (TandemHeart or Impella RP_1): This solution appears of interest when moderate dysfunction appears largely reversible during a short-term period. This has the rationale to replace and protect right ventricle during the first vulnerable phase of postoperative management
LVAD Implantation + Temporary CF-RVAD (Levitronix): Encouraging data exist regarding the use of Levitronix and weaning from RVAD during the first 15 days. Surgical solutions to leave the sternum closed have been adopted to reduce the need of further surgical procedures. An interesting approach is by cannulating femoral vein and pulmonary trunk with a tunneled interposition prosthesis that can be ligated through a left minimal access without resternotomy
LVAD Implantation + Pulsatile Temporary RVAD: This is probably the solution warranting the higher probability of right ventricular myocardial recovery during the midterm but paying a lower quality of life and the need of reoperation when parameters for weaning are met
BiVAD Implantation with 2 CF-LVADs: Off-label choice warranting lower survival with respect to LVAD implantation and carrying a high rate of complications
TAH: It is today the simplest to manage and safest solution to assist both ventricles with >50% survival at 1 year

This solution however still carries a great simplicity of management and the highest number of patients gaining HTx (looking at the seventh ISHLT report 56% versus less than 20%), thus appearing an effective solution in the setting of BTT. The safety of the transplant procedure when respecting the rule for a safe sternal closure of such patients is another additional argument in favor of TAH implantation [62]. The noise and the quality of life with this approach are one of the major concerns regarding the future development of this technology.

The choice between these possible approaches should be always debated with the patient, keeping in mind that right ventricular dysfunction is a marker of illness as well as an indicator of poor survival; thus it should be always anticipated trying to preserve patient survival and quality of life. Therefore, when an outpatient in INTERMACS classes IV–VII begins to show minimal right ventricular dysfunction, it should be immediately referred to an MCS center to warrant the best outcome, avoiding whenever possible to replace a supportable heart.

4.7 Patient Comorbidities and Reversibility

Many patients with advanced HF have mild to moderate abnormalities of renal function. The serum creatinine concentration may often exceed 2 mg/dl with a creatinine clearance below 50 ml/min, which both have been shown to adversely impact survival after transplantation [63–66]. While renal dysfunction secondary to systemic congestion/impaired perfusion may improve with diuretics or inotropic agents, underlying intrinsic renal disease may represent a significant comorbidity. If cardiac insufficiency is the primary cause of renal dysfunction, it improves after LVAD implant or transplant. During the first 6 months of LVAD support, generally a significant improvement of renal function is observed [67, 68].

When intrinsic renal disease is suspected, a careful nephrologic evaluation is needed, and patients should undergo 24-h urine collection for proteinuria and creatinine clearance, renal ultrasonography looking at kidney size and structure, and possibly evaluation of the renovascular system (sequential SPECT and/or vascular Doppler). Severe renal impairment with GFR lower than 30 ml/min represents a relative contraindication to LVAD, where a high potential recovery should be weighted with an increased hazard of perioperative CRRT, RVF, and mortality. Chronic hemodialysis remains a contraindication for long-term VADs as there are few dialysis centers that accept patients with an LVAD, due to the complex hemodynamic management. Risk of infection is an issue in LVAD patients, and the need of a permanent vascular is an additional risk; few data on safety of peritoneal dialysis exists, but a renal function so profoundly compromised represents a clear risk of complications.

Right HF with hepatic congestion may lead to high transaminase levels, with or without elevated bilirubin, with associated coagulation disorders, but these may be reversible. On the contrary, primary liver diseases and cirrhosis need to be excluded through imaging studies and even a parenchymal biopsy in search of hepatic fibrosis.

Evidence of hepatic synthetic dysfunction with an elevated INR in the absence of warfarin therapy, as disclosed by a high MELD (model for end-stage liver disease) score, is of concern prior to MCS, and attempts should be made to correct this prior to the procedure.

Pulmonary diseases increase the risk of poor outcomes after LVAD implantation, so patients with severe chronic obstructive pulmonary disease or restrictive lung disease are generally excluded. Preoperative mechanical ventilation is one of the driving risk factors leading to the increased risk of mortality of INTERMACS I patients.

Anemia, thrombocytopenia, and coagulopathies have been correlated with poor outcomes following VAD implantation. The use of antiplatelet agents should be discontinued several days prior to surgery whenever possible to prevent perioperative bleeding that could impact perioperative renal dysfunction and right ventricular failure. Heparin-induced thrombocytopenia in patients coming out from ECMO is common. Bleedings are a frequent adverse event following continuous-flow VAD implantation whose pathophysiology is primarily related to angiodysplasia and the development of acquired von Willebrand syndrome. Understanding and management of coagulation before LVAD implantation are pivotal to experience a low rate of complications.

Stroke remains a devastating adverse event following LVAD implantation, and checkup for carotid artery disease is a standard pre-LVAD evaluation in patients at risk for atherosclerotic vascular disease. Severe stenosis may be treated prior to LVAD implantation whenever possible. Interesting data on peripheral circulation in patients undergoing second-generation LVAD implantation disclose that those patients experience a greater loss of pulsatility than those treated with OMM, differently from first-generation devices that showed to restore a normal peripheral circulation. These effects on the peripheral circulation have always to be considered because they may potentially increase the incidence of complications due to the higher shear stress and to the opening of arteriovenous shunts [69].

There are conflicting data about the influence of obesity on transplant outcomes. Obesity may be associated with increased morbidity, complications such as infection, and poor perioperative survival and difficulty identifying an appropriately sized donor heart. Obesity may increase 5-year mortality up to twofold, but the same degree of obesity may not be a contraindication to LVAD implantation and represent an indication to a bridge to candidacy policy to be considered carefully giving the low number of patients experiencing a significant weight-loss and gaining heart transplant candidacy. Infections significantly more frequently occur in the overweight, primarily because of drivelines, which rest within skinfolds. Extremely obese patients had higher rates of device-related infection and re-hospitalization. Bariatric surgery to improve weight loss and reduce potential complications has been suggested, but no sufficient data support this strategy.

Patients with the lowest BMI (<22.9) had the worst prognosis. Cardiac cachexia documented by poor nutrition status and low albumin and total protein concentrations (<3.5 and 6 mg/dl, respectively) is a common and deemed risk factor for patients undergoing MCS, that may be or not related with reversible or not reversible frailty [70], and associated with altered immune function, impaired wound healing, and muscle atrophy, lowering the chance to recovery and increasing the risk of prolonged hospitalizations. Prealbumin and total cholesterol are even more sensitive markers of nutritional status and should be routinely evaluated in all candidates for LVAD therapy.

Patients who have severe fixed pulmonary hypertension (defined as pulmonary arterial systolic pressure greater than 60 mmHg, transpulmonary gradient greater than 15 mm Hg, or pulmonary vascular resistance greater than 6 Wood units while unresponsive to treatment with pulmonary vasodilators) are very high-risk candidates for cardiac transplantation because of the high likelihood of postoperative right ventricular failure. When right ventricular function is still preserved, LVADs joke a pivotal role to reverse the pulmonary hypertension by unloading the left ventricle.

By convention, history of malignancy within 5 years is a contraindication for heart transplant, with rare exceptions. However, if the overall prognosis is good from an oncologic standpoint, there is no reason not to consider the patient for LVAD DT or as BTC when young.

Diabetes is a risk factor for complications of LVADs as for every cardiac surgery procedure; however a growing evidence is developing showing that LVAD implantation with subsequent hemodynamic and metabolic optimization can improve the course of diabetes mellitus.

Congenital heart disease in adults produces more complex physiology than simple ischemic or nonischemic cardiomyopathy. Congenital abnormalities can alter the chest anatomy as can prior surgeries performed for palliations and surgical repairs. Adhesions, conduits, shunts, patches, and anastomoses create multiple surgical challenges. Many centers avoid transplanting these patients because their outcomes are frequently worse than those patients who have "straightforward" advanced HF. Given the young age of many patients with adult congenital heart disease, it is especially important to find options to prolong their lives with MCS and possibly to make HTx outcome predictable. Also in this setting the timing plays a major role as patients having end-stage protein losing enteropathy are not amenable of successful implantation.

4.8 Risk Scores

Risk models, or a statistically derived framework to predict outcomes from robust datasets, can be particularly helpful in patients' selection process [71, 72]. Clinical decision support tools are computational systems that aid healthcare decision making. A robust model will have the power to discriminate (i.e., correctly stratify patients by risk) and calibrate (i.e., the degree of agreement between the predicted and observed risk) and will be broadly applicable, with minimal complexity and good external validation. In advanced HF, risk models are useful for predicting mortality from HF and for predicting survival after VAD therapy, thereby allowing one to better gauge when the risks of MCS therapy outweigh the risks of death from continued medical therapy of HF. The magnitude of such tools cannot be understated when it comes to aiding in the informed consent and shared decision-making process for patients, families, and the healthcare team. In the last 2 years, interesting models to predict with a Bayesian analysis have been conducted to try to have a more accurate prediction (▶ http://www.mycora.org). Recently it has been pointed out that the evolution of decision making in this field depends strictly from the feasibility to use such a score bedside [73]. Incorporating such scores in the clinical charts the clinician uses for the clinical management of the patients could help to implement the use of scores in the clinical arena and to validate those.

4.9 Assessment of Hemorrhagic and Thromboembolic Risk

Bleeding has been one of the most common complications since the introduction of LVAD therapy, with a fourfold increased risk of reoperation for bleeding over standard open-heart surgery [74]. This is caused by multiple factors including abnormal coagulation at time of surgery, often because of preoperative use of warfarin and/or antiplatelet agents or hepatic congestion, poor nutrition, high venous pressures, and adhesions frequently occurring in patients with previous sternotomy [75]. It has been also recognized in about 25% of patients a second phase at risk of bleeding that develops beginning 1 month after the implant of the VAD. Increasing age seems to be mostly correlated with an increased risk of bleeding [76]. A common site of bleeding is in the upper gastrointestinal tract, and this is typically caused by the development of arteriovenous malformations, primarily located in the stomach or early portions of the small bowel. This seems to be a unique sequela of continuous-flow physiology, as it was not seen with the first generation of pulsatile-flow devices. Patients with prior history of gastrointestinal bleeding should have upper and lower endoscopy before LVAD. Recent attention has been directed at the uniform reduction in multimers of von Willebrand factor in the serum in response to nonpulsatile flow as one possible explanation for the increased bleeding associated with continuous-flow VADs [77]. The presence of bleeding diathesis may be a serious contraindication to LVAD unless coagulopathy is caused by a reversible hepatic dysfunction [78]. Low platelet count before implantation also predicts poor outcomes [79].

4.10 Frailty, Nutritional Status, and Risk of Infections

Frailty is a biological syndrome that reflects a state of decreased physiologic reserve and can be diagnosed if three or more of the following criteria are present: unintentional weight loss (10 pounds in the past year), self-reported exhaustion, weakness (typically measured as grip strength), slow gait, and low physical activity [70]. The definition of frailty used in the Cardiovascular Health Study [80] has pointed out many markers of frailty and claims a high accuracy. Whatever the definition of frailty, it is prevalent among patients with HF and is associated with an increased risk for emergency department visits and hospitalizations, independently of comorbidities.

A patient in advanced HF may be frail due to illness related to extracardiac factors (aging, cancer, lung disease, diabetes, cirrhosis, peripheral vascular disease, neurological disease) or due to primarily LVAD-responsive frailty. In this case the frail patient is likely to have a good outcome and a low incidence of adverse events after LVAD implantation. LVAD implantation may discriminate patients in LVAD-responsive frailty (reversible frailty) with primarily LVAD-independent frailty. LVAD-independent frailty implies a greater risk of death, complications (e.g., stroke, gastrointestinal bleed, or chronic hemolytic anemia), and/or persistently poor functional status after LVAD placement. Distinguishing frail patients from non-frail patients and within frail patients LVAD responsive from LVAD independent is one of the most relevant tasks to reduce the burden of adverse event after LVAD implantation and increase the perception of the clinical benefit of an MCS program.

Patients with HF experience an excess burden of frailty and could greatly benefit from interventions aimed at preventing or managing frailty. Frailty incidence varies according to NYHA class being uncommon in patients with NYHA class III patients but affecting almost 50% of patients with NYHA class IV heart failure and patients with higher intracardiac filling pressures and particularly with advanced right heart failure. Frail patients also had higher levels of bilirubin and lower levels of serum albumin secondary to the effect of right heart failure on liver function.

A common pathophysiological pathway including elevated levels of inflammatory mediators such as IL-6, TNF-α, and C-reactive protein and common clinical features such as anorexia, sarcopenia, weakness, and reduced physical activity may help to distinguish illness-related cachexia and age-related frailty. Heart failure-related frailty is largely limited to those with advanced symptomatic heart failure. For older CHF patients such as destination VADs, the distinction between different kinds of frailty may be really challenging. Many studies of frailty within elderly surgical populations including heart failure patients undergoing implantation of destination VADs have identified frailty as an independent predictor of increased adverse events: higher postoperative complications, prolonged hospital stay, increased hospital readmission rate, and mortality. Postoperative complications are adversely affected by frailty, and handgrip has been shown to be a particularly effective predictor of survival. Five variables have been independently associated with the syndrome of physical frailty, particularly the objective measures of physical performance, such as grip strength and gait speed [81]. Both weakened handgrip strength and slow gait speed have been previously assessed as a single-item marker of frailty within a cardiac surgical population. Other components of Fried's frailty phenotype (unintentional weight loss, exhaustion, and physical activity) may be of utmost importance and should equally enter frailty assessment performed from clinicians in their "end of the bed" assessment of potential MCS recipients.

Regarding its reversibility, [82] reported improved grip strength over 6 months after destination VAD implantation and two single-center studies have reported that cachexia is reversible after heart or lung transplantation.

4.11 Surgical Issues and Need of Eventual Concomitant Procedures

There are no data clearly in favor of one surgical approach on another; however many data seems to dissuade from a full sternotomy access in BTT patients with the aim to reduce the surgical challenge of the subsequent HT. The most common solutions in this setting are left thoracotomy with small right thoracotomy for the outflow-graft anastomosis and left thoracotomy alone with anastomosis on the left subclavian artery [83]. Until now no clear advantages emerged for one solution over another. The solution with anastomosis on the descending aorta has been almost abandoned due to the complex emo-rheology of this approach [84].

It is not clear if the claimed benefit of such an approach is related to a real superiority or if it is due to a selection bias leading to avoid such approaches in severely ill patients. Authors in favor of minimal invasive techniques claim also a lower incidence of RVF due to the protective role of the integrity of pericardium and of the lower incidence of bleeding [85]. Redo patients are more commonly treated through thoracotomy to avoid bleedings.

Another relevant surgical task is the need of concomitant procedures:

- Atrial septum defect should be always resolved in the same surgical time. Beating heart treatment is generally preferred to avoid aortic cross clamping.
- CABG is generally avoided if not performed with the aim of myocardial recovery. Right coronary CABG may be necessary to preserve right ventricular function.
- Aortic valve regurgitation: The progression of mild aortic valve regurgitation has been addressed from many studies in the latest period and the only concerns are about the management of pulsatility and the risk of hemolysis. In case of aortic root dilatation, care should be taken to perform the outflow-graft anastomosis distant from the aortic root to avoid distortion and earlier progression of aortic root dilation due to the increased shear stress on a diseased aortic wall. In case of moderate (more than 3+) aortic valve regurgitation aortic valve should be treated with a biological prosthesis. The risk of a suboptimal result should be always weighted with the need of a longer cross-clamping time. TAVI implantation before surgery may be a solution in selected patients.
- Mitral valve regurgitation: Some data exist regarding the utility of mitral valve repair associated to LVAD implantation. Secondary

mitral valve regurgitation is reduced by LVAD implantation but not completely resolved especially if mitral annulus is dilated. The reverse remodeling of left ventricle is not predictable and in the era cf-LVAD appears less common; moreover, mitral regurgitation appears a risk factor for delayed right ventricle failure. The increased bleeding risk and the need of aortic cross clamping associated with mitral valve repair in patients undergoing LVAD implantation should be always weighted with the awaited benefit of the patient.

- Aortic or mitral valve stenosis: This should be addressed surgically with biological prostheses.
- Tricuspid regurgitation: Tricuspid repair in case of annular dilation and sufficient ventricular function is supported by limited evidences, but a strong rationale emerges beside it from the knowledge of surgical literature.

4.12 Psychosocial Evaluation and Quality of Life

Prior to implant an LVAD, an accurate evaluation of the capacity to cope with therapy and rules to manage correctly an LVAD should be always performed. The adequacy of the caregivers and their education are an equally important factor to be considered. Social systems to warrant a support to LVAD candidates and to families depend from the capacity of the center to interact with other physicians and specialists and from the further expansion of the MCS field. Dedicated chapter in the book extensively addresses this important topic.

4.13 Durable Biventricular Support

Implantation of biventricular support carries a higher risk of complications and a lower survival compared to LVAD implantation. The high incidence in such a population of hepatorenal syndrome with the pro-inflammatory status related to prolonged gut ischemia appears the principal causes of this increased risk. Surgical solutions for biventricular support will be extensively reported in other chapters in this book.

4.13.1 Technical Feasibility of Intracorporeal Implantation

Until the release of the 50 cc SynCardia TAH, one of the more common factors to implant a BiVAD in a patient with a biventricular dysfunction was the dimensions (BSA<1.7 m^2 and AP diameter at T10 < 10 cm) of the patient [86]. In this setting BiVAD implantation was preferentially paracorporeal with pulsatile devices (for pediatric population) or intracorporeal (for DT of the elderly patient) using an LVAD as right ventricular support. The HVAD has been more commonly used in this configuration also if approximately every LVAD has been adopted to try to support failing right ventricles. Future solutions with cf-LVAD will be discussed in other sections.

4.13.2 Pulsatility

It's the opinion of the authors that in such patients, whose biventricular dysfunction is really advanced, pulsatility still play an important role for recovery of organ dysfunction and to prevent adverse events due to low pulsatility, but the need of a lower biological impact of the surgical procedure may be a factor pushing toward a BiVAD implantation (on ECMO or on beating heart). TAH appears the safest solution in this setting and probably will be increasingly adopted in the future with the miniaturization obtained in the 50 cc TAH. However, surgeon and cardiologist have to deal with frail patients whose recovery may be difficult to predict and have to deem with patient frailty aiming to keep the right balance between risks and benefit of every surgical solution.

4.13.3 Policy of Implantation

Nowadays in the setting of BTT, TAH appears the solution more commonly achieving the target. Looking at the data from the seventh INTERMACS and of the first IMACS registry report, TAH is capable to bridge the patient to HTx nearly in the 50% of the cases.

4.14 Quality of Life and Recovery of Native Ventricular Dysfunction

Even if TAH is the unique device accepted and licensed for biventricular support as destination therapy, most cardiologist and surgeon believe that the quality of life is heavily prejudged from its noise and from the large cannulas of this device. This explains why the technology is working to search new solutions for this large population.

The BiVAD appears to many authors more acceptable in terms of quality of life and absence of noise, and the aim of a possible recovery of right ventricular function seems to justify BiVAD implantation also if its ideal configuration is still not well defined and its results are still suboptimal. In a recent study on BiVAD implantation, the patients implanted with atrial cannulation of right sections had lower thrombotic risk and higher mortality leaving unresolved the question about the best surgical solution to support right sections.

4.14.1 Need to Explant the Heart

TAH appears the best solution in all the cases in which leaving the native heart appears a source of problems. The more common situations in which native heart has to be replaced completely are:

- Transplant graft failure: The native heart often has a restrictive pattern and some authors claim an immunological need to replace the heart. Also if data coming from kidney re-transplant don't seem to support such a theory, in transplant graft failure TAH appears the best solution as a bridge to a second transplant [87].
- Treated or untreated congenital cardiomyopathies: The native heart has zones of stasis and low flows that could be amenable of thrombosis, and the removal of the large number of biological conduits needed in the patients with multiple redo may justify the implantation of a TAH [88].
- Hypertrophic, ischemic, or restrictive cardiomyopathies in which the dysfunction of the failing myocardium may impede correct positioning of inflow cannulas and or increase the risk of intracavitary thrombi.

4.14.2 Patient choice and informed consent

Patients' informed consent and beliefs have to always be taken in consideration. Giving the low survival and the high incidence of complications, all the possible solutions have to be discussed with the patient aiming to the best outcome both in terms of quality of life and in terms of length of life. Being completely dependent from a machine maybe difficult to tolerate and poses the patient and the caregivers in front to a huge responsibility that they have to understand and share with the physicians.

4.15 Temporary Circulatory Support

Temporary circulatory support in impending shock represents a parachute, no data coming from RCSs support its adoption, but when the patient is going to shock, it is lifesaving and gives the time to reason on the best durable solution for the patient.

The concept of "bridging" a patient with temporary circulatory support (TCS) to stabilize hemodynamics and improve end-organ function prior to the implantation of a durable VAD is increasingly being employed. During the last period, implants of durable VAD in patients in critical cardiogenic shock decreased steeply, while the use of TCS devices between 2008 and 2013 has increased at least tenfold [47]. This bridge strategy allows for varying degrees of ventricular support through rapidly deployable TCS devices. The aim is to stabilize hemodynamics, improve end-organ function, and reduce the risk of mortality and of perioperative complications like RVF whose incidence may increase up to 40% in this setting. The most commonly employed TCS device is an intra-aortic balloon pump (IABP), which has limited ability to augment cardiac output [6]. However when the patient is really critical and residual cardiac power (publication from SHOCK trial) is lower, an active system of TCS is needed. Extracorporeal circulatory membranous oxygenation (ECMO) is the most commonly and safely adopted bridge strategy capable to replace both the heart and the lung function but complicated by many different drawbacks. The principal complications due to ECMO implantation are suboptimal unloading of the heart and lung reducing the likelihood of cardiac and lung recovery, bleedings, infections, and problems due to cannulation (surgical bleedings, limb ischemia, etc.). Anecdotal cases are reported without anticoagulation, but the presence of the membrane oxygenator drives the need of a stricter management of the coagulation cascade. Many centers are rapidly shifting toward implantation of BiVADs (i.e., Levitronix BiVAD) when oxygenator is no longer needed. To reduce complications of TCS and possibly ameliorate the outcome both of TCS and of durable VAD implantation, extracorporeal VADs placed in the operating room have been more recently replaced from percutaneous extracorporeal VADs (i.e., Impella and TandemHeart on the basis of the desired amount of cardiac output) aiming to evolve toward ambulatory percutaneous TCS (i.e., Procyrion) [87].

The aim of a TCS is to favorably change the risk associated with VAD implant in a patient presenting with critical cardiogenic shock (INTERMACS profile 1) to the risk of VAD implant associated with a patient with profile 2 or 3 characteristics.

Unfortunately recent data from Shah [19] et al. show that, although TCS was able to successfully stabilize patients prior to durable VAD implantation, post-dVAD outcomes paralleled profile 1 patients without TCS but not with profiles 2–3 patients, and the incidence of right ventricular failure necessitating RVAD implantation, renal failure requiring renal replacement therapy, and mortality following VAD implantation were consistently higher in patients with TCS and profile 1 patients without TCS compared to profile 2–3 patients.

Clinical criteria for initiation of TCS are hard to determine. There are certain absolute indications (cardiac arrest, circulatory compromise despite inotropes, elevated lactate, vasopressor support) and contraindications (severe peripheral arterial disease, advanced age, frailty) that most clinicians would agree upon [13, 89].

In the setting of myocardial infarction, the clinical profile often doesn't allow to bridge the patient toward LVAD due to many cardiac and extracardiac reasons [90]. In this setting bridge to TAH has to be balanced with the feasibility of a recovery of a sufficient clinical stability [29].

In many cases, a longer duration of support may allow complete end-organ recovery, but this aim should always be weighed against the risks of concomitant therapies (ventilator, catheters, heparin infusion, etc.) and risks of immobility/deconditioning [91]. A recent article by Durinka et al. showed that patients supported with ECMO were supported for an average of 12 days [18] and reported a 92% survival to discharge for ECMO patients transitioned to a VAD in less than 14 days, but reported inferior survival for patients supported > 14 days, indicating that a prolonged support is associated with increased mortality risk.

References

1. Fleischmann KE, Beckman JA, Buller CE et al (2009) 2009 ACCF/AHA Focused Update on Perioperative Beta Blockade: A Report of the American College of Cardiology Foundation/American Heart Association Task Force on Practice Guidelines. Circulation 120(21):2123–2151. http://dx.doi.org/10.1161/CIRCULATIONAHA.109.192689. ISSN 1524-4539
2. Kirklin JK et al (2015) Seventh INTERMACS annual report: 15,000 patients and counting. JHLT 34(12):1495–1504. doi:10.1016/j.healun.2015.10.003. ISSN 1053-2498
3. Patel CB, Cowger JA, Zuckermann A (2014) A contemporary review of mechanical circulatory support. J Heart Lung Transplant 33(7):667–674. https://doi.org/10.1016/j.healun.2014.02.014. ISSN 1557-3117
4. Lund LH, Edwards LB, Kucheryavaya, AY, Dipchand AI, Benden C, Christie JD, et al. The registry of the International Society for Heart and Lung Transplantation: Thirtieth Official Adult Heart Transplant Report—2013; Focus Theme: Age for the International Society for Heart and Lung Transplantation. 2013. doi: 10.1016/j.healun.2013.08.006
5. Kirklin JK, Cantor R, Mohacsi P, Gummert J, De By T, Hannan MM et al (2016) First annual IMACS report: a global International Society for Heart and Lung Transplantation Registry for Mechanical Circulatory Support. J Heart Lung Transplant 35(4):407–412. doi:10.1016/j.healun.2016.01.002
6. Khazanie P, Rogers JG (2011) Patient selection for left ventricular assist devices. Congest Heart Fail 17(5):227–234. doi:10.1111/j.1751-7133.2011.00236.x
7. Slaughter MS, Meyer AL, Birks EJ (2011) Destination therapy with left ventricular assist devices: patient selection and outcomes. Curr Opin Cardiol 26(3):232–236. doi:10.1097/HCO.0b013e328345aff4
8. Miller LW, Guglin M (2013) Patient selection for ventricular assist devices: a moving target. J Am Coll Cardiol 61(12):1209–1221. doi:10.1016/j.jacc.2012.08.1029
9. Lund LH, Matthews J, Aaronson K (2010) Patient selection for left ventricular assist devices. Eur J Heart Fail 12(5):434–443. doi:10.1093/eurjhf/hfq006
10. Angelo LD, Bovolo V, Frigerio M (2014) Ventricular assist devices for heart failure: a focus on patient

selection and complications. Res Rep Clin Cardiol 5:199–211. doi:10.2147/RRCC.S48886
11. Long EF, Swain GW, Mangi AA (2014) Comparative survival and cost effectiveness of advanced therapies for end-stage heart failure. Circ Heart Failure. doi:10.1161/CIRCHEARTFAILURE.113.000807
12. Kirklin JK, Naftel DC, Kormos RL, Stevenson LW, Pagani FD, Miller MA et al (2012) The Fourth INTERMACS Annual Report: 4,000 implants and counting. J Heart Lung Transplant 31(2):117–126
13. Gilotra NA, Stevens GR (2015) Temporary mechanical circulatory support: a review of the options, indications, and outcomes. Clin Med Insights Cardiol 8(Suppl 1):75–85. doi:10.4137/CMC.s15718
14. Cowger J, Shah P, Stulak J, Maltais S, Aaronson KD, Kirklin JK et al (2016) INTERMACS profiles and modifiers: heterogeneity of patient classification and the impact of modifiers on predicting patient outcome. J Heart Lung Transplant 35:440–448. doi:10.1016/j.healun.2015.10.037 ISSN 1053-2498
15. Copeland JG, Copeland H, Gustafson M, Mineburg N, Covington D, Smith RG, Friedman M (2012) Experience with more than 100 total artificial heart implants. J Thorac Cardiovasc Surg 143(3):727–734. doi:10.1016/j.jtcvs.2011.12.002. Epub 2012 Jan 14. PMID: 22245242
16. Riebandt J, Haberl T, Mahr S, Laufer G, Rajek A, Steinlechner B, Schima H, Zimpfer D (2014) Preoperative patient optimization using extracorporeal life support improves outcomes of INTERMACS Level I patients receiving a permanent ventricular assist device. Eur J Cardiothorac Surg 46(3):486–492. ; discussion 492. doi: 10.1093/ejcts/ezu093. Epub 2014 Mar 18. PMID: 24648428
17. Young JB (2007) Heart failure's near dead and dying. J Am Coll Cardiol 50(13):1291–1293. doi:10.1016/j.jacc.2007.07.008
18. Durinka JB, Bogar LJ, Hirose H, Brehm C, Koerner MM, Pae WE, Cavarocchi NC (2014) End-organ recovery is key to success for extracorporeal membrane oxygenation as a bridge to implantable left ventricular assist device. ASAIO J (American Society for Artificial Internal Organs : 1992) 60(2):189–192. doi:10.1097/MAT.0000000000000043
19. Shah P, Smith S, Haft JW, Desai SS, Burton NA, Romano MA, Cowger JA (2016) Clinical outcomes of advanced heart failure patients with cardiogenic shock treated with temporary circulatory support before durable lvad implant. ASAIO J 62(1):20–27. doi:10.1097/MAT.0000000000000309
20. Schumer EM, Ising MS, Trivedi JR, Slaughter MS, Cheng A (2015) Early outcomes with marginal donor hearts compared with left ventricular assist device support in patients with advanced heart failure. Ann Thorac Surg 100:522–527. doi:10.1016/j.athoracsur.2015.02.089
21. Stewart GC, Kittleson MM, Cowger JA, Johnson FL, Patel CB, Mountis MM et al (2015) Who wants a left ventricular assist device for ambulatory heart failure? Early insights from the MEDAMACS screening pilot. J Heart Lung Transplant 34(12):1630–1633. doi:10.1016/j.healun.2015.07.009
22. Estep JD, Starling RC, Horstmanshof DA, Milano CA, Selzman CH, Shah KB, et al., for the ROADMAP Study Investigators. Risk assessment and comparative effectiveness of left ventricular assist device and medical management in ambulatory heart failure patients. J Am Coll Cardiol. 2016;66(16):1747–1761. doi:10.1016/j.jacc.2015.07.075
23. Miller LW, Guglin M, Rogers J (2013) Cost of ventricular assist devices can we afford the progress? Circulation 127(6):743–748. doi:10.1161/CIRCULATIONAHA.112.13982
24. Slaughter MS (2010) Advances in LVAD patient management: clinical strategies to minimize adverse events. PARADIGM Adv Heart Fail Technol 3:1–2
25. Pulikottil-Jacob R, Suri G, Connock M, Kandala NB, Sutcliffe P, Maheswaran H, Banner NR, Clarke A. Comparative cost-effectiveness of the HeartWare versus HeartMate II left ventricular assist devices used in the United Kingdom National Health Service bridge-to-transplant program for patients with heart failure J Heart Lung Transplant 2014;33(4):350–358. doi:10.1016/j.healun.2014.01.003. Epub 2014 Jan 19. PMID: 24582838
26. Liao L, Allen LA, Whellan DJ (2008) Economic burden of heart failure in the elderly. PharmacoEconomics 26:447–462
27. Uriel N, Jorde UP, Woo Pak S, Jiang J, Clerkin K, Takayama H, Mancini DM (2013) Impact of long term left ventricular assist device therapy on donor allocation in cardiac transplantation. J Heart Lung Transplant 32(2):188–195. doi:10.1016/j.healun.2012.11.010
28. Fang JC, Stehlik J (2013) Moving beyond "bridges"*. JACC Heart Failure 1(5):379–381. doi:10.1016/j.jchf.2013.08.003
29. Drakos SG, Kfoury AG, Stehlik J, Selzman CH, Reid BB, Terrovitis JV, Li DY (2012) Bridge to recovery: understanding the disconnect between clinical and biological outcomes. Circulation 126(2):230–241. doi:10.1161/CIRCULATIONAHA.111.040261
30. Ammirati E et al (2014) Current indications for heart transplantation and left ventricular assist device: a practical point of view. Eur J Intern Med 25(5):422–429. doi:10.1016/j.ejim.2014.02.006
31. Tsipouras MG, Karvounis EC, Tzallas AT, Katertsidis NS, Goletsis Y, Frigerio M, Verde A, Trivella MG, Fotiadis DI (2013) Adverse event prediction in patients with left ventricular assist devices. Conf Proc IEEE Eng Med Biol Soc 2013:1314–1317. doi:10.1109/EMBC.2013.6609750
32. Akhter SA, Badami A, Murray M, Kohmoto T, Lozonschi L, Osaki S, Lushaj EB (2015) Hospital readmissions after continuous-flow left ventricular assist device implantation: incidence, causes, and cost analysis. Ann Thorac Surg 100(3):884–889. doi:10.1016/j.athoracsur.2015.03.010. Epub 2015 Jun 19
33. Meyns BP, Simon A, Klotz S, Wittwer T, Schlensak C, Rega F, Burkhoff D. Clinical benefits of partial circulatory support in New York Heart Association Class IIIB and Early Class IV patients.Eur J Cardiothorac Surg 2011;39(5):693–698. doi: 10.1016/j.ejcts.2010.07.049. Epub 2010 Oct 8. PMID: 20934882
34. Zucchetta F, Tarzia V, Bottio T, Gerosa G (2014) The Jarvik-2000 ventricular assist device implantation: how we do it. Ann Cardiothorac Surg 3(5):525–531. doi:10.3978/j.issn.2225-319X.2014.09.09
35. Frazier OH, Myers TJ, Westaby S, Gregoric ID (2003) Use of the Jarvik 2000 left ventricular assist system as a

bridge to heart transplantation or as destination therapy for patients with chronic heart failure. Ann Surg 237(5):631–636; discussion 636–637. doi:10.1097/01.SLA.0000064359.90219.44
36. Westaby S, Siegenthaler M, Beyersdorf F, Massetti M, Pepper J, Khayat A, Frazier OH (2010) Destination therapy with a rotary blood pump and novel power delivery. Eur J Cardiothorac Surg 37(2):350–356. doi:10.1016/j.ejcts.2009.03.071
37. Wever-Pinzon O, Selzman CH, Drakos SG, Saidi A, Stoddard GJ, Gilbert EM, Labedi M, Reid BB, Davis ES, Kfoury AG, Li DY, Stehlik J, Bader F (2013) Pulsatility and the risk of nonsurgical bleeding in patients supported with the continuous-flow left ventricular assist device HeartMate II. Circ Heart Fail 6(3):517–526. doi:10.1161/CIRCHEARTFAILURE.112.000206. Epub 2013 Mar 11
38. Moazami N, Dembitsky WP, Adamson R, Steffen RJ, Soltesz EG, Starling RC, Fukamachi K (2015) Does pulsatility matter in the era of continuous-flow blood pumps? J Heart Lung Transplant 34(8):999–1004. doi:10.1016/j.healun.2014.09.012. Epub 2014 Sep 28
39. Imamura T, Kinugawa K, Nitta D, Hatano M, Kinoshita O, Nawata K, Ono M. Advantage of pulsatility in left ventricular reverse remodeling and aortic insufficiency prevention during left ventricular assist device treatment Circ J 2015;79(9):1994–9. doi: 10.1253/circj.CJ-15-0419. Epub 2015 Jun 25 PMID: 26118343
40. Tolpen S, Janmaat J, Reider C, Kallel F, Farrar D, May-Newman K (2015) Programmed speed reduction enables aortic valve opening and increased pulsatility in the LVAD-assisted heart. ASAIO J 61(5):540–547. doi:10.1097/MAT.0000000000000241
41. Ising MS, Sobieski MA, Slaughter MS, Koenig SC, Giridharan GA. Feasibility of pump speed modulation for restoring vascular pulsatility with rotary blood pumps ASAIO J 2015;61(5):526–532. doi: 10.1097/MAT.0000000000000262. PMID: 26102173
42. Bourque K, Cotter C, Dague C, Harjes D, Dur O, Duhamel J, Spink K, Walsh K, Burke E (2016) Design rationale and preclinical evaluation of the HeartMate 3 left ventricular assist system for hemocompatibility. ASAIO J 62(4):375–383. doi:10.1097/MAT.0000000000000388
43. Kimura M, Kinoshita O, Nawata K, Nishimura T, Hatano M, Imamura T, Endo M, Kagami Y, Kubo H, Kashiwa K, Kinugawa K, Kyo S, Komuro I, Ono M (2015) Midterm outcome of implantable left ventricular assist devices as a bridge to transplantation: Single-center experience in Japan. J Cardiol 65(5):383–389. doi:10.1016/j.jjcc.2014.06.007. Epub 2014 Jul 14. PMID: 25034705
44. Jabbar HR, Abbas A, Ahmed M, Klodell CT Jr, Chang M, Dai Y, Draganov PV (2015) The incidence, predictors and outcomes of gastrointestinal bleeding in patients with left ventricular assist device (LVAD). Dig Dis Sci 60(12):3697–3706. doi:10.1007/s10620-015-3743-4. Epub 2015 Jun 14
45. Jorde UP (2016) Relative preservation of high molecular weight von Willebrand factor multimers during HM 3 support-plain physics or a matter of clinical consequence? J Heart Lung Transplant 35(7):857–859. doi:10.1016/j.healun.2016.06.007
46. Cheng A, Williamitis CA, Slaughter MS (2014) Comparison of continuous-flow and pulsatile-flow left ventricular assist devices: is there an advantage to pulsatility? Ann Cardiothorac Surg 3(6):573–581. doi:10.3978/j.issn.2225-319X.2014.08.24
47. John R, Aaronson KD, Pae WE, Acker MA, Hathaway DR, Najarian KB, Slaughter MS, HeartWare Bridge to Transplant ADVANCE Trial Investigators (2014) Drive-line infections and sepsis in patients receiving the HVAD system as a left ventricular assist device. J Heart Lung Transplant 33(10):1066–1073. doi:10.1016/j.healun.2014.05.010. Epub 2014 Jun 4.PMID: 25087103
48. Gray BW, Haft JW, Hirch JC, Annich GM, Hirschl RB, Bartlett RH, Support EL (2015) ASAIO J 61:2–7. doi:10.1097/MAT.0000000000000150
49. Chang CH, Chen HC, Caffrey JL et al (2011) Survival analysis after extracorporeal membrane oxygenation in critically ill adults: a comparison with conventional cardiopulmonary resuscitation. Crit Care Med 39:1. doi:10.1097/CCM.0b013e3181feb339
50. Hacking DF, Best D, d'Udekem Y, Brizard CP, Konstantinov IE, Millar J, Butt W (2015) Elective decompression of the left ventricle in pediatric patients may reduce the duration of venoarterial extracorporeal membrane oxygenation. Artif Organs 39(4):319–326. doi:10.1111/aor.12390. Epub 2014 Oct 20
51. Lee M, Akashi H, Kato TS, Takayama H, Wu C, Xu K, Collado E, Weber MP, Kennel PJ, Brunjes DL, Ji R, Naka Y, George I, Mancini D, Farr M, Christian Schulze P (2016) Vascular inflammation and abnormal aortic histomorphometry in patients after pulsatile- and continuous-flow left ventricular assist device placement. J Heart Lung Transplant. pii: S1053-2498(16)00022-X. doi:10.1016/j.healun.2015.12.027 [Epub ahead of print]
52. Topilsky Y, Pereira NL, Shah DK, Boilson B, Schirger JA, Kushwaha SS, Joyce LD, Park SJ (2011) Left ventricular assist device therapy in patients with restrictive and hypertrophic cardiomyopathy. Circ Heart Fail 4:266–275. doi:10.1161/CIRCHEARTFAILURE.110.959288
53. Ammash NM, Seward JB, Bailey KR, Edwards WD, Tajik AJ (2000) Clinical profile and outcome of idiopathic restrictive cardiomyopathy. Circulation 101:2490–2496
54. Frazier OH, Gregoric ID, Messner GN (2005) Total circulatory support with an LVAD in an adolescent with a previous Fontan procedure. Tex Heart Inst J 32(3):402–404. PMID: 16392230
55. Weinstein S, Bello R, Pizarro C, Fynn-Thompson F, Kirklin J, Guleserian K, Woods R, Tjossem C, Kroslowitz R, Friedmann P, Jaquiss R (2014) The use of the Berlin Heart EXCOR in patients with functional single ventricle. J Thorac Cardiovasc Surg 147(2):697–704; discussion 704–705. doi:10.1016/j.jtcvs.2013.10.030. Epub 2013 Nov 28
56. Ryan TD, Jefferies JL, Zafar F, Lorts A, Morales DL (2015) The evolving role of the total artificial heart in the management of end-stage congenital heart disease and adolescents. ASAIO J 61(1):8–14. doi:10.1097/MAT.0000000000000156. Review
57. Takeda K, Naka Y, Yang JA, Uriel N, Colombo PC, Jorde UP, Takayama H (2014) Outcome of unplanned right ventricular assist device support for severe right heart failure after implantable left ventricular assist device insertion. J Heart Lung Transplant 33(2):141–148. doi:10.1016/j.healun.2013.06.025. Epub 2013 Aug 6. PMID: 23932442

58. Patlolla B, Beygui R, Haddad F (2013) Right-ventricular failure following left ventricle assist device implantation. Curr Opin Cardiol 28(2):223–233. doi:10.1097/HCO.0b013e32835dd12c
59. Lampert BC, Teuteberg JJ (2015) Right ventricular failure after left ventricular assist devices. J Heart Lung Transplant 34(9):1123–1130. doi:10.1016/j.healun.2015.06.015
60. Dandel M et al (2015) Left ventricular vs. biventricular mechanical support: decision making and strategies for avoidance of right heart failure after left ventricular assist device implantation. Int J Cardiol 198:241–250. doi:10.1016/j.ijcard.2015.06.103
61. Reichenspurner H (2015) When is the patient sick enough to implant MCS ? – importance and assessment of RV function ISHLT number of transplants by year, 2014–2015
62. Ihnken KA, Ramzy D, Esmailian F, Trento A, Arabía FA (2016) Surgical technique to facilitate explanation of mechanical circulatory support devices: LVADs, BiVADs, and TAHs before heart transplantation. ASAIO J 62(2):211–213. doi:10.1097/MAT.0000000000000318. PMID: 26692405
63. Slaughter MS, Pagani FD, Rogers JG, Miller LW, Sun B, Russell SD et al (2010) Clinical management of continuous-flow left ventricular assist devices in advanced heart failure. J Heart Lung Transplant 29(4 SUPPL):S1–S39. doi:10.1016/j.healun.2010.01.011
64. Cowger, J., Romano, M.A, Stulak, J., Pagani, F. D., & Aaronson, K.D. (2011). Left ventricular assist device management in patients chronically supported for advanced heart failure. Curr Opin Cardiol, 26(2), 149–154. doi:10.1097/HCO.0b013e3283438258
65. Danchin N, Puymirat E (2011) 1980–2010: the three glorious decades of cardiology. A comprehensive and collective effort rewarded by outstanding clinical results. Rev Española Cardiología (English Ed) 64(11):959–961. doi:10.1016/j.rec.2011.08.001
66. Lee S, Fukamachi K, Golding L, Moazami N, Starling RC (2013) Left ventricular assist devices: from the bench to the clinic. Cardiology 125(1):1–12. doi:10.1159/000346865. PMID: 10831523
67. Patel AM, Adeseun G a, Ahmed I, Mitter N, Rame JE, Rudnick MR (2013) Renal failure in patients with left ventricular assist devices. Clin J Am Soc Nephrol CJASN 8:484–496. doi:10.2215/CJN.06210612
68. Kirklin JK et al (2013) Quantifying the effect of cardiorenal syndrome on mortality after left ventricular assist device implant. J Heart Lung Transplant 32(12):1205–1213
69. Nguyen PH, Tuzun E, Quick CM (2016) Aortic pulse pressure homeostasis emerges from physiologic adaptation of systemic arteries to local mechanical stresses. Am J Physiol Regul Integr Comp Physiol 311(3):R522–R531. doi:10.1152/ajpregu.00402.2015
70. Flint KM, Matlock DD, Lindenfeld J, Allen LA (2012) Frailty and the selection of patients for destination therapy left ventricular assist device. Circ Heart Fail 5(2):286–293. doi:10.1161/CIRCHEARTFAILURE.111.963215
71. Ravichandran AK, Cowger J (2015) Left ventricular assist device patient selection: do risk scores help? J Thorac Dis 7(12):2080–2087. doi:10.3978/j.issn.2072-1439.2015.11.02
72. Scandroglio AM, Pieri M, Zangrillo A, Kaufmann F, Falk V, Potapov E, Krabatsch T (2016) Role of survival scores before left ventricular assist device implantation. ASAIO J 62(4):438–441. doi:10.1097/MAT.0000000000000376
73. Yang Q, Zimmerman J, Steinfeld A, Carey L, Antaki JF (2016) Investigating the heart pump implant decision process: opportunities for decision support tools to help. In: Proceedings of the 2016 CHI conference on human factors in computing systems (CHI '16). ACM, New York, pp 4477–4488. doi: http://dx.doi.org/10.1145/2858036.2858373
74. Kilic A, Acker MA, Atluri P (2015) Dealing with surgical left ventricular assist device complications. Journal of Thoracic Disease. AME Publications. doi:10.3978/j.issn.2072-1439.2015.10.64
75. Himmelreich G, Ullmann H, Riess H, Rosch R, Loebe M, Schiessler A, Hetzer R (1995) Pathophysiologic role of contact activation in bleeding followed by thromboembolic complications after implantation of a ventricular assist device. ASAIO J 41:M790–M794. PMID: 8573916
76. Atluri P, Goldstone AB, Kobrin DM, Cohen JE, MacArthur JW, Howard JL, Jessup ML, Rame JE, Acker MA, Woo YJ (2013) Ventricular assist device implant in the elderly is associated with increased, but respectable risk: a multi-institutional study. Ann Thorac Surg 96(1):141–147. doi:10.1016/j.athoracsur.2013.04.010
77. Crow S, Chen D, Milano C, Thomas W, Joyce L, Piacentino V, Sharma R, Wu J, Arepally G, Bowles D, Rogers J, Villamizar-Ortiz N (2010) Acquired von Willebrand syndrome in continuous-flow ventricular assist device recipients. Ann Thorac Surg 90:1263–1269. doi:10.1016/j.athoracsur.2010.04.099
78. Munoz SJ, Stravitz RT, Gabriel DA (2009) Coagulopathy of acute liver failure. Clin Liver Dis 13(1):95–107. doi:10.1016/j.cld.2008.10.001
79. Uriel N, Pak SW, Jorde UP, Jude B, Susen S, Vincentelli A, Ennezat PV, Cappelman S, Naka Y, Mancini D (2010) Acquired von Willebrand syndrome after continuous-flow mechanical device support contributes to a high prevalence of bleeding during long-term support and at the time of transplantation. J Am Coll Cardiol 56:1207–1213. doi:10.1016/j.jacc.2010.05.016. Epub 2010 Jul 2
80. Kulminski AM, Ukraintseva SV, Culminskaya IV et al (2008) Cumulative deficits and physiological indices as predictors of mortality and long life. J Gerontol A Biol Sci Med Sci 63:1053–1059. PMID: 18948555 PMCID: PMC2684458
81. Chung CJ, Wu JM, Kato TS, Dam TT, Givens RC, Templeton DL, Maurer MS, Naka Y, Takayama H, Mancini DM, Schulze PC (2014) Reduced handgrip strength as a marker of frailty predicts clinical outcomes in patients with heart failure undergoing ventricular assist device placement. J Card Fail 20(5):310–315. doi:10.1016/j.cardfail.2014.02.008. Epub 2014 Feb 22
82. Kobrin DM, Donnelly JP, Acker AL, Howard JL, Zalewski CM, Walsh SL, Hill CE, O'Hara ML, Marble JF, Atluri P, Wald JW, Goldberg LR, Woo YJ, Acker MA, Rame JE (2013) Dynamic BMI changes in patients implanted with continuous flow left ventricular assist devices: evidence for reversibility of cardiac cachexia and impact on survival. J Heart Lung Transplant 32(4S):S90–S91

83. Sileshi B, O'Hara BK, Davis ME, Haglund NA, Meng X, Deegan R et al (2016) Outcomes of patients implanted using a left thoracotomy technique for a miniaturized centrifugal continuous-flow pump. ASAIO J. doi:10.1097/MAT.0000000000000407
84. Sileshi B, Haglund NA, Davis ME, Tricarico NM, Stulak JM, Khalpey Z et al (2015) In-hospital outcomes of a minimally invasive off-pump left thoracotomy approach using a centrifugal continuous-flow left ventricular assist device. J Heart Lung Transplant 34(1):107–112. doi:10.1016/j.healun.2014.09.023
85. Hanke JS, Haverich A, Schmitto JD (2016) Right heart failure after left ventricular assist devices: surgical considerations. J Heart Lung Transplant 35(3):395–396. doi:10.1016/j.healun.2015.12.013
86. Leprince P et al Patients with a body surface area less than 1.7 m2 have a good outcome with the cardiowest total artificial heart. J Heart Lung Transplant 24(10):1501–1505. doi: http://dx.doi.org/10.1016/j.healun.2005.01.016
87. Kalya A, Jaroszewski D, Pajaro O, et al (2013) Role of total artificial heart in the management of heart transplant rejection and retransplantation: case report and review. Clin Transplant. 2013;27(4):E348–50. doi:10.1111/ctr.12146. Epub 2013 May 31
88. Wells D, Villa CR, Simón Morales DL. (2017) The 50/50 cc Total Artificial Heart Trial: Extending the Benefits of the Total Artificial Heart to Underserved Populations. Semin Thorac Cardiovasc Surg Pediatr Card Surg Annu. 2017;20:16–19. doi:10.1053/j.pcsu.2016.09.004
89. Saffarzadeh A, Bonde P (2015) Options for temporary mechanical circulatory support. J Thorac Dis AME Publications. doi:10.3978/j.issn.2072-1439.2015.09.14
90. Acharya D, Loyaga-Rendon RY, Pamboukian SV, Tallaj JA, Holman WL, Cantor RS et al (2016) Ventricular assist device in acute myocardial infarction. J Am Coll Cardiol 67(16):1871–1880. doi:10.1016/j.jacc.2016.02.025.
91. Raman L, Dalton HJ (2016) Year in review 2015: Extracorporeal membrane oxygenation. Respir Care 61(7):986–991. doi:10.4187/respcare.04985

Preoperative Assessment and Clinical Optimization

Maria Frigerio, Manlio Cipriani, Fabrizio Oliva, and Federico Pappalardo

© Springer International Publishing Switzerland 2017

A. Montalto et al. (eds.), *Mechanical Circulatory Support in End-Stage Heart Failure*,
DOI 10.1007/978-3-319-43383-7_5

5.1 Introduction

Indications for short- or long-term mechanical circulatory support (MCS) in patients with acute or chronic severe disease, of various degrees of urgency, and with different probabilities of myocardial recovery are presented and discussed in details in other chapters.

Short-term mechanical support is generally a rescue therapy and can be applied in almost all the patients, due to the variety of available devices, some of which can also be implanted percutaneously. The goal is to maintain perfusion and oxygenation, thus gaining time, while hopefully there would be some improvement in myocardial, lung, and end-organ function. The predicted duration goes from days to weeks.

On the other side, long-term mechanical support therapy (most often provided with a left ventricular assist device, LVAD) is now intended for accompanying patients for months to years. Comparing INTERMACS reports published in 2010 and 2015, which include about 1000 and over 15,000 cases, respectively, there is an increasing proportion of patients who received LVAD as permanent treatment (destination therapy, DT) from <10% to >45% and a decreasing 1-year transplant rate, from >50% to 20%, in patients who received LVAD with bridge-to-transplant (BTT) strategy [1, 2]. Currently, indication for LVAD therapy is considered earlier in the course of the disease, in order to avoid the sum of procedure- and device-related adverse events and patient-related risk factors [3]. Despite improvements regarding device duration, portability, user interface, and may be thrombogenicity, relevant morbidity is still associated with long-term LVAD, even when functional improvement without excess mortality is simultaneously obtained [4].

For these reasons, it is recommended to perform a comprehensive patient evaluation before the operation, to assess baseline status, and to identify pre-existing or new comorbid conditions that may influence postoperative survival and the probability of adverse events and complications, or may compromise the expected improvement in functional status and quality of life [5, 6]. In practice, this work-up is similar to what is usually done for HTX candidate selection. As for HTX listing, the border between contraindications, unacceptable or acceptable risk factors is not clear-cut in many situations. However, the objectives of these screening processes are not exactly the same, both in terms of specific goals and of underlying principles. Regarding HTX listing, besides beneficiality versus risk in the individual patient, the best use of a scarce, fixed resource must be taken into account also from the perspective of the community. Another difference with respect to HTX is that in many patients, except those with INTERMACS profile 1 and 2, LVAD implant is an elective or semi-elective procedure. Thus, in most cases, there are some days/weeks for addressing patient-specific risk factors, to minimize their burden on patient outcome or at least to set up in advance a strategy to monitor and approach expected complications. On the contrary, HTX cannot be planned, and generally there is a very short time – if any – for preoperative patient assessment and treatment. This chapter will summarize briefly the preoperative evaluation process before LVAD implantation; then some of the issues that may deserve attention, to reduce the probability of unfavorable outcome and/or complications, will be specifically discussed. The interplay between long-term MCS and HTX is discussed elsewhere (▶ Chaps. 8, 10, and 13).

5.2 Long-Term LVAD: Preoperative Work-Up

◻ Table 5.1 provides a summary of what, ideally, should be done in patients under evaluation prior to long-term LVAD implant [5, 6]. Several aspects are taken into account: prognosis on medical therapy [7–11]; global status, including psychosocial aspects and quality of life [12–15], hemodynamic and morphological aspects [16, 17], kidney and liver function [11], coagulation and hematology [18–20], diabetes, nutritional status [21], respiratory function, peripheral vessels, neurological status, and infections [22]; and screening for cancer or other comorbidities, some of which are discussed later. The depth, extent, and degree of details of preoperative evaluation should be adapted to individual patients' characteristics, including age, diagnosis, pathophysiological profile, and severity of the clinical picture (◻ Table 5.2). For details, see also ▶ Chaps. 1, 2, 3, and 5.

Table 5.1 Long-term MCS/VAD – preoperative work-up

Section	What to do	In which patient and when	Why and how: rationale, scope, mode
Cardiology	Echocardiography	All	Standard comprehensive evaluation of advanced heart failure Special attention to LV dimensions, wall thickness, thrombosis RV dimension and function (in non-inotrope-dependent pts with RV dilation/ dysfunction, consider DSE) *see* Tables 5.3 and 5.4 Aortic valve (regurgitation 2+ or more may require correction) Aortic root (for dilation, calcium, thrombosis)
	Cardiopulmonary exercise test	Non-inotrope dependent, INTERMACS ≥4	Evaluation of functional status and prognosis [7, 8]
	6-min walking test	Non-inotrope dependent, INTERMACS ≥4	Evaluation of functional status and exercise tolerance as perceived by the patient. Monitor arterial oxygen saturation besides heart rate, rhythm, and blood pressure
	Right heart catheterization	All	RAP, PAP (s,d,mean), PCWP, cardiac output, SVR, PVR, systemic AP, RVSWI
	Coronary angiography or CT scan	Known IHD or no prior screening for CAD	Diagnosis of CAD Concomitant, prior, alternative revascularization Bypass position and patency
Score	Heart failure scores	See notes	For prognosis on medical therapy HFSS or MECKI scores preferred in ambulatory pts [7, 8] ADHF-NTproBNP score suggested in hospitalized pts [9, 10] SHFM may also be used, but could underestimate mortality
	LVAD risk scores	See notes	For prognosis with LVAD. No validated score with contemporary devices and outcome available
	RVF risk scores	See notes	For estimating the risk of RVF after LVAD. No validated score available. *See* Tables 5.3 and 5.4
	MELD score	See notes	For prognosis. Validated in chronic liver disease to evaluate the need and risk of liver transplantation. Correlates with risk and with any therapy (medical, LVAD, HTX, etc.). Limited value on warfarin [11]
	Quality of life	All	For preoperative assessment and serial evaluation after implant [12, 13] EuroQoL-5d (nonspecific for HF, included in INTERMACS database) recommended for feasibility and pre-/post-op comparisons MLWHFQ or KCCMQ, specific for HF, may also be used
	Frailty	See notes	Complex, holistic concept may be evaluated with various parameters and their combinations. May be useful to estimate post-implant prognosis and functional recovery. Further studies are needed prior to recommended systematic assessment of frailty for decision making [14, 15]

(continued)

Table 5.1 (continued)

Section	What to do	In which patient and when	Why and how: rationale, scope, mode
Psychosocial evaluation	Psychologist consultation	All (+/– relatives)	Understand patients' and families' expectations and preferences, evaluate adherence to therapy, increase self-empowerment
	Psychiatric consultation	Pertinent history or status	In case of symptoms, or history of psichiatrico or psychiatric disorder, tobacco use, alcohol consumption, illicit substance use, dependences
	Socioeconomic conditions	All	Adequacy with respect to postoperative management, need for assistance
Kidney and liver function	Blood test	All	Use GFR to estimate renal function BUN and uric acid are related to HF severity AST/ALT increase mostly in acute HF Bilirubin increases mostly in chronic HF, especially when decompensated Reduced albumin and pseudocholinesterase are associated with chronic conditions Kidney and liver dysfunction correlates with prognosis with any therapy Recent onset HF and young age may be associated with superior probability of recovery of end-organ dysfunction if CO is restorated
	Ultrasounds	All	Rule out/evaluate chronic disease (primary), lithiasis, tumors, degenerative disease, etc.
	CMR, CT scan	As per specific indications	If needed on the basis of medical history, symptoms, signs, and other examinations
Hematology	Hct, Hb, WBC and formula, RBC and volume, iron, transferrin, ferritin, platelets	All	Check the presence and etiology of anemia: hemoglobinopathies, bleeding, infection, chronic disease, etc. Screen for signs of inflammatory or oncohematologic conditions
	Specialist consultation	Pertinent history or status	If suspected oncohematologic or other complex conditions
Coagulation and platelets	AP-INR, PTT, platelets count	All	Evaluate current conditions and postoperative risk
	Thrombophilia evaluation	Pertinent history or status	Thrombophilia may increase postoperative risk, but no specific guidelines are available [19–21]
	Antiplatelets, antibodies, others	As above	Thrombocytopenia, heparin-induced or due to other causes, for risk estimation and perioperative strategy [20, 21]

Table 5.1 (continued)

Section	What to do	In which patient and when	Why and how: rationale, scope, mode
Diabetes	Rest blood glucose	All	Diagnosis of diabetes and prediabetes
	Hb glycated	Pertinent history or status	As above
	Fundus oculi	As above	Estimate diabetes-related end-organ damage, vessels
	EMG, ENG	As above	Estimate diabetes-related end-organ damage, peripheral neuropathy
	Specialist consultation	Unsatisfactory blood glucose control	Therapy adjustment, preop optimization
Nutritional status	BMI	All	Estimate status and postop risk
	Blood test	Cholesterol, PT, proteins, albumin, prealbumin	Estimate status and postop risk
	Specialist consultation	Hyponutrition, cachexia Obesity, severe	Rule out behavioral disturbances, nutritional plan for preop optimization Rule out behavioral disturbances, dietary plan, possible role of bariatric surgery [22]
Respiratory function	Chest X-ray	All	Screen for concomitant disease/infection/pleural effusion, etc.
	Spirometry	All	Evaluate respiratory function. Rule out lung disease as major determinant of functional limitation
	CT scan	As per specific indications	Evaluate interstitial disease, pulmonary embolism, emphysema, tumors, etc.
Extracardiac vascular disease	Doppler ultrasound – carotid and vertebral system	All, after 40 years* of age	Peri- and postoperative risk. Reference in case of subsequent control.
	Doppler ultrasound – lower limbs	All, after 50 years* of age	Peri- and postoperative risk. Reference in case of subsequent control.
Neurological status	Focused neurologic examination	Pertinent history or status	
	Neurological consultation	As above	Evaluate current conditions and postoperative risk
	Brain CT scan, magnetic resonance	As above	As above

(continued)

Table 5.1 (continued)

Section	What to do	In which patient and when	Why and how: rationale, scope, mode
Infections	Nasal swab	All	Evaluate *Staphylococcus* colonization. Consider preop local treatment [23]
	Others	Hospitalized pts	Routine cultures as per local protocols for surveillance of nosocomial infection
	Specialist consultation	Pertinent history or status	Plan pre/periop antimicrobial strategy
Other	Hemoccult	All	Check for gastrointestinal bleeding
	Screening for cancer	As per protocol	Screen for breast, colorectal, prostatic, or lung cancer as per local protocols in general population according to age and gender
	EGDS	All	Estimate risk of bleeding; treat preop peptic ulcer
	Colonoscopy	>50 years* or pertinent history/status	Screen for diverticulosis, cancer, and other lesions, to estimate postop risk. Consider CT "virtual" colonoscopy or miniaturized camera in "frail" pts

ADHF-NTproBNP acute decompensated heart failure-N-terminal B-type natriuretic peptide, *ALT* aspartate alanine transferase, *AP* arterial pressure, *AP-INR* prothrombin activity-international normalized ratio, *AST* aspartate amino transferase, *BMI* body mass index, *BUN* blood urea nitrogen, *CAD* coronary artery disease, *CMR* cardiac magnetic resonance, *CO* cardiac output *CT* computed tomography, *CPET* cardiopulmonary exercise test, *DSE* dobutamine stress echocardiography, *EGDS* esophago-gastric-duodenoscopy, *EMG* electromyography, *ENG* electroneurography, *EuroQoL-5D* European quality of life 5-dimensional score, *GFR* glomerular filtration rate, *Hb* hemoglobin, *Hct* hematocrit, *HF* heart failure, *HFSS* heart failure survival score, *HTX* heart transplantation, *IHD* ischemic heart disease, *INTERMACS* Interagency Registry of Mechanically Assisted Circulatory Support, *KCCMQ* Kansas City Cardiomyopathy Questionnaire, *LV* left ventricle, *LVAD* left ventricular assist device, *MECKI* metabolic exercise cardiac kidney index, *MELD* model for end-stage liver disease, *MLWHFQ* Minnesota Living With Heart Failure Questionnaire, *PAP* pulmonary artery pressure, *PCWP* pulmonary capillary wedge pressure, *PT* prothrombin time, *pts* patients, *PTT* partial thromboplastin time, *PVR* pulmonary vascular resistance, *RAP* right atrial pressure, *RBC* red blood cell, *RV* right ventricle, *RVF* right ventricular failure, *RVSWI* right ventricular stroke work index, *s,d,mean* systolic, diastolic, mean, *SHFM* Seattle Heart Failure Model, *SVR* systemic vascular resistance, *WBC* white blood cell

*To be considered also at younger age, if there are pertinent history, risk factors, symptoms, or signs

Table 5.2 Clinical setting, INTERMACS profile, and type of preoperative work-up

Clinical setting	INTERMACS profile	Time frame	Preoperative work-up
High urgency , new onset HF/ shock	1, 2	Hours	Basic
Urgent implant, new diagnosis/shock	2, 3	Hours to days	Basic
Urgent implants, chronic HF	3 (2)	Days to hours	Intermediate to complete
Semi-elective implant	3, 4	Days to weeks	Complete
Elective implant	4+	Weeks	Complete

HF heart failure, *INTERMACS* Interagency Registry of Mechanically Assisted Circulatory Support; for details

5.3 Considerations for Preoperative Optimization

5.3.1 Hemodynamic and Volume Status Optimization

- **Right Ventricular Failure**

Right ventricular failure (RVF) following LVAD therapy is associated with a greater risk of death and complications such as bleeding or renal insufficiency and with longer hospital stay and reduced survival to transplantation [24–26]. Delayed, unplanned (RVAD) support for RVF ensuing in patients which entered the operating room to receive an isolated LVAD implant has been associated with high in-hospital mortality up to 50%, superior to that observed with planned biventricular assist device (BiVAD) implantation strategy [25]. Thus, preoperative estimate of the risk for RVF is essential in LVAD candidates.

In patients enrolled in trials with continuous-flow LVAD (HeartMate II, Thoratec, or HVAD, HeartWare) and in observational patient cohorts, the reported incidence of RVF ranged from less than 20% to more than 40% [27–30]. This variability is partly due to the absence of a uniform definition of RVF: the main criteria for diagnosis are the need for RVAD implant, and/or prolonged (>14 days) inotropic support, need and duration of nitric oxide inhalation, and length of stay in the intensive care. Numerous preoperative parameters and various scores have been proposed to estimate the probability of RVF in LVAD candidates [16, 27–34]. Most studies are based on relatively small cohorts, with BTT indication, and some of them include patients receiving pulsatile-flow LVAD. Thus, reliable scores for estimating with good prospective accuracy the probability for RVF in contemporary CF-LVAD patients are lacking. Clinical decision must be made on the basis of a comprehensive evaluation, including echocardiography (Echo) and right heart catheterization. Hemodynamic and clinical factors associated with an increased risk for RVF after LVAD implant are summarized in ◻ Table 5.3, while Echo parameters are listed in ◻ Table 5.4 [16, 26, 28–34].

A comprehensive review on Echo in LVAD patients has been published by the American Society of Echocardiography in 2015 [16]. Echo is the primary imaging modality for studying

◻ **Table 5.3** Hemodynamic and clinical assessment of the risk for right ventricular failure after left ventricular assist device implantation

Hemodynamic parameters predictor of RVF	
CVP >15 mmHg	Normal value: 0–7 mmHg
RVSWI <300 mmHg/mL/m^2	RVSWI = (MAP-RAP) × SVI = 300–900 mmHg × mL/m^2 SVI = CI/Heart Rate × 1000 = 33–47 ml/m^2/beat
RAP/PCWP > 0.63	
PAPi < 1.85	(PAS– PAD)/RAP
Patient frailty for RVF	
Biochemical parameters	Bilirubin >2 mg/dL Transaminase: AST >45 mg/dL Albumin <3.5 g/dL Low total cholesterol Renal function: (BUN >50 mg/dL or creatinine >2.3 mg/dL) NGAL > 100 ng/ml

CVP central venous pressure, mmHg, *RAP* right atrial pressure, mmHg, *MAP* pulmonary artery mean pressure, mmHg, *PCWP* pulmonary capillary wedge pressure, mmHg, *Cindex* ml/min/m2, *SVI* stroke volume index, ml, *RVSWI* right ventricular stroke work index, *PAPi* pulmonary artery pulsatility index, *sPAP* systolic pulmonary artery pressure, mmHg, *dPAP* diastolic pulmonary artery pressure, mmHg, *NGAL* neutrophil gelatinase-associated lipocalin, *BMI* body mass index

Table 5.4 Echocardiographic assessment of the risk for right ventricular failure after left ventricular assist device implantation

Echocardiographic predictors of post-LVAD RVF		
Parameter	**Limitations**	**References**
Altered RV geometry		
RV fractional area change (FAC) RV/LV end-diastolic diameter ratio (>0.75) RV volumes (3D)	Reproducibility Overstated by significant TR and low PVR Standardization of views Technically challenging and not widely available	[16, 28–30]
TAPSE	Sensitive to afterload Less reliable if prior cardiac surgery	[16]
Tissue Doppler imaging (TDI)	Dependent on transducer angle Confounded by cardiac motion and tethering	[31]
RV strain Global longitudinal Free wall longitudinal Global systolic strain rate	Limited validation and reliability Requires adequate views of RV free wall	[16, 31, 32]
RV contractile reserve Dobutamine stress echocardiography	Feasibility and tolerance	[33, 34]

FAC fractional area contraction, *LV* left ventricle, *PVR* pulmonary vascular resistance, *RV* right ventricle, *TAPSE* tricuspid annular plane systolic excursion, *TR* tricuspid regurgitation

the right ventricle, but the results may be influenced by poor image quality, especially in patients in intensive care unit. Moreover, some parameters mainly related to RV wall motion may be less reliable in case of prior cardiac surgery. Novel approaches such as three-dimensional echocardiography, measurement of RV strain, and, in patients not dependent on continuous inotropic therapy, INTERMACS profile >3, dobutamine-stress echocardiography may be useful to evaluate RV contractility and contractile reserve [28, 31–34].

Among the various hemodynamic parameters that have been proposed so far, those reflecting persistent RV volume overload despite aggressive medical therapy (and possibly IABP) may indicate irreversible RV dysfunction. On the other side, persistently high pulmonary artery (PA) systolic pressure (sPAP) after diuretic and vasodilator treatment may be considered as a surrogate of preserved RV contractile function: in this case, an LVAD may be implanted with a reasonably low probability of RVF and may serve also as a bridge to candidacy for HTX, which is precluded by pulmonary hypertension (▶ see Chap. 8). Since optimal loading conditions may not always be reached before operation, the search for load-independent parameters has been undertaken. PA pulsatility index (PAPi) is a simple hemodynamic variable calculated as the ratio between pulmonary artery (PA) pulse pressure (sPAP – PA diastolic pressure, dPAP) and right atrial (RA) pressure that could help to identify patients at high risk of developing RVF [35]. This index provides an insight on RV mechanics corrected for both left and right heart preload, represented, respectively, by dPAP and RAP, and is independent from stroke volume.

Clinical factors that may predict an increased risk for RVF after LVAD are those related to the characteristic and evolution of the underlying disease and to signs of severity and chronicity of RV dysfunction. Chemotherapy-induced cardiomyopathy is often characterized from the beginning by biventricular dysfunction, "restrictive" pathophysiology, and mildly dilated left ventricle, defining a suboptimal condition for LVAD therapy [36]. Dilated idiopathic or ischemic cardiomyopathy is generally characterized by significant, severe left ventricular dysfunction preceding both echocardiographic and clinical phenotypes of RV dysfunction; in this condition, the development of overt RV dysfunction is a negative prognostic sign on medical therapy and should be anticipated or approached at the very beginning in order to obtain better outcomes after LVAD implant. In HTX candidates with pulmonary hypertension undergoing serial right heart catheterization, a reduction of PAP values associated with normal or high RAP and low or very low cardiac output may be the hemodynamic hallmark of evolving RV dysfunction. Several clinical and biochemical parameters, most of them included among negative prognostic factors in patients with advanced heart failure and in those undergoing LVAD or HTX, have been also associated with an increased risk for RVF [37, 38]. Among markers of renal function, creatinine may be influenced also by coexisting conditions (e.g., diabetic nephropathy), while increased urea nitrogen reflects the use of excessive diuretic to limit congestive symptoms. Regarding liver dysfunction, high transaminase levels generally reflect acute/subacute congestion, but their value may be normal in chronic severe HF, when bilirubin is more often elevated.

Much attention has been devoted to predicting early RVF after LVAD implantation. Another adverse event possibly correlated with preoperative conditions is the late occurrence of RVF that has been defined as RVF requiring readmission after discharge from index hospitalization; diabetes mellitus, body mass index >29 kg/m^2, and blood urea nitrogen level >41 mg/dl were reported as significant predictors for late RHF [39]. Clinical profile, incidence, and approaches to prevention and treatment of this condition are not well defined. Current knowledge is summarized in ▶ Chap. 28.

▪▪ Other Issues in Hemodynamic and Volume Optimization

Whenever possible, LVAD implant should be preceded by optimization of volemia and correction of end-organ damage resulting from acute/subacute congestion and low-output state. In this phase, the principles of treatment are those of advanced to refractory heart failure. Unfortunately, evidence-based recommendations are neither abundant nor strong in this field [5, 40, 41]. Moreover, these goals cannot be achieved in all the patients, even in those considered relatively stable (INTERMACS profile 3 or more), and the side effects and risks of increased levels of inotropic support and/or high-dose diuretics must be weighted against the risk of operation in a decompensated status. The use of levosimendan to improve end-organ perfusion and hemodynamics prior to LVAD implant has been explored in small, non-conclusive, observational studies. The most interesting observation was that patients who were unresponsive to levosimendan, in terms of natriuretic peptide level and hemodynamic changes, were at high risk for the occurrence of RVF and unfavorable outcome [42]. Preserving or restoring renal function is even more important in patients at risk for renal failure due to comorbidities such as diabetes or nephrovascular disease. Non-pharmacological therapy, e.g., renal replacement therapy or mechanically assisted ventilation, may improve renal function indexes and oxygenation, but the need for such therapies is a hallmark of very advanced disease and is associated with reduced probability of survival.

▪▪ Infections

While typical device-related infections, i.e., driveline infections, are commonly a late complication and are scarcely influenced by preoperative conditions, early infections such as pneumonia and sepsis may complicate post-LVAD course as generally observed after cardiac surgery, with the additional risks related to the need for hemodynamic adaptation and the presence of prosthetic, non-biological material [43, 44].

General measures for preventing early infections are removal of unnecessary intravenous lines and catheters, dental assessment, and aggressive treatment of existing infections [5]. Delay in the implant after complete resolution of major infections may be appropriate if allowed by the hemodynamic status. Recent infection may require a modified antimicrobial prophylaxis, targeted to specific agents besides standard care [45]. Perioperative care and complications are discussed in ▶ Chaps. 24, 25, and 28. Patients with chronic obstructive pulmonary disease (COPD) must be evaluated not only in terms of respiratory function and potential for symptomatic improvement after LVAD implant but also regarding the risk for postoperative infections. A peculiar challenge is represented by patients with abdominal conditions that may develop inflammation and infections, such as cholelithiasis or diverticulosis. Abdominal surgery before LVAD implant does not appear justified in most asymptomatic patients, but special attention should be paid after the operation, with a low alarm threshold in face of even subtle symptoms.

▪▪ Thrombosis and Bleeding

Thrombotic and bleeding complications are two major clinical issues in patient requiring circulatory support devices. Continuous flow (CF) generates an unique physiologic interaction with the hematological system and vascular surfaces [46, 47]. The activation of the coagulation system may cause thrombus formation within the device itself or in the aortic root and may cause embolism to the brain or coronary arteries, leading to ischemic stroke, transient ischemic attack, and myocardial infarction. Thus, anticoagulation is required to prevent thrombosis but must be balanced with the risk of bleeding, that is, a common complication during device support and a major cause of morbidity and rehospitalization, with a mortality rate of 9–10% [48, 49]. Gastrointestinal (GI) bleeding is a hallmark of CF support, occurring more frequently than observed previously with pulsatile devices (19–25% according to recent estimates) [50]. It is most often derived from angiodysplasia (microvascular malformations related to increased angiogenesis), with or without acquired von Willebrand disease, developed as a consequence of high shear stress and turbulence generated by the pump apparatus. GI bleeding is obstinate and characterized by high recurrence rate.

Finding the right balance between thrombosis and bleeding is of utmost importance particularly in the setting of long-term LVAD therapy. Preoperative assessment of propensity for thrombosis or bleeding is important to estimate the early and long-term risk of LVAD implant [19, 20, 51].

It is recommended to obtain a detailed personal and family history regarding venous thromboembolic disease, including history of deep vein thrombosis, pulmonary embolism, sudden death, cerebral sinus, and splanchnic vein thrombosis. Moreover, any history of an abnormality of blood cell lines should be assessed, with special attention for leukopenia and thrombocytopenia that may indicate an underlying hematologic condition. Several hematologic disorders and a history of unprovoked thrombotic events are risk factors for early complications and mortality: Fried evidence that patients with a history of prior hematologic condition (idiopathic thrombocytopenic purpura (ITP), Factor V Leiden, elevated Factor VIII, heparin-induced thrombocythemia (HIT), or undefined hypercoagulable state) have a high frequency of bleeding, thrombotic, and neurologic events (6- and 12-month actuarial rates were both 81.1% but fell to 49% at 2 years) [18]. In case of positive hematological history, a further work-up is needed, testing protein C, protein S, cardiolipin antibody (IgG and IgM), lupus anticoagulant (LAC), prothrombin, antithrombin III, RPR, and JAK2 mutation. Unfortunately, therapeutic anticoagulation, frequently used in advanced heart failure patients, may be a confounding factor when trying to ascertain abnormalities like antithrombin, protein C and protein S deficiency, or antibody-mediated disorders. Moreover, some of these conditions (e.g., positive LAC) reduce the reliability of standard laboratory test for monitoring therapeutic anticoagulation. It is also important to ascertain the history of drug intolerance, e.g., allergy to acetylsalicylic acid. A peculiar condition is represented by the presence of anti-heparin antibodies that may cause thrombocytopenia in case of heparin rechallenge (heparin-induced thrombocytopenia, HIT) [19, 20]. These issues are discussed in details in ▶ Chaps. 27 and 28.

The presence of gastrointestinal lesions at risk for bleeding should be ascertained and treated prior to LVAD implant. Intracardiac thrombosis demonstrated by Echo can be addressed at the time of the operation, although it could imply a more invasive surgical approach [16]. History of prior peripheral or cerebral embolism must be excluded and, if present, must be evaluated accurately with respect to carotid, aortic, or other vessel diseases.

5.3.2 Nutritional, Endocrine, and Metabolic Considerations

Heart failure (HF) and other chronic or critical illnesses are associated with metabolic, endocrine, and nutritional disturbances: usually, the pathophysiological basis is not a primary deficiency of hormones, rather a complex interplay between the primary disease and the subsequent adaptive or maladaptive changes. In this perspective, the approach with substitutive therapy is neither straightforward nor uniformly useful.

▪ Thyroid Function

Non-thyroidal illness syndrome (NTIS) is characterized by low plasma triiodothyronine (T3), low plasma thyroxin (T4), increased reverse T3 (rT3), and normal or slightly decreased thyroid-stimulating hormone (TSH). NTIS is frequent in critically ill patients, with a prevalence of 18% in moderate-to-severe HF, and has a negative prognostic role. In patients with heart diseases, low T3 status is a strong predictor of mortality [52]. In a cohort of HTX recipients, the early postoperative finding of low T3 syndrome was associated with higher mortality and complication rates [53]. However, four randomized controlled trials (RCTs) have addressed the role of thyroid hormone administration in such patients and showed no benefit on mortality. Moreover, thyroid hormone replacement might further suppress TSH levels. The possible role of thyroid hormone replacement in HF with low T3 syndrome remains an unresolved question, especially in the specific subgroup of advanced HF patients.

▪▪ Testosterone

Metabolic derangements associated with advanced HF include a tendency toward a catabolic state, secondary to alterations in neuroendocrine and cytokine pathways, among which reduced testosterone levels seem to play a key role [54]. The administration of testosterone in HF patients is aimed to counteract maladaptive mechanisms leading to muscle wasting, weakness, hyporexia, and anemia. Testosterone has also direct cardiovascular effects, determining an acute increase of cardiac output and a decrease in systemic vascular resistance. Low levels of testosterone have been consistently associated with exercise intolerance in HF patients. A meta-analysis by Toma et al. [55] evaluated four studies in which testosterone supplementation showed a significant improvement in exercise capacity in patients with heart failure, without changes in myocardial structure or function. Improvement in exercise capacity might be attributed to improved oxygen delivery to muscles secondary to peripheral vasodilation, acute increase of cardiac output, anti-inflammatory properties, and increase in muscle mass. The available evidences, including the safety profile, seem to encourage future studies on administration of testosterone in patients with advanced HF in which LVAD implant is planned.

▪▪ Anemia

Anemia and the amount of red blood cell transfusions have been recognized as strong predictors of perioperative morbidity and mortality in cardiac and noncardiac surgery. A retrospective study on 65 patients who received a long-term LVAD showed a 6-month survival two times higher in non-anemic (Hb > 12 g/dL) than in anemic patients [56]. Iron deficiency and reduced erythropoiesis are the main features of anemia in chronic/advanced illness; thus treatment may include the administration of iron and/or erythropoiesis-stimulating agents (ESA). Iron is involved in many physiologic processes, as intellectual functioning, oxygen uptake and transport, thyroid hormone effects, and cardiovascular function. Iron deficiency in patients with HF has a variable reported prevalence, much higher (up to 80%) in patients in NYHA class III or IV. Pathophysiology of anemia in LVAD patients is similar to that of chronic illnesses: an inflammatory milieu, sustained by the altered cytokine pattern of advanced heart failure and by the immune reaction against the foreign surface of LVAD materials, may both suppress erythropoietin production and reduce its effects on tissue targets. The role of iron replacement therapy in HF patients with iron deficiency is now well established. Two recent trials showed a symptomatic improvement up to 6–12 months and a tendency toward reduced rehospitalizations, in patients with HF, reduced ejection fraction, iron deficiency, and anemia, who received intravenous iron (ferric carboxymaltose) versus placebo [57, 58]. On the contrary, concerning ESA, the RED-HF study demonstrated that administration of darbepoetin alpha did not improve clinical outcomes in patients with systolic heart failure and mild-to-moderate anemia, whereas thromboembolic events were more frequent in the treatment group [59]. Indeed, a retrospective, observational cohort study on 221 patients receiving HeartMate II LVAD with a mean follow-up of 14.2 ± 11.9 months [60] showed significantly higher rates of suspected pump thrombosis and all-cause mortality in patients who received ESA during index admission with respect to those who did not.

Vitamin D

The protective effect of vitamin D in HF includes its antiproliferative action on cardiac myocytes, suppression of plasma renin activity, a regulatory action on blood pressure (BP) and on anti-thrombotic homeostasis, and a reduction of the transcription of genes encoding for inflammatory cytokines. Hypovitaminosis D (irrespective with sun exposure) is highly prevalent and is associated with a poor prognosis in HF patients [61]. A recent study on 154 end-stage HF patients who received LVAD implantation showed a high prevalence of vitamin D deficiency [25(OH)D < 25 nmol/L] and its independent association with higher risk for stroke (HR 2.44, 95% CI 1.09–5.45, $p = 0.03$) and mortality (HR 2.78 95% CI 1.52–5.09, $p = 0.001$) [62]. However, whether administration of vitamin D could improve outcomes in LVAD patients remains to be demonstrated.

Nutritional Status

Approximately 50% of HF patients experience weight loss, muscular atrophy, weakness, and reduced immune function, sustained by low-grade systemic inflammation, determining metabolic shift toward catabolism, and nutritional deficit due to anorexia, delayed gastric emptying, reduced intestinal motility, and liver congestion. A smaller percentage of advanced HF patients develop a condition termed "cardiac cachexia." Cachexia is defined as "a complex metabolic syndrome characterized by loss of muscle with or without loss of fat mass, which prominent clinical feature is weight loss in adults (corrected for fluid retention) or growth failure in children (excluding endocrine disorders)." In chronic patients, albumin deficiency and coagulation abnormalities (typically, spontaneously increased INR) reflect reduced liver synthesis and are not rarely accompanied by weight loss and ultimately cachexia [38]. Fat loss is a predictor of unfavorable outcome, but it is unclear whether it is a surrogate of enhanced catabolism or if the adipose tissue is cardioprotective in the setting of HF [37]. In unselected HF patients, the presence of cachexia is a strong predictor of mortality at 18 months (50% versus 17% in non-cachectic subjects) [63]. However, the relation between body mass index (BMI) and mortality in LVAD patient is not linear, showing increased risk in both severely underweight and overweight patients [2]. Hyponutrition, as estimated with the Mini Nutritional Assessment (MNA), is an independent predictor of mortality in patients with advanced HF candidate to LVAD implantation [64]. In a study on 590 LVAD recipients, Musci et al. demonstrated a worse early prognosis for patients with BMI < 20 kg/m^2, but at 30 days from the operation and thereafter, underweight patients had similar survival rates as patients with normal weight [65]. Thus, cachexia "per se" should not represent a contraindication to MCS/LVAD implant, but must be taken into account within a comprehensive patient evaluation.

Nutritional challenges in LVAD patients include a preoperative nutritional assessment, an individualized preoperative and postoperative nutritional strategy, and the prevention and management of complications associated with enteral and parenteral nutrition. In fact, while enteral nutrition may be limited in low-output state, total parenteral nutrition is associated with increased risk of fungal infections. Moreover, overfeeding must be avoided, especially in the early and/or complicated postoperative phase, because carbon dioxide production is mainly linked to the amount of delivered calories, thus negatively interfering with early respiratory weaning and extubation.

Respiratory Considerations [66]

Dyspnea is a common symptoms of both heart and lung disease. Prevalence of concomitant COPD is high among HF patients and is associated with worse prognosis either with or without surgery. Lung infection and pulmonary embolism are major complications of "natural" and perioperative patient course. Thus, measurement of pulmonary function is recommended as part of patient work-up: severe obstructive disease may be considered a contraindication for heart transplantation (HTX), but is most often a risk factor for LVAD that may be implanted with DT strategy. Restrictive abnormalities and/or altered alveolocapillary transfer may be a consequence of heart chambers dilation and chronic pulmonary congestion; thus reevaluation after volume status correction may be useful. Differential diagnosis with drug-induced interstitial disease must be remembered in patients on long-term amiodarone therapy.

Thoracic CT scan may be useful according to specific indications: prior cardiac and/or thoracic surgery, calcifications at chest X-ray, or other diagnostic tests, for anatomical assessment and surgical planning, and known/suspected actual or recent infection, pulmonary embolism, pleural effusion, and cancer, as part of overall risk/benefit evaluation. Polysomnography is recommended in case of suspected sleep apnea, drowsiness, periodic breathing, and desaturation episodes, although the role of noninvasive ventilation in HF patients with sleep disorders – especially central apnea– has been recently questioned.

When LVAD implant is planned, respiratory exercises and training, and/or noninvasive ventilation, possibly with the help of specialized technicians, could be useful in patients with COPD, pulmonary congestion, or other respiratory disorders, to improve lung capacity and also pulmonary hemodynamics. In the lack of evidences for general recommendations, choices should be done on patient-specific basis, taking into account patient history, adaptation to ventilatory equipment (that depends also on general functional status and muscular strength), and observed effects on respiratory rate and blood gas exchange.

▪▪ Psychosocial Considerations

Short-term MCS therapy is applied to very critically ill, sometimes unconscious patients, is intended for temporary/rescue treatment, and, despite inherent risks and limitations regarding mobilization and quality of life, is generally accepted in the hope of myocardial recovery or further therapeutic solutions. Thus, psychosocial assessment and prediction of patient's capability to cope with his or her new condition are relevant when long-term MCSD (or TAH) implantation is under evaluation. Adaptation to living with a portable MCSD relates to patient expectations, cognitive function, awareness of expected outcomes, symptomatic benefits, complications with the device and alternative therapies, propensity to learn new competences, self-confidence, familiarity with electronic devices, attitudes toward new technologies, and so on [67]. Physical and medical conditions, depending on preoperative status and postoperative course – including, when it happens, adverse events – obviously interfere with subjective appreciation of the value and limitations of therapy. Similar considerations may be applied to relatives and caregivers. Efforts to make living with the device easier (familiarization with the device regarding technical issues, training for care of the driveline exit site, basic knowledge of medications, and adherence to drug schedule and appropriate lifestyle – all included in the broad concept of patient empowerment) are of great importance and may begin in the preoperative period, with possibly favorable impact on postoperative quality of life and outcomes. Psychological and ethical issues are addressed in ▶ Chap. 31. Baseline evaluation should allow room for conversations between the patient and multidisciplinary staff (cardiologists, cardiac surgeon, nurses and technicians, psychologist, etc.). Psychiatric and/or social worker evaluations are needed when specific concerns arise, as in case of prior/recent/actual psychiatric disorders; attempted suicide; substance abuse (including alcohol) or addiction (including tobacco); nonadherence to the therapeutic program, including lifestyle beyond drug regimen; serious economic and/or housing problems, and social deprivation. Denial of treatment is justified in the face of patient nonadherence and major or multiple psychosocial difficulties, or some difficulties on top of medical concerns [5,15,66]. In fact, as for HTX, nonadherence to treatment and to recommended lifestyle is a risk factor for complications and inferior postoperative survival. How low or high the threshold for psychosocial contraindications would be set, it depends also on local principles and policies governing healthcare organization and delivery, including the interrelationship between healthcare and social services; the amount and criteria for funding these services; the role and strength of nonprofit, charitable organizations; and the value of this therapy as perceived by the medical community and at societal level. Economic issues are discussed in ► Chap. 32. Confounding factors may be reactive depression and frustration due to severe illness, difficulties in realizing functional limitation, and bad prognosis as may happen in patients with recent onset of disease, deteriorated cognitive status as a consequence of low-output state and/or hyponatremia, and a reticent attitude regarding behavioral problems, especially if perceived to reduce the probability to get a lifesaving treatment.

References

1. Kirklin JK, Naftel DC, Kormos RL et al (2010) Second INTERMACS annual report: more than 1,000 primary left ventricular assist device implants. J Heart Lung Transplant 29:1–10
2. Kirklin JK, Naftel DC, Pagani FD et al (2015) Seventh INTERMACS annual report: 15,000 patients and counting. J Heart Lung Transplant 34:1495–1504
3. Mancini D, Colombo P (2015) Left ventricular assist devices: a rapidly evolving alternative to transplant. J Am Coll Cardiol 65:2542–2555
4. Estep JD, Starling RC, Horstmanshof DA et al (2015) Risk assessment and comparative effectiveness of left ventricular assist device and medical management in ambulatory heart failure patients: results from the ROADMAP Study, for the ROADMAP Study Investigators. J Am Coll Cardiol 66:1747–1761
5. Feldman D, Pamboukian SV, Teuteberg JJ et al (2013) The 2013 International Society of Heart and Lung Transplantation Guidelines for Mechanical Circulatory Support. Executive Summary. J Heart Lung Transplant 32:157–187. (See Lietz K, Deng M, Feldman D et al. Task Force 1: Selection of candidates for Mechanical Circulatory Support and risk management prior to implantation for fixed comorbidities.)
6. Peura JL, Colvin-Adams M, Francis GS et al (2012) AHA Scientific Statement. Recommendations for the use of Mechanical Circulatory Support: device strategy and patient selection. A scientific statement from the American Heart Association. Circulation 126:2648–2667
7. Goda A, Lund LH, Mancini DM (2011) The Heart Failure Survival Score outperforms the peak oxygen consumption for heart transplantation selection in the era of device therapy. J Heart Lung Transplant 30: 315–325
8. Cattadori G, Agostoni P, Corrà U et al (2013) Severe heart failure prognosis evaluation for transplant selection in the era of beta-blockers: role of peak oxygen consumption. Int J Cardiol 168:5078–5081
9. Scrutinio D, Ammirati E, Passantino A et al (2015) Predicting short-term mortality in advanced decompensated heart failure – role of the updated acute decompensated heart failure/N-terminal pro-B-type natriuretic Peptide risk score. Circ J 79: 1076–1083
10. Scrutinio D, Ammirati E, Guida P et al (2014) The ADHF/NT-proBNP risk score to predict 1-year mortality in hospitalized patients with advanced decompensated heart failure. J Heart Lung Transplant 33:404–411
11. Bonde P, Ku NC, Genovese EA et al (2012) Model for end-stage liver disease score predicts adverse events related to ventricular assist device therapy. Ann Thorac Surg 93:1541–1547
12. Grady KL, Naftel DC, Myers S et al (2015) Change in health-related quality of life from before to after destination therapy mechanical circulatory support is similar for older and younger patients: analyses from INTERMACS. J Heart Lung Transplant 34:213–221
13. Kiernan MS, Sundareswaran KS, Pham DT et al (2016) Preoperative determinants of quality of life and functional capacity response to left ventricular assist device therapy. J Card Fail 22:797–805
14. Dunlay SM, Park SJ, Joyce LD et al (2014) Frailty and outcomes after implantation of left ventricular assist device as destination therapy. J Heart Lung Transplant 33:359–365
15. Bruce CR, Delgado E, Kostick K et al (2014) Ventricular assist devices: a review of psychosocial risk factors and their impact on outcomes. J Card Fail 20:996–1003
16. Stainback RF, Estep JD, Agler DA et al (2015) Echocardiography in the management of patients with Left Ventricular Assist Devices: recommendations from the American Society of Echocardiography. J Am Soc Echocardiogr 28:853–909
17. Atluri P, Goldstone AB, Fairman AS et al (2013) Predicting right ventricular failure in the modern, continuous flow left ventricular assist device era. Ann Thorac Surg 96:857–863 ; discussion 863–864
18. Fried J, Levin AP, Mody KM et al (2014) Prior hematologic conditions carry a high morbidity and mortality in patients supported with continuous-flow left ventricular assist devices. J Heart Lung Transplant 33:1119–1125
19. Benken ST, Tillman N, Dajani S, Shah A, Thomas T (2014) A retrospective evaluation of fondaparinux for confirmed or suspected heparin-induced thrombocytopenia in left-ventricular-assist device patients. J Cardiothorac Surg 9:55
20. Morshuis M, Boergermann J, Gummert J, Koster A (2013) A modified technique for implantation of the HeartWare™ left ventricular assist device when using bivalirudin anticoagulation in patients with acute heparin-induced thrombocytopenia. Interact Cardiovasc Thorac Surg 17:225–226
21. Chaudhry UI, Kanji A, Sai-Sudhakar CB, Higgins RS, Needleman BJ (2015) Laparoscopic sleeve gastrectomy in morbidly obese patients with end-stage heart failure and left ventricular assist device: medium-term results. Surg Obes Relat Dis 11:88–93

22. Schweizer ML, Chiang HY, Septimus E et al (2015) Association of a bundled intervention with surgical site infections among patients undergoing cardiac, hip, or knee surgery. JAMA 313:2162–2171
23. Patlolla B, Beygui R, Haddad F (2013) Right-ventricular failure following left ventricle assist device implantation. Curr Opin Cardiol 28:223–233
24. Dandel M, Potapov E, Krabatsch T et al (2013) Load dependency of right ventricular Performance Is a Major Factor to be Considered in Decision Making Before Ventricular Assist Device Implantation. Circulation 128(26 Suppl 1):S14–S23
25. Takeda K, Naka Y, Yang J et al (2014) Outcome of unplanned right ventricular assist device support for severe right heart failure after implantable left ventricular assist device insertion. J Heart Lung Transplant 33:141–148
26. Kormos RL, Teuteberg JJ, Pagani FD et al (2010) Right ventricular failure in patients with the HeartMate II continuous-flow left ventricular assist device: incidence, risk factors, and effect on outcomes. J Thorac Cardiovasc Surg 139:1316–1324
27. Drakos SG, Janicki L, Horne BD et al (2010) Risk factors predictive of right ventricular failure after left ventricular assist device implantation. Am J Cardiol 105:1030–1035
28. Raina A, Seetha Rammohan HR, Gertz ZM, Rame JE, Woo YJ, Kirkpatrick JN (2013) Postoperative right ventricular failure after left ventricular assist device placement is predicted by preoperative echocardiographic structural, hemodynamic, and functional parameters. J Card Fail 19:16–24
29. Potapov EV, Stepanenko A, Dandel M et al (2008) Tricuspid incompetence and geometry of the right ventricle as predictors of right ventricular function after implantation of a left ventricular assist device. J Heart Lung Transplant 27:1275–1281
30. Vivo RP, Cordero-Reyes AM, Qamar U et al (2013) Increased right-to-left ventricle diameter ratio is a strong predictor of right ventricular failure after left ventricular assist device. J Heart Lung Transplant 32:792–799
31. Kato TS, Jiang J, Schulze PC, Jorde U, Uriel N, Kitada S et al (2013) Serial echocardiography using tissue Doppler and speckle tracking imaging to monitor right ventricular failure before and after left ventricular assist device surgery. JACC Heart Fail 1:216–222
32. Grant ADM, Smedira NG, Starling RC, Marwick TH (2012) Independent and incremental role of quantitative right ventricular evaluation for the prediction of right ventricular failure after left ventricular assist device implantation. J Am Coll Cardiol 60:521–528
33. Ammirati E, Cipriani M, De Chiara B et al (2014) Left ventricular or Bi-ventricular assist device? How dobutamine stress echocardiography can untie the dilemma of right ventricular dysfunction. Int J Cardiol 5:7–9
34. Deswarte G, Kirsch M, Lesault P-F, Trochu J-N, Damy T (2010) Right ventricular reserve and outcome after continuous-flow left ventricular assist device implantation. J Heart Lung Transplant 29:1196–1198
35. Morine KJ, Kiernan MS, Pham DT, Paruchuri V, Denofrio D, Kapur NK (2016) The Pulmonary Artery pulsatility index is associated with right ventricular failure following left ventricular assist device surgery. J Cardiac Fail 22:110–116
36. Oliveira GH, Dupont M, Naftel D et al (2014) Increased need for right ventricular support in patients with chemotherapy-induced cardiomyopathy undergoing mechanical circulatory support: outcomes from the INTERMACS Registry (Interagency Registry for Mechanically Assisted Circulatory Support). J Am Coll Cardiol 63:240–248
37. Melenovsky V, Kotrc M, Borlaug B et al (2013) Relationships between right ventricular function, body composition, and prognosis in advanced heart failure. J Am Coll Cardiol 62:1660–1670
38. Horwich TB, Kalantar-Zadeh K, MacLellan RW, Fonarow GC (2008) Albumin levels predict survival in patients with systolic heart failure. Am Heart J 155:883–889
39. Takeda K, Takayama H, Colombo PC, Jorde UP, Yuzefpolskaya M, Fukuhara S et al (2015) Late right heart failure during support with continuous-flow left ventricular assist devices adversely affects post-transplant outcome. J Heart Lung Transplant 34:667–674
40. Yancy CW, Jessup M, Bozkurt M et al (2013) The ACC/AHA HF 2013 ACCF/AHA guideline for the management of heart failure. A report of the American College of Cardiology Foundation/American Heart Association Task Force on Practice Guidelines. Circulation 128:e240–e327
41. Gheorghiade M, Vaduganathan M, Ambrosy A et al (2013) Current management and future directions for the treatment of patients hospitalized for heart failure with low blood pressure. Heart Fail Rev 18:107–122
42. Sponga S, Ivanitskaia E, Potapov E, Krabatsch T, Hetzer R, Lehmkuhl H (2012) Preoperative treatment with levosimendan in candidates for mechanical circulatory support. ASAIO J 58:6–11
43. Schaffer JM, Allen JG, Weiss ES et al (2011) Infectious complications after pulsatile-flow and continuous-flow left ventricular assist device implantation. J Heart Lung Transplant 30:164–174
44. Zierer A, Melby SJ, Voeller RK et al (2007) Late-onset driveline infections: the Achilles' heel of prolonged left ventricular assist device support. Ann Thorac Surg 84:515–520
45. Acharya MN, Som R, Tsui S (2012) What is the optimum antibiotic prophylaxis in patients undergoing implantation of a left ventricular assist device? Interact Cardiovasc Thorac Surg 14:209–214
46. Eckman PM, John R (2012) Bleeding and thrombosis in patient with continuous-flow ventricular assist devices. Circulation 125:3038–3047
47. Najjar SS, Slaughter MS, Pagani FD et al (2014) An analysis of pump thrombus events in patient in the HeartWare ADVANCE bridge to transplant and continuous access protocol trial. J Heart Lung Transplant 33:23–34
48. Tsirious A, Paone G, Nemeh HW et al (2014) Factors determining post-operative readmissions after left ventricular assist device implantation. J Heart Lung Transplant 33:1041–1047
49. Kirklin JK, Naftel DC, Kormos RL et al (2014) Third INTERMACS Annual Report: the evolution of

destination therapy in the United States. J Heart Lung Transplant 30:115–123
50. Aggarwall A, Pant R, Kumar S et al (2012) Incidence and management of gastrointestinal bleeding with continuous flow assist device. Ann Thorac Surg 93:1534–1540
51. Boyle AJ, Jorde UP, Sun B et al (2014) Pre-operative risk factors of bleeding and stroke during left ventricular assist device support: an analysis of more than 900 HeartMate II outpatients. J Am Coll Cardiol 63:880–888
52. Gerdes AM, Iervasi G (2010) Thyroid replacement therapy and heart failure. Circulation 122:385–393
53. Kowalczuk-Wieteska A, Baranska-Kosakowska A, Zakliczynski M, Lindon S, Zembala M (2011) Do thyroid disorders affect the postoperative course of patients in the early post-heart transplant period? Ann Transplant 16:77–81
54. Oskui PM, French WJ, Herring MJ, Mayeda GS, Burstein S, Kloner RA (2013) Testosterone and the cardiovascular system: a comprehensive review of the clinical literature. J Am Heart Assoc 2:e000272
55. Toma M, McAlister FA, Coglianese EE et al (2012) Testosterone supplementation in heart failure a meta-analysis. Circ Heart Fail 5:315–321
56. Vrtovec B, Radovancevic R, Delgado RM, Radovancevic B, Bracey AW, Gregoric ID et al (2009) Significance of anaemia in patients with advanced heart failure receiving long-term mechanical circulatory support. Eur J Heart Fail 11:1000–1004
57. Anker SD, Comin Colet J, Filippatos G, Willenheimer R, Dickstein K, Drexler H et al (2009) Ferric carboxymaltose in patients with heart failure and iron deficiency. N Engl J Med 361:2436–2448
58. Ponikowski P, van Veldhuisen DJ, Comin-Colet J et al (2015) Beneficial effects of long-term intravenous iron therapy with ferric carboxymaltose in patients with symptomatic heart failure and iron deficiency. Eur Heart J 36:657–668
59. Swedberg K, Young JB, Anand IS et al (2013) Treatment of anemia with darbepoetin alfa in systolic heart failure. N Engl J Med 368:1210–1219
60. Nassif ME, Patel JS, Shuster JE et al (2015) Clinical outcomes with use of erythropoiesis stimulating agents in patients with the HeartMate II left ventricular assist device. JACC Heart Fail 3:146–153
61. Gotsman I, Shauer A, Zwas DR et al (2012) Vitamin D deficiency is a predictor of reduced survival in patients with heart failure; vitamin D supplementation improves outcome. Eur J Heart Fail 14:357–366
62. Zittermann A, Morshuis M, Kuhn J, Pilz S, Ernst JB, Oezpeker C et al (2015) Vitamin D metabolites and fibroblast growth factor-23 in patients with left ventricular assist device implants: association with stroke and mortality risk. Eur J Nutr 55:305–313
63. Doehner W, Frenneaux M, Anker SD (2014) Metabolic impairment in heart failure: the myocardial and systemic perspective. J Am Coll Cardiol 64: 1388–1400
64. Holdy K, Dembitsky W, Eaton LL, Chillcott S, Stahovich M, Rasmusson B et al (2005) Nutrition assessment and management of left ventricular assist device patients. J Heart Lung Transplant 24:1690–1696
65. Musci M, Loforte A, Potapov EV et al (2008) Body mass index and outcome after ventricular assist device placement. Ann Thorac Surg 86:1236–1242
66. Birks E, Feldman D, Hryniewicz K et al (2013) The 2013 International Society of Heart and Lung Transplantation guidelines for mechanical circulatory support. Task Force 2: patient optimization, consent, and appropriate timing for mechanical circulatory support: modifiable risk management prior to implantation. J Heart Lung Transplant 32:157–187
67. Modica M, Ferratini M, Torri A et al (2015) Quality of life and emotional distress early after left ventricular assist device implant: a mixed-method study. Artif Organs 39:220–227

Preoperative Evaluation of Right Ventricular Function

Michael Dandel, Evgenij V. Potapov, and Nader Moazami

© Springer International Publishing Switzerland 2017
A. Montalto et al. (eds.), *Mechanical Circulatory Support in End-Stage Heart Failure*,
DOI 10.1007/978-3-319-43383-7_6

6.1 Introduction

Left ventricular assist devices (LVADs) are safer and provide better quality of life than biventricular assist devices (BVADs), but end-stage heart failure (HF) often involves both ventricles, even if left-sided heart disease was its initial cause. Although LVADs can facilitate RV improvement, severe right ventricular failure (RVF) can persist after LVAD implantation inducing high risks for death even if LVAD implantation is later followed by additional RV assist device (RVAD) implantation. The incidence of RVF requiring a RVAD after LVAD implantation is ~10% [1, 2]. Thus, it is crucial to identify preoperatively or at latest intraoperatively those patients who definitely need a BVAD. The decision between LVAD and BVAD is challenging and involves many clinical, hemodynamic, biochemical, and echocardiographic criteria [3]. Preoperative evaluation of RV function is a cornerstone for that decision making.

This chapter provides an overview of the main tools for preoperative RV evaluation aiming to avoid both unnecessary BVAD implantations and post-LVAD irreversible RVF. Special attention is focused on assessment of RV size, geometry, and function in relation to loading conditions, aiming to predict preoperatively the potential RV changes inducible by LVAD-promoted reduction of RV afterload.

6.2 RV Dysfunction in Patients Who Necessitate MCS

Etiopathogenetically, RVF which may necessitate MCS can be divided into:

1. Primary (intrinsic) RVF due to myocardial alterations affecting either the RV alone (RV infarction, arrhythmogenic cardiomyopathy) or both ventricles (ischemia/infarction, genetic/acquired cardiomyopathies)
2. Secondary (hemodynamic) RVF due to increased afterload (pulmonary hypertension) induced by high postcapillary and/or precapillary pulmonary vascular resistance (PVR)

Patients who need an RVAD in addition to an LVAD are those with severe irreversible RV remodeling and functional alterations, either due to excessive chronic pressure overload induced by primary impaired LV function or those with primary biventricular failure induced by global myocardial damage (infarction, cardiomyopathies). In most cases, temporary RVADs have been used with the goal of eventual removal as the initial hemodynamic load improves. In case of irreversible RVF, the use of current LVADs for chronic RVAD use has been reported, but this is not widely practiced.

6.2.1 Particularities of RV Failure Induced by a Failing Left Ventricle

Although congestive heart failure (CHF) usually emerges from a failing LV, secondary RV myocardial alterations also contribute to the CHF syndrome. Association of severe LV and RV failure is usually found in end-stage CHF and the most common cause of right-sided HF is left-sided HF [3, 4].

During LV failure progression, with ongoing cardiac output (CO) reduction, the imbalanced neurohumoral changes responsible for generalized arterial vasoconstriction and increase in venous tone also increase the renal sodium and water retention responsible for circulatory overload (intravascular congestion). Increased water retention with subsequent edema formation, hepatomegaly, and ascites may become misleading for evaluation of RV function because it can occur also with pure left-sided HF, without any hemodynamic evidence of right-sided HF [4]. However, since both ventricles are in a circuit, their stroke volume (SV) must be equal. Thus, any LV-SV reduction necessitates a corresponding RV-SV reduction to prevent fatal pulmonary edema. Initially, before any alteration in RV myocardial contractility, the high pulmonary venous pressure and contraction of small pulmonary arteries induced by LV-SV reduction will increase the PVR, which reduces the highly afterload-dependent RV pump function and consequently also the RV-SV. Early RV exhaustion by the excessive high afterload is prevented by RV myocardial hypertrophy followed by additional dilation (adaptive remodeling). LV failure also increases the RV preload by excessive renal fluid retention which increases the venous return. The high preload and afterload accentuate RV dilation

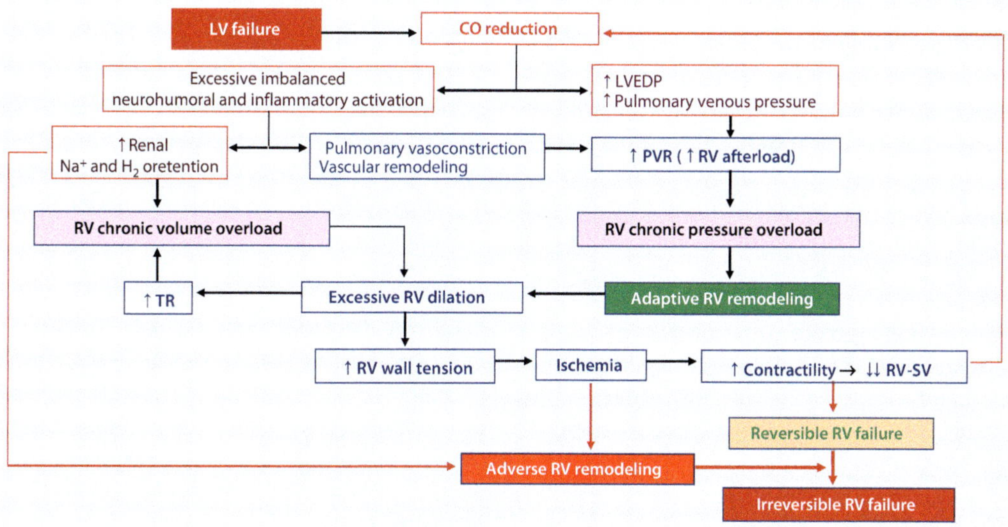

Fig. 6.1 Pathophysiology of chronic pressure overload-induced right ventricular (RV) dysfunction and irreversible failure in patients with congestive heart failure due to primary impaired left ventricular (LV) function. *CO* cardiac output, *LVEDP* left ventricular end-diastolic pressure, *PVR* pulmonary vascular resistance, *RV-SV* right ventricular stroke volume, *TR* tricuspid regurgitation

with progressive increase of tricuspid valve regurgitation (TR). By increasing the RV wall tension, both pulmonary hypertension (PH) and RV dilation will also progressively impair RV coronary blood flow and induce myocardial ischemia which finally reduces RV myocardial contractility. Optimally timed LVAD implantation can reverse all those alterations in RV size, geometry, and function. However, delay of LVAD implantation reduces the ability of the RV to improve after LVAD implantation because chronic excessive afterload and preload with massive RV myocyte stretch and hypertrophy can induce myocyte death (especially by apoptosis) and irreversible pathologic RV remodeling with increased wall stiffness and reduced pump function [5]. Severe irreversible RV remodeling can be sufficient for persistence and also progression of RVF independent of the neurohumoral status of the patient, and in such cases, there will be a high probability for persistence of right-sided HF even after LVAD implantation [3–5]. Impaired LV function before and after LVAD implantation also affects RV geometry and function via the shared septum and other features of ventricular interdependence and may also affect RV recovery after LVAD implantation. An overview on the pathophysiology of chronic pressure overload-induced RV changes in patients with congestive heart failure due to primary impaired LV function is shown in Fig. 6.1.

6.2.2 Particularities of Primary RV and LV Failure: True Biventricular Failure

There are relevant pathophysiologic and hemodynamic differences between CHF due to primary impaired LV function and global HF due to heart muscle diseases with impaired biventricular systolic and/or diastolic function. In patients with biventricular dysfunction due to genetic or acquired myocardial alterations, the impaired LV function is usually associated with less increase in left-sided heart filling pressures (consequently also less LV and LA dilation) and induces less pulmonary intravascular congestion because of the low SV ejected by the failing RV and also because the intravascular congestion due to increased renal sodium and water retention secondary to CO reduction involves mainly the systemic circulation. Their PVR is also lower than in patients with CHF due to primary impaired LV function, and their pulmonary artery pressure

(PAP) can be normal or is only moderately elevated. Clinically this may suggest a predominantly right-sided heart failure and can lead to false therapeutic decisions. In certain patients with primary biventricular failure due to severe myocardial systolic and diastolic dysfunction, the absence of relevant RV dilation due to increased myocardial stiffness, which also impedes a massive reduction of RVEF despite of the low SV of the failing RV, may suggest a predominantly LV failure. Because such a primarily damaged RV will not improve during LV support, LVAD implantation alone is useless and highly risky, especially in patients with normal PVR and low velocity of tricuspid regurgitation jets.

6.2.3 Reversibility of RV Failure by RV Afterload Reduction

Acting more as a volume pump, the RV tolerates less pressure than volume overload and has higher sensitivity to afterload changes than the LV. The distinctly load sensitivity of RV size, geometry, and performance explains its ability for reverse remodeling and functional improvement after normalization of loading conditions [6]. LVAD implantation often induces acute PVR reduction accompanied by acute changes in RV geometry with TR reduction and improvement of RV pump function [7]. In certain patients, starting of LV mechanical unloading induces acute RV dilation suggesting that the failing RV may not be able to handle the acute extra volume load induced by the LVAD-promoted increase of the CO. However, such LVAD-promoted RV volume overloading is limited because after removal of the excessive blood volume from the pulmonary vessels, the output of the LVAD into the systemic circulation will decrease correspondingly to the decrease of failing RV output. Long-term LVAD support usually further reduces the PVR facilitating RV reverse remodeling and functional recovery [3]. However, LVAD support in patients with CHF is rarely followed by complete RV recovery, and severe postoperative RVF associated with high patient mortality is more frequent than persistence of RVF after PVR reduction by lung transplantation for precapillary PH or by pulmonary endarterectomy in patients with chronic thromboembolic PH [3]. The less predictable RV improvement in CHF patients receiving an LVAD is mainly related to differences in the etiology of myocardial injury which induced the CHF, differences in duration of RVF before VAD implantation, and differences in the direct impact of the initial myocardial injury on RV myocardium and also to the impact of ventricular interdependence changes induced by LV unloading on RV geometry and function.

6.3 Main Tools for Assessment of Right Ventricular Function

Echocardiography, right heart catheterization (RHC), and cardiac magnetic resonance imaging (MRI) are the standard clinical methods for preoperative evaluation of RV function.

6.3.1 Echocardiography

Challenges and Limits in RV Echo-Assessment

There are particular challenges and limits in RV echo-assessment. RV volume and ejection fraction (EF) measurements are less reliable, and therefore, 2D echo-derived RV volume and EF calculations are not anymore recommended by the American Society of Echocardiography (ASE) for clinical use [8]. 3D echo is more useful for estimation of RV volumes and EF, but it is technically challenging and not widely available. However, the more reliable RVEF calculation by 3D echo does not change the fact that due to its afterload dependency, RVEF cannot be used as an index of myocardial contractility [8]. Nevertheless, 2D echo is still preferentially used for assessment of RV function because it allows easy measurements of RV fractional area change (FAC_{RV}) and tricuspid annulus peak systolic excursion (TAPSE), which can provide similar information to RVEF [9]. However, FAC_{RV} measurements showed high interobserver and intra-observer variability, whereas TAPSE measurements are angle dependent and influenced by both LV function and overall heart motion [9]. Recently only a poor correlation between magnetic resonance imaging (MRI)-derived RVEF and TAPSE ($r = 0.45$) [10] was also found. It must be also emphasized that, because of their load dependency, RVEF, FAC_{RV}, and TAPSE can change without changes in myocardial contractility. Thus, they will decrease with increasing PVR even if myocardial contractility remains unaltered. Additionally, TR can induce RVEF, FAC_{RV}, and TAPSE changes which can be misleading for assessment of RV contractile function and estimation of RV myocardial contractility.

Also Doppler-derived indices of RV function, such as the myocardial performance index (MPI) and the TR-derived rate of RV pressure rise (dp/dt), which are unaffected by RV geometry, are increasingly used for RV echo-assessment. The clinical value of RV dp/dt ratio is limited by the angle and load dependency of measurements [8–10]. RV dp/dt measurements are also less accurate in severe TR [6]. Afterload dependence and unreliability of measurements in patients with elevated RA (including severe TR) limit the diagnostic value of MPI, and the ASE does not recommend MPI as the sole quantitative method for evaluation of RV function [8]. The time interval between onset and cessation of TR flow corrected for heart rate (TRDc), a surrogate for early systolic equalization of RV and RA pressure, appeared also useful for evaluation of RV function. A decreased TRDc in CHF patients before LVAD implantation was identified as a risk factor for postoperative RVF [11].

RV wall motion assessment by TDI-derived velocity measurements is also useful because velocity appeared less load dependent than displacement. A major limitation of TDI is the angle dependency of measurements. Nevertheless, especially the tricuspid lateral annulus peak systolic wall motion velocity (TAPS'), which correlates with TAPSE but is less load dependent, the RV isovolumic contraction peak velocity (IVC_V) and the RV isovolumic acceleration (IVA) appeared suited for evaluation of RV contractile function [12].

Strain imaging is also useful for RV evaluation because myocardial strain (deformation) is not affected by the movement of the entire heart, and deformation analysis (strain and strain rate imaging) allows discrimination between active and passive myocardial tissue movement. Angle-independent speckle-tracking-derived strain imaging parameters like the RV longitudinal peak systolic strain (PSSL) and strain rate (PSSrL) appeared particularly useful for assessment of RV contractile function [13]. Main limitations of speckle-tracking strain imaging are dependency on image quality plus relatively low temporal resolution and segmental reproducibility of measurements (especially for 3D speckle tracking), as well as the influence of RV loading conditions especially on myocardial strain values [13].

Pressure overload-induced RVF in CHF due to primary impaired LV function is finally the result of both systolic and diastolic RV dysfunctions. However, only RV systolic dysfunction was identified as a predictor of mortality in CHF [8]. Echo assessment of RV diastolic function is also challenging because it cannot be described by a single parameter, and the influence of respiration, heart rate, and preload changes on trans-tricuspid velocities can induce misleading diastolic parameter changes [8].

RV Echo Evaluation in Relation with Its Loading Conditions

Distinctly load dependency of RV size, geometry, and function indicates the necessity for RV evaluation in relation with its loading conditions, especially in patients with CHF due to primary impaired LV function where RVF is induced by pathological loading conditions, which are potentially reversible during LVAD support. The usefulness of integrative approaches for RV evaluation, using combinations of parameters which include RV afterload, was increasingly investigated during the last years [3–14]. Very promising appeared to be the RV stroke work index (SWI_{RV}) because its calculation from RHC-derived data (i.e., $SWI_{RV} = \{ [\text{mean PAP} - \text{mean RAP}] \cdot SV \}/\text{body surface area}$) appeared more useful than any echo variable used individually for evaluation of RV function in end-stage CHF [15]. However, because echo-estimations of right atrial (RA) and mean PAP are less reliable than their direct measurements during RHC, the poor correlation between echo-derived and RHC-derived SWI_{RV} calculations is not surprising and therefore echo-derived SWI_{RV} is rarely used for assessment of RV function. However, recently, two simplified composite echo-derived variables which incorporate either TAPSE and load or SV and load were identified as more easy calculable surrogates for the SWI_{RV} [16]. One of them is the "simplified RV contraction-pressure index" (sRVCPI), which incorporates TAPSE and load, and is derived as $sRVCPI = TAPSE \cdot \Delta P_{RV-RA}$, where ΔP_{RV-RA} is the pressure gradient between RV and RA [17]. sRVCPI showed a close correlation with RHC-derived SWI_{RV} ($r = 0.68$; $p < 0.001$) [15]. The other is the "RV stroke work" (RVSW), which incorporates SV and load RVSW = (pulmonary valve-area · VTI_{PV}) · (4 · peak TR velocity) [2], where VTI_{PV} is the velocity-time integral of the systolic trans-pulmonary jet, which also showed a close correlation with the RHC-derived SWI_{RV} ($r = 0.74$; $p < 0.0001$) [16].

Also recently, composite echo variables which incorporate either longitudinal displacement and load (i.e., TAPSE/systolic PAP and TAPSE/PVR) or velocity of myocardial shortening and load (i.e., afterload-corrected peak systolic longitudinal strain rate) were also found suited for assessment of RV contractile function [14, 18, 19]. The TAPSE/systolic PAP ratio is a simplified approach to assess RV contraction by plotting fiber longitudinal shortening versus the force generated for overcoming the imposed load [18]. This allows estimations of RV performance status which in turn might facilitate the decision-making process and prognosis assessments in clinical praxis. The limitations of this index are related to the well-known limitations of TAPSE and systolic PAP echo measurements. Nevertheless, in a larger study, this index appeared as a strong and independent predictor of mortality in patients with HF due to primary impaired LV function [11]. Because PVR is a critical determinant of RV systolic function, its inclusion into echo-derived composite variables can also be beneficial for RV assessment. Echo-derived RV ejection efficiency (RVEe), defined as RVEe = TAPSE/PVR, is such a composite variable which reflects that relationship in a simplified manner [19]. However, there is controversy on the reliability of echo-derived PVR estimations in patients with PVR >6 Wood units [8–19]. Future studies are necessary to determine if echo-derived RVEe is indeed able to predict patient outcome.

The afterload-corrected peak systolic longitudinal strain rate, a reproducibly and easy obtainable combined variable for assessment of RV adaptability to load, defined as PSSrL · $\Delta P_{RV\text{-}RA}$, where PSSrL is the peak global systolic longitudinal strain rate and $\Delta P_{RV\text{-}RA}$ the pressure gradient between RV and RA, is based on the relationship between RV myocardial shortening velocity and RV load [16]. Because myocardial shortening velocity is load dependent, RV systolic pressure increase reduces the PSSrL. Nevertheless, as long as RV contractile function remains unchanged, due to the $\Delta P_{RV\text{-}RA}$ increase, the RV load-corrected PSSrL will remain relatively stable. However, if RV afterload increase overwhelms RV ability to adapt its contractile function correspondingly, in addition to PSSrL reduction, there will be also a $\Delta P_{RV\text{-}RA}$ reduction due to the increase of RA pressure, even before the RV systolic pressure finally also becomes lower due to progressive impairment of RV contractility. The load-corrected PSSrL will be therefore more useful for the evaluation of RV adaptability to loading conditions than the PSSrL alone.

A distinctly different approach for assessment of RV contractile function is provided by the recently introduced "RV load-adaptation index" (LAI_{RV}). The LAI_{RV}, a composite echo-derived variable based on the relationship between RV load and RV dilation, also taking the RA pressure into account, is reflected by the ratio between the systolic mean pressure gradient between the RV and RA ($\Delta P_{RV\text{-}RA}$) and RV end-diastolic volume per long-axis length (EDV/L_{ED}):

$$\begin{aligned} LAI_{RV} &= \frac{\Delta P_{RV-RA}}{EDV / L_{ED}} \approx \frac{VTI_{TR}}{A_{ED} / L_{ED}} \\ &= \frac{VTI_{TR}\left(cm\right) \cdot L_{ED}\left(cm\right)}{A_{ED}\left(cm^2\right)} \end{aligned}$$

Thus, using the TR velocity-time integral (VTI_{TR}) instead of $\Delta P_{RV\text{-}RA}$ and the easily measurable RV end-diastolic area (A_{ED}) instead of the RV end-diastolic volume (EDV), a dimensionless index of similar value for RV evaluation can be obtained (■ Fig. 6.1) [3, 6, 14]. Because $\Delta P_{RV\text{-}RA}$ is calculated from the mean velocity of the TR jet, the use of VTI_{TR} instead of $\Delta P_{RV\text{-}RA}$ is unrestricted possible and has the advantage to include also the duration of systolic loading. The use of A_{ED} instead of EDV is justified by the good correlation between the echo-derived RV-A_{ED} and the MRI-derived RV-EDV [20]. Thus, a small RV area relative to long-axis length (size and geometry unaltered) in a patient with high VTI_{TR} (i.e., high RV systolic pressure and relatively low RA pressure) yields a high LAI_{RV} which indicates good adaptation to load (RV ability to increase systolic pressure without relevant RV dilation and without RA pressure increases suggesting good RV contractile function) and the potential of RV to improve its performance after reduction of loading conditions. A large area relative to long-axis length (spherical dilation) despite a relatively

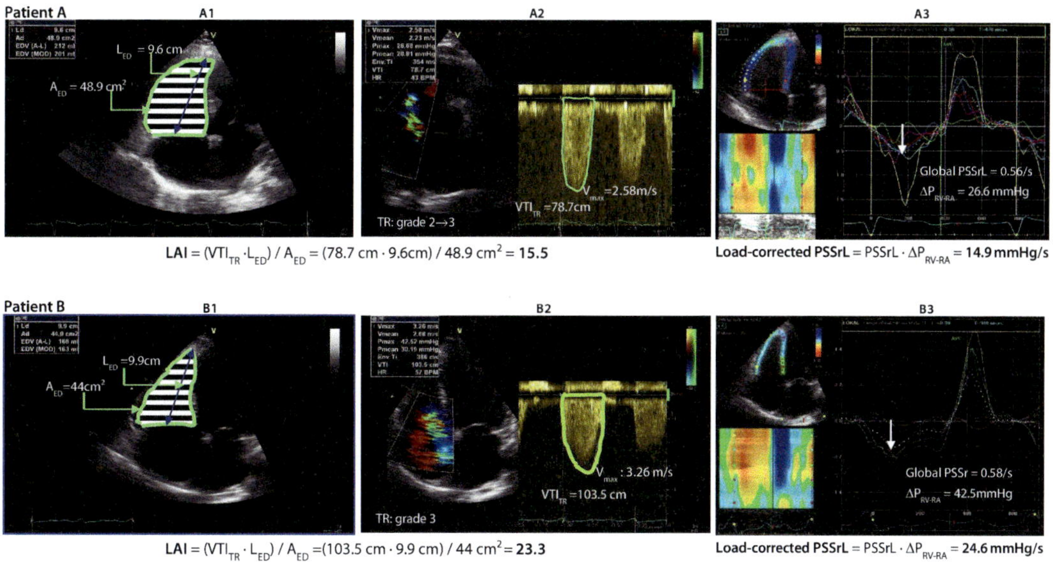

Fig. 6.2 Right ventricular (RV) load adaptation index (LAI) and load-corrected global peak systolic longitudinal strain rate (PSSrL) in two patients with end-stage congestive heart failure due to primary impaired left ventricular function. In patient A, the more dilated RV (A1) with a lower pressure gradient between RV and right atrium (A2) and a lower velocity of RV myocardial shortening (A3) yield a 33.5% and 39.4% lower LAI and load-corrected PSSrL, respectively, in comparison with patient B (B1, B2, B3). The low LAI and load-corrected PSSrL in patient A indicate a high risk for RV failure after LVAD implantation (need for temporary or even permanent mechanical support also for the RV). The relatively high LAI in patient B indicates RV ability to improve during LVAD support. *TR* tricuspid regurgitation, VTI_{TR} TR velocity-time integral, V_{max} maximum (peak) velocity, $\Delta P_{RV\text{-}RA}$ pressure gradient between RV and right atrium

low VTI_{TR} yields a low LAI_{RV} indicating poor adaptation to load (excessive RV dilation despite low RV pressure-load indicating impaired RV systolic function) suggesting a reduced myocardial contractility. LAI_{RV} values <15 indicate low RV adaptability to load which is insufficient to prevent RVF even at normal PVR [3–6]. Thus, RV evaluation in relation to its actual loading conditions can be helpful in proper decision making especially before VAD implantation (Fig. 6.2).

Recently, also 3D echo data were used for assessment of the relationship between RV remodeling and afterload. Regression analysis between 3D echo-derived RV end-systolic volume-index and systolic PAP appeared able to distinguish between adapted, adapted-remodeled, and adverse-remodeled RV [21].

6.3.2 Right Heart Catheterization

RHC which provides valuable direct hemodynamic data, also allowing calculations of PVR and certain composite variables which allow RV assessment in relation to loading conditions, is another cornerstone for RV evaluation.

Invasive measurements of certain hemodynamic variables like CVP (central venous pressure), PCWP (pulmonary capillary wedge pressure), PAP, and CI (cardiac index) are essential for preoperative RV evaluation because high CVP and CVP/PCWP ratio and low CI and mean PAP decrease were often identified as risk factors for RVF after LVAD implantation [3, 6, 22]. However, CVP, PAP, PCWP, and CI measured before LVAD implantation were not found in all studies significantly different in patients with and without postoperative RVF, and alone none of them appeared able to predict RVF or freedom from RVF after LVAD implantation [3]. For certain hemodynamic variables like CI and PCWP, this might be in part also due to the lower accuracy of measurements. Particularly concerning for RVF after LVAD implantation is high CVP in the setting of low PAP [3–6]. The ratio of RA pressure and PCWP can help to differentiate patients with relevant intrinsic RV dysfunction from those with a congested right-sided heart (without altered RV contractility) due to elevated left-sided filling pressures. A high CVP/PCWP ratio (>0.63) reflects inherent RV dysfunction, whereas a low CVP/PCWP ratio reflects right-sided congestion as a result of high left-sided filling pressures.

Among the RHC-derived composite variables for RV evaluation, the SWI_{RV}, which allows RV assessment in relation to its afterload, can be particularly suited for preoperative decision making between LVAD and BVAD implantation because SWI_{RV} appeared more reliable than any echo variable used individually for evaluation of RV function in end-stage CHF [15]. SWI_{RV} values <300 mmHg/mL/m^2 usually reflect significant RV dysfunction, and patients with the need for RVAD support after LVAD implantation showed preoperatively significantly lower SWI_{RV} values than those without post-LVAD RVF [22]. A weakness of the SWI_{RV} is its less precise calculation in patients with higher degree of TR or in those with low CI because of the less reliable CO measurements by the thermodilution method in such patients.

Composite variables derived from both RHC and echo measurements can also be useful for RV evaluation before VAD implantation. Thus, composite variables which incorporate longitudinal displacement and load like TAPSE/systolic PAP and TAPSE/PVR or velocity of myocardial shortening and load (afterload-corrected PSSrL) already appeared suited for assessment of RV contractile function even if their calculation was exclusively based on echo measurements, although echo-derived estimation of PAP and especially that of PVR is not very accurate [14, 18, 19]. However, those composite variables might become more reliable by a combined use of echo-derived TAPSE or PSSrL measurements and RHC-derived PAP measurements or PVR calculations, respectively.

Analysis of RV function by pressure-volume loops, possible with conductance catheters, allows quantification of various parameters like $\Delta P/\Delta t$, stroke work, elasticity, and compliance which can be helpful for preoperative decision making before VAD implantation. However, RV conductance measurements by pressure-volume loops are more challenging than LV conductance measurements (difficulties in obtaining reliable ventricular volumes), and to date the clinical usefulness of these measurements for preoperative prediction of RV function after LVAD implantation is not established.

6.3.3 Cardiac Computed Tomography and Magnetic Resonance Imaging

Both cardiac computed tomography (CCT) and MRI allow reliable and reproducible assessment of RV size, geometry, SV, and EF without geometric assumptions about the RV. Multi-slice spiral CCT and MRI measurements of RV volumes, mass, SV, and EF also show high correlations ($r \geq 0.91$) [23]. Major limitations like nephrotoxicity, ionizing radiation, low temporal resolution, and especially the difficulties in the examination of patients with inotropic-dependent end-stage CHF make CCT less useful than echocardiography for preoperative RV evaluation in VAD candidates. However, after LVAD implantation, when RV assessment by transthoracic echocardiography becomes more difficult, especially due to device-related artifacts, CCT can be considered as a useful imaging modality for RV evaluation.

Although MRI is increasingly used for RV evaluation because it is particularly suited for assessing RV volume and for calculation of SV, RVEF, and tricuspid valve regurgitant volumes and, in combination with RHC-derived hemodynamic data, also able to assess independently RV function, remodeling, afterload, and contractile properties, there are yet no published data on its usefulness and safety for preoperative RV evaluation in MCS candidates. The main limitation for the use of MRI to evaluate RV function before final decision making between LVAD and BVAD implantation is the restriction of MRI use only to hemodynamic stable patients without implanted defibrillators and/or devices for biventricular pacing. In addition, MRI cannot be used postoperatively for RV assessment because the method is contraindicated in the presence of an LVAD.

6.4 Prediction of RV Improvement and Anticipation of RV Failure After LVAD Implantation

Like LV performance, RV performance is a reflection of contractility, preload, and afterload, also being influenced by valvular function, heart rhythm, synchrony of ventricular contraction, and ventricular interdependence. Nevertheless, in comparison with the LV, size, geometry, and performance of the RV are definitely more sensitive to changes in loading conditions, especially to afterload changes. This explains RV ability to improve during its afterload reduction inducible by mechanical LV support.

However, RV reverse remodeling with TR reduction and improvement of myocardial function after LVAD implantation depend not only on the reversibility of myocardial alterations by reduction of RV loading conditions but also on the reversibility of pathologic circulatory and metabolic changes induced by both imbalanced neurohumoral and inflammatory reactions to the low CO- and CHF-related end-organ failure (especially the kidney and liver). Additionally, changes of interventricular interactions induced by sudden LV unloading and potential intraoperative and early postoperative complications can impair the initial ability of the RV to improve after LVAD implantation. Prediction of RV improvement during LVAD support is therefore a highly complex and challenging issue.

6.4.1 Risk Factors for Postoperative RV Failure

RVF with and without the necessity of additional RVAD support complicates 10–40% of LVAD implants. Patients with different post-LVAD course of RV function show already preoperatively significant differences in certain laboratory data reflecting relevant pathophysiological consequences of severe CHF (especially hepatic and renal dysfunction), echo variables (especially those for RV assessment), and invasively obtained hemodynamic parameters [7, 11, 22–24]. RV end-diastolic S/L axis ratio > 0.57, TR > 2nd degree, FAC_{RV} < 31%, $\Delta P_{RV\text{-}RA}$ < 35 mmHg, RV/LV diameter ratio ≥ 0.75, TAPS' < 8 cm/s, PSSL < −9.6%, PSSrL<0.6/s, LA volume index <38 mL/m^2, CVP >15 mmHg, elevated serum bilirubin, creatinine and lactic dehydrogenase (LDH) levels, plus elevated markers of inflammation were identified by univariate analysis as the most relevant risk factors [6, 11, 19, 22, 25–34]. TR ≥ moderate to severe, CVP/PCWP ratio >0.63, CVP > 15 mmHg, RV/LV diameter ratio ≥ 0.75, blood urea nitrogen >39 mg/dL, and ventilatory support were revealed as risk factors for postoperative RVF also by multivariate analysis (◘ Tables 6.1 and 6.2) [6, 11, 22, 24, 27, 31, 34]. However, these variables were not identified in all studies as significant risk factors for RVF. This might be mainly due to the differences between centers with regard to defining RVF and their selection criteria for VAD support. With only few exceptions, the numerous risk factors for RVF after LVAD implantation appeared alone unable to predict reliably RVF or freedom from RVF.

◘ Table 6.1 Univariate logistic regression data on the relevance of selected generally accepted preoperative risk factors for RV failure after LVAD implantation

Selected risk factors for RHF	Odds RVF	95% CI	P value
High serum creatinine [22, 29]	1.68	1.30–2.18	< 0.01
	1.42	0.66–3.10	0.36
High blood urea nitrogen [11, 22]	1.03	1.01–1.04	< 0.01
	1.0	0.98–1.04	0.3
Renal replacement therapy [22]	9.93	2.72–36.24	< 0.01
Bilirubin (total) increase [11, 22]	1.68	1.29–2.29	< 0.01
	1.1	0.6–2.2	0.7
Aspartate aminotransferase (AST) increase [22, 29]	1.00	1.000–1.003	< 0.01
	1.00	1.00–1.01	0.57

(continued)

Table 6.1 (continued)

Selected risk factors for RHF	Odds RVF	95% CI	P value
AST ≥ 80 IU/l [19]	3.20	1.64–6.25	< 0.01
High lactic acid dehydrogenase (LDH) [6, 22]	1.34	1.09–1.64	< 0.01
	1.001	0.999–1.002	< 0.01
High N-terminal prohormone brain natriuretic peptide (NT-proBNP) [6]	2.33	1.27–4.27	< 0.01
High BNP [30]	1.001	1.00–1.001	0.04
RV end-diastolic diameter (RVEDD) increase [6]	1.25	1.13–138	< 0.01
RV short-/long-axis ratio increase [25]	4.4	1.4–13.7	0.01
Reduced RV ejection fraction (RVEF) [6]	0.87	0.80–0.95	< 0.01
Severe RV dysfunction [22]	2.21	1.20–4.07	0.01
Reduced tricuspid annulus peak systolic excursion (TAPSE) [6, 29]	0.98	0.82–1.00	< 0.01
	0.26	0.06–1.05	0.06
Lateral RV peak longitudinal strain [29]	0.84	0.75–0.92	< 0.01
Left ventricle end-diastolic diameter (LVEDD) reduction [30]	0.91	0.84–0.98	0.02
LVEDD ≤ 62 mm [30]	12.6	1.38–115.4	0.02
Tricuspid regurgitation (TR) severity			
≥ Grade II [29]	1.04	0.69–1.56	0.84
> Grade II [6]	2.40	1.13–5.13	< 0.01
≥ Grade III [25]	4.7	1.26–17.6	0.01
Pulmonary capillary wedge pressure (PCWP) [6, 28]	0.61	0.50–0.76	< 0.01
	0.91	0.81–1.02	0.125
Pulmonary artery mean pressure (PAPm) decrease [6, 22]	0.66	0.58–0.76	< 0.01
	0.97	0.94–0.99	0.04
PAPm < 36 mmHg [27]	1.7	1.00–3.00	< 0.05
Central venous pressure (CVP) increase [6]	4.0	2.42–6.73	< 0.01
CVP > 15 mmHg [27]	2.1	1.20–3.60	< 0.01
CVP/PCWP > 0.63 [27]	2.5	1.37–4.60	< 0.05
Cardiac index (CI) decrease [6, 22]	0.90	0.67–0.97	< 0.01
	0.61	0.37–1.00	0.049
Preoperative ventilator support [22]	3.18	1.62–6.26	< 0.01
Preoperative need for intravenous vasopressor therapy [22]	4.80	2.02–11.41	< 0.01
Preoperative need for intravenous anti-arrhythmic therapy [22]	2.56	1.22–5.33	0.02

Table 6.2 Multivariate analyses data on the relevance of selected preoperative risk factors for RV failure after LVAD implantation

Selected risk factors for RHF	Odds ratio	95% CI	P value
Serum creatinine			
≥ 2.3 mg/dl [22]	2.9	1.1–7.7	<0.01
≥ 1.9 mg/dl [31]	4.8	1.9–12.0	<0.01
> 1.7 mg/dl [27]	1.6	0.9–2.9	>0.05
Blood urea nitrogen > 39 mg/dl [27]	2.1	1.1–4.1	0.02
Bilirubin (total) ≥ 2 mg/dl [22]	2.4	1.1–5.2	<0.01
Aspartate aminotransferase (AST) ≥ 80 IU/l [22]	2.1	0.96–4.5	<0.01
Lateral RV peak longitudinal strain (PSSL) < – 9% [29]	0.84	0.75–0.92	<0.01
Severe RV dysfunction [31, 34]	3.7	1.7–8.1	<0.01
	5.0	2.0–12.5	<0.01
Left ventricle end-diastolic diameter (LVEDD) ≤ 62 mm [30]	12.8	1.39–118.4	0.03
High RV/LV end-diastolic diameter ratio [30]	5.4	2.4–12.4	0.01
Reduced TR flow time corrected for heart rate (TRDc) [ms] [11]	0.82	0.69–0.93	<0.01
Pulmonary artery mean pressure (PAPm) < 36 mmHg [27]	1.7	1.0–3.0	<0.05
PAPm decrease [6]	0.5	0.41–0.62	<0.01
Cardiac index (CI) ≤ 2.2 l/min/m^2 [31]	5.7	1.3–24.4	0.02
Central venous pressure (CVP) increase [6]	6.2	3.13–8.35	<0.01
CVP > 15mmHg [34]	2.0	0.9–4.2	0.09
CVP/PCWP > 0.63 [27]	2.3	1.2–4.3	0.01
Severe tricuspid regurgitation (TR) [34]	4.1	1.4–12.4	0.01
Systemic blood pressure ≤ 96 mmHg [31]	2.9	1.2–6.9	0.02
Nonischemic etiology of heart failure [24]	3.3	1.3–8.4	0.01
Preoperative need for intravenous vasopressor therapy [22]	3.9	1.5–9.8	<0.01
Previous cardiac surgery [31]	4.5	1.7–11.8	<0.01
Preoperative circulatory support [24, 28]	5.3	2.0–14.0	<0.01
	3.9		<0.01
Preoperative ventilator support [27, 34]	5.5	2.3–13.2	<0.01
	4.3	1.9–9.6	<0.01

6.4.2 Prediction of RV Function After LVAD Implantation

RVF after LVAD implantation can be classified into three major types:

(a) RVF due to preoperatively underestimated irreversible RV alterations (often predictable)
(b) RVF which becomes manifest only intraoperatively or early postoperatively (less predictable)
(c) RVF which develops late after LVAD implant (preoperatively most difficult predictable)

Only few of the significant risk factors for post-LVAD RVF appeared alone sufficiently predictive for postoperative RV function. Even highly relevant risk factors like RA pressure and PA systolic pressure appeared alone unable to correctly classify patients with and without the potential to become and/or remain free from RVF after LVAD implantation (area under the curve [AUC]: 0.53 and 0.59, respectively) [22]. Among the investigated echo variables, only TAPS' and PSSrL (i.e., variables reflecting RV wall motion velocity and myocardial shortening velocity, respectively) plus S/L_{ED} revealed high predictive values for postoperative RV function (AUC≥ 0.87) [6].

For decision making between LVAD and BVAD implantation, it appeared more reliable to use both complex quantitative scoring systems which incorporate measures of different risk factors for post-LVAD RVF and composite variables which include RV geometry, function, and load [6, 26, 30]. The AUC values of 63% and 68% for the composite variables SWI_{RV} and CVP/PCWP, respectively, which incorporate invasively obtainable hemodynamic measures, indicate useful risk discrimination capacities of those variables for post-LVAD RVF [22–27]. Post-LVAD RVF occurred in only 10% and 11%, respectively, of patients with preoperative SWI_{RV} > 300 mmHg · mL/m^2 and CVP/PCWP < 0.63 [27]. Scoring systems using weighted scales that incorporate preoperative laboratory measurements, clinical data (intubation, vasopressor and/or inotrope requirement, previous cardiac surgery, etc.), and hemodynamic measurements showed higher risk discrimination capacities for postoperative RVF (AUC: 0.73–0.91) and are considered particularly useful for decision making before VAD implantation [26–34]. At certain cutoff values, different scoring systems revealed positive and negative predictive values for post-LVAD RVF between 71–83% and 69–80%, respectively (◘ Table 6.3). However, the majority of those scoring systems are based rather on variables which reflect the preoperative severity of HF-related multiorgan dysfunction than on measurements directly related to RV contractile performance including its potential reversibility. This might explain the different risk discrimination capacities for post-LVAD RVF found in different studies using the same scoring system not containing data on RV size, geometry, and function.

More recently, several echo-derived measurements also appeared able to predict post-LVAD RVF if they were used in combination, as part of an algorithm or scoring system or as composite variables [6, 25, 32, 33]. ◘ Figure 6.3 shows an algorithm for device selection, used since 2008 in the German Heart Institute Berlin, which uses RV echo data in combination with RHC-data (for PVR calculation) and is based on measurements of right-sided heart anatomy (RV and RA size, RV geometry) and function (RVEF, TR) in relation with RV afterload [25].

At certain cutoff values, different echo-derived composite variables and scoring systems revealed positive and negative predictive values for post-LVAD RVF of between 75–97% and 64–97%, respectively (◘ Table 6.1). To date, the highest predictive values (≥87%) for both RVF and freedom from RVF after LVAD implantation were found for the composite echo variables LAI_{RV} and RV load-corrected PSSrL which reflect RV adaptability to load [6]. However, it is difficult to compare the results of studies aiming to find the most useful predictors for freedom from RVF after LVAD implantation in patients with end-stage CHF because of relevant differences in the evaluated populations and investigated variables.

Certain post-LVAD RVF risk scores appeared also able to stratify the risk for death after LVAD implantation [22, 26, 28]. The highest ability to

Table 6.3 Overview of the risk discrimination capacity for RVF of combined variables which incorporate major risk factors for RVF after LVAD implantation

Variables [units]	Components of the combined variables	AUC (95% CI)	Cutoff values	Predictive value for RVF	
				Positive (%)	Negative (%)
SWI_{RV} [mmHg • ml/m²] [22, 27]	SV × (PAPm – CVP)/BSA	**0.63** (0.55–0.72)	450 300	42.6 72.2	75.8 54.9
CVP/PCWP [27, 30]	Central venous pressure/pulmonary capillary wedge pressure	**0.68** **0.82** (0.68–0.96)	0.63	64.5	53.3
Michigan RVFRS [points (p)] [22]	Vasopressor requirement; AST ≥80 IU/L; bilirubin ≥2 mg/dL; creatinine ≥2.3 mg/dL	**0.73** (0.65–0.81)	≤ 3 ≥ 5	70.9 80.0	79.6 73.7
Michigan RVFRS + RV/LV [points (p)] [2]	Michigan RVFRS components + RV/LV diameter ratio	**0.74**	–	–	–
Michigan RVFRS + $PSSL_{RV}$ [points (p)] [29]	Michigan RVFRS components + RV systolic peak longitudinal strain	**0.77**	–	–	–
RVF risk score for RVAD need [points (p)] [31]	CI ≤2.2 mg/dL; SWI_{RV} ≤0.25 mmHg • liter/m²; SBP ≤96 mmHg; creatinine ≥1.9 mg/dL; severe pre-VAD RV dysfunction; Previous cardiac surgery	–	< 30 ≥ 65 50[a]	45.3 89.5 –	96.2 71.5 –
RVF risk score [points (p)] [28]	Destination therapy; obesity; PVR; inotrope dependency; ACE inhibitor and/or AT II receptor blocker therapy; β-blocker	**0.74** ± 0.04	≤ 5 ≥ 12	56.0 83.3	88.9 69.3
Quantitative preoperative risk score (CRITT score) [points (p)] [34]	CVP; RV dysfunction; intubation; TR tachycardia	**0.80** (0.72–0.88)	≥ 2 ≥ 4	– 80.0	93.0 –
Total RVF score for BVAD need [points (p)] [30]	CVP/PCWP >0.5;BSA ≤1.4 m;BNP≤1200 pg/ml; LVEDD ≤62 mm; preoperative hemofiltration	**0.91** (0.80–1.00)	20[b]	–	–
Modified LV-echo-for-RVF score [points (p)] [33]	LVEDD; LVEF; LAD/LVEDD; SWI_{RV}; bilirubin (serum); albumin (serum)	**0.79**	≤ 3 ≥ 7	– 93.4	97.1 –
TTE score [points (p)] [32]	FAC_{RV}; RAP (estimated); LAV index;	**0.73**	≥ 5[c]	75	64
RV load-corrected PSSrL [6] PSSrL • $\Delta P_{RV\text{-}RA}$ [mmHg/s]	Peak systolic longitudinal strain rate Pressure gradient between RV and RA	**0.95** (0.93–1.00)	24	97 (84–99)	87 (77–93)

(continued)

Table 6.3 (continued)

Variables [units]	Components of the combined variables	AUC (95% CI)	Cutoff values	Predictive value for RVF	
				Positive (%)	Negative (%)
Load adaptation index (LAI) [4]	TR velocity time integral; RV end-diastolic area and long-axis length	**0.97** (0.97–0.99)	14	**83** (73–88)	**97** (95–99)

[a]At this threshold: 85% sensitivity and 80% specificity for prediction of BVAD need
[b]At this threshold: 80% sensitivity and specificity for prediction of RVF and a score >20 indicated high probability of BVAD requirement (odds ratio: 16, $p = 0.02$)
[c]At this threshold: 63% sensitivity and 78% specificity for prediction of RVF
RVF RV failure, *AUC* area under the curve, *RVAD, LVAD, and BVAD* right ventricular, left ventricular, and biventricular assist device; respectively, *SWI* stroke work index, *PAPm* mean pulmonary arterial pressure, *SV* stroke volume, *BSA* body surface area, *AST* aspartate aminotransferase, *TR* tricuspid regurgitation, *RVFRS* RV failure risk score, *PVR* pulmonary vascular resistance, *FAC* fractional area change, *RAP* right atrial pressure, *LVEDD* left ventricular end-diastolic diameter, *LAV* left atrial volume, *LVEF* LV ejection fraction, *LAD* left atrial diameter

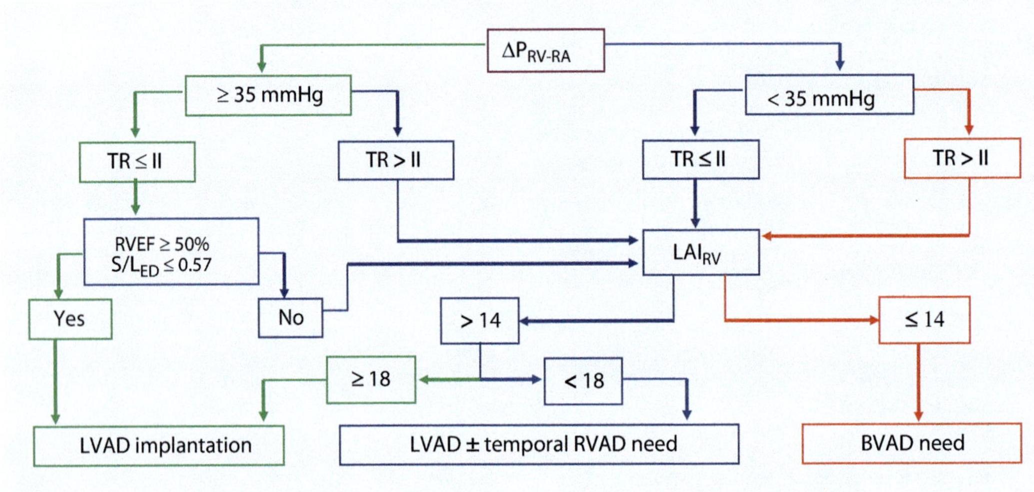

Fig. 6.3 Algorithm for device selection based on transthoracic echocardiography data. Patients without relevantly impaired RV systolic function (EF ≥50%) plus not more than moderate RV dilation ($S/L_{ED} \leq 0.57$) and tricuspid regurgitation (TR ≤ grade II) associated with a high pressure gradient between right ventricle and right atrium ($\Delta P_{RV\text{-}RA}$ ≥35 mmHg), indicating high RV afterload without relevantly increased RA pressure, need only a left ventricular assist device (LVAD). In patients with low $\Delta P_{RV\text{-}RA}$ (<35 mmHg) as well as in those with high $\Delta P_{RV\text{-}RA}$ associated with RV dilation (± EF reduction) and high TR (> grade II), the RV load adaptation index (LAI_{RV}) allows the differentiation between those who need only a left ventricular assist device (LVAD) and those who necessitate also mechanical support for the RV, either as temporal or permanent right ventricular assist device (RVAD). *BVAD,* biventricular assist device

identify patients at higher risk for postoperative death was shown by the complex scoring systems that incorporate preoperative clinical, hemodynamic, and laboratory data reflecting not only cardiac dysfunction but also end-organ dysfunction which can remain a high risk for mortality even after right-sided heart function improvement during LVAD-support [3, 22, 28]. Thus, composite echo variables for assessment of RV function in relation to loading conditions and several complex scoring systems for prediction RV function and patient survival appear able to facilitate earlier decision making for LVAD implantation before RV dysfunction and/or end-

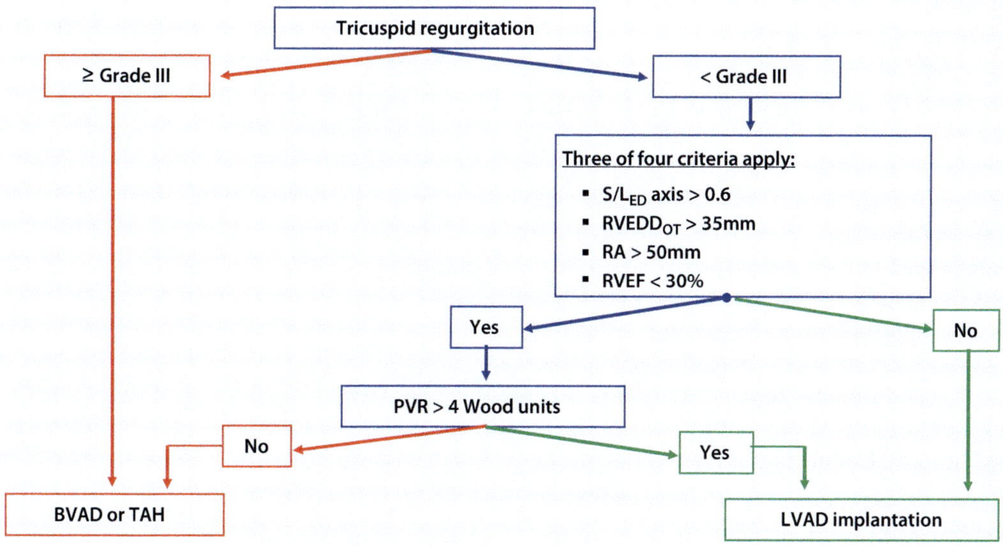

Fig. 6.4 Algorithm for device selection based on right ventricular (RV) echocardiographic evaluation in combination with right heart catheterization data for calculation of pulmonary vascular resistance (PVR) after optimization of volume status and inotropic support. *S/L$_{ED}$* end-diastolic short/long axis ratio, *RVEDD$_{OT}$* RV outflow tract end-diastolic diameter, *BVAD* biventricular assist device, *TAH* total artificial heart, *LVAD* left ventricular assist device

organ damage becomes irreversible [3]. Figure 6.4 shows an algorithm for device selection more recently developed in the German Heart Institute Berlin, which is exclusively based on transthoracic echo data evaluating the RV and the tricuspid valve competence in relation with RV loading conditions. In CHF due to primary impaired LV function, several strategies aimed to optimize RV function before VAD implantation can avoid the need of a permanent BVAD even in the presence of RVF associated with multiorgan dysfunction. However, delaying LVAD implantation in rapidly deteriorating patients aiming to improve adverse or unfavorable risk factors instead of immediate biventricular mechanical support implantation has serious limitations, because such patients are at imminent risk of death. Nevertheless, careful preoperative RV evaluation allowing a distinction between reversible and irreversible RV alterations can spare many patients unnecessary implantation of a permanent BVAD. In patients with severe RV dilation (±TR>grade II) and reduced systolic function, RV echo-assessment in relation to its loading conditions enables a distinction between those who need only a temporary RVAD in addition to an LVAD and those who definitely need a permanent BVAD implantation.

6.5 Conclusions

In patients who necessitate MCS, association between severe LV failure and RV dysfunction is usually found, even if left-sided heart disease was the initial cause of CHF. To avoid, not only post-LVAD irreversible RVF but also unnecessary permanent BVAD implantation, both often associated with worse postoperative patient outcome, preoperative proper decision between BVAD and LVAD is crucial.

Reliable assessment of RV function, prediction of RV potential to improve during LVAD support, and anticipation of postoperative persistence of RVF plus preoperative optimization of RV function and optimal timing of LVAD implantation in relation to risk factors for postoperative RVF are paramount for avoidance of unnecessary permanent BVADs. Preoperative echocardiography, RHC, clinical data, and certain laboratory tests are the main tools for identification of patients at high risk of post-LVAD RVF. The relative importance of the numerous risk factors for RVF after LVAD implantation remains controversial and incompletely known.

Certain composite variables which incorporate measures of RV geometry, function, and loading conditions plus several quantitative scoring systems which incorporate measures of different risk factors for post-LVAD RVF can predict the need for an RVAD in addition to an LVAD. Complex scoring systems that incorporate mainly preoperative clinical, laboratory, and hemodynamic data reflecting global cardiac dysfunction, including also consecutive end-organ dysfunction, showed higher ability to predict post-LVAD patient survival, whereas measurements reflecting right-sided heart function appeared more suited to predict post-LVAD RVF if they are used in combination, either as composite variables or as part of algorithms which focus mainly on evaluation of RV in relation to its loading conditions. Unfortunately, the fact that the preoperative risk assessments cannot account for undesired intra-operative events (blood transfusion, arrhythmias, air embolism, deleterious effects of excessive LV unloading on RV and tricuspid valve geometry function, etc.) that may injure a previously adequate RV remains a weakness of all attempts to predict the freedom from RVF after LVAD implantation.

References

1. Vivo RP, Cordero-Reyes AM, Qamar U et al (2013) Increased right-to-left diameter ratio is a strong predictor of right ventricular failure after left ventricular assist device. J Heart Lung Transplant 32:792–799
2. Potapov E, Meyer D, Swaminathan M et al (2011) Inhaled nitric oxide after left ventricular assist device implantation: a prospective, randeomized, double-blind, multicenter, placebo- controlled trial. J Heart Lung Transplant 30:870–878
3. Dandel M, Krabatsch T, Falk V (2015) Left ventricular vs. biventricular mechanical support: decision making and strategies for avoidance of right heart failure after left ventricular assist device implantation. Int J Cardiol 198:241–250
4. Mann DL (2012) Pathophysiology of heart failure. In: Bonow R, Mann DL, Zipes DP, Libby P (eds) Braunwald's heart disease. A textbook of cardiovascular medicine, 9th edn, pp 487–504
5. Cheng W, Kajstura J, Li P, Wolin MS, Sonnenblick EH et al (1995) Stretch-induced programmed myocyte cell death. J Clin Invest 96:2247–2259
6. Dandel M, Potapov E, Krabatsch T et al (2013) Load dependency of right ventricular performance is a major factor to be considered in decision making before ventricular assist device implantation. Circulation 128(11):S14–S23
7. Kukucka M, Potapov E, Stepaneko A et al (2011) Acute impact of left ventricular unloading by left ventricular assist device on right ventricle geometry and function: effect of nitric oxide inhalation. J Thorac Cardiovasc Surg 141:1009–1014
8. Rudski LG, Lai WW, Afilalo J et al (2010) Guidelines for echocardiographic assessment of right heart in adults: a report of the American Society of Echocardiography. J Am Soc Echocardiogr 23:685–713
9. Anavekar NS, Gerson D, Skali H et al (2007) Two-dimensional assessment of right ventricular function. An echocardiographic-MRI correlative study. Echocardiography 24:452–456
10. Focardi M, Cameli M, Carbone SF et al (2015) Traditional and innovative echocardiographic parameters for the analysis of right ventricular performance in comparison with cardiac magnetic resonance. Eur Heart J Cardiovasc Imaging 16:47–52
11. Topilsky Y, Oh JK, Dipesh KS et al (2011) Echocardiographic predictors of adverse outcomes after continuous left ventricular assist device implantation. J Am Coll Cardiol Imaging 4:211–222
12. Lindqvist P, Waldenström A, Wikström G, Kazzam E (2005) The use of isovolumetric contraction velocity to determine right ventricular state of contractility and filling pressures. A pulsed Doppler tissue imaging study. Eur J Echocardiogr 6:264–270
13. Dandel M, Hetzer R (2009) Echocardiographic strain and strain rate imaging – Clinical applications. Int J Cardiol 132(1):11–24
14. Dandel M, Knosalla C, Kemper D et al (2015) Assessment of right ventricular adaptability to loading conditions can improve the timing of listing to transplantation in patients with pulmonary arterial hypertension. J Heart Lung Transplant 34(3):319–328
15. Cameli M, Bernazzali S, Lisi M et al (2013–2015) Right ventricular longitudinal strain and right ventricular stroke work index in patients with severe heart failure: Left ventricular assist device suitability for transplant candidates. Transplant Proc 2012:44
16. Di Maria MV, Burkett DA, Youoszai MD et al (2015) Echocardiographic estimation of right ventricular stroke work in children with pulmonary arterial hypertension. Comparison with invasive methods. JASE online 23
17. Frea S, Bovolo V, Bergerone S et al (2012) Echocardiographic evaluation of right ventricular stroke work index in advanced heart failure: A new index? J Card Fail 18(12):886–893
18. Guazzi M, Bandera F, Pelissero G et al (2013) Tricuspid annular systollic excursion and pulmonary artery pressure relationship in heart failure: An index of right ventricular function and prognosis. Am J Physiol Heart Circ Physiol 305(9):H1373–H1381
19. Lopez-Candales A, Lopez FR, Trivedi S, Elwing J (2014) Right ventricular ejection efficiency: A new echocardiographic measure of mechanical

performance in chronic pulmonary hypertension. Echocardiography 31:516–523

20. Shiran H, Zamanian RT, McConnell MV et al (2014) Relationship between echocardiographic and magnetic resonance derived measures of right ventricular size and function in patients with Pulmonary Hypertension. Am Soc Echocardiogr 27(4): 405–412
21. Ryo K, Goda A, Onishi T (2015) Pulmonary hypertension associated with patient outcomes by 3-dimensional wall motion tracking Echocardiography. Circ Cardiovasc Imaging 8:e003176
22. Matthews JC, Koelling T, Pagani F, Aaronson K (2008) The right ventricular failure risk score a preoperative tool for assessing the risk of right ventricular failure in left ventricular assist device candidates. J Am Coll Cardiol 51:2163–2172
23. Lembcke A, Dohmen PM, Dewey M et al (2005) Multislice computed tomography for pre-operative evaluation of right ventricular volumes and function: comparison with magnetic resonance imaging. Ann Thorac Surg 79(4):1344–1351
24. Ochiai Y, McCarthy P, Smedira N et al (2002) Predictors of severe right ventricular failure after implantable assist device insertion: analysis of 245 patients. Circulation 106(Suppl):1198–1202
25. Potapov EV, Stepanenko A, Dandel M et al (2008) Tricuspid incompetence and geometry of the right ventricle as predictors of right ventricular function after implantation of a left ventricular assist device. J Heart Lung Transplant 27:1275–1281
26. Kukucka M, Stepanenko A, Potapov E et al (2011) Right-to-left ventricular end-diastolic diameter and prediction of right ventricular failure with continuous-flow left ventricular assist devices. J Heart Lung Transplant 30:64–69
27. Kormos RL, Teutenberg JJ, Pagani FD et al (2010) Right ventricular failure in patients with the HeartMate II continuous flow left ventricular assist device: incidence, risk factors and effect on outcomes. J Thorac Cardiovasc Surg 139(5):1316–1324
28. Drakos SG, Janicki L, Horne BD et al (2010) Risk factors of right ventricular failure after left ventricular assist device implantation. Am J Cardiol 105:1030–1035
29. Grant ADM, Smedira GN, Starling RC, Marwick TH (2012) Independent and incremental role of quantitative right ventricular evaluation for prediction of right ventricular failure after ventricular assist device implantation. J Am Coll Cardiol 60:521–528
30. Shiga T, Kinugawa K, Imamura T et al (2012) Combination evaluation of preoperative risk indices predicts requirement of biventricular assist device. Circ J 76:2785–2791
31. Fitzpatrick JR III, Frederick JR, Hsu VM et al (2008) Risk score derived from preoperative data analysis predicts the need for biventricular mechanical circulatory support. J Heart Lung Transplant 27(12):1286–1292
32. Raina A, Harish R, Rammohan S et al (2013) Postoperative right ventricular failure after left ventricular assist device placement is predicted by preoperative echocardiographic structural, hemodynamic and functional parameters. J Card Fail 19:16–24
33. Kato ST, Farr M, Schulze PC et al (2012) Usefulness of two-dimensional echocardiographic parameters of the left side of the heart to predict right ventricular failure after left ventricular assist device implantation. Am J Cardiol 109:246–251
34. Atluri P, Goldstone AB, Fairman AS et al (2013) Predicting right ventricular failure in the modern, continuous flow left ventricular assist device era. Ann Thorac Surg 96:857–864

High INTERMACS Profiles: Medical Versus MCS Treatment

A. Barbone and Bart P. Meyns

© Springer International Publishing Switzerland 2017
A. Montalto et al. (eds.), *Mechanical Circulatory Support in End-Stage Heart Failure*,
DOI 10.1007/978-3-319-43383-7_7

Therapy with a left ventricular assist device (LVAD) is an established treatment for patients with advanced heart failure (HF). Past clinical trials evaluating LVADs for bridge to transplant and destination therapy (DT) were designed to assess safety and effectiveness in patients with the most advanced stage of HF. The guidelines today recommend consideration of LVAD support when patients have progressed to stage D heart failure, the point at which therapeutic options have been exhausted and the projected benefits in quality of life and survival outweigh the risks [1]. Consequently, the majority of LVAD implantations are performed in patients who are hospitalized and dependent on intravenous inotropic support. It has to be reminded that the initiation of inotropic therapy and its continuation are subjective clinical decisions and, therefore, the somewhat arbitrary decision of whether or not to initiate inotropic therapy; thus it does not necessarily identify a sicker population of patients. Anyhow INTERMACS classes IV–VII are expected to be a less sick population and consequently at a lower heart failure life-threatening risk. By definition these are stage D heart failure patients, NYHA classes III–IV, thus highly symptomatic for heart failure but not yet dependent on inotropic drug to preserve end-organ function.

The prevalence of symptomatic heart failure has increased, including a prolongation of the advanced phase of the disease. The American Heart Association characterizes the far end of the heart failure continuum as stage D or "refractory end-stage heart failure" as further defined by the European Society of Cardiology [2]. These overlapping definitions describe a group of patients for whom symptoms limit daily life, despite usual recommended therapies, and for whom lasting remission into less symptomatic disease is unlikely. The increasing prevalence, high symptom burden, and possible disease-exchanging therapies (i.e., transplantation and mechanical circulatory support) for patients living with advanced heart failure mandate a systematic and thoughtful approach to decision making.

7.1 Estimating Prognosis in Heart Failure

To begin with, the assessment of prognosis is the foundation for selection among therapies for life-threatening disease, but this is particularly challenging for heart failure. The clinical course varies dramatically across the spectrum of disease severity and is relatively unpredictable for individual patients. This contrasts with the more linear decline of patients with advanced cancer, which has traditionally been the model for approaches to end-stage disease. Even late in heart failure, patients often enjoy "good days" and brief interludes of apparent stability, which can lull them and their care providers into postponing vital decisions. Prognosis is further clouded by the unique contrast between unexpected sudden death (i.e., lethal arrhythmia) and lingering death with congestive symptoms (i.e., progressive pump failure).

Most prognostic models in heart failure focus on mortality, which is easily determined and highly relevant; however, other clinical outcomes also might rank high in importance to individual patients. Multiple studies have documented patients' willingness to sacrifice survival in exchange for symptom relief, a trade-off that varies between patients and within the same patient over time and is correlated loosely with disease severity but strongly with do-not-resuscitate status.

Even under these idealized circumstances, most models designed to predict mortality have only modest accuracy. Further complicating practical use, prediction models represent the average survival for a population of patients with characteristics similar to those of the individual patient. A 70% chance of 2-year survival does not directly translate to an individual who will instead be 100% alive or dead at any point in time. For patients with advanced disease, interest often focuses instead on the expected length of time remaining; patients ask the question, "How long do I have?" This point prediction of survival time is even more difficult to estimate even if a model fits well for a cohort.

Ultimately, the stochastic nature of heart failure conveys a high level of prognostic uncertainty for most patients. Future events have a certain degree of unpredictability, such that improved understanding of risk tends to add incrementally less prognostic information to existing models. Even a perfect model that includes all possible measurements describes only what has already happened. The trajectory can often be steepened by new conditions or life events, such as myocardial infarction, a serious fall, or the death of a spouse. It is vital to acknowledge uncertainty in discussions about future care [3].

7.2 The Historical INTERMACS Perspective

The INTERMACS allowed some preliminary evaluation of indication broadening and LVAD implant anticipation to classes IV–VII. In a revision of the initial experience with the continuous-flow devices [4], followed for 24 months, it showed how the severity of advanced heart failure impacts length of stay, survival to discharge, and actuarial survival. Compared to lower INTERMACS class, the less sick patients in classes IV–VII reported shorter hospital lengths of stay at the implant, greater survival to discharge, and superior long-term actuarial survival. Although classes IV–VII had statistically similar survival to discharge in comparison to classes II–III, the mean length of stay for classes IV–VII was more than 3 weeks shorter than that for classes II–III. These findings suggest that LVADs are not only effective but also less resource intensive in stable advanced heart failure patients, particularly if they are electively implanted prior to inotrope dependence. Those preliminary data suggested the need for further studies to better evaluate the clinical and economic outcomes of VAD therapy in less severely ill heart failure patients.

Although in the latest INTERMACS data report, at the tenth year of the registry [5], it appears evident that the rate of implant in the higher classes is not raising as it could be foreseen 10 years ago, barely leveling below a 20% of the overall population. This might be explained by the general feeling for the MCS, the complication rate and type that this therapy involves. It's not a case, if the increase in Thoratec® HeartMate II pump thrombosis risk that was reported in 2013 [6] also led directly to the indefinite suspension of the National Heart, Lung, and Blood Institute (NHLBI)-sponsored Randomized Evaluation of VAD Intervention before Inotropic Therapy (REVIVE-IT) trial of LVAD therapy in earlier-stage, non-inotrope-dependent patients. The trial was suspended after equipoise was lost, due to device complication rate, and not accepted to randomize New York Heart Association Functional Classification III patients to the HM II device or optimized medical management (OMM). Indeed this clinical trial was advocated by a joint experts and authority panel to further investigate the clinical benefit of a wider MCS usage [7]. Despite subsequent attempts to restart enrollment in a modified protocol after the device thrombosis case was addressed, this study has been turned in a registry that (from the https:\\ clinicaltrials.gov) will establish a prospective, observational, multicenter patient cohort in ambulatory patients with chronic, advanced, systolic heart failure that will provide a greater understanding of their clinical trajectory (rates of hospitalizations, transplantation, MCSD use, and death) and better inform the selection of appropriate candidates for a future study of a strategy of early LVAD therapy versus optimal medical management in this population. The study will continue until up to 400 eligible heart failure subjects have been enrolled (estimated length of accrual is 12 months).

Relatively high adverse event (AE) rates associated with LVADs may be at the base of the limited adoption of the therapy. Furthermore, there are limited prospective data comparing the relative risks (AEs) and benefits (functional capacity and quality of life improvement) of LVAD treatment versus OMM. The intent of REVIVE-IT was to examine LVAD versus OMM in patients with even less advanced HF (NYHA III symptoms/INTERMACS profile 7) than another observational sponsored trial in high INTERMACS class, the ROADMAP [8], that we'll address further in this chapter.

7.3 From Survival to Quality of Life (QoL)

It's now accepted that the need for inotropic therapy (sliding into INTERMACS class II) modifies prognosis and significantly reduces life expectancy rewarding MCS as survival benefit; this is not granted in the not bedbound advanced chronic heart failure (ACHF) population. In the INTERMACS [6], the overall survival rate at 1 year reaches 80%, matching the 1-year survival of an average class D ACHF patient not inotropic dependent [9]. In this same registry, despite the burden of a late emergency implant is evident (class I survival at 1 year drops to 75%), so far it could not be proven a survival benefit of an early implant in a higher functional class. Indeed the initial burden for the lowest class melts down in the longer follow-up, all the classes matching practically the same survival at the fourth year, suggesting a primary role of the MCS device complications as life-threatening parameter.

Although survival considerations might strongly apply to patients in impending death risk, further concerns might rise once we move to the quality of life (QoL). Despite multiple statistical analyses have been developed to assess QoL for patient in ACHF, it is very hard to render the bargain of trading one disease (ACHF in OMM) with another disease (MCS).

Health-related quality of life (HRQOL) might benefit by LVAD support in all INTERMACS profiles, including IV–VII [10]. Indeed in this study, the benefit in terms of QoL is reported across all the pre-implant INTERMACS classes. Despite the enthusiastic reports, some punctuations are needed: the overall QoL is perceived very poor by all ACHF patients, independently from their functional status - INTERMACS classes IV–VII reported very low QoL similarly to lower classes, suggesting an insufficient statistical sensitivity of the questionnaire. Some of the specific fields are less rewarded by MCS than others, for example, anxiety/depression, self-care, and pain-related field showing how some aspects of everyday life are not "normalized" in this patient population. Overall the QoL event scores after long period of support never equalize the age-matched population, further proving the limiting burden by the MCS despite hemodynamical and functional normalization of the supported patients.

7.4 The ROADMAP Study

On this background, a sponsor-based, large observational clinical study was planned with the HMII continuous-flow LVAD in advanced, ambulatory HF patients who were not dependent on intravenous inotropic support and who meet US Food and Drug Administration - approved indications for LVAD as destination therapy (DT): the ROADMAP study [8]. This is the first study that tried to systematically approach the high INTERMACS [IV–VII] population; as we have previously anticipated for the REVIVE-IT trial, despite long discussions, it was not felt that equipoise exists for LVAD versus OMM in this population class, thus a randomized trial was still not justified, and observational studies could still be considered a valid source of clinical relevant information.

In the ROADMAP Trial, a total of 200 patients were enrolled for LVAD DT support ($n = 97$) or continuing on the ongoing OMM ($n = 103$). This study reports a registry; thus a large baseline enrollment bias exists given that probably motivation to accept a surgical implanted device is clearly involved in the patient selection. Consequently, patients in the LVAD group were more severely ill compared with the OMM group (NYHA functional class IV, 52% versus 25%; INTERMACS profile 4, 65% versus 34%), had lower baseline HRQOL, had more severe depression (87% versus 60% [at least mild depression]), and had lower predicted Seattle Heart Failure Model 12-month survival rates.

Patient questionnaires at baseline demonstrated that more LVAD patients reported how they were not satisfied or only slightly satisfied with their quality of life on baseline medical therapy (79%) compared with those who remained on OMM (48%). Significantly more LVAD patients at baseline also reported a perception that they were going to live <1 year (53% versus 9%). Of the 103 OMM patients, 18 died and 18 received a delayed LVAD at least 1 month after enrollment (including 1 patient receiving a total artificial heart), leaving 58 patients alive on original OMM therapy at 12 months (9 patient withdrawal). For the 97 patients in the LVAD arm, 17 died, 3 received a heart transplant (2 urgent and 1 elective), and 3 withdrew from the study within 30-day enrollment before receiving an LVAD, leaving 74 patients on LVAD support at 12 months. More patients who received LVAD support achieved the primary composite end point than patients who received OMM (39% versus 21%): the main difference between the two groups was the delayed LVAD implant in OMM patients. One of the most interesting outcomes recorded is the 30-day operative mortality after LVAD implantation that hit 1%, the same as the mortality rate in the OMM group within 30 days after enrollment. Although using an intention-to-treat analysis, Kaplan-Meier survival (freedom from death) at 12 months was similar in both groups.

In the study the clinical and functional efficacy of LVAD was largely proven both on direct comparison that compared to control group: 77% of LVAD patients improved to NYHA functional class I (25%) or II (52%) at 12 months compared with 0% before implantation, while 29% of OMM patients alive at 12 months had NYHA functional class II (no class I). Similarly, the average 6MWD improved significantly in LVAD patients (187–263 m) compared with no significant change in OMM patients (214–249 m). The composite measures combining survival on original therapy with improvements in NYHA functional class, HRQOL, and depression all showed significantly greater change for LVAD than OMM.

The downside of LVAD therapy is shown in the adverse event (AE) report: bleeding was the primary driver of LVAD AEs (bleeding accounted for 65% of LVAD events) while worsening HF, accounted for 82% of OMM events. Pump thrombosis occurred in six LVAD patients, four requiring pump exchange, with only one early event within 90 days of implantation. The composite AE rate for bleeding, driveline infection, pump thrombosis, stroke, ventricular arrhythmias, and worsening HF was 1.89 EPPY (LVAD) versus 0.83 EPPY (OMM); without bleeding, the composite AE rates were similar. More LVAD patients (80%) than OMM patients (62%) had re-hospitalizations within 1 year of enrollment; leading causes of re-hospitalizations were bleeding for LVAD patients and worsening HF for OMM patients.

As expected the study's observational nature resulted in an imbalance in the severity of illness between the OMM and LVAD patients; thus the comparisons of the study arms can't leave aside that these two cohorts probably had different underlying disease severity. Survival was similar in both groups in the intention-to-treat analysis. As treated, the event-free actuarial survival over a 12-month period was significantly better with LVAD (80%) than OMM. Thus, the risk/benefit analyses in the ROADMAP study might underestimate the benefit and overestimate the risk of LVAD versus OMM, and despite these differences, more LVAD patients still met the primary endpoint.

7.5 Will New Technologies Expand the Indication?

This is the great question that has been challenging the MCS world since the beginning. On regular basis new technologies, promising higher performance at lower biological costs, are expected to move the equipoise between MCS and OMM toward the VADs to further improve survival and moreover QoL of NHYA class IIIb patients.

Lately a new device approached the CE mark clinical trial to start its clinical career [11]: the HeartMate 3 showing in the initial experience a substantial reduction in adverse event rate, in particular pump thrombosis. This device is designed for intrapericardial placement, with an inflow conduit inserted into the LV and the outflow graft attached to the ascending aorta as any standard VAD. A fully magnetically levitated (Full MagLev) rotor with large blood flow paths (0.5 mm along the side and 1.0 mm above and below the rotor) is supposed to minimize shear forces, reducing the detrimental effects on blood components. This rotor design avoids the need for mechanical bearings, reducing wear of the moving component and heat generation within the pump. The device's internal surfaces are textured with titanium microspheres, like the previous device of the family, to promote adhesion of patient's cells to further reduced thrombogenicity. All patients enrolled in the trial were NYHA functional class IIIB or IV before implantation, functional class that improved significantly ($p < 0.0001$) at 6 months. Peculiarly, when revising the INTERMACS class, 48% of the patients ($n = 24$) are classes IV–VII showing an attitude of the investigators toward higher INTERMACS profiles. Improvement in 6-min walk distance was demonstrated by comparison of individual patient paired data. QoL assessment by the Visual Analog Score paired by individual patients improved at 6 months ($p < 0.0001$). Survival rates of 98% at 30 days and 92% at 6 months compare well with the reported survival in prior studies involving bridge-to-transplant (BTT) or DT indications. Additionally, compared with a Seattle Heart Failure Model (SHFM)-predicted 6-month survival of 78%, the support with this new device was associated with a mortality risk reduction of 66%. The most frequent adverse event following LVAD implantation, bleeding, varies by patient-defined variables such as age, sex, body mass index, and etiology of HF. Overall bleeding frequency and the need for reoperation due to bleeding in this study appear considerably less than reported in prior BTT and DT studies. Placement of the Full MagLev LVAS in the thorax, as with other previously implanted devices, eliminates the need to surgically create an abdominal pocket, thereby reducing the amount of surgical dissection required. Other significant AE to be reported is the overall infection rate that in this study reached 36% within the 6 months of follow-up, with 10% of patients reporting a driveline infection. Also the 12% stroke rate (8% debilitating stroke) observed in this study was higher than expected.

Thus the initial overall experience can be considered as positive as it could, but, as previously happened in other trials, the very limited patient population in the high selective setting of a clinical trial might not be able to fully represent the real-world experience.

Furthermore the device tests in the high INTERMACS profile, despite a clear implementation in QoL and functional data, have been associated with a relative high rate of complications in terms of bleeding and strokes. As previously mentioned the high AE rate remains the real challenge to overcome for this technology to further expand in higher INTERMACS class.

7.6 New Dedicated Technology

A new device was especially intended to be used in the high INTERMACS patient class, with the idea to decrease the surgical, neurological, and infective complication rate and to provide a step forward in the MCS world. The CircuLite Synergy® (◘ Fig. 7.1) device was designed with the purpose of providing a smaller, less invasively implantable assist device that would benefit patients with severe symptomatic heart failure with no other treatment option, who were not yet sick enough to justify implantation of a full-support ventricular support device. In brief, the CircuLite Synergy pump is the size of an AA battery, weighing 25 g and having an outer body diameter of 14 mm and a length of 49 mm. The inflow cannula is made of silicone reinforced with nitinol with a length of 20.5 cm and an inner diameter of 6 mm and has a Dacron cuff on the tip made of titanium to enhance healing. The outflow graft is a 1 mm thick polytetrafluoroethylene (PTFE) prosthesis with an inner diameter of 8 mm and is trimmed to fit during the implant. A percutaneous lead connects the micro-pump to a rechargeable dual battery pack system and controller. The surgical implant procedure requires a 4 cm subclavicular incision to allow the right subclavian artery isolation. A subcutaneous pocket is formed anterior to the right pectoralis muscle similar to a pacemaker pocket. Thereafter, an anterolateral thoracotomy in the fourth right intercostal space is performed. The pericardium is opened with respect to the phrenic nerve, and, after full heparinization, two 4/0 polypropylene purse-string sutures are placed in the left atrium between the insertions of the right upper and lower pulmonary veins. After insertion of a guidewire, the nitinol-reinforced silicone-inflow cannula is inserted on a trocar over the guidewire using the Seldinger technique and secured with the two purse-string sutures. The proximal end of the inflow cannula is tunneled through the second intercostal space to exit the thorax in the area of the subcutaneous pocket. PTFE outflow graft is anastomosed to the subclavian artery. The micro-pump percutaneous lead is then tunneled to exit the body over the right upper quadrant of the abdomen.

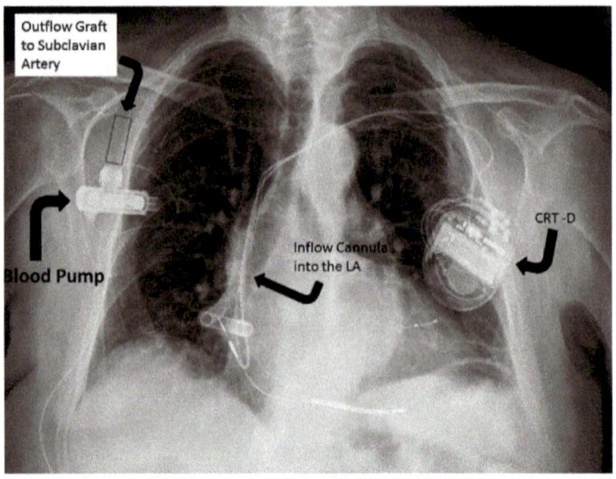

◘ **Fig. 7.1** Thoracic X-ray of CircuLite implanted for partial support (With permission by Dr. Barbone Alessandro)

In the initial published experience [12], hospital discharge has occurred in as little as 10 days but has generally been between 14 and 20 days (median of 17 days). Patients were anticoagulated with aspirin (100 mg day^{-1}) and warfarin with a goal to achieve an international normalized ratio (INR) value of 2.5–3.0.

Given that the surgical procedure is not requiring sternotomy, prior cardiac operations [coronary artery bypass grafting (CABG), valve surgery, or Dor procedure] are not considered at higher risk compared to previously not-operated chest.

Patients were selected as on the cardiac transplant waiting list with a predicted waiting time >6 months and in the New York Heart Association (NYHA) class IIIB or IVA despite appropriate treatment with diuretics, angiotensin-converting enzyme (ACE) inhibitor, or angiotensin receptor blockade and beta blocker as tolerate, ambulatory, not inotropic dependent, and with limitations in the activities of daily living (INTERMACS classes IV–VII). Exclusion criteria included acute decompensated heart failure, acute postcardiotomy heart failure, existing thrombus in the left atrium, mechanical mitral or aortic valve, significant aortic regurgitation, severe depressed renal function (serum creatinine > 2.5 mg dl/1), elevated liver enzymes >2 times the upper limit of normal, and contraindication to anticoagulation.

Medication in the implanted patients was supposed to be appropriate for end-stage heart failure with the main differences with respect to the general MCS population that the treated patients should still be treated with beta blockers, ACE inhibitors or angiotensin receptor blockers, and less frequently treated with inotropic agents.

Acute and chronic hemodynamic effects for partial mechanical support 24 h after surgery were reported [12] as estimated pump flow was with a range of 2.3–3.5 l min/1. With this additional pump output, hemodynamic improvements assessed at 24 h following surgery included an increase of the total cardiac index (CI) (from 2.0 ±0.4 to 3.3 ±0.9 l min/1 m^2, $p < 0.001$) and the decrease of the pulmonary systolic pressure (from 55 ±15 to 53 ±14 mmHg, $p = 0.34$) and pulmonary diastolic pressure (from 27 ±9 to 21 ±5 mmHg, $p = 0.002$). At an average follow-up of 9.5 ±5.5 weeks, sustained improvements in all parameters, including clinically and statistically significant reductions in pulmonary and arterial resistances, are found.

Given the baseline characteristics for patients entering this trial, severe adverse events (SAEs) were expected and have been similar in nature to those reported for LVADs. However, at this initial point, it is encouraging that the frequency of SAEs experienced by the Synergy patients, particularly in the first 30 days following surgery, appears to occur at a significantly reduced rate to those reported for other LVADs. Reported SAEs have included bleeding requiring transfusion or return to the operating room, infections (including sepsis from any cause, driveline or pocket infections, and infections not necessarily related to the device), and strokes. Overall, including all reports for Synergy patients, SAEs during the first 30 days occurred at approximately half the rate as that reported for other MCS [8]. The Achilles's heel of this technology was the pump thrombosis or exchange for any reason, which accounted for about a third of the events reported after the first 30 days of support.

The comparison of the CircuLite patients to those implanted with other MCS bridge-to-transplant study is very interesting. The patients had similar baseline demographic characteristics and, most surprisingly, almost identical hemodynamic profiles and end-organ function. The major difference was that these baseline hemodynamic characteristics were observed in the Synergy patients with greater use of standard heart failure therapy (i.e., more ACE inhibitor, angiotensin receptor blockade (ARB), and beta blocker use) and less inotropic support than in regular MCS population. This is consistent with the notion that development of intolerance to standard heart failure medical therapy (which usually manifests as a gradual reduction of drug dosing by the treating clinician), along with worsening symptoms, may identify patients who are approaching a stage where early intervention with a device such as the Synergy device should be considered. Early clinical experiences [13] supported the hypothesis that, when applied prior to significant end-organ dysfunction and becoming inotrope dependent, even in the elderly and more fragile population, partial support with the Synergy device can indeed provide adequatesupport and interrupt the progressive hemodynamic deterioration characteristic of severe heart failure.

The other important hypothesized feature of the Synergy device was that its lesser invasive nature (small size, no sternotomy, and no cardiopulmonary bypass) would be associated with less adverse events in the short and long term.

One more interesting finding of CircuLite use in the clinical setting regards the development of right-heart failure: interestingly, preoperative pulmonary artery systolic pressures have ranged between 26 and 90 mmHg, indicating a wide range of right ventricular function at baseline. It could be argued that, in contrast to a full-support VAD, which can abruptly increase cardiac output to 6–7 l/min and acutely overload the right ventricle, the acute increase in cardiac output resulting from the Synergy system is of the order of only 1.0–1.5 l/min. Thus, it could be that concerns about development of right- heart failure will be less with a partial-support device.

Unfortunately the CircuLite Synergy® device in the clinical setting proved to have too many device-related adverse events, and its clinical experience has been withheld to allow a full reengineering of its main components, although it was able to prove the concept that partial support is sufficient to allow improvement in hemodynamics and QoL in the INTERMACS 4–7 end-stage heart failure population, sparing the patients of major surgery and allowing even the most fragile patients to approach the MCS world.

7.7 Conclusions

First, we must reaffirm that LVADs can be a lifesaving and life-sustaining therapy for appropriately selected patients with advanced HF in INTERMACS profiles I–IV. Extending implants into a less sick advanced HF population (profiles V–VI) requires a more precise indication. Gradual deterioration of the renal function, increasing pulmonary artery pressures, and decrease of quality of life are the most frequent reasons why patients with INTERMACS profiles V–VII are advanced to mechanical support [12].

Secondly, reducing adverse events of LVADs will expand the indications in the less sick patient. Engineering progress, along with a better understanding of hemocompatibility, will undoubtedly help to reduce the problem of pump thrombosis and will allow the expansion of mechanical circulatory support into broader groups of patients. Until then, we must redouble our efforts to ensure that today's patients live longer and better with approved pump technology even as we look with hope to the future.

Thirdly, early MCS implant might play a role in slowing progression of ACHF further improving survival and QoL throughout two different mechanisms: improving OMM tolerance (especially beta blockers, ACEi, and anti-neurohormonal therapy) that constantly needs to be downgraded with the disease progression and cardiac performance decrement; indeed each acute heart failure event further compromises the end-organ function and organ reserves slowly, each time reaching a new level of hemodynamic compensation at a lower functional level [14].

For patients requiring an "unconventional" treatment for end-stage heart failure, highly symptomatic but yet not dying (INTERMAC IV–VII), the unchallenged treatment is still not available. MCS placement in this population is a highly preference-sensitive decision; it involves a number of risk-benefit trade-offs among mortality, adverse events, and functionality that require robust clinician-patient dialogue early in the course of patients' illnesses to allow for preference-congruent decisions. In weighing these three trade-offs, some patients may elect to delay or decline LVAD therapy to avoid LVAD-related adverse events [15].

Shared decision making for advanced heart failure has become both more challenging and more crucial as duration of disease and treatment options have increased. High-quality decisions are chosen from medically reasonable options and are aligned with values, goals, and preferences of an informed patient. Providers have an ethical and legal mandate to involve patients in medical decisions. Shared decision making recognizes that there are complex trade-offs in the choice of medical care. Shared decision making also addresses the ethical need to fully inform patients about the risks and benefits of treatments. In the setting of multiple reasonable options for medical care, shared decision making involves clinicians working with patients to ensure that patients' values, goals, and preferences guide informed decisions that are right for each individual patient [3]. A major purpose of a high-functioning healthcare system is to provide the resources with which an activated, informed patient can engage in productive discussions with a proactive, prepared healthcare team. Shared decision making moves beyond informed consent. It asks that clinicians and patients share information with each other and work toward patient-centered decisions about treatment [16]. Shared decision making incorporates the perspective of the patient, who is responsible for articulating goals, values, and preferences as they relate to his or her healthcare. Shared decision making incorporates the perspective of the clinician, who is responsible for narrowing the diagnostic and treatment options to those that are medically reasonable. Shared decision making is most easily applied to preference-sensitive decisions, in which both clinicians and patients agree that equipoise exists, and decision support helps patients think through, forecast, and deliberate their options. However, in situations in which clinicians hold the view that scientific evidence for benefit strongly outweighs harm, behavioral support (e.g., smoking cessation counseling) designed to describe, justify, and recommend specific behavior may also be appropriate and complementary to decision support. Finally, certain therapeutic options may be considered unreasonable and therefore independent of patient demands. Although not all patients will be able to clearly articulate decisions that are congruent with their stated goals, shared decision making aims to ensure that patients' values, goals, and preferences are explored and incorporated into the medical decision-making process. Shared decision making puts into practice the principle of "patient-centered care."

The approach to decision takes the perspective of the individual patient rather than that of society in general. Although individual medical decisions taken collectively have implications for distributive justice and resource allocation, it is not the responsibility of clinicians, patients, or families to directly factor these global considerations into individual decisions. Rather, discussions regarding alternative treatment options, including no treatment, should be focused on meeting a specific individual's values, goals, and preferences within the context of societal rules and regulations.

References

1. McMurray JJV, Adamopoulos S, Anker SD, Auricchio A, Böhm M, Dickstein K, Falk V, Filippatos G, Fonseca C, Gomez-Sanchez MA, Jaarsma T, Køber L, Lip GYH, Maggioni AP, Parkhomenko A, Pieske BM, Popescu BA, Rønnevik PK, Rutten FH, Schwitter J, Seferovic P, Stepinska J, Trindade PT, Voors AA, Zannad F, Zeiher A (2012) ESC Guidelines for the diagnosis and treatment of acute and chronic heart failure 2012. Eur Heart J 33:1787–1847
2. Metra M, Ponikowski P, Dickstein K, McMurray JJV, Gavazzi A, Bergh CH, Fraser AG, Jaarsma T, Pitsis A, Mohacsi P, Böhm M, Anker S, Dargie H, Brutsaert D, Komajda M, on behalf of the Heart Failure Association of the European Society of Cardiology (2007) Advanced chronic heart failure: a position statement from the Study Group on Advanced Heart Failure of the Heart Failure Association of the European Society of Cardiology. Eur J Heart Fail 9:684–694
3. Allen LA, Stevenson LW, Grady KL, Goldstein NE, Matlock DD, Arnold RM, Cook NR, Felker GM, Francis GS, Hauptman PJ, Havranek EP, Krumholz HM, Mancini D, Riegel B, Spertus JA (2012) Decision making in advanced heart failure: a scientific statement from the American Heart Association. Circulation 125: 1928–1952
4. Boyle AJ, Ascheim DD, Russo MJ, Kormos RL, John R, Naka Y, Gelijns AC, Hong KN, Teuteberg JJ (2010) Clinical outcomes for continuous-flow left ventricular assist device patients stratified by pre-operative INTERMACS classification. J Heart Lung Transplantat 30:402–407
5. Kirklin JK, Naftel DC, Kormos RL, Pagani FD, Myers SL, Stevenson LW, Acker MA, Goldstein DL, Silvestry SC, Milano CA, Baldwin JT, Pinney S, Eduardo Rame J, Miller MA (2014) Interagency Registry for Mechanically Assisted Circulatory Support (INTERMACS) analysis of pump thrombosis in the HeartMate II left ventricular assist device. J Heart Lung Transplant 33:12–22
6. Kirklin JK, Naftel DC, Pagani FD, Kormos RL, Stevenson LW, Blume ED, Myers SL, Miller MA, Baldwin JT, Young JB (2015) Seventh INTERMACS annual report: 15,000 patients and counting. J Heart Lung Transplant 34(12):1495–1504
7. Baldwin JT, Mann DL (2010) NHLBIGÇÖs program for VAD therapy for moderately advanced heart failure: The REVIVE-IT pilot trial. J Card Fail 16:855–858
8. Estep JD, Starling RC, Horstmanshof DA, Milano CA, Selzman CH, Shah KB, Loebe M, Moazami N, Long JW, Stehlik J, Kasirajan V, Haas DC, O'Connell JB, Boyle AJ, Farrar DJ, Rogers JG (2015) Risk assessment and comparative effectiveness of left ventricular assist-device and medical management in ambulatory heart failure patients results from the ROADMAP Study. J Am Coll Cardiol 66:1747–1761
9. Levy WC, Mozaffarian D, Linker DT, Sutradhar SC, Anker SD, Cropp AB, Anand I, Maggioni A, Burton P, Sullivan MD, Pitt B, Poole-Wilson PA, Mann DL, Packer M (2006) The seattle heart failure model: prediction of survival in heart failure. Circulation 113:1424–1433
10. Grady KL, Naftel D, Stevenson L, Amanda Dew M, Weidner G, Pagani FD, Kirklin JK, Myers S, Baldwin T, Young J (2014) Overall quality of life improves to similar levels after mechanical circulatory support regardless of severity of heart failure before implantation. J Heart Lung Transplant 33:412–421
11. Netuka I, Sood P, Pya Y, Zimpfer D, Krabatsch T, Garbade J, Rao V, Morshuis M, Marasco S, Beyersdorf F, Damme L, Schmitto JD (2015) Fully magnetically levitated left-ventricular assist system for treating-advanced HFA multicenter study. J Am Coll Cardiol 66:2579–2589
12. Meyns BP, Simon A, Klotz S, Wittwer T, Schlensak C, Rega F, Burkhoff D (2011) Clinical benefits of partial circulatory support in New York Heart Association class IIIB and early class IV patients. Eur J Cardiothorac Surg 39:693–698
13. Barbone A, Pini D, Rega F, Ornaghi D, Vitali E, Meyns B (2013) Circulatory support in elderly chronic heart failure patients using the CircuLite(R) Synergy(R) system. Eur J Cardiothorac Surg 44:207–212

14. Gheorghiade M, De Luca L, Fonarow GC, Filippatos G, Metra M, Francis GS (2005) Pathophysiologic targets in the early phase of acute heart failure syndromes. Am J Cardiol 96:11–17
15. Bruce C, Blumenthal-Barby JS, Meyers D (2015) Benefits and challenges of early introduction of left ventricular assist-device placement. A patient-centered perspective. J Am Coll Cardiol 66:1762–1765
16. Charles C, Gafni A, Whelan T (1997) Shared decision-making in the medical encounter: what does it mean? (or it takes at least two to tango). Soc Sci Med 44: 681–692

Low INTERMACS Profiles: Temporary ECMO or TAH Support

V. Tarzia, G. Bortolussi, Lorenzo Bagozzi, T. Bottio, and G. Gerosa

© Springer International Publishing Switzerland 2017
A. Montalto et al. (eds.), *Mechanical Circulatory Support in End-Stage Heart Failure*,
DOI 10.1007/978-3-319-43383-7_8

8.1 Introduction

According to the INTERMACS registry, "low profiles" define the highest severity in the spectrum of advanced heart failure.

Profile 1, the so-called "crash and burn", refers to patients in cardiogenic shock, with critical hypotension despite inotropic support and established organ hypoperfusion.

Profile 2 includes those with declining hemodynamics and perfusion despite intravenous inotropic therapy, while profile 3 identifies patients where inotropes achieve to stabilize blood pressure and organ function, but weaning is not possible.

It is important to note that the passage from one category to another is all but infrequent, and rapid deterioration may occur in the space of minutes to hours.

These critically ill patients, beyond conventional therapy, often require mechanical circulatory support (MCS) to survive until the definitive treatment becomes available.

MCS includes extracorporeal life support (ECLS), temporary mono- or biventricular assist device (VAD), long-term VAD, and total artificial heart (TAH).

8.2 Which Device in INTERMACS 1 Patients?

In the present chapter, we aim to outline the choice of the ideal MCS device in INTERMACS profile 1 patients.

This setting describes patients in cardiogenic shock, with a decreased cardiac function, but also at risk of developing a multiorgan dysfunction syndrome (MODS) as a result of peripheral hypoperfusion.

Once established, MODS strongly increases mortality regardless of mechanical support; hence the key to success after MCS implantation resides in patient selection, choice of timing, and optimal level of support.

In fact, according to INTERMACS registry, long-term LVAD has been associated with lower survival when offered to patients in profile 1; therefore over the years LVAD implants in the sickest patients have decreased from 40% to 14%.

One of the main reasons of poorer outcome is thought to be the higher incidence of post-implant severe right ventricular failure observed with INTERMACS profile 1. This may induce to consider and manage these patients as affected by or at high risk for biventricular failure, thus requiring a system able to replace the function of both ventricles.

Currently available devices with such characteristic, which supply full flow, at least equal to the minimum cardiac index of 2.4 l/min, are:

- Extracorporeal life support (ECLS) – also known as venoarterial extracorporeal membrane oxygenation (ECMO)
- Biventricular VAD (BiVAD)
- Total artificial heart (TAH)

These devices differ considerably among them: ECLS can be deployed rapidly, at the bedside, and bears a relatively low complication rate. The main limits lie in the fact that it is a short-term support and it provides a *non-physiological* flow.

For these reasons, in INTERMACS profile 1 patients, where intervention is demanded within hours when not minutes, ECLS represents the first-line treatment, a "bridge-to-life" to keep the patient alive, while the optimal therapeutic strategy is determined.

ECLS can even be implanted using a percutaneous route, at the bedside under local anesthesia whenever the patient's condition allows. This microinvasive approach provides several advantages over the techniques currently used.

First of all, simplicity, therefore it can be carried out regardless of where the patient is admitted – even in outlying hospitals – and does not necessarily require the presence of a cardiac surgeon and an anesthetist.

Secondly, implantation with local anesthesia, instead of sedation/general anesthesia, minimizes the risk of further compromising the already unstable patient's hemodynamics.

Lastly, the minimal invasivity of this approach avoids open surgery, in particular sternotomy, thus reducing the risk of hemorrhage and infection. This is an extremely important consideration with ECLS as sepsis and bleeding are the two commonest complications.

Also, it's worth noting how major complications, which have traditionally deterred the indications for ECLS, have decreased with the availability of newer circuits and thinner cannulae as with increasing clinical experience.

8.3 Post-implant Management

After implant, at first all patients need full-flow support (patient's estimated required cardiac output, calculated as BSA*2.4 l/min). In this phase stabilization is obtained, with cardiac function totally replaced by ECLS, which guarantees circulatory support and organ perfusion.

At this point some pulsatility may be observed, and this would be a sign of some residual cardiac function. In this second phase, inotropic support is maintained, as is IABP when already present prior to ECLS implantation; awakening is fostered to guarantee sympathetic tone, and extubation achieved as soon as possible, to reduce pulmonary resistance. Support is reduced, monitoring pulsatility and organ perfusion (lactate, urine output, central venous pressure, pulmonary capillary wedge pressure).

Inotrope therapy is maintained to help the native heart opening the aortic valve and emptying the left ventricle (LV), thus eliminating the need for a vent. Otherwise, LV dilatation usually occurs, forewarning pulmonary edema. An option in this case is to insert an apical vent cannula, via left anterior mini-thoracotomy, and connect it to the venous line. The main disadvantage of this technique is the difficult monitoring and balancing of flows in the venous line, where blood from right atrium and left ventricle merge.

8.4 Weaning from Temporary Support

If the patient remains stable, the third phase is commenced, which consists of a weaning protocol. After obtaining hemodynamic stabilization and improvement of organ function (either neurologic, respiratory, renal, and hepatic), ECLS support is progressively decreased to 1 l/min. The persistence of satisfactory hemodynamics on low-to-medium dose inotropes supports the feasibility of weaning from ECLS. In detail, assessment includes echocardiographic evaluation of ventricular function (LVEF >35%, good RV contractility) and volume (absence of excessive ventricular distension or severe tricuspid regurgitation), as well as clinical parameters such as normal systemic pressure (systolic >85 mmHg) and central venous pressure, normal blood lactate level, and urine output.

The strategy after ECLS implant depends on etiology of the shock: it has been demonstrated that acute causes, such as myocardial infarction or myocarditis, achieve recovery in a very high percentage of cases, near 50%, while chronic cardiomyopathies do not.

Therefore, in "acute" patients the first objective to pursue is recovery, which can be predicted by some parameters:

- Blood pressure: mean > 60 mmHg, systolic > 85 mmHg
- Presence of arterial pulsatility
- Left ventricular ejection fraction >30%
- Satisfactory right ventricular contractility
- Tricuspid regurgitation less than severe
- EDVi < 100 ml
- Aortic velocity-time integral (VTI) ≥10 cm
- Spectral tissue Doppler lateral mitral annulus peak systolic annular velocity (TDSa) ≥6 cm/s
- Female gender

In our experience, successful weaning is normally associated with required flow less than 60% of the calculated full support.

It is reasonable to follow this path within the first 9 days, since mortality in the subgroup of patients with acute etiologies increases sensibly afterward.

Conversely, in decompensated chronic etiologies, ECLS still plays a role as a lifesaving tool, but from the onset it should be considered as a bridge to decision. *In view of the absence of reasonable chances of recovery, and of the constantly increasing mortality since the beginning of support, the plan about subsequent treatment should be taken within hours to a few days.*

Options include heart transplant, bridging to a long-term intracorporeal VAD, to a short-term paracorporeal LVAD or BiVAD, or to a TAH.

8.5 Multiple Organ Failure: Temporary ECMO or TAH Support?

Despite ECLS support, patients may develop organ failure, generally renal, hepatic, and respiratory. In this situation, ECLS is insufficient to revert the ongoing multiorgan dysfunction syndrome, and a device with higher output is needed.

Both TAH and BiVAD are an option, although evidence from the INTERMACS registry seems to favor the former.

The currently available SynCardia TAH, pumping up to 6.5 l/min with the 50 cc and 9 l/min with the 70 cc ventricle, provides higher, more physiological flows and is able to overcome elevated vascular resistances, either in the systemic and the pulmonary district.

The traditional limitation in implanting the SynCardia TAH in patients with less than 11 cm anteroposterior distance between sternum and T10 has been overcome by the introduction of the 50 cc model. This allowed to extend the indication to patients with more than 7.5 cm anteroposterior distance, BSA > 1.35.

Data on the role of TAH implantation in INTERMACS profile 1 patients are very limited, but recent experiences suggest good results, particularly when compared to VAD implantation in similar populations.

However, it is reasonable to directly implant TAH only when certain conditions are met:

- Absence of reasonable chances of recovery
- Biventricular failure, with associated end-organ damage
- In cases where BiVAD is contraindicated:
  - Refractory malignant arrhythmias
  - Large left ventricular thrombosis
  - Acquired ventricular septal defect
  - Restrictive cardiomyopathies
  - Complex congenital heart disease
  - Aortic regurgitation or the presence of mechanical aortic prosthesis

Finally, the TAH has historically been intended as a bridge to transplant, but as experience increases, its use as bridge-to-candidacy (recent history of cancer, elevated pulmonary vascular resistances) grows, and it has also recently been FDA approved for destination therapy.

Bibliography

1. Stevenson LW, Pagani FD, Young JB, Jessup M, Miller L, Kormos RL, Naftel DC, Ulisney K, Desvigne-Nickens P, Kirklin JK (2009) INTERMACS profiles of advanced heart failure: the current picture. J Heart Lung Transplant 28(6):535–541
2. Kirklin JK, Naftel DC, Pagani FD, Kormos RL, Stevenson LW, Blume ED, Myers SL, Miller MA, Baldwin JT, Young JB (2015) Seventh INTERMACS annual report: 15,000 patients and counting. J Heart Lung Transplant 34(12):1495–1504
3. Kirklin JK, Naftel DC, Kormos RL, Stevenson LW, Pagani FD, Miller MA, Baldwin JT, Young JB (2012) The fourth INTERMACS annual report: 4,000 implants and counting. J Heart Lung Transplant 31(2):117–126
4. Abrams D, Combes A, Brodie D (2014) Extracorporeal membrane oxygenation in cardiopulmonary disease in adults. J Am Coll Cardiol 63:2769–2778
5. Aissaoui N, Luyt CE, Leprince P, Trouillet JL, Léger P, Pavie A, Diebold B, Chastre J, Combes A (2011) Predictors of successful extracorporeal membrane oxygenation (ECMO) weaning after assistance for refractory cardiogenic shock. Intensive Care Med 37(11):1738–1745
6. Tarzia V, Bortolussi G, Bianco R, Buratto E, Bejko J, Carrozzini M, De Franceschi M, Gregori D, Fichera D, Zanella F, Bottio T, Gerosa G (2015) Extracorporeal life support in cardiogenic shock: impact of acute versus chronic etiology on outcome. J Thorac Cardiovasc Surg 150(2):333–340
7. Cook JA, Shah KB, Quader MA, Cooke RH, Kasirajan V, Rao KK, Smallfield MC, Tchoukina I, Tang DG (2015) The total artificial heart. J Thorac Dis 7(12):2172–2180
8. Kirklin JK, Naftel DC, Pagani FD, Kormos RL, Stevenson LW, Blume ED, Miller MA, Baldwin JT, Young JB (2014) Sixth INTERMACS annual report: a 10,000-patient database. J Heart Lung Transplant 33(6):555–564
9. Copeland JG, Smith RG, Arabia FA, Nolan PE, Sethi GK, Tsau PH, McClellan D, Slepian MJ, CardioWest Total Artificial Heart Investigators (2004) Cardiac replacement with a total artificial heart as a bridge to transplantation. N Engl J Med 351(9):859–867
10. Shah KB, Thanavaro KL, Tang DG, Kasirajan V (2013) Clinical outcomes for INTERMACS profile 1 patient implanted with the total artificial heart. J Heart Lung Transplant 32(4):S236

Low INTERMACS Profiles: Temporary Midterm Paracorporeal VAD Support

Steven Tsui, Colleen Pietras, and David L. Joyce

© Springer International Publishing Switzerland 2017
A. Montalto et al. (eds.), *Mechanical Circulatory Support in End-Stage Heart Failure*,
DOI 10.1007/978-3-319-43383-7_9

9.1 Introduction

Low INTERMACS profiles encompass a clinical spectrum which ranges from patients on intravenous inotropes with acceptable hemodynamics but deteriorating end-organ function (INTERMACS II) at one end to those in extremis requiring immediate circulatory support (INTERMACS I) at the other end. In all cases, the primary goal is prompt restoration of end-organ perfusion and oxygen delivery, with the aim of bridging patients to myocardial recovery or, in cases with no potential for cardiac recovery, more permanent forms of cardiac replacement therapy.

In the acutely unstable patient (e.g., those undergoing cardiopulmonary resuscitation or those with uncertain neurology following cardiac arrest), peripheral extracorporeal membrane oxygenation (ECMO) has become the temporary mechanical circulatory support (MCS) of choice in most institutions. This is due to its low cost and relative ease of insertion by the bedside in an emergency situation.

9.2 Why Not Use ECMO?

Mindful of the limitations of peripheral ECMO and its adverse event profile with extended duration of use, many physicians would prefer to deploy temporary ventricular assist devices (VADs) in the less unstable, low INTERMACS profile patients. Furthermore, some patients already supported with peripheral ECMO exhibit worrying clinical features that predispose to a poor outcome. They may benefit from the use of temporary VADs in addition to or instead of ECMO. These include patients with severe pulmonary edema resulting in upper body hypoxia and those with nonejecting ventricles (e.g., secondary to profound ventricular systolic dysfunction or intractable ventricular arrhythmias). A heart that is unable to eject adequately often leads to ventricular distension and stagnation of blood inside the cardiac chambers, pulmonary vasculature, and aortic root. These, in turn, predispose to in situ thrombosis, which is difficult to manage at the best of times and is often fatal. Therefore, before the situation becomes irretrievable, temporary VAD support may be deployed to decompress the left ventricle, enabling forward flow through the pulmonary circulation and to wash out the aortic root [1]. Selected temporary VAD systems may also permit the addition of an oxygenator to relieve upper body hypoxia until pulmonary edema resolves.

9.3 Why Not Use Durable VAD?

Although more durable MCS may be deployed in low INTERMACS profile patients, implantation of long-term VADs in acute cardiogenic shock patients is accompanied by higher perioperative risks and significantly reduced survival compared with their use in patients with higher INTERMACS profiles. The 2015 INTERMACS annual report on implantable VAD support revealed 6-month survivals of 82% in level 1, 87% in levels 2 and 3, and 89% in levels 4 through 7 patients ($P = 0.0001$) [2]. In all likelihood, patients who do not recover from the shock state with temporary MCS will probably not survive with longer-term VADs from the outset. Due to a tenfold difference in device cost, the primary use of temporary VADs to triage low INTERMACS profile patients would appear to be more cost-effective than using longer-term VADs in these situations.

The 2013 International Society of Heart and Lung Transplantation guidelines for mechanical circulatory support have provided recommendations of a limited number of scenarios in which long-term VAD may be considered in acute cardiogenic shock (Table 9.1) [3].

Table 9.1 2013 International Society of Heart and Lung Transplantation guidelines for mechanical circulatory support: indications for durable VADs in acute cardiogenic shock

A. Patients whose ventricular function is deemed unrecoverable or unlikely to recover without long-term device support
B. Patients who are deemed too ill to maintain normal hemodynamics and vital organ function with temporary MCS or who cannot be weaned from temporary MCS or inotropic support
C. Patients with the capacity for meaningful recovery of end-organ function and quality of life
D. Patients without irreversible end-organ damage

9.4 Rationale for Temporary VAD Support

In low INTERMACS profile patients in whom cardiac recovery is a possibility (e.g., patients with myocardial stunning following acute ischemia and reperfusion and those with fulminant myocarditis), it would probably be more appropriate to consider using temporary VAD support. A recent or evolving stroke is considered at least a temporary contraindication for implantable VAD. In emergency cases with uncertain neurology, a short-term VAD may be considered to allow for proper assessment of the neurologic status of the patient. In countries where temporary VAD support is an eligible criterion for the urgent heart transplant waiting list, even chronic heart failure patients with acute decompensation may be better off being supported with a temporary VAD, thus avoiding the long wait for a transplant once an implantable VAD is in place and its associated adverse events. If the waiting time for an urgent heart transplant is short in terms of days or weeks, temporary VAD support under these circumstances may actually prove to be more cost-effective as well (◘ Table 9.2).

◘ **Table 9.2** Indications for temporary VAD support in low INTERMACS profiles patients

Opportunity of myocardial recovery
Myocardial stunning following acute ischemia and reperfusion
Postcardiotomy
Fulminant myocarditis
Primary graft dysfunction post-heart transplant
Ominous features while on ECMO support
Severe pulmonary edema resulting in upper body hypoxia
Nonejecting ventricles with stasis
Unsuitable for primary durable VAD support
Recent or evolving stroke
Uncertain neurology following cardiac arrest
Severe end-organ dysfunction with uncertain capacity for recovery
Inadequate psychosocial support for home discharge

9.5 Types of Temporary VAD Systems

Temporary VADs are being used more frequently in order to normalize cardiac output in patients struggling with severe heart failure and, often times, patients in cardiogenic shock. There is a shift in pharmacologic therapy to a more hybrid approach incorporating MCSD. Bridge to decision is an option that utilizes temporary methods not only to stabilize the patient but to bide time until more definitive therapy has been decided. Some of the more common options include both percutaneous and surgical approaches(◘ Table 9.3).

TandemHeart system (CardiacAssist, Inc.) is an extracorporeal continuous-flow centrifugal pump which acts as a left atrial-to-femoral artery bypass (◘ Fig. 9.1). It consists of transseptal and arterial cannulae and a centrifugal blood pump which delivers flow rates up to 4 L/min at a maximum speed of 7500 rpm. Clinical trials [4–11] in the United States and Europe have provided evidence supporting an increase in cardiac index and mean arterial pressure and a subsequent decrease in pulmonary capillary wedge pressure.

Impella (Abiomed) is another extracorporeal device used for partial circulatory support and for determining intravascular pressure. Available in 2.5, 3.5, and 5.0 L options, the Impella is a short-term axial flow device that draws blood from the left ventricle and empties it into the aortic root (◘ Fig. 9.2). Benefits include reducing end-diastolic volume and pressure, mechanical work, myocardial wall tension, oxygen demand, and overall cardiac output.

HeartMate PHP (percutaneous heart pump) (Thoratec Corporation) is a low profile, rapid

◘ **Table 9.3** Examples of temporary ventricular assist devices

Percutaneous devices
TandemHeart
Impella
HeartMate PHP
Surgical options
Berlin EXCOR
CentriMag

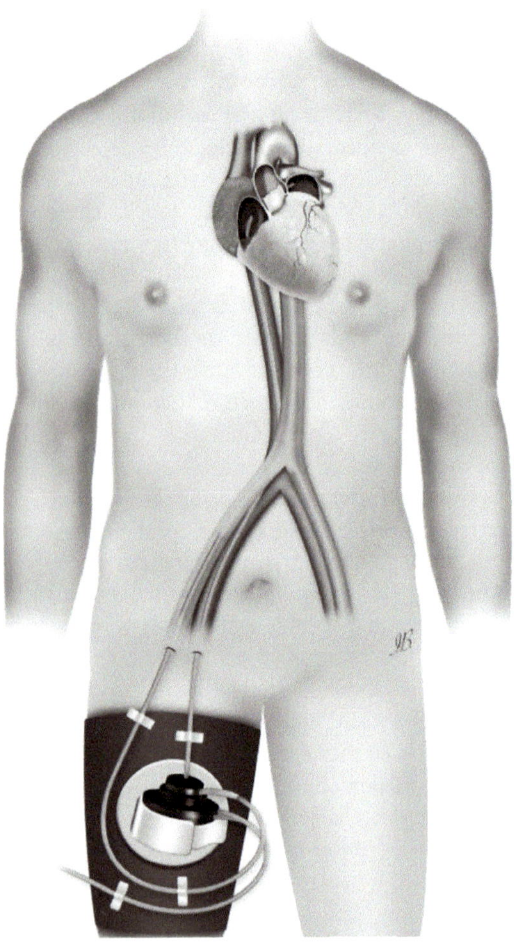

◘ **Fig. 9.1** TandemHeart system (CardiacAssist, Inc.) (Illustration by Ilaria Bondi's Peppermint Advertising)

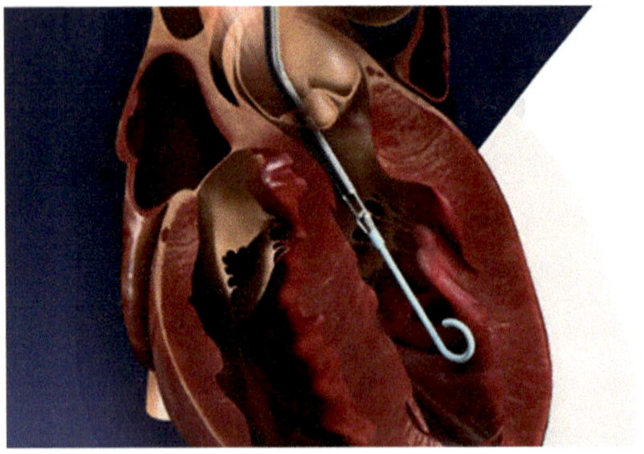

◘ **Fig. 9.2** Impella (Abiomed)

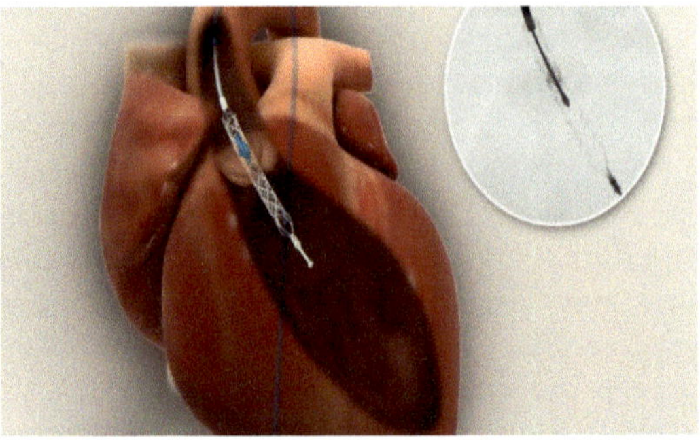

◘ **Fig. 9.3** HeartMate PHP (percutaneous heart pump)

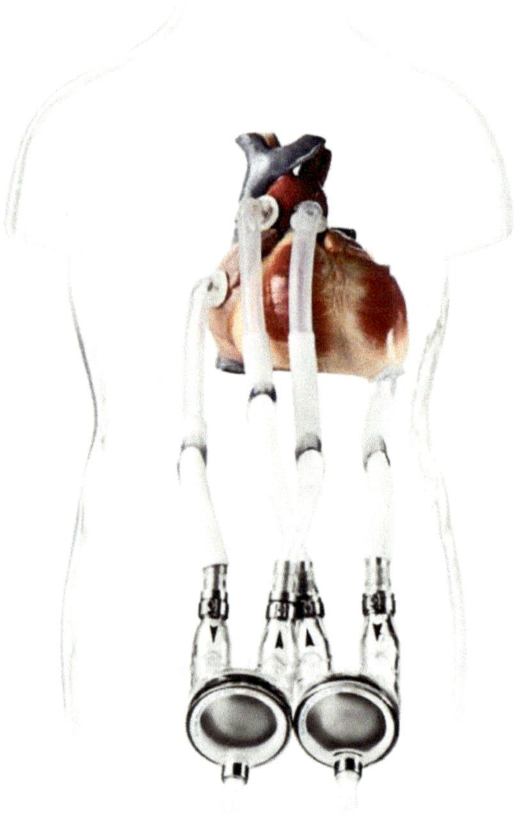

◘ **Fig. 9.4** Berlin EXCOR (Berlin Heart Inc.)

insertion, catheter-based heart pump designed to provide 4–5 L/min of high forward flow to unload the left ventricle and fulfill end-organ perfusion. It is inserted through the femoral artery using a 14 French sheath and, once through the aortic valve, expands to 24 French for maximal flow (◘ Fig. 9.3). This device is currently under investigation in postcardiotomy patients weaning from cardiopulmonary bypass.

Berlin EXCOR (Berlin Heart Inc.) is a pediatric VAD used as a bridge to transplant in eligible patients with severe isolated left ventricular or biventricular dysfunction in need of circulatory support (◘ Fig. 9.4). As an extra-

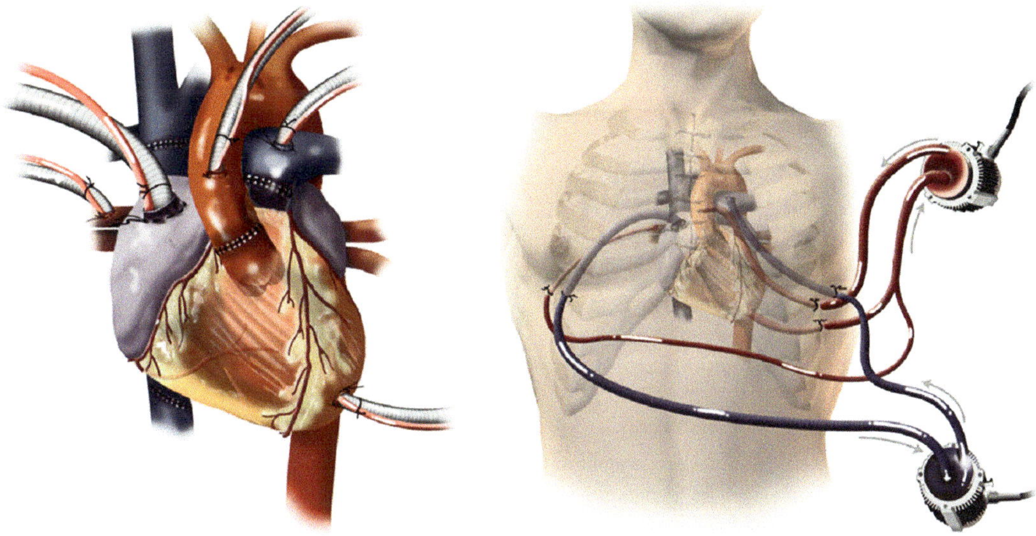

■ **Fig. 9.5** CentriMag (Thoratec Corporation)

corporeal, pneumatically driven, pulsatile VAD, it is designed for long-term support of the right and/or left ventricle when the heart is unable to sustain perfusion or pressure. It consists of one or two extracorporeal pumps, cannulas connecting them to the atrium or ventricle and great arteries, and an IKUS driving unit. The driving unit provides air pressure to the blood pump which moves the membrane and either fills or empties the chambers. The pumps are available in five sizes based on stroke volume (10, 25, 30, 50, and 60 mL). A multicenter prospective cohort study suggests its use has risen dramatically over the past decade wherein three-quarters of children survived to transplant or recovery.

CentriMag (Thoratec Corporation) is a continuous-flow extracorporeal centrifugal-type rotary blood pump that is magnetically levitated. It includes a single-use pump, reusable motor, and a monitoring console. The impeller floats freely and is held centrally in the flow path by a magnetic field (■ Fig. 9.5). The motor controls speed and checks its position 50,000 times/s. It is capable of delivering flows up to 9.9 L/min. It is designed for temporary left, right, or biventricular support. It is authorized to provide temporary circulatory support up to 30 days for patients in cardiogenic shock secondary to acute right ventricular failure. This contact-free environment minimizes hemolysis. It is simple to implant, easy to manage, and has excellent reliability and a low risk of thrombosis.

The ideal MSCD in the acute setting would allow percutaneous access, enable hemodynamic support and myocardial protection, and be associated with a low-complication rate. Cardiogenic shock complicates 5–8% of all admissions associated with myocardial infarction. The intra-aortic balloon pump (IABP) continues to be the most commonly used device worldwide. Retrospective studies show some mortality benefit, but randomized prospective studies show no benefit between devices. Recent advances in MCS are optimistic, but more randomized trials are needed to define clear indications for implantation preference.

In regard to the percutaneous approaches to cardiogenic shock, there are several ongoing studies which compare IABP to either standard treatments or to percutaneous left ventricular assist device (LVAD). Evidence supporting the use of IABP points toward a beneficial effect on hemodynamics, but there was no convincing randomized data supporting the use of IABP in infarct-related cardiogenic shock. When IABP was compared with percutaneous LVAD, there was no doubt that LVAD provided superior hemodynamic support in these patients, but their use did not improve early survival.

The Impella-EUROSHOCK registry looked at the same scenario requiring left ventricular support with the Impella 2.5 VAD. Results highlighted a reduction of lactate levels, suggesting improved organ perfusion. Patient selection appeared to be an important factor in that these patients maintained high 30-day mortality.

A multi-institutional study evaluated the safety, effectiveness, and outcomes of CentriMag in patients with cardiogenic shock. This preliminary study provided a short-term support for patients with cardiogenic shock and found a low incidence of device-related complications with no device failures. Results from the nationwide registry suggest that VADs can restore normal hemodynamics and support recovery of native cardiac function in the majority of patients when alternative options have been tried and failed.

The 2015 SCAI/ACC/HFSA/STS Clinical Expert Consensus Statement reviews the physiologic impact on the circulation of devices such as Impella, TandemHeart, and ECMO and their use in clinical situations, such as acute decompensated heart failure and cardiogenic shock. The consensus is that percutaneous devices are superior to pharmacologic therapy. IABP is thought to be less beneficial than Impella or TandemHeart. Devices may be considered when oxygenation remains impaired or for failure to wean off cardiopulmonary bypass. Univentricular or biventricular devices may be considered in severe biventricular failure, specifically with acute right ventricular failure associated with cardiogenic shock.

There is a consensus that randomized controlled trials involving all of these devices in a variety of clinical scenarios would be beneficial. In our experience at Mayo Clinic in Rochester, Minnesota, we recently came across a clinical situation involving a 55-year-old female with biventricular systolic and diastolic heart failure, dilated cardiomyopathy, and ejection fraction of 15–20%, who failed medical management.

Right heart catheterization showed severe pulmonary hypertension with a mean pulmonary artery pressure of 54 mmHg in the setting of massively elevated right and left heart filling pressures. Right atrial pressure was 25 mmHg, and wedge pressure was 25–30 mmHg. Cardiac index was 1.7 L/min/m^2, and pulmonary artery saturation was consistent with a low-output state (see Fig. 9.6). Nipride challenge was performed to a dose of 4.5 mcg/kg/min. Pulmonary artery pressure was subsequently stable, but wedge pressure went up, indicating a reduction in pulmonary vascular resistance. Pulmonary saturation did increase with the nitroprusside, suggesting a significant improvement in forward flow with vasodilatation (see Fig. 9.7).

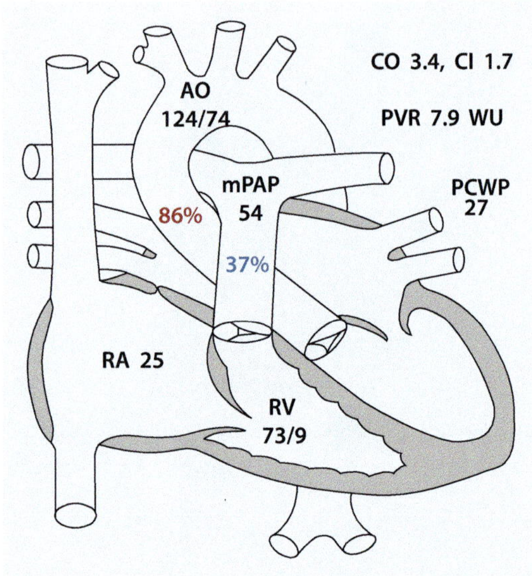

Fig. 9.6 Right atrial pressure was 25 mmHg, and wedge pressure was 25–30 mmHg. Cardiac index was 1.7 L/min/m^2, and pulmonary artery saturation was consistent with a low-output state

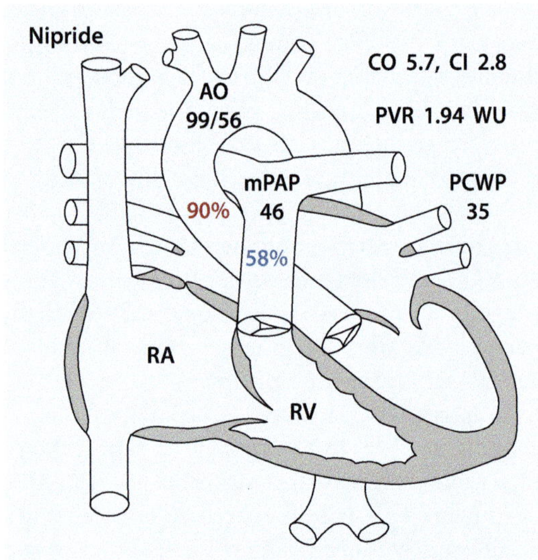

Fig. 9.7 Effect of Nipride. Wedge pressure went up, indicating a reduction in pulmonary vascular resistance. Pulmonary saturation did increase with the nitroprusside, suggesting a significant improvement in forward flow with vasodilatation

Our patient had advanced end-stage heart failure complicated by renal failure due to cardiorenal syndrome with an acute kidney injury. With the degree of right-sided heart failure and severe pulmonary hypertension, she initially was not believed to be a good LVAD candidate.

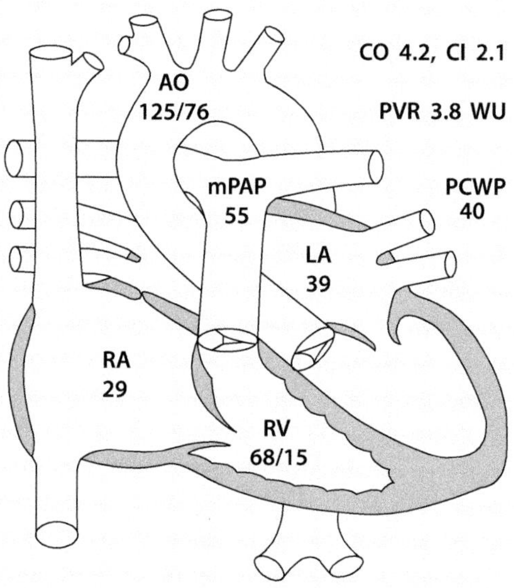

Fig. 9.8 Hemodynamic condition with 1 week of temporary MCS and milrinone therapy

Worsening renal function with diuretics despite extremely high filling pressures suggested she would not be a viable candidate for advanced therapies. However, she did tolerate a high dose of nitroprusside suggesting she might benefit from further afterload reduction. She continued on elevated doses of both hydralazine and isosorbide dinitrate.

In the interim, we considered short-term solutions to allow time for improved hepatorenal function in the setting of cardiogenic shock. We ultimately instituted short-term MCS with a TandemHeart device.

Following 1 week of temporary MCS, milrinone therapy, and diuresis, she remained hemodynamically stable with improved renal and hepatic function (see Fig. 9.8). She successfully underwent HeartMate II LVAD implantation as destination therapy with potential bridge to candidacy.

References

1. Narain S, Paparcuri G, Fuhrman TM, Silverman RB, Peruzzi WT (2012) Novel combination of impella and extra corporeal membrane oxygenation as a bridge to full recovery in fulminant myocarditis. Case Rep Critical Care 2012:459296
2. Feldman D, Pamboukian SV, Teuteberg JJ, Birks E, Lietz K, Moore SA et al (2013) The 2013 international society for heart and lung transplantation guidelines for mechanical circulatory support: executive summary. J Heart Lung Transplant 32:157–187
3. Kirklin JK, Naftel DC, Pagani FD, Kormos RL, Stevenson LW, Blume ED et al (2015) Seventh INTERMACS annual report: 15,000 patients and counting. J Heart Lung Transplant 34:1495–1504
4. Burkhoff D, Cohen H, Brunckhorst C, O'Neill W (2006) A randomized multicenter clinical study to evaluate the safety and efficacy of the tandemheart percutaneous ventricular assist device versus conventional therapy and intra-aortic balloon pumping for treatment of cardiogenic shock. Amer Heart J 152(3):469e1–469e8
5. Anderson M, Smedira N, Samuels L, Madani M, Naka Y et al (2010) Use of the AB5000 ventricular assist device in cardiogenic shock after acute myocardial infarction. Ann Thorac Cardiovasc Surg 90(3): 706–712
6. Rihal C, Naidu S, Givertz M, Szeto W, Burke J, Kapur N et al (2015) The 2015 SCAI/ACC/HFSA/STS clinical expert consensus statement on the use of percutaneous mechanical circulatory support devices in cardiovascular care. J Card Fail 21(6):499–518
7. Thiele H, Sick P, Boudriot E, Diederich KW, Hambrecht R et al (2005) Randomized comparison of intra-aortic balloon support with a percutaneous left ventricular assist device in patients with revascularized acute myocardial infarction complicated by cardiogenic shock. Eur Heart J 26(13):1276–1283
8. Seyfarth M, Sibbing D, Bauer I, Frohlich G, Bott-Flugel L (2008) A randomized clinical trial to evaluate safety and efficacy of a percutaneous left ventricular assist device versus intra-aortic balloon pump for treatment of cardiogenic shock caused by myocardial infarction. J Amer Coll Cardiol 52(19):1584–1588
9. John R, Long JW, Massey HT, Griffith BP, Sun BC et al (2011) Outcomes of a multicenter trial of the levitronix centrimag ventricular assist system for short-term circulatory support. J Thorac Cardiovasc Surg 141(4): 932–939
10. Lauten A, Engstrom AE, Jung C, Empen K, Erne P et al (2013) Percutaneous left ventricular support with the impella-2.5-assist-device in acute cardiogenic shock: results of the impella-EUROSHOCK-registry. Circ Heart Fail 6(1):23–30
11. Cheng J, den Uil C, Hoeks S, van der Ent M, Jewbali L et al (2009) Percutaneous left ventricular assist devices vs intra-aortic balloon pump counterpulsation for treatment of cardiogenic shock: a meta- analysis of controlled trials. J Eur Heart 30(17):2102–2108

Low INTERMACS Profiles: One-Stage Durable LVAD Implantation for INTERMACS Level 1: Indications and Contraindications

Daisuke Yoshioka, Koji Takeda, Hiroo Takayama, and Yoshifumi Naka

© Springer International Publishing Switzerland 2017
A. Montalto et al. (eds.), *Mechanical Circulatory Support in End-Stage Heart Failure*, DOI 10.1007/978-3-319-43383-7_10

10.1 Introduction

Left ventricular assist devices (LVADs) have become the standard of care for patients with end-stage heart failure as a bridge-to-transplant (BTT) therapy [1] and as a destination therapy (DT) [2]. Over the past decade, numbers of LVAD implants in North America have grown exponentially, with over 15,000 patients undergoing LVAD implantation with continuous-flow LVAD. Approval of DT and other studies have accelerated the shift of timing of LVAD implantation to more ambulatory patients with heart failure in several years [3]. However, in the seventh annual Interagency Registry for Mechanically Assisted Circulatory Support (INTERMACS) report, about 15% of all patients with INTERMACS profile 1 underwent LVAD implantation, and this rate has not changed in the past several years [4]. Therefore, it is important to discuss about the treatment strategy for patients at the INTERMACS level 1. The major problems of patients at the INTERMACS level 1 include not only decompensated hemodynamic condition but also other organ dysfunction or uncertified neurological status. At the first encounter for patients with cardiogenic shock, candidacy for DT or BTT LVAD is often unclear. In addition, because of the severity of their illness, the time to make a decision is very limited. Therefore, an alternative approach instead of primary implantable LVAD insertion may be considered using short-term mechanical circulatory support (MCS) for patients at the INTERMACS level 1. This treatment strategy is considered as a bridge-to-decision therapy. The merit of this strategy is that stabilization of hemodynamics and improvement of organ function can be achieved before long-term durable LVAD implantation. We reported favorable outcomes with CentriMag (Thoratec Co., Pleasanton, CA) VAD usage in patients with cardiogenic shock [5]. Moreover, recent advances in technology enable us to implant percutaneous short-term VADs such as extracorporeal membrane oxygenation (ECMO) and Impella (Abiomed, Danvers, MA). Percutaneous MCS devices can be less invasively implanted and are especially applicable for salvage treatment in critically ill cases [6]. This staged procedure has potential benefits to restore hemodynamic instability and end-organ function and may improve outcomes following definitive surgeries [7]. On the other hand, there remain several concerns in the bridge-to-decision strategy. Patients require a second intervention in cases which require subsequent implantable LVAD insertion. The second surgery after surgical short-term VAD requires adhesive dissection and more transfusions. Moreover, bridge-to-bridge surgery imposes increasing risk of device infection on patients [8]. In addition, bridging strategy using multiple MCS devices could increase medical cost and impose prolonged hospital stay. Thus, one-stage durable LVAD implantation is possibly advantageous with regards to cost and adverse consequences associated by multiple interventions. No studies have been conducted comparing outcomes between two strategies in INTERMACS 1 patients. Nonetheless, utmost careful attention must be paid for appropriate patient selection.

10.2 Indications

INTERMACS profile 1, which is defined as "crash and burn" or critical cardiogenic shock, includes a wide range of patients. Their etiologies can include acute myocardial infarction (AMI), acute decompensated cardiac myopathy, postcardiotomy shock, and fulminant myocarditis. All these patients do not necessarily need durable LVAD. Patients with fulminant myocarditis often rapidly deteriorate and require MCS; however, prognosis of fulminant myocarditis is much better than other etiologies, and many patients with fulminant myocarditis achieve myocardial recovery within 1 month [9–12]. Then, it is reasonable to implant temporary MCS rather than one-stage durable LVAD. The advantage of one-stage durable LVAD insertion is also quite limited in the setting of postcardiotomy shock. Temporary MCS such as ECMO should be considered in this situation. In patients with acute decompensating heart failure, it seems feasible to implant durable LVAD if they are already listed on a heart transplant list or are obvious candidates for DT therapy. Acute myocardial infarction (AMI) requires more complicated strategies. Almost all patients with AMI would never be listed for heart transplantation, and they are often obscure for BTT/DT candidacy because of coexistent multiple comorbidities. Moreover, these patients always receive antiplatelet therapy before and after percutaneous coronary intervention or other causes. There have been very few reports on one-stage implantation for AMI [13, 14]. However, the number of implantable LVAD patients included in this study was very limited; therefore, further studies are mandatory to analyze the efficacy of one-stage implantation in AMI patients.

INTERMACS level 1 patients have variable end-organ function from end-stage failure to normal limit. Pre-existing renal dysfunction with a cutoff creatinine value of 1.96 mg/dL was an independent risk factor for early mortality after durable VAD implantation for patients at the INTERMACS level 1 [15]. Several studies have also reported on the relationship between renal function and mortality [16–19]. Although preoperative renal dysfunction can improve after LVAD implantation, patients in profound cardiogenic shock often require perioperative renal replacement therapy, resulting in prolonged ICU stay, increased risks of other complications, and eventual death. Early interventions to restore end-organ perfusion should be considered without delay. If renal function progressively declines despite optimal medical therapy, bridge-to-decision strategy might be considered to see reversibility of renal function. These patients often have simultaneous hepatic dysfunction. Hepatic dysfunction usually accompanies coagulation disorder and platelet dysfunction. The one-stage implantation of durable LVAD will bring the risk of intra- and postoperative bleeding complications in these patients. It would be reasonable to use the less invasive temporal MCS to avoid more invasive one-stage LVAD implantation in those with coagulopathy.

INTERMACS 1 patients usually have pulmonary edema due to an increase of pulmonary venous system pressure. Pulmonary edema can dramatically improve after left ventricular unloading by LVAD. However, for patients complicated with severe acute pulmonary injury, simultaneous implantation of a temporary right ventricular assist device (RVAD) with membrane oxygenator can be considered as an option [20].

Unknown neurological status is also a common complication in INTERMACS 1 patients because of their acuity of illness. In these patients, predicting the neurological prognosis in the acute phase is difficult, and it will usually take several days to weeks to recover. Unknown neurological status should be a contraindication for durable LVAD; thus, it is reasonable to bridge them with a short-term MCS before durable LVAD insertion.

Because of these baseline patient illnesses, mortality after primary LVAD implantation in INTERMACS 1 is significantly higher than that of patients in other INTERMACS profile [4]. The INTERMACS data showed 82, 76, and 58% of survival at 6, 12, and 36 months, respectively. The contributed hazard ratio of INTERMACS level 1 for early cause mortality was 1.55 in this report. The careful decision-making for one-stage implantation of durable LVAD for patients at the INTERMACS level 1 should be warranted considering high-risk patient profiles. The HeartMate II risk score (HMRS), which is calculated using patients' age, albumin, serum creatinine, international normalized ratio (INR), and center volume, has been reported to be useful to predict the mortality after LVAD implantation in INTERMACS level 2 or more ambulant patients [21]. Recently, Adamo et al. reported that HMRS was also useful to predict the mortality of patients at the INTERMACS level 1 [22]. In this report, the 90-day mortality was 6.9%, 11.8%, and 39.1% in low, mild, and high HMRS groups, respectively. Considering these results, one-stage durable LVAD implantation might be a feasible option for patients in the low to mild HMRS groups within the INTERMACS level 1.

10.3 Surgical Procedure

Implantation of durable LVAD in patients at the INTERMACS level 1 can be done in a similar manner to that of patients in other INTERMACS profiles. Meticulous attention should be paid to reduce surgical invasion and to salvage patients. One major concern during the perioperative period is worsening of right-sided heart failure. Patients in cardiogenic shock often show some degree of biventricular dysfunction. The INTERMACS annual report revealed that patients with INTERMACS profile 1 developed postoperative right-sided heart failure more frequently than those in other profiles. Others showed that INTERMACS level 1 was one of the risk factors for requirement of postoperative RVAD [4, 23, 24]. Sustained right-sided heart failure after LVAD surgery imposes further end-organ damage. Timely insertion of RVAD is necessary before end-organ malperfusion progresses. An aggressive use of concomitant temporary RVAD insertion might be warranted to facilitate end-organ recovery in patients with profound shock.

10.4 Conclusion

Because of lack of previous studies, it remains unclear whether one-stage implantation of durable LVAD is superior to bridge-to-decision strategy for patients at the INTERMACS level 1 in terms of mortality, morbidity, and medical cost. Currently, decision making for treatment strategy for patients in INTERMACS level 1 mainly depends on each institution and/or surgeon's preference. More importantly, INTERMACS 1 profile includes a variety range of patients' cohort. Therefore, current profiles system does not adequately stratify the risk for one-stage durable LVAD implantation. From the limited available data, one-stage durable LVAD implantation seems feasible in certain cohort of patients within INTERMACS 1 profile. However, further clinical studies should be demanded to reveal a better comprehensive strategy in patients within INTERMACS 1 profile.

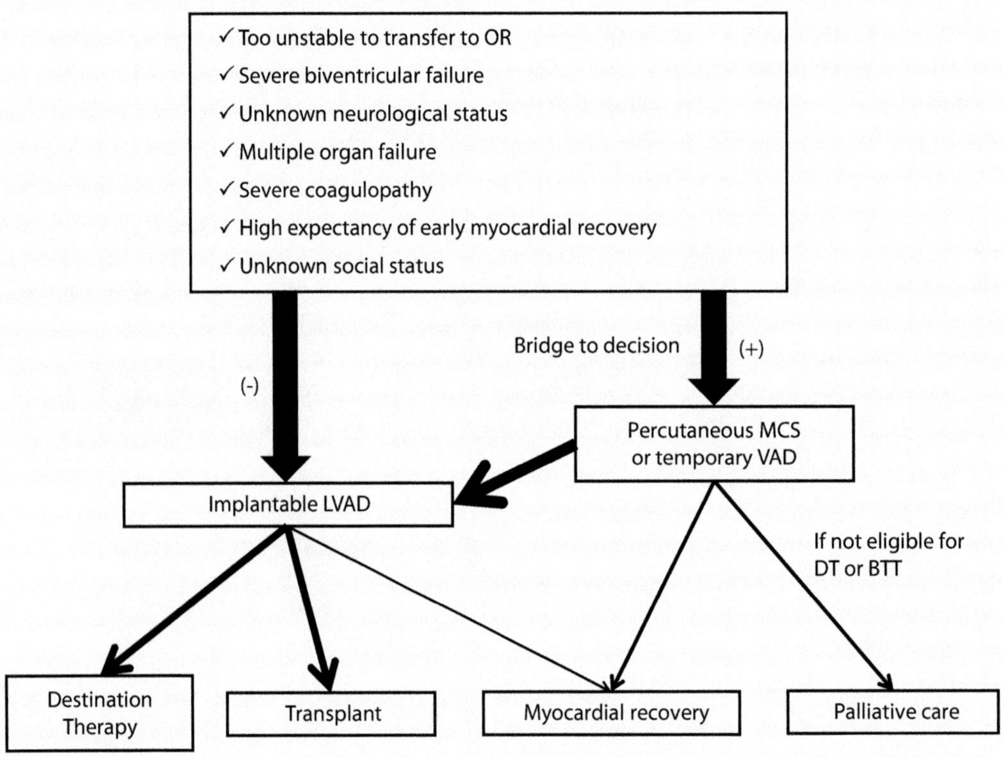

References

1. Miller LW, Pagani FD, Russell SD, John R, Boyle AJ, Aaronson KD et al (2007) Use of a continuous-flow device in patients awaiting heart transplantation. N Engl J Med 357:885–896
2. Rose EA, Gelijns AC, Moskowitz AJ, Heitjan DF, Stevenson LW, Dembitsky W et al (2001) Long-term use of a left ventricular assist device for end-stage heart failure. N Engl J Med 345:1435–1443
3. Estep JD, Starling RC, Horstmanshof DA, Milano CA, Selzman CH, Shah KB et al (2015) Risk assessment and comparative effectiveness of left ventricular assist device and medical management in ambulatory heart failure patients: results from the ROADMAP study. J Am Coll Cardiol 66:1747–1761
4. Kirklin JK, Naftel DC, Pagani FD, Kormos RL, Stevenson LW, Blume ED et al (2015) Seventh INTERMACS annual report: 15,000 patients and counting. J Heart Lung Transp 34:1495–1504
5. Takayama H, Soni L, Kalesan B, Truby LK, Ota T, Cedola S et al (2014) Bridge-to-decision therapy with a continuous-flow external ventricular assist device in refractory cardiogenic shock of various causes. Circ Heart Fail 7:799–806
6. Truby L, Mundy L, Kalesan B, Kirtane A, Colombo PC, Takeda K et al (2015) Contemporary outcomes of venoarterial extracorporeal membrane oxygenation

for refractory cardiogenic shock at a large tertiary care center. ASAIO J 61:403–409
7. Takayama H, Soni L, Kalesan B, Truby LK, Ota T, Cedola S et al (2014) Bridge-to-decision therapy with a continuous-flow external ventricular assist device in refractory cardiogenic shock of various causes. Circ Heart Fail. 7:799–806
8. Yoshioka D, Sakaguchi T, Saito S, Miyagawa S, Nishi H, Yoshikawa Y et al (2012) Initial experience of conversion of Toyobo paracorporeal left ventricular assist device to DuraHeart left ventricular assist device. Circ J 76:372–376
9. McCarthy RE 3rd, Boehmer JP, Hruban RH, Hutchins GM, Kasper EK, Hare JM et al (2000) Long-term outcome of fulminant myocarditis as compared with acute (nonfulminant) myocarditis. N Engl J Med 342:690–695
10. Diddle JW, Almodovar MC, Rajagopal SK, Rycus PT, Thiagarajan RR (2015) Extracorporeal membrane oxygenation for the support of adults with acute myocarditis. Crit Care Med 43:1016–1025
11. Lorusso R, Centofanti P, Gelsomino S, Barili F, Di Mauro M, Orlando P et al (2015) Venoarterial extracorporeal membrane oxygenation for acute fulminant myocarditis in adult patients: a 5-year multi-institutional experience. Ann Thorac Surg 27:S0003-S4975. (15)01375-2
12. Mody KP, Takayama H, Landes E, Yuzefpolskaya M, Colombo PC, Naka Y et al (2014) Acute mechanical circulatory support for fulminant myocarditis complicated by cardiogenic shock. J Cardiovasc Transl Res 7:156–164
13. Pawale A, Pinney S, Ashley K, Flynn R, Milla F, Anyanwu AC (2013) Implantable left ventricular assist devices as initial therapy for refractory postmyocardial infarction cardiogenic shock. Eur J Cardiothorac Surg 44:213–216
14. Dang NC, Topkara VK, Leacche M, John R, Byrne JG, Naka Y (2005) Left ventricular assist device implantation after acute anterior wall myocardial infarction and cardiogenic shock: a two-center study. J Thorac Cardiovasc Surg 130:693–698
15. Yoshioka D, Sakaguchi T, Saito S, Miyagawa S, Nishi H, Yoshikawa Y et al (2012) Predictor of early mortality for severe heart failure patients with left ventricular assist device implantation: significance of INTERMACS level and renal function. Circ J 76:1631–1638
16. Klotz S, Vahlhaus C, Riehl C, Reitz C, Sindermann JR, Scheld HH (2010) Pre-operative prediction of post-VAD implant mortality using easily accessible clinical parameters. J Heart Lung Transplant. 29(1):45–52
17. Lietz K, Long JW, Kfoury AG, Slaughter MS, Silver MA, Milano CA et al (2007) Outcomes of left ventricular assist device implantation as destination therapy in the post-REMATCH era: implications for patient selection. Circulation 116:497–505
18. Sandner SE, Zimpfer D, Zrunek P, Rajek A, Schima H, Dunkler D, Grimm M, Wolner E, Wieselthaler GM (2009) Renal function and outcome after continuous flow left ventricular assist device implantation. Ann Thorac Surg 87:1072–1078
19. Butler J, Geisberg C, Howser R, Portner PM, Rogers JG, Deng MC et al (2006) Relationship between renal function and left ventricular assist device use. Ann Thorac Surg 81:1745–1751
20. Leidenfrost J, Prasad S, Itoh A, Lawrance CP, Bell JM, Silvestry SC (2016) Right ventricular assist device with membrane oxygenator support for right ventricular failure following implantable left ventricular assist device placement. Eur J Cardiothorac Surg 49: 73–77
21. Cowger J, Sundareswaran K, Rogers JG, Park SJ, Pagani FD, Bhat G et al (2013) Predicting survival in patients receiving continuous flow left ventricular assist devices: the HeartMate II risk score. J Am Coll Cardiol 61(3):313–321
22. Adamo L, Nassif M, Tibrewala A, Novak E, Vader J, Silvestry SC et al (2015) The heartmate risk score predicts morbidity and mortality in unselected left ventricular assist device recipients and risk stratifies INTERMACS class 1 patients. JACC Heart Fail 3: 283–290
23. Saito S, Matsumiya G, Sakaguchi T, Miyagawa S, Yoshikawa Y, Yamauchi T et al (2010) Risk factor analysis of long-term support with left ventricular assist system. Circ J 74:715–722
24. Kormos RL, Teuteberg JJ, Pagani FD, Russell SD, John R, Miller LW et al (2010) Right ventricular failure in patients with the HeartMate II continuous-flow left ventricular assist device: incidence, risk factors, and effect on outcomes. J Thorac Cardiovasc Surg 139:1316–1324

Bridge to Transplant and Destination Therapy Strategies in the United States

Yasuhiro Shudo, Hanjay Wang, Andrew B. Goldstone, and Y. Joseph Woo

© Springer International Publishing Switzerland 2017
A. Montalto et al. (eds.), *Mechanical Circulatory Support in End-Stage Heart Failure*,
DOI 10.1007/978-3-319-43383-7_11

11.1 Introduction

Heart disease is the leading cause of death in the United States. Advanced or medically refractory heart failure represents the end-stage form of heart disease, and carries a life expectancy of less than 2 years [1]. Many treatments have been developed for patients with end-stage heart failure, among which heart transplantation remains the standard [2]. However, the persistent shortage of available donor organs has resulted in an ever-increasing waitlist for transplantation, as well as longer waiting periods prior to surgery.

Within the last 15 years, major strides have been made in the area of mechanical circulatory support (MCS), allowing patients with medically refractory heart failure a number of exciting and practical alternatives to heart transplantation. In the REMATCH trial, investigators prospectively randomized 129 patients ineligible for heart transplant to optimal medical therapy or left ventricular assist device (LVAD) implantation, and demonstrated a 48% reduction in the risk of death from any cause in the LVAD group. Published in 2001, this landmark trial not only illustrated the dismal prognosis for patients with end-stage heart failure who are managed with medical therapy alone, but also demonstrated the relative superiority of LVAD therapy, with benefits achieved in both survival and quality of life (◘ Fig. 11.1) [3]. Since that time, we have witnessed significant technological advancements in MCS, including a transition from pulsatile to continuous-flow pumps, and a progressive miniaturization of increasingly durable MCS devices. Following approval by the US Food and Drug Administration (FDA) in 2008–2010, continuous-flow LVADs are now employed for both transplant-eligible patients as bridge to transplant (BTT) and transplant-ineligible patients as destination therapy (DT) [4–6]. Overall, a total of 2,431 long-term MCS devices were implanted in the year 2014 alone [6].

This chapter will focus on the use of implantable long-term MCS devices as BTT and DT for adult patients with advanced heart failure. Specifically, we will review the landscape of BTT and DT in the United States, as well as describe considerations for device selection.

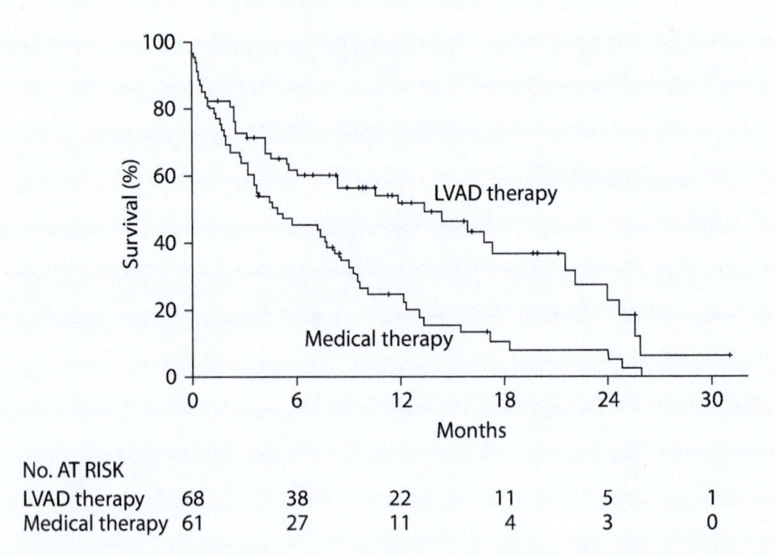

◘ **Fig. 11.1** Kaplan-Meier analysis of survival for transplant-ineligible patients who received a left ventricular assist device (LVAD) versus optimal medical therapy (Reproduced, with permission, from Rose et al. [3])

11.2 Strategies for Mechanical Circulatory Support

The strategies underlying the use of implantable MCS devices in patients with end-stage heart failure are stratified based on transplant eligibility, and include bridge to transplant (BTT) as well as destination therapy (DT) [3–9]. BTT is a strategy for patients actively listed for heart transplantation, utilizing MCS to prevent death or progressive end-organ dysfunction in the setting of low cardiac output while awaiting transplant. In contrast, DT is a strategy for patients requiring lifelong circulatory support, who are not eligible for heart transplantation because of relative or absolute contraindications. There exist additional MCS strategies including bridge to candidacy (i.e., for patients who are not currently listed for heart transplantation and have no absolute contraindications to transplant, but who have medical, social, or financial barriers to transplant candidacy at the time of evaluation) and bridge to recovery (i.e., for patients who may expect sufficient recovery of native myocardial function after temporary MCS device implantation to unload the recovering ventricle), although these will not be within the scope of our discussion below.

It is important to note that, although distinct strategies (BTT or DT) can be defined with regard to clinical intent at the time of MCS device implantation (◘ Fig. 11.2), these strategies can also evolve as a patient's condition changes over time. For example, a DT patient who was previously ineligible for transplant may experience improvement in comorbidities after LVAD implantation and become transplant-eligible with MCS. Alternatively, a BTT patient awaiting transplant after LVAD implantation may become transplant-ineligible because of device-related complications or progression of coexistent comorbidities. Therefore, patient assignment to BTT or DT may be dynamic and is dependent on the clinical situation. Decisions about candidacy for each strategy should be made collaboratively by an experienced heart failure team, including both surgeons and cardiologists, and reassessed as dictated by the patient's clinical course. This process is particularly important in order to ensure appropriate patient selection, proper device selection, and optimal timing for device placement.

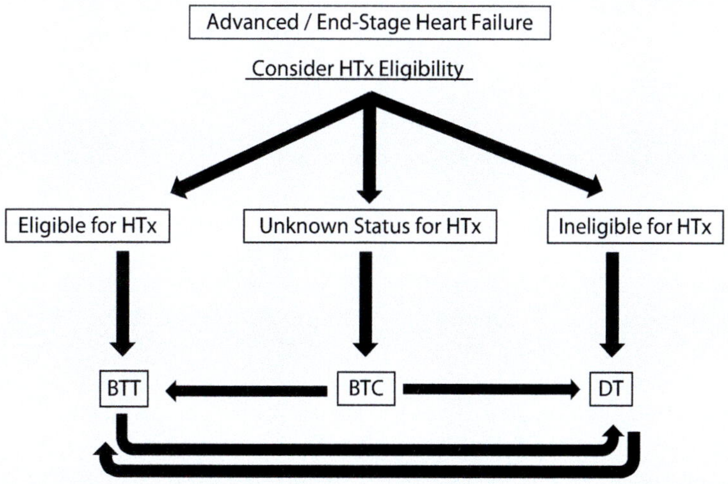

◘ **Fig. 11.2** Strategies for mechanical circulatory support implantation. *HTx* indicates orthotopic heart transplant; *BTT*, bridge to transplant; *BTC*, bridge to candidacy; and *DT*, destination therapy

The selection of patients for MCS device implantation requires careful evaluation of heart failure history and severity. The general indicators of advanced heart failure leading to referral for MCS device implantation include New York Heart Association (NYHA) class IIIb–IV symptoms, failure of optimal medical therapies, frequent hospitalizations for heart failure exacerbation, inotrope dependence, recurrent or refractory ventricular tachyarrhythmia, unresponsiveness to cardiac resynchronization therapy, end-organ dysfunction due to low cardiac output, peak oxygen consumption less than 14 ml/kg/min, and 6 minute walk distance less than 300 meter [10]. To aid in the identification of patients who might benefit from LVAD support, the Seattle Heart Failure Model can be used to estimate a heart failure patient's expected mortality over the subsequent 1 to 2 years [11]. A thorough assessment of operative risk and potential complications must also be performed to determine whether a patient is an appropriate surgical candidate for an implantable MCS device.

Another critical component of the preoperative evaluation for MCS involves determining the potential need for biventricular support. Previous work has clearly demonstrated a significant mortality benefit when patients at risk of failing isolated LVAD therapy and requiring biventricular support receive early, planned biventricular assist device (BiVAD) therapy instead of an LVAD followed by later conversion to BiVAD therapy. In one study of 99 patients who ultimately received BiVAD support, the survival at 1 year post-implantation was 48% among patients who were planned for direct BiVAD implantation, versus 25% for patients who received an LVAD initially and were later converted to BiVAD therapy [12]. To assist in determining which patients may ultimately require biventricular support, the 5-point CRITT score may be utilized, in which a binary scoring system (i.e., 0 or 1 point) is applied for each of five criteria identified by multivariable analysis to be associated with increased risk of requiring biventricular support: central venous pressure > 15 mmHg (C), severe right ventricular dysfunction (R), preoperative mechanical ventilation or intubation (I), severe tricuspid regurgitation (T), and tachycardia (T) [13]. According to this model, 93% of patients with a total CRITT score of 0 or 1 successfully tolerated isolated LVAD therapy, whereas 80% of patients with a score of 4 or 5 required biventricular support. As such, isolated LVAD therapy may be recommended for patients with a CRITT score of 0–1, and BiVAD therapy may be recommended for a score of 4–5. Patients with a CRITT score of 2-3 have less predictable outcomes, and may tolerate isolated LVAD therapy with appropriate pharmacologic support, or may require temporary right ventricular support.

11.2.1 Bridge to Transplant (BTT)

Historically, BTT once represented the predominant strategy for patients receiving an implantable MCS device, with 42.4% of patients in the 2006–2007 INTERMACS registry actively listed for heart transplant at the time of device implantation [5]. Although the proportion of MCS strategies declared as BTT decreased to 21.7% by 2011–2013 (with a concomitant increase seen in the use of DT), BTT continues to serve as an invaluable option for patients for whom heart transplantation remains the ideal ultimate therapy.

It is well established that patients actively awaiting heart transplant experience improved survival, functional status, and quality of life through the use of a long-term durable LVAD as BTT therapy [14–15]. In a study of 133 patients who received a continuous-flow LVAD as BTT, Miller et al. observed survival at 180 days post-implant to be 75%, including those who received a heart transplant, those who recovered native cardiac function, and those with continued survival on MCS [14]. Based on more recent data from the INTERMACS registry in 2014, the actuarial survival of BTT patients at 1 year is now expected to be >80% [5]. Miller et al. also observed recovery in renal and hepatic function after LVAD implantation, measured by significant improvements in serum creatinine, blood urea nitrogen, and transaminase levels at 3 months post-implant. Functional status improved by at least two NYHA classes in 83% of patients by 3 months post-implant.

The percentage of BTT patients receiving a heart transplant by 1 year after device implantation is currently 20–30% [6]. In light of the continued organ shortage, the BTT strategy is perhaps most beneficial in patients who are expected to have an extended time on the waiting list for heart transplantation. Reasons for an extended waiting time commonly include ABO blood type, large body habitus, or the presence of anti-HLA antibodies. However, for any patient under consideration for BTT therapy, the overall operative risk combines those associated with two surgeries instead of one. The initial LVAD implantation procedure is typically approached through a median sternotomy and performed with cardiopulmonary bypass, and the potential postoperative complications (e.g., bleeding, infection, stroke, thrombosis, and LVAD failure) can in some cases affect a patient's ultimate transplant eligibility. The eventual transplant operation would involve a redo sternotomy and repeat cardiopulmonary bypass, both of which are associated with increased operative risk. For heart failure patients with a previous history of cardiac surgery prior to LVAD implantation, commonly including coronary artery bypass grafting, valve surgery, or congenital repairs, the operative risk is greater still, and may even be prohibitive. Furthermore, the transfusion of blood products during or after the initial LVAD implantation procedure can result in increased sensitization to HLA antibodies, which ultimately may increase the difficulty of finding a suitable donor match [16]. All of the above must be carefully considered in order to appropriately select patients for successful BTT therapy.

11.2.2 Destination Therapy (DT)

Over the past decade, LVAD therapy as DT has become a well-established option for end-stage heart failure patients with contraindications to heart transplantation [3–6, 9]. As introduced previously, the prospectively randomized REMATCH trial first illustrated the superiority of LVAD therapy (using the HeartMate XVE) over optimal medical therapy alone among transplant-ineligible patients in 2001. Survival at 1 year was 52% among LVAD recipients versus 23% among patients medically-managed [3]. Later in 2009, the pulsatile-flow HeartMate XVE was compared to the newer continuous-flow HeartMate II in a randomized study of 200 advanced heart failure patients who were ineligible for transplant [7]. Survival at 1 year was 68% in the HeartMate II group versus 52% for the HeartMate XVE group, and at 2 years, 58% compared to 24%, respectively. For reference, the 2-year survival among medically-managed, transplant-ineligible patients in the REMATCH trial was just 8% [3]. Thus, for end-stage heart failure patients with contraindications to heart transplantation, commonly including those with advanced age (over 72 years old), morbid obesity (body mass index greater than 35 kg/m^2), active infection, severe diabetes mellitus, severe peripheral vascular disease, psychosocial instability, recent drug/alcohol/tobacco abuse (within 6 months), and irreversible pulmonary hypertension [15], the survival benefit associated with MCS use as DT is well established. These patients also experience significant improvements in quality of life based on assessments such as the Minnesota Living with Heart Failure Questionnaire and Kansas City Cardiomyopathy Questionnaire, as well as considerable recovery of functional status, with 80% of patients who received a HeartMate II having NYHA class I or II symptoms at 2 years after LVAD implantation [7].

Given the advancements in technology and the parallel improvements in patient care and selection, the use of MCS as DT has rapidly grown over the past decade. In the 2006–2007 INTERMACS registry, only 14.7% of patients who received an LVAD were declared for DT, but by 2011–2014, the DT proportion had increased dramatically to 46%, becoming the predominant strategy among all LVAD implantations [5–6]. In fact, because DT LVADs have demonstrated such effectiveness under its original indication (i.e., for transplant-ineligible patients with less than 2 years life expectancy on maximal heart failure medication), some surgeons and cardiologists have advocated expanding the use of LVAD therapy as DT to include heart failure patients who are less ill and who have not yet developed sequelae of end-stage cardiac insufficiency. To this end, the Randomized Evaluation of VAD InterVEntion before Inotropic Therapy (REVIVE-IT) trial has been designed to evaluate all-cause mortality, functional status, and quality of life among heart failure patients who are not dependent on inotropes and who do not exhibit end-organ dysfunction due to heart failure. Patients will be randomized to early LVAD therapy or optimal medical therapy [17]. Overall, with further optimizations in patient care and selection strategy moving forward, and continued innovations in MCS device technology to enhance durability, safety, and convenience, DT LVADs have the potential to reduce the burden of the current donor organ shortage, and eventually may even challenge heart transplantation as the standard of care for patients with end-stage heart failure [18].

11.3 Device Selection for Mechanical Circulatory Support

Currently in the United States, several different durable MCS devices are FDA approved and actively used either as BTT or DT (◘ Table 11.1). As previously discussed regarding selection of a specific MCS strategy (BTT versus DT), the selection of a specific device for MCS should also be made collaboratively by an experienced heart failure team, and only after careful evaluation of the patient's heart failure history. Patient-specific factors that should be considered include the patient's overall prognosis, the desired MCS strategy (BTT versus DT), the expected duration of MCS, and the need for left, right, or biventricular support. Practical considerations, such as the patient's body habitus and anticoagulation status, the surgeon's preference and familiarity with various devices, or MCS device availability, may all impact the ultimate choice of device as well.

11.3.1 Devices for Bridge to Transplant

The HeartMate II (Thoratec Corporation, Pleasanton, CA, USA) is a continuous, axial-flow rotary pump, which was approved as an LVAD for BTT therapy by the FDA in 2008. With a total displaced volume of 63 mL and weight of 290 g, the HeartMate II is implanted in a surgically-created, extraperitoneal pocket in the abdomen just below the diaphragm. The pump can generate flows up to 10 L/min, operating at pump speeds of 6,000 rpm to 15,000 rpm. The HeartMate II's continuous, axial-flow design is regarded as the device's greatest advantage compared to earlier pulsatile models (e.g., the now-retired HeartMate XVE), as the simplified pump mechanism allows for a single internal moving part (i.e., the pump rotor) and eliminates the blood-pumping chamber that is required in older pulsatile models. These modifications theoretically increase the durability of the pump and also allow for a reduction in the size and weight of the device. Early data suggested excellent results for the HeartMate II as BTT therapy, with 91% of patients reaching heart transplant, cardiac recovery, or continued survival on LVAD support at 6 months, and 85% of those on continued LVAD support surviving beyond 1 year post-implantation [4]. Functional status improvement by at least two NYHA classes has been reported in 83% of patients by 3 months after receiving a HeartMate

◘ Table 11.1 Mechanical circulatory support devices approved by the FDA and currently in use

MCS Device	Manufacturer	Mechanism	Implants in 2014 (% total)	Strategy (FDA approval date)	References
Thoratec HeartMate II	Thoratec Corporation	Continuous, axial flow	1625 (66.8%)	BTT (2008), DT (2010)	[4, 7, 14, 19, 24]
HeartWare HVAD	HeartWare Inc.	Continuous, centrifugal flow	728 (29.9%)	BTT (2012)	[20]
Thoratec PVAD	Thoratec Corporation	Pulsatile, pneumatic	24 (1.0%)	BTT (1995)	[21]
CardioWest TAH	SynCardia Systems	Pulsatile, pneumatic	54 (2.2%)	BTT (2004)	[23]

MCS mechanical circulatory support, *FDA* food and drug administration, *TAH* total artificial heart, *BTT* bridge to transplant, *DT* destination therapy (Implant data from Kirklin et al. [6])

II, and the rate of pump replacement over a period of 6 months was 4%, attesting to the enhanced durability of the device [14]. More recently, however, data published collectively by three institutions in 2014 demonstrated a sudden, unexplained increase in pump thrombosis rate, specific to the HeartMate II, from 2.2% to 8.4% at 3 months post-implantation [19]. Affected patients treated with pump exchange or transplant did not have an increased risk of mortality compared to patients without pump thrombosis, but in the absence of treatment, mortality within 6 months was 48%. Studies to better understand and manage this phenomenon are ongoing.

The HeartWare HVAD (HeartWare International, Inc., Framingham, MA, USA) is a miniaturized, continuous centrifugal-flow pump, which was approved as an LVAD for BTT therapy by the FDA in 2012. With a total displaced volume of 50 mL and weight of 160 g, the HeartWare HVAD is implanted solely within the pericardial space and does not require the abdominal pocket needed for HeartMate II implantation. Using a magnetically and hydrodynamically levitated rotor, which represents the single internal moving part of the device, the HeartWare HVAD can generate flows up to 10 L/min, operating at pump speeds of 2,000 rpm to 3,000 rpm. The replacement of mechanical bearings by the frictionless, levitated rotor system theoretically further increases the durability of the device. A multicenter prospective study of 140 patients receiving the HeartWare HVAD for BTT demonstrated non-inferiority at 6 months with regard to reaching heart transplant, cardiac recovery, or continued survival on LVAD support compared to contemporaneous LVAD recipient controls drawn from the INTERMACS registry, with 91% of the HeartWare HVAD BTT group achieving the successful outcomes described above at 6 months [20]. Quality of life scores and functional status as measured by 6-minute walking distance were also significantly improved at 6 months post-HVAD implantation. The rate of device replacement was similar to that for the HeartMate II.

The Thoratec PVAD (Thoratec Corporation, Pleasanton, CA, USA) is a pulsatile, pneumatic pump, which was approved for BTT therapy by the FDA in 1995. The device consists of a 65 mL stroke volume pump placed in a paracorporeal position outside of the body on the abdomen anteriorly, with inflow and outflow cannulas surgically placed internally and across the chest wall to connect the pump to the patient's circulation. The external pump is most commonly regulated using the full-to-empty control mode, allowing for automatic tuning of the pump's beat rate (20–110 bpm) and flow output (up to 7.2 L/min) according to venous return and therefore the body's physiologic needs. For left ventricular support, the inflow and outflow cannulas may be placed at the left ventricle apex and ascending aorta, respectively. For right ventricular support, the right atrium and pulmonary artery may be cannulated. As such, the highly-versatile Thoratec PVAD can provide univentricular support to the left or right ventricle separately, or provide biventricular support if two pumps are used together. Additionally, because of the pump's position outside of the body, the device is compatible with patients of almost any body size. According to a review of 797 patients who received the Thoratec PVAD for BTT therapy, 60% survived to transplantation, with 86% of transplanted patients surviving to hospital discharge [21]. Those receiving isolated left ventricular support had the highest survival-to-transplantation rate of 68%, whereas those receiving isolated right ventricular support and biventricular support had survival-to-transplantation rates of 41% and 55%, respectively. Currently, the use of the Thoratec PVAD is declining, although its versatility in providing left, right, or biventricular support for patients of almost any body size continues to prove useful in select cases.

The total artificial heart (TAH) is a MCS option typically reserved for end-stage heart failure patients with severe, irreversible biventricular failure, as LVAD implantation is contraindicated in these patients due to the decompensated right ventricle's intolerance of full LVAD flows. Heart failure patients with other contraindications to LVAD or biventricular assist device implantation, including intractable arrhythmias, may also benefit from TAH implantation [22]. Instead of being surgically attached to the failing heart, the TAH completely replaces both ventricles and all four native heart valves. As a result, the TAH assumes total responsibility for driving the pulmonary and systemic circulations. Implantation of a TAH also eliminates any other abnormalities of the native heart, including valve dysfunction and arrhythmias.

The CardioWest Total Artificial Heart (SynCardia Systems, Inc., Tucson, AZ, USA) is a biventricular pneumatic pump, which was approved for BTT therapy by the FDA in 2004. With a total displaced volume of 400 mL and weight of 160 g, the device is designed to completely replace the native heart in orthotopic position, and provide pulsatile blood flow to both the pulmonary and systemic circulations. The CardioWest TAH can generate a cardiac output up to 9 L/min. Although the early generation of this TAH system required patients to remain in the hospital and connected to large, bulky power sources, patients with the CardioWest TAH are now able to be discharged home while awaiting transplant. A recent report of 101 LVAD-ineligible, critically ill heart failure patients who received the CardioWest TAH revealed a survival-to-transplantation rate of 68%, and an overall survival at 1 year of 55% [23]. Although 24.7% of cases required mediastinal exploration for concern of hemorrhage, 63.4% had infections (e.g., lung, urinary tract) that warranted treatment, and 8% had documented stroke, cardiac replacement with a TAH nevertheless offered these patients who may have otherwise received hospice care a reasonable chance of continued survival to heart transplantation. Post-transplant survival at 1 year was 77%.

11.3.2 Devices for Destination Therapy

Currently, the Thoratec HeartMate II is the only continuous-flow LVAD actively used for DT in the United States, having attained FDA approval for DT in 2010. As previously discussed, an early randomized study of 200 transplant-ineligible heart failure patients found survival at 1 and 2 years after HeartMate II implantation for DT to be 68% and 52%, respectively [7]. A continuation of this study more recently demonstrated updated 1- and 2-year survival rates to be 73% and 63%, respectively [24]. For reference, the 2-year survival among medically-managed, transplant-ineligible patients in the REMATCH trial was 8% [3], clearly illustrating the effectiveness of permanent LVAD support for these critically ill patients with no other options for management.

11.3.3 Future Devices

Several devices are currently under FDA-approved clinical investigation for long-term MCS. For BTT, the HeartAssist5 (ReliantHeart, Inc., Houston, TX, USA) is a continuous axial-flow LVAD that weighs 92 g and is designed to be implanted into the pericardial space. Indeed, this device is a modified version of the MicroMed DeBakey VAD Child, which was previously approved by the FDA for use in pediatric patients. The HeartAssist5 utilizes an inducer-impeller to generate flows up to 10 L/min, and is uniquely able to perform direct flow measurements using a built-in ultrasonic flow probe. The device also monitors pump motor speed and electric current, and transmits these data to a secure data center such that physicians can remotely monitor the device's status. Recruitment for the HeartAssist5 BTT clinical trial is now underway.

For DT, the HeartWare HVAD clinical trial was completed by April 2015, with preliminary data reportedly showing 55% survival free from disabling stroke at 2 years, which was non-inferior to that (57.4%) of existing FDA-approved LVADs for DT [25]. The FDA approval process for the HeartWare HVAD for DT indication will commence following completion of a supplemental trial, which is now underway. In addition, DT clinical trials focused on the CardioWest TAH and Jarvik 2000 (Jarvik Heart, Inc., New York, NY, USA) are both currently recruiting patients. Briefly, the Jarvik 2000 is a continuous axial-flow LVAD that weights 90 g and is also designed to be implanted into the pericardial space. The device uses a vaned impeller to generate flows up to 7 L/min.

Finally, the Thoratec HeartMate III is a new device currently undergoing feasibility trials in the United States. The device weighs 200 g and is implanted into the pericardial space. Using a magnetically levitated centrifugal pump and impeller, the HeartMate III generates flows up to 10 L/min and also features pump speed modulation, allowing for antithrombotic cycling to prevent thrombosis of the pump.

11.4 Conclusion

Mechanical circulatory support represents an invaluable surgical therapy for patients with end-stage heart failure. Strategies for durable MCS device implantation may be classified as bridge to transplant or destination therapy. Over the past decade, significant progress has been made with regard to patient selection and management, surgical technique, and optimization of devices. As technology continues to rapidly improve and new devices arrive on the clinical scene, the role of MCS is likely to expand and perhaps one day even challenge heart transplantation as the standard of care for advanced heart failure.

References

1. Hunt SA, Abraham WT, Chin MH et al (2005) ACC/AHA 2005 guideline update for the diagnosis and management of chronic heart failure in the adult: a report of the American College of Cardiology/American Heart Association Task Force on Practice Guidelines (Writing Committee to Update the 2001 Guidelines for the Evaluation and Management of Heart Failure). Circulation 112(12):e154–e235
2. Mulligan MS, Shearon TH, Weill D, Pagani FD, Moore J, Murray S (2008) Heart and lung transplantation in the United States, 1997-2006. Am J Transplant 8(4p2):977–987
3. Rose EA, Gelijns AC, Moskowitz AJ et al (2001) Randomized Evaluation of Mechanical Assistance for the Treatment of Congestive Heart Failure (REMATCH) Study Group. Long-term mechanical left ventricular assistance for end-stage heart failure. N Engl J Med 345(20):1435–1443
4. Starling RC, Naka Y, Boyle AJ et al (2011) Results of the post-U.S. Food and Drug Administration-approval study with a continuous flow left ventricular assist device as a bridge to heart transplantation: a prospective study using the INTERMACS (Interagency Registry for Mechanically Assisted Circulatory Support). J Am Coll Cardiol 57(19):1890–1898
5. Kirklin JK, Naftel DC, Pagani FD et al (2014) Sixth INTERMACS annual report: a 10,000-patient database. J Heart Lung Trans 33(6):555–564
6. Kirklin JK, Naftel DC, Pagani FD et al (2015) Seventh INTERMACS annual report: 15,000 patients and counting. J Heart Lung Transplant 34(12):1495–1504
7. Slaughter MS, Rogers JG, Milano CA et al (2009) Advanced heart failure treated with continuous-flow left ventricular assist device. N Engl J Med 361(23):2241–2251
8. Pagani FD, Miller LW, Russell SD et al (2009) Extended mechanical circulatory support with a continuous-flow rotary left ventricular assist device. J Am Coll Cardiol 54(4):312–321
9. Park SJ, Tector A, Piccioni W et al (2005) Left ventricular assist device as destination therapy; a new look at survival. J Thorac Cardiovasc Surg 129(1):9–17
10. Peura JL, Colvin-Adams M, Francis GS et al (2012) Recommendations for the use of mechanical circulatory support: device strategies and patient selection: a scientific statement from the American Heart Association. Circulation 126(22):2648–2667
11. Anand I, Maggioni A, Burton P et al (2006) The seattle heart failure model: prediction of survival in heart failure. Circulation 113(11):1424–1433
12. Fitzpatrick JR, Frederick JR, Hiesinger W et al (2009) Early planned institution of biventricular mechanical circulatory support results in improved outcomes compared with delayed conversion of a left ventricular assist device to a biventricular assist device. J Thorac Cardiovasc Surg 137(4):971–977
13. Atluri P, Goldstone AB, Fairman AS et al (2013) Predicting right ventricular failure in the modern, continuous flow left ventricular assist device era. Ann Thorac Surg 96(3):857–864
14. Miller LW, Pagani FD, Russell SD et al (2007) Use of a continuous-flow device in patients awaiting heart transplantation. N Engl J Med 357(9):885–896
15. Mancini D, Lietz K (2010) Selection of cardiac transplantation candidates in 2010. Circulation 122(2):173–183 Review
16. Freudenberger RS, Tawfik I, Shinnar M, Pendergast T (2009) Panel-reactive screening and treatment practices following bridge to transplantation ventricular assist device placement. Transplant Proc 41(5):1813–1815
17. Baldwin JT, Mann DL (2011) NHLBI's program for VAD therapy for moderately advanced heart failure: the REVIVE-IT pilot trial. J Card Fail 16(11):855–858
18. Kirklin JK, Naftel DC, Pagani FD et al (2012) Long-term mechanical circulatory support (destination therapy): on track to compete with heart transplantation? J Thorac Cardiovasc Surg 144(3):584–603
19. Starling RC, Moazami N, Silvestry SC et al (2014) Unexpected abrupt increase in left ventricular assist device thrombosis. N Engl J Med 370(1):33–40
20. Aaronson KD, Slaughter MS, Miller LW et al (2012) Use of an intrapericardial, continuous-flow, centrifugal pump in patients awaiting heart transplantation. Circulation 125(25):3191–3200
21. Farrar DJ (2000) The Thoratec ventricular assist device: a paracorporeal pump for treating acute and chronic heart failure. Semin Thorac Cardiovasc Surg 12(3):243–250
22. Copeland JG, Smith RG, Arabia FA et al (2004) Cardiac replacement with a total artificial heart as a bridge to transplantation. N Engl J Med 351(9):859–867
23. Copeland JG, Copeland H, Gustafson M et al (2012) Experience with more than 100 total artificial heart implants. J Thorac Cardiovasc Surg 143(3):727–734
24. Park SJ, Milano CA, Tatooles AJ et al (2012) Outcomes in advanced heart failure patients with left ventricular assist devices for destination therapy. Circ Heart Fail 5(2):241–248
25. Pagani FD, Milano CA, Tatooles AJ, et al (2015) HeartWare HVAD for the treatment of patients with advanced heart failure ineligible for cardiac transplantation: results of the ENDURANCE destination therapy trial. Presented at the International Society for Heart and Lung Transplantation 35th Annual Meeting and Scientific Sessions, 15–18 Apr, Nice

Mechanical Circulatory Support as Bridge to Recovery

Michael Dandel and Stephan Schueler

© Springer International Publishing Switzerland 2017

A. Montalto et al. (eds.), *Mechanical Circulatory Support in End-Stage Heart Failure*,
DOI 10.1007/978-3-319-43383-7_12

12.1 Introduction

Long-term MCS with ventricular assist devices (VADs) allows end-stage failing hearts to recover and, occasionally, even reverse remodeling with functional improvement allowing VAD removal followed by years of freedom from heart failure (HF) recurrence is possible [1–3]. Although myocardial recovery at the cellular and subcellular level has been often observed after VAD implantation, translation of these changes into functional recovery at organ level was observed less frequently, and stable cardiac improvement which might allow long-term HF-free outcome after VAD removal has occurred only rarely. Acute HF can completely reverse during left ventricular assist device (LVAD) support [4]. Outcome data for patients with chronic end-stage HF who were electively weaned from VADs are few but are encouraging.

The possibility of cardiac recovery during long-term MCS gives rise to three major challenges: (1) assessment of recovery after VAD implantation and decision making in favor of or against VAD explantation; (2) search for additional recovery-facilitating and/or regenerative therapy, aiming to increase the number of weaning candidates; and (3) preimplantation prediction of possible cardiac recovery during MCS, aiming to provide the basis for possible future use of VADs as a therapeutic strategy for cardiac recovery.

This chapter summarizes the knowledge about myocardial recovery during long-term VAD support and reviews the knowledge on its clinical relevance, its stability after VAD explantation, and its assessment before decision making in favor of or against VAD explantation.

12.2 Myocardial Reverse Remodeling and Functional Recovery During MCS

Pathological remodeling of failing hearts includes (1) myocyte defects (hypertrophy, β-adrenoreceptor changes, alterations in excitation-contraction coupling and contractile properties, mytochondrial abnormalities with altered myocardial energetics, loss and/or disarray of the cytoskeleton, etc.), (2) myocyte death (necrosis, apoptosis, autophagy), and (3) extracellular matrix (ECM) alterations (degradation, replacement fibrosis, angiogenesis). These changes induce alterations in ventricular size, geometry, and function. The high wall stress due to ventricular dilation leads to coronary flow alterations (aggravated by stroke volume reduction), increased oxidative stress with activation of genes sensitive to free-radical generation (tumor necrosis factor, interleukin-1β), sustained expression of stretch-activated genes (endothelin, angiotensin II, tumor necrosis factor), and/or activation of hypertrophic signaling pathways which all additionally worsen the ventricular function [5]. Ongoing myocardial injury is also facilitated by activation of the inflammatory system with production and release of inflammatory cytokines and by release of autoantibodies (AABs) against cardiac proteins. High AAB levels against the β_1-adrenoreceptor were detectable in over 80% of patients with end-stage idiopathic dilated cardiomyopathy (IDCM), and patients who required MCS also showed high intracardiac expression for inflammatory cytokines [6, 7].

Prolonged MCS can induce reverse remodeling by reversal of myocyte and ECM abnormalities. By reducing also the serum levels of cardiac AABs and the myocardial levels of inflammatory cytokines (tumor necrosis factor-α, interleukin-8) which are involved in the development and progression of HF, VADs can reverse both ventricular dilation and functional alterations [6, 8]. Reverse remodeling is necessary for functional recovery but only rarely results in clinically relevant cardiac recovery [5]. Today, neither the components of the process of reverse remodeling which are necessary for myocardial recovery nor the minimum levels of reverse remodeling necessary for cardiac recovery allowing VAD removal are reliably known.

Myocardial recovery during MCS occurs at the different levels with different rates. At cellular, molecular, and genomic level, there is a high probability of relevant recovery, but clinically adequate and stable cardiac recovery which allows VAD removal occurs in only few patients. Patients who were successfully weaned from their VAD often showed only incomplete recovery at the time of VAD removal, and HF recurred in about one half of them during the first 10 post-weaning years [9]. In many patients who become eligible for VAD explantation, HF reversal is based on myocardial "remission" rather than on real "recovery" with freedom from future heart events [5]. Nevertheless, as long as post-explant cardiac function remains normal, it is clinically not possible to differentiate between recovery and remission.

12.2.1 Recovery at Cellular, Molecular, and Genomic Levels

During prolonged MCS, the failing myocardium shows different degrees of reversal in genomic, molecular, and histological alterations. However, the few studies on reverse remodeling at cellular and subcellular level in weaned patients, differences in etiology and severity of HF in weaned patients, and also differences in the pharmacological regimes used by different centers in VAD-supported patients all make it still difficult to understand even the basic mechanisms responsible for cardiac recovery which allows successful weaning of some patients from their VAD.

Myocyte Size, Structure, and Function

Myocardial hypertrophy is a characteristic change in failing hearts with relevant contribution to cardiac remodeling and contractile dysfunction. VADs usually induce regression of hypertrophy but its relationship with unloading-promoted cardiac recovery remained unclarified [8]. In patients with IDCM as the underlying cause for HF before LVAD implantation, regression of hypertrophy appeared not predictive for recovery, which allows LVAD explantation [3].

Pre-LVAD alterations in myocyte structure and function showed different degrees of reversibility during MCS. LVADs often improved both developed tension and relaxation rates at the myocyte level, but in most cases without evidence of cardiac recovery that would allow LVAD removal [6, 10]. Myocardial recovery in patients who were successfully weaned from LVADs appeared associated with specific changes in sarcomeric, non-sarcomeric, and membrane-associated proteins plus improvement of myocyte contractile function [10, 11]. In weaned patients with nonischemic cardiomyopathy as the underlying cause of HF, comparisons of myocardial samples collected at VAD implantation and explantation showed increases of certain sarcomeric (i.e., myosin heavy chain, troponin T and C, β-actin, sarcomeric actinin, α-tropomyosin, and α-filamin A) and non-sarcomeric proteins (nuclear laminar protein lamin A/C, cytoskeletal actinin, spectrin, integrin β5 and α5) [11]. Improvement in calcium handling, mitochondrial function, and response to β-AR stimulation was also observed during MCS, and it appeared often associated with improvement in myocyte contraction and relaxation [6, 10, 12].

During VAD support also relevant changes in myocardial gene expression with major role in improvement of Ca^{2+}-handling were found, and sarcoendoplasmic reticulum (SR) function can also recover [6, 12]. Improved SR uptake activity appeared associated with an increased SR Ca^{2+}-ATPase2A protein and mRNA expression [13, 14]. By restoration of calcium-handling proteins, VAD support results in faster sarcolemmal Ca^{2+} entry and higher Ca^{2+} concentration in the SR, and an association between clinically relevant cardiac recovery and improvement of sarcoplasmic calcium homeostasis was also found. It was observed that the beneficial effect of MCS on Ca^{2+}-handling reaches its maximum during the first 4 post-implant months, afterwards returning, with prolongation of unloading, to pathological levels [13]. This finding corresponds to the clinical observation that the probability of long-term cardiac stability after LVAD removal is higher for patients who necessitate shorter ($\leq$6 months) LVAD support before LVAD explantation [3].

Chronic HF is characterized by impaired myocardial β-adrenoreceptor (β-AR) signaling due to β-AR downregulation and desensitization which seems to be mainly due to phosphorylation of agonist-occupied β-ARs by the upregulated G protein-coupled receptor kinase 2 (GRK2) [12].

VADs can improve β-AR signaling by inducing normalization of β-AR density and improvement in response to β-AR stimulation which appeared associated with a decrease in myocardial GRK2 expression and activity [6, 12, 14]. However, LVADs can restore myocardial β-AR signaling to near normal even in patients without clinically relevant recovery, and thus restoration of β-AR signaling alone does not induce recovery of adequate ventricular function to allow weaning from LVAD [12, 14]. Ventricular unloading can also improve cellular responses to oxidative stress [15].

Apoptosis and Myocardial Regeneration

MCS can reduce apoptosis. VADs induce an improvement in altered expression of the anti-apoptotic protein Bcl-2 and the repair-proliferation marker "proliferating cell nuclear antigen," an increase in transcription of certain anti-apoptotic genes, and a reduction of DNA fragmentation [6, 10, 12, 16].

The increase in circulating bone marrow progenitor cells after LVAD implantation and the indirect detection of cell division or progenitor cell proliferation in myocardial specimens obtained at LVAD explantation also suggest possible facilitation of myocardial regeneration inducible by ventricular unloading [17, 18].

Extracellular Matrix and Microvascular Density

Myocardial fibrosis and reduced microvascular density are characteristic changes in failing hearts that make a relevant contribution to cardiac remodeling and contractile dysfunction [5, 10]. Regression of LV dilation during reduction of mechanical stretch by LVAD support facilitates ECM changes, and the restoration of collagen networks in turn can facilitate improvement in ventricular geometry and function [6, 10]. ECM changes related to ventricle dilation during HF development appeared related to upregulation of matrix metalloproteinases that cleave matrix components and to downregulation of their inhibitors [10]. LVADs can reverse this process and thus restore the collagen networks [6]. Available data suggest that the beneficial response of the ECM to LVAD support might be a critical component of clinical recovery, but the exact mechanisms involved in that process are not yet fully understood [6]. It is also still controversial whether VAD support always results in an increase or decrease of interstitial fibrosis. In a study on 35 weaned patients with IDCM as the underlying cause for MCS, LVAD implantation was followed by reduction in cardiac fibrosis, and the degree of fibrosis was smaller in patients who recovered to levels allowing LVAD explantation [8]. However, reduction in cardiac fibrosis was found only in 82% of the successfully weaned patients. A study on rats with dilated cardiomyopathy showed that prolonged ventricular unloading has the tendency to increase both myocardial stiffness (by increase in fibrosis) and apoptosis [19]. This might partially explain the higher HF recurrence rate observed in weaned patients with VAD support times of >6 months before explantation in comparison with those who underwent explantation after less than 6 months of ventricular unloading [3]. Unloading also results in increased microvascular density accompanied by endothelial cell activation [20]. The increase in microvascular density during prolonged LVAD support also appeared associated with upregulation of angiogenesis related genes [5, 20]. However, the functional significance of these changes is unclear because coronary flow reserve remained impaired after LVAD support [5].

12.2.2 Recovery at Organ Level Allowing VAD Explantation

Cardiac recovery allowing VAD explantation occurs definitely less frequently than myocardial recovery at the cellular level and appeared related to the etiology of myocardial damage, the duration of heart disease, and the amount of fibrosis before VAD implantation. Acute myocarditis showed higher recovery rates than nonischemic chronic cardiomyopathy (CCM), while recovery from ischemic CCM allowing VAD explantation is a rarity [3, 21–24]. The overall recovery rate allowing adult patient weaning from VAD, regardless of the etiology of the underlying cardiac disease before VAD implantation, is between 1% and 9% [9, 24]. The high discrepancy between the reported recovery rates reflects the difficulty of decision making in favor or against VAD removal and suggests that the weaning experience gained by individual centers is essential for the detection of potential weaning candidates.

Acute myocarditis and postcardiotomy HF can completely reverse during MCS, and therefore elective weaning from VADs was initially performed almost exclusively in such patients [4, 10, 24]. In acute HF where reversible causes of HF can play a major role, the contribution of VADs to recovery processes might be mainly indirect (lifesaving MCS only providing the necessary time for spontaneous and/or pharmacologically facilitated myocardial recovery). However, in chronic life-threatening HF unresponsive to any medical treatment, long-term ventricular wall tension reduction by mechanical unloading appeared to have a relevant facilitating impact on myocardial recovery.

Recovery from chronic HF is often incomplete. Nevertheless, the probability for HF recurrence during the first year after LVAD explantation is usually less than 15% [1, 3, 4, 21, 22, 25–27]. However, only few cardiothoracic centers have performed higher numbers of elective VAD explantations in such patients. For nonischemic CCM, recovery rates varying between 8% and 70% were reported. The high range might be in part due to differences in experience of individual heart centers with evaluation of cardiac recovery and medical therapy during VAD support, but is probably mainly due to the different selection criteria for VAD implantation and explantation used by different centers. In the Harefield study, using a specific pharmacological regimen which included the β_2-adrenergic agonist clenbuterol, 11 (73%) of 15 patients with nonischemic cardiomyopathy were weaned from LVAD [21]. More recently, using the same therapeutic regimen, the same group weaned 12 (60%) of the 20 enrolled patients [28]. However, these high recovery rates were not reproducible in the multicenter "US Harefield Recovery-Protocol Trial" [25]. According to the largest studies on this topic, recovery rates of between 10% and 20% are probably realistic for nonischemic CCM, whereas recovery rates reported for ischemic CCM were rarely above 1% [8, 22, 25]. Unloading-promoted cardiac recovery rates might also depend on the type of VADs implanted. Higher recovery rates were found with pulsatile devices in comparison to continuous-flow pumps, and it was presumed that pulsatile systems may provide better unloading conditions for recovery [8, 29]. However, those differences in recovery rates might also be related to the more restrictive weaning criteria which were used during the last years which coincides with the preferentially use of non-pulsatile VADs [22].

VAD use in infants and children was introduced more recently, and data on unloading-promoted cardiac recovery in pediatric patients are relatively scarce. Studies on children who received a Berlin Heart EXCOR system reported recovery rates which allowed successful weaning from the mechanical support of between 5.1% and 16.5% [30, 31]. Thus, as in adults, cardiac recovery allowing VAD removal is also quite rare in children. However, for those who can be weaned from their VAD, the chances for long-term freedom from HF recurrence are good.

12.3 Weaning from VADs

After long controversy about the clinical relevance of VAD-promoted recovery from chronic HF and on the feasibility of elective weaning of patients from their VAD, taking into account the risk of early post-weaning HF recurrence, this topic gained increasing interest during the past 10 years, especially after the publication of the first long-term weaning results in patients with chronic HF reversal after LVAD implantation [2, 3, 27]. Post-weaning survival for patients with end-stage nonischemic chronic HF before VAD implantation was found comparable with that of patients who recovered from acute HF where reversible causes of HF can play major roles (◘ Table 12.1).

Table 12.1 Main studies assessing recovered patient outcome after VAD explantation

Study (year)	Pre-implant diagnosis (number of patients)	Follow-up [months]	HF recurrence [number (%)]	Deaths [number (%)]	Post-explant patient survival rates (%)				
					1 year	3 years	5 years	7 years	10 years
Müller et al. (1997) [1]	IDCM (5)	2–20	0	0	–	–	–	–	–
Hetzer et al. (1999) [2]	IDCM (19)	1–31	5 (26.7%)	2 (10.5%)	81.8	–	–	–	–
Hetzer et al. (2001) [27]	IDCM (28)	1–66	9 (32.1%)	5 (17.8%)	88.0	81.7	–	–	–
Ferrar et al. (2002) [4]	Nonischemic HF (22)[a]	14–120[e]	3 (15.8%)	3 (15.8%)	91.0	85.0	–	–	–
Dandel et al. (2005) [3]	IDCM (32)	3–111	14 (43.7%)	6 (18.7%)	87.0	78.3	78.3	–	–
Simon et al. (2005) [23]	Acute + chronic HF (11)[b]	3–43	2 (20.0%)	0	–	–	–	–	–
Birks et al. (2006) [21]	Nonischemic cardiomyopathy (11)	59 ± 5 (max 67.5)	1 (9.1%)	3 (27.3%)	90.9	81.8 at 4 years		–	–
Dandel et al. (2008) [8]	IDCM (35)	4–156	16 (45.7%)	8 (22.9%)	88.5	83.5	79.1	75.3	75.3
Dandel et al. (2011) [22]	Nonischemic CCM (47)[c]	1–178	17 (36.2%)	14 (29.8%)	82.5	72.0	71.5	65.7	65.7
Dandel et al. (2012) [9]	Nonischemic CCM (53)[c]	1–204	20 (37.7%)	15 (28.3%)	82.0	77.9	72.8	67.0	67.0
Birks et al. (2012) [26]	DCM (37)[d] Myocarditis (3)	46 ± 39	7 (17.5%)	8 (20.0%)	89.9	73.9	73.9	73.9	–

[a] 12 myocarditis, 7 postpartum cardiomyopathy, 1 viral cardiomyopathy, 2 idiopathic dilated cardiomyopathy (IDCM)
[b] 4 postpartum cardiomyopathy, 3 myocarditis, 2 postcardiotomy, 1 IDCM
[c] *CCM* chronic cardiomyopathy
[d] *DCM* dilated cardiomyopathy
[e] Only one patient with pre-implant acute HF remained stable for 120 months after explantation

12.3.1 Long-Term Results After VAD Explantation

In patients with nonischemic CCM, the study with the largest number of weaned patients and the longest post-weaning follow-up revealed probabilities of 67.1 ± 7.6% and 47.3 ± 9.2% for 5-year and 10-year freedom from HF recurrence after VAD explantation, respectively, without differences between patients weaned from pulsatile and non-pulsatile VADs [9]. These good results were possible although before explantation, only 8,7% of the weaned patients had an LV ejection fraction (LVEF) >50% [9]. Thus VAD explantation can be successful even after incomplete cardiac recovery. In another study, the post-explant rate of freedom from death or HTx reached 69% at both 5 and 7 years [26]. A recent evaluation of 53 weaned patients with nonischemic CCM as the underlying cause for VAD implantation revealed 5- and 10-year post-explant survival probabilities (including post-HTx survival for those with HF recurrence) of 72.8 ± 6.6% and 67.0 ± 7.2%, respectively [9]. Assessment of post-weaning survival only from HF recurrence or weaning-related complications revealed higher probabilities for 5- and 10-year survival (87.8 ± 5.3% and 82.6 ± 7.3%, respectively) [9]. In a study which compared long-term outcomes of patients bridged to recovery versus patients bridged to HTx, the actuarial survival rate at 5 years after LVAD explantation was 73.9%, whereas in the group bridged to HTx where all patients were finally transplanted, the actuarial post-HTx survival rate at 5 years was 78.3% [26]. Thus, patients weaned from VADs were not at a higher risk for death in comparison to those who underwent HTx, even if the recovery was incomplete and the underlying cause for VAD implantation was a chronic cardiomyopathy. For patients with nonischemic CCM as the underlying cause for MCS, the 5-year survival probability of VAD-explanted patients was also higher than that of patients who could not be weaned from their VAD (73% versus 52%, $p < 0.01$) [7]. The good long-term survival data of weaned patients with IDCM as the underlying cause for MCS, a disease that long time was considered to be almost irreversible, also suggest that VAD explantation should be considered in all VAD recipients with relevant cardiac improvement, not only in those with potentially more reversible cardiac diseases [3].

12.3.2 Assessment of Cardiac Recovery After VAD Implantation

Assessment of recovery, either at rest or during exercise, necessitates temporary interruptions of mechanical unloading ("off-pump trials"). Short off-pump trials allow evaluations of the heart under the same circumstances which will exist after VAD removal. However, whereas pulsatile VADs allow optimal cardiac assessment during complete pump stops, complete stops of axial-flow pumps lead to retrograde flow into the LV followed by reduction of the diastolic arterial pressure which, reducing the LV afterload, can generate overestimations of LV systolic function. The misleading retrograde blood flow into the LV during off-pump trials can impede correct weaning decisions. Therefore, for such pumps, rotor speed reduction to values which result in close to zero flow in one cardiac cycle (3000–6000 rpm) is better than complete pump stop [3]. Before off-pump trials heparin must be given (60–100 IU/kg according to the prothrombin time) to prevent thrombus formation inside the pump [8, 22]. Patients with heparin-induced thrombocytopenia should receive argatroban (synthetic thrombin inhibitor) infusions (2 μg/kg/min started 1 h before off-pump trials) [22]. Duration of individual off-pump periods can vary between 3 and 15 min [8, 22]. In patients with a BVAD, it is appropriate to stop both pumps (RV pump 30 s earlier than the LV pump) [22]. In patients with insufficient recovery, as already shown during the first 3 min, the off-pump trial should be stopped [9]. With appropriate caution, the risk of off-pump trials is low [9, 22]. In patients with cardiac recovery, it appeared useful to conduct such trials weekly or every 2 weeks and to make the final decision for elective LVAD explantation only after cardiac improvement has reached its maximum (no further improvement in at least two consecutive off-pump trials) [9]. During recovery it appears useful to change the working mode of the pumps in order to intensify the unloading if the ventricle size needs further reduction or to exert moderate load on the ventricular muscle after maximum improvement [1, 2, 8].

The main diagnostic methods to assess cardiac recovery are echocardiography, heart catheterization, and cardiopulmonary exercise testing.

Role of Echocardiography

Echocardiography is the cornerstone for both selection of potential weaning candidates and evaluation of clinically relevant recovery. After VAD implantation, repeated transthoracic echocardiography (TTE) screenings with normal VAD function are necessary for selection of potential weaning candidates. Weaning candidates are patients with LV end-diastolic diameter (LVEDD) <55 mm (or 55–60 mm at BSA $\geq$1.8m^2) and fractional shortening (FS) >15%, no or $\leq$grade I mitral and/or aortic regurgitation, no RV dilation, and TR $\leq$grade II [22]. Before the first off-pump trial, it is useful to perform stepwise pump rate reductions under TTE monitoring to verify whether complete interruption of unloading is possible and also makes sense. Thus, if incomplete interruption of unloading already provokes symptoms (dizziness, sweating, etc.), complete interruption of unloading is risky and senseless. If the patient remains asymptomatic but the LVEDD increases beyond 60 mm, a complete interruption, although possible, is senseless, because such a patient is not yet a weaning candidate (◘ Table 12.2).

The actual echo-assessment of recovery in weaning candidates is usually based on the results of repeated off-pump trials at rest. After long-term VAD support, even short periods of physiological loading by interruption of unloading may represent a challenge for a possibly incomplete recovered ventricle. It therefore appears reasonable to avoid at least initially any risk of myocardial exhaustion which might interfere with possibly still ongoing recovery. For this reason, all 116 adults who were weaned in the German Heart Institute Berlin between 1995 and 2015 from long-term VADs underwent assessments of cardiac recovery exclusively at rest [9, 22]. Although echo-assessment at rest is limited by the lack of information about inotropic reserves and cardiac adaptation to stress, the weaning results appeared

◘ Table 12.2 Transthoracic echocardiographic measurements for evaluation of cardiac recovery during off-pump trials

Echocardiographic methods	Measurements
2D echocardiography	LV end-diastolic and end-systolic diameters (LVEDD and LVESD, respectively) LV end-diastolic short/long axis ratio (S/L_{ED}) LV end-diastolic relative wall thickness (RWT_{ED})[a] LV fractional shortening (FS) LV ejection fraction (LVEF) measured by biplane Simpson's method RV end-diastolic dimensions (on parasternal and apical views) RV fractional area change (FAC) and ejection fraction (RVEF)
PW and color Doppler	Doppler indices of LV diastolic function (transmitral flow, isovolumetric relaxation time) LV stroke volume (SV)[b] Regurgitation on mitral, aortic, tricuspid, and pulmonary valves
CW Doppler	Pulmonary arterial systolic pressure estimation in patients with tricuspid valve regurgitation
Tissue Doppler imaging	LV systolic wall motion peak velocity (Sm) at the basal posterior wall measured with the pulsed-wave tissue Doppler (PW-TD) Tricuspid lateral annulus peak systolic wall motion velocity (TAPS') measured on apical four-chamber views with the PW-TD
Speckle tracking 2D strain imaging	LV radial, circumferential, and longitudinal strain and strain rate LV synchrony and synergy of contraction

[a]RWT_{ED} = [interventricular septum thickness + posterior wall thickness]/LVEDD
[b]Product of time velocity integral measured with pulsed-wave Doppler at the LV outflow tract (LVOT) and cross-sectional area of the LV outflow tract

relevantly unaffected by that, insofar as the results reported by groups who used stress echocardiography and/or exercise testing were not better [9, 25]. Nevertheless, dobutamine stress echocardiography (DSE) can provide valuable information for weaning decisions. Conventionally, an absolute EF increase by 5% during dopamine infusion indicates preservation of contractile reserve [25]. A possible limitation of DSE might be the risk of myocardial exhaustion with negative impact on an ongoing myocardial recovery process. Further studies are therefore necessary to establish the real value of DSE for weaning decisions.

In principle, off-pump TTE at rest should be as comprehensive as possible, including tissue Doppler and strain imaging. Unfortunately not all recommended parameters are measurable in all weaning candidates because of poor image quality in some patients with VAD support.

Importance of Right Heart Catheterization

Off-pump right heart catheterization (RHC) is another cornerstone for recovery assessment [9, 25]. RHC is paramount for final decisions in favor of or against VAD explantation. A final off-pump trial of ≥15 min in the operation room, with repeated hemodynamic measurements under continuous echo-monitoring, is indispensable before explantation surgery [9]. RHC is also necessary before any preliminary decision making in weaning candidates with borderline TTE data and/or relevant cardiac improvement only after >6 months of unloading and/or long history length of HF [9, 22]. In patients with axial-flow pumps, such preliminary RHCs are more reliable if off-pump measurements are preceded by occlusion of the outlet cannula with a balloon [9]. Balloon occlusion allows complete stops of these pumps without any misleading retrograde flow into the ventricle [7]. Normal and stable hemodynamics during off-pump RHC trials is a necessary condition for a decision in favor of VAD removal, but not sufficiently predictive for long-term post-explant cardiac stability [9, 22].

Exercise Testing

Recovered patients showed after the 6 min walk (6 MW) no correlation between heart rate (HR) and mean arterial pressure (MAP), suggesting that HR increase was independent of MAP change (true inotropic reserve response) [25]. Unlike non-recovered patients, those with unloading-promoted recovery also showed significant LVEF increase after the 6 MW [25]. Harefield Hospital (UK) developed an algorithm for testing recovery that includes a 6 MW test with repeated measurements afterward to determine the inotropic reserve [25]. The same group also uses cardiopulmonary exercise testing using oxygen uptake (VO_2) for weaning decisions [25].

12.3.3 Optimizing Unloading-Promoted Cardiac Recovery

Whereas renin, angiotensin II (Ang-II), and aldosterone plasma levels usually decrease after LVAD implantation, in the unloaded myocardium, both norepinephrine (NE) and Ang-II tissue levels are elevated and promote cardiac interstitial fibrosis with increase in myocardial stiffness [32]. Angiotensin-converting enzyme (ACE) inhibitors, being able to reduce myocardial Ang-II and also the Ang-II-induced myocardial sympathetic activation, can prevent the progression of extracellular matrix remodeling, and in combination with MCS, ACE inhibitors might be able to reverse, at least partially, that remodeling [32]. Additionally, also Ang-II receptor antagonists, aldosterone antagonists, and β-blockers are recommended to promote recovery during VAD support [8, 25]. Medication doses should be individually adapted with the goal of reducing HR toward 55–60 bpm and blood pressure to the lowest optimally tolerated value, as well as to maintain optimal renal function [9].

More recently, clenbuterol (selective β_2-adrenergic receptor agonist) appeared able to promote myocardial recovery during VAD support [21, 25]. With clenbuterol as additional therapy, the weaning rate from VADs increased beyond 60% (Harefield study) [21, 25]. To confirm these results, a multicenter trial using the Harefield protocol was initiated in the USA (Harp trial) [25]. Unfortunately, only one of the 17 patients enrolled in the HARP study finally underwent explantation.

A potential tool for facilitation of unloading-promoted myocardial recovery might in the future be the development of automatic control strategies for the LV afterload impedance allowing optimization of unloading and a controlled "myocardial training" [7].

12.3.4 Pre-explant Prediction of Long-Term Stability of Cardiac Recovery

After VAD implantation, TTE parameters of "off-pump" cardiac function, ventricular size and geometry, their stability between and during off-pump trials after maximum improvement, and HF duration before VAD implantation allow detection of patients with the potential to remain stable for >5 post-weaning years [8, 9, 22]. Final off-pump LVEF of ≥45% at rest showed a predictive value of 74% for post-explant cardiac stability of ≥5 years, but together with either HF history length of ≤5 years, or final off-pump LV end-diastolic diameter (LVEDD) ≤55 mm, or LV end-diastolic relative wall thickness (RWT_{ED}) ≥0.38, or LV systolic peak wall motion velocity (Sm) ≥8 cm/sec that predictive value can increase to 86% [8, 22]. Taking into consideration also the pre-explant stability of LVEF, LV size and LV geometry during the time between maximum improvement and VAD explantation, as well as during the final off-pump trial before VAD removal, the predictive value of TTE for post-explant cardiac stability of ≥5 years increases beyond 93% [9]. In patients with stable off-pump LVEF ≥45% at rest plus normal and stable LV size (LVEDD ≤55 mm) and/or geometry (RWT_{ED} ≥0.38), even the predictive value for post-explant cardiac stability of ≥10 years can reach 90% [9]. Exercise testing also appeared predictive for recovery. Stable or increased MAP and pulse pressure, as well as LVEF ≥53% after the 6 MW, appeared to be strong predictors of recovery [25].

12.3.5 Protocols for Decision Making in Favor of VAD Explantation

The "Berlin weaning criteria" which have evolved during 20 years of weaning experience are shown in ◻ Table 12.3. Essential criteria are, in addition to a stable off-pump LVEF ≥45%, normal and stable LV size and shape, as well as high stability of hemodynamic parameters measured during the off-pump RHC trials [9, 22]. Even in patients with good recovery, it appears useful to explant VADs only after the recovery has reached its maximum (no further improvement during the next 2–4 weeks) [9]. If a relevant LVEF reduction and/or LV enlargement occurs during the next 2–4 weeks after maximum cardiac recovery, it can be risky to explant the VAD, even if the LVEF did not fall below 45% and the LVEDD did not increase beyond 55 mm [22]. The Harefield weaning criteria include fewer TTE parameters; instead they use the 6 MW test and the peak VO_2 (optimal, >16 mL/kg/min or >65% predicted) [25]. However, both weaning protocols do not recommend LVAD explantation in patients with LVEF <45% [9, 22, 25].

For more reliable evaluation of cardiac recovery, since 2005 the Berlin group also used speckle tracking-derived 2D strain imaging. The advantages of this method are its ability to differentiate between active and passive movement of myocardial segments, the angle independency of deformation-velocity measurements, and the possibility to quantify intraventricular asynchrony and dyssynergy and to evaluate components of myocardial function, such as longitudinal myocardial shortening, that are not visually assessable. Unfortunately, the available off-pump 2D strain imaging data are yet insufficient for reliable assessment of their predictive value for long-term post-explant cardiac stability. However, in borderline cases, off-pump data on deformation velocity as well as on intraventricular synchrony and synergy of contraction, including their stability after maximum improvement, can be useful for weaning decisions. The major limitation of this method is its dependence on image quality.

Table 12.3 Main left ventricular assist device (LVAD) explantation criteria[a]

Examination	Parameters and parameter-derived measurements during the last off-pump trial before LVAD explantation[b]
Echocardiography[c]	LV end-diastolic diameter (LVEDD) ≤ 55 mm
	LV ejection fraction (LVEF) ≥ 45%
	Stable pre-explant LVEF after maximum improvement
	Stable pre-explant LVEDD after maximum improvement and during the final off-pump trial
	Stable stroke volume (SV) during the final off-pump trial
	Systolic wall motion peak velocity (Sm) ≥ 8 cm/s, stable after maximum improvement and during the final off-pump trial
	No or less than grade II regurgitation at mitral and/or aortic valve
	No RV dilation (RVOT[d] diameter <35 mm, end-diastolic short/long axis ratio <0.6)
	No or maximum grade II regurgitation at the tricuspid and/or pulmonary valve
RH catheterization	Cardiac index (CI) >2.6 L/min/m^2
	Pulmonary capillary wedge pressure <13 mmHg
	Right atrial pressure (mean) <10 mmHg
Electrocardiography	Sinus rhythm Heart rate (HR) <90/min No more than 25% HR increase during off-pump trials
Artrial pressure	Mean pressure ≥65 mmHg

[a]These criteria used at present at the Deutsches Herzzentrum Berlin have evolved from a weaning experience of 18 years after explantation of 100 long-term VADs, primarily designed as bridge-to-HTx or permanent therapy [9, 22]
[b]Measurements at rest, without inotropic support
[c]Since 2005 also speckle tracking-derived 2D strain imaging parameters (global longitudinal strain and strain rate, intraventricular synchrony and synergy, including pre-explant stability of all these parameters after maximum improvement and during the final off-pump trial) were taken into consideration for weaning decisions [22]
[d]*RVOT* right ventricular outflow tract

12.3.6 Risk Factors for Recurrence of Heart Failure After Weaning

Off-pump LVEF <45% showed 88% predictive value for HF recurrence during the first 3 years after VAD removal, and values <40% even appeared nearly 100% predictive for early recurrence of HF [8, 9]. Nearly 100% predictive for early recurrence of HF is also an off-pump LVEF < 45% in patients with a history of HF > 5 years [22]. In patients with LVEF <50%, an LVEDD >55 mm and/or unstable LV geometry and/or history length of >5 years is a relevant risk factor for HF recurrence (predictive values 83%–100%) [22].

Table 12.4 Major risk factors for recurrence of heart failure after LVAD explantation

Risk factors for post-weaning recurrence of HF	Higher risk for HF recurrence	Predictive value for HF recurrence during the first 3 post-explant years
Patient age at explantation	Higher patient age	Patient age not predictive for outcome
History length of HF before LVAD implantation	Longer history of HF	88.9% pv for >5 years history length
Duration of unloading until recovery	Longer unloading	77% pv for >6 months of unloading
Incomplete LV reverse remodeling and/or insufficient functional recovery[a]		
Reduced pre-explant LVEF	Lower LVEF and/or its Higher instability[b]	87.5% pv for LVEF <45%[c] 90% pv for LVEF ≥45% with pre-explant alteration of >10% (interval change)
Pre-explant LV dilation	Higher LVEDD and/or its Higher instability[b]	88.9% pv for LVEDD >55 mm[c]
High pre-explant LV wall tension (reduced RWT)	Lower RWT and/or its Higher instability[b]	81.8% pv for RWT_{ED} <0.38[c] 87% pv for RWT_{ED} reduction of >8% during the final off-pump trial
Altered pre-explant LV geometry (high sphericity) expressed by a high S/L_{ED}	Higher S/L_{ED} and/or its Higher instability[b]	84.6% pv for S/L_{ED} increase of >10% during the final off-pump trial
Reduced pre-explant wall motion velocity (Sm)	Lower Sm and/or its Higher instability[b]	83.3% pv for Sm <8 cm/s[c] 90% pv for Sm pre-explant alteration of >10%

PV predictive value
[a]Transthoracic echocardiography
[b]Parameter changes during the time between maximum improvement and LVAD explantation ("interval change") and/or during the final off-pump trial ("pre-explant change")
[c]Parameters measured during the final off-pump trial

Unstable "off-pump" LVEF alone is a risk factor for early recurrence of HF even if pre-explant LVEF is >45%, the LV size and geometry are normal, and the history length of HF is <5 years [9, 22]. Also altered and/or unstable LV geometry and low and/or unstable peak wall motion velocity (Sm) are relevant risk factors for HF recurrence even in patients with LVEF ≥45% [9].

In addition to the definitely proved risk factors for post-weaning HF recurrence mentioned above (see also Table 12.4), there are also other risk factors detectable by TTE or RHC during the off-pump trials with potential relevance for weaning decisions (Table 12.5).

12.4 Unloading-Promoted Myocardial Recovery: A Treatment Goal

Long-term VADs are to date used as lifesaving support which later becomes either a bridge-to-HTx or a definitive therapy for patients who cannot receive HTx. However, possibly the most attractive potential indication for VADs in the future might be their elective use as a therapeutic strategy for cardiac recovery. This will be possible only if the potential for recovery during VAD support becomes predictive before VAD implantation. Unfortunately the low rates of

Table 12.5 Additional risk factors detectable during "off-pump" trials at rest with relevance for weaning decisions

Examination	Parameters and parameter-derived measurements performed during off-pump trials
TTE	Progressive velocity-time-integral (VTI) reduction in the LV outflow tract reflecting stroke volume reduction
	Transmitral flow pattern alteration (new appearance or accentuation of pre-existent restrictive flow profile)
	New appearance or accentuation of tricuspid regurgitation (TR)
	Pulmonary arterial pressure increase (TR flow velocity increase)
	RV diameter increase and/or RV geometry alteration
	Reduction of systolic peak wall motion velocity at lateral tricuspid annulus (TAPS′)
	Relevant LV synchrony and synergy alterations (strain imaging) or accentuation of LV asynchrony and dyssynergy during off-pump trials
RH catheterization	Cardiac output reduction of >15% after pump stop
	Pulmonary capillary wedge pressure (PCWP) >13 mmHg
	Right atrial mean pressure >10 mmHg or increase of >50% during pump stops
Electrocardiography	More than 25% HR increase during off-pump trials and/or new appearance or increase in number of extrasystolic beats
Arterial pressure	Diastolic systemic arterial pressure <50 mmHg during off-pump trials (risk for misleading overestimation of LV function)

clinically relevant cardiac recovery during VAD support and the lack of reliable methods to predict recovery before VAD implantation, on the one hand, and the highly invasive procedure of VAD implantation with possibly serious complications after surgery, on the other hand, do not today allow VAD implantations primarily designed as a therapeutic option for cardiac recovery.

Recovery occurred more often in patients with less LV dilation, and it was also suggested that pre-implant LV size can predict the potential for VAD-promoted myocardial recovery. However, it was found that even preoperative LVEDD of >70 mm does not exclude reverse remodeling and LVEF increase beyond 45% during LVAD support allowing long-term cardiac stability after LVAD removal [8, 22]. Even in the largest series of patients with DCM as the underlying cause for MCS who underwent LVAD removal after recovery, it was not possible to identify any echo-parameter measured before implantation which was able to predict recovery during LVAD support [8, 22]. Thus, to date standard echocardiography cannot predict cardiac recovery during mechanical unloading. The possible superiority of strain imaging in this matter needs to be assessed in the future.

In DCM patients, histological examination of myocardial tissue obtained before VAD implantation showed that less fibrosis and myocyte hypertrophy are related to more cardiac recovery during VAD support, and fibrosis was found to be a predictor of sustained myocardial recovery [33]. Weaned patients with ≥5-year post-explant cardiac stability showed less fibrosis before VAD implantation than those with early post-weaning

HF recurrence [22]. Nevertheless, more information is necessary before any elective LVAD implantation with the aim of cardiac recovery can be considered only on the base of reduced pre-implant fibrosis. History length of HF ≥5 years does not exclude reverse remodeling with EF increase beyond 45%, but such patients are at higher risk for HF recurrence during the first 3 post-weaning years than those with history of HF <5 years (probability of HF recurrence 89%) [22]. However, short history of HF alone is not predictive for cardiac recovery during MCS [9, 22].

12.5 Conclusion and Future Directions

Stable cardiac recovery which allows a long-term HTx/VAD-free outcome after VAD removal is relatively rare and appears to be related to the etiology, severity, and duration of myocardial damage. Weaning from VADs is a feasible clinical option with potential successful results for >15 years even if nonischemic CCM was the underlying cause for MCS and even if cardiac recovery remains incomplete. Echocardiography and RHC are the cornerstone methods to assess cardiac recovery. Many parameters have proved to be useful for assessment of recovery and for prediction of long-term weaning success. Nevertheless, to date there is no "golden standard" for recovery assessment. Off-pump LVEF ≥45% and LVEDD ≤55 mm, at rest, are generally accepted as basic criteria for LVAD explantation, and their stability for 2–4 weeks after maximum improvement is an important requirement. Other off-pump echo-parameters of cardiac function (including tissue Doppler and strain imaging data) and LV geometry, as well as their pre-explant stability (between and during off-pump trials after maximum improvement), are helpful for weaning decisions (◘ Figs. 12.1, 12.2, and 12.3).

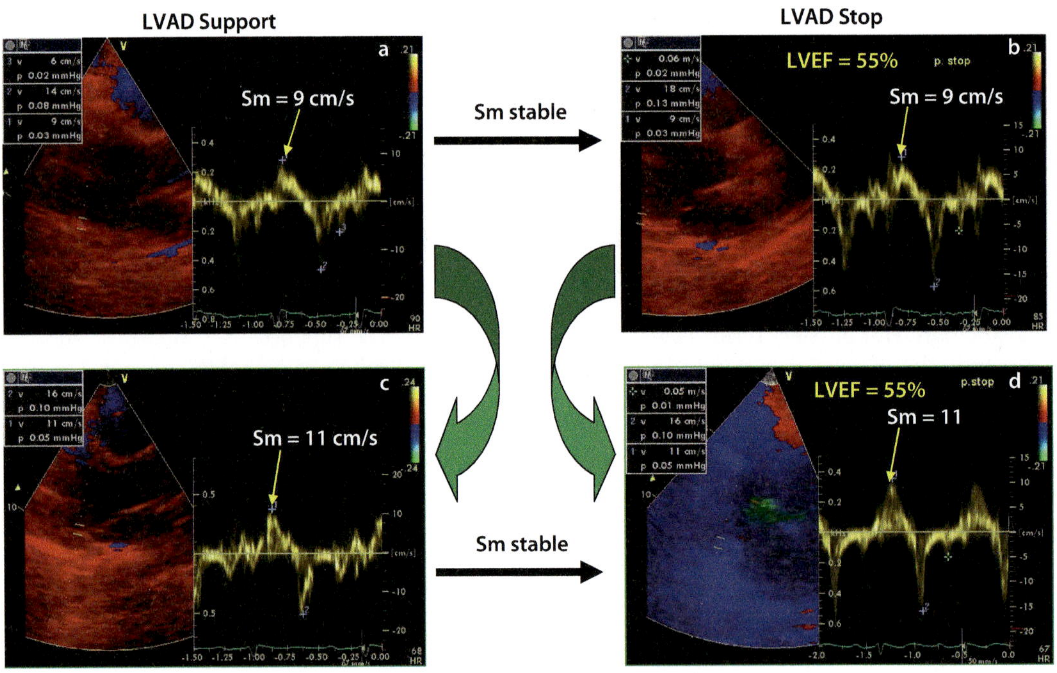

◘ **Fig. 12.1** Usefulness of left ventricular (*LV*) peak systolic wall motion velocity (*Sm*) measurements at the basal posterior wall by pulsed-wave tissue Doppler to assess the stability of LV contractile function during and between off-pump trials and for detection of further cardiac improvement after LVEF has reached its peak value. At the time when LVEF reached its maximum value (55%), Sm was 9 cm/s during full LVAD support (**a**) and remained stable during the off-pump trial (**b**). Although the LVEF remained unchanged, the Sm values with (**c**) and without(**d**) LVAD support increased during the next 3 weeks of unloading up to 11 cm/s (+22%). Thereafter, there was no further Sm improvement and the LVAD was successfully explanted

Stable normal hemodynamics during off-pump RHC trials is necessary for weaning decisions, but not sufficiently predictive for long-term cardiac stability after VAD explantation. Off-pump CI >2 L/min/m^2 and PCWP <14 mmHg are major requirements for VAD explantation. HF history length ≥5 years is one of the major risk factors for HF recurrence after VAD explantation.

There are two major limitations for a potential future use of VADs as therapeutic strategy aimed to reverse HF. First, the low probability of relevant cardiac recovery even after combination of unloading with drugs known to enhance reverse remodeling and second, the fact that recovery is not predictable before VAD implantation.

There are still several open questions on myocardial recovery after VAD implantation, which need to be answered in the future:

1. What causes the great discrepancy between the high recovery rates on cellular and molecular levels and the low rate of functionally stable cardiac recovery allowing VAD explantation?
2. Can future research on molecular and cellular levels provide a platform for additional adjunctive therapies (pharmacologic and/or cell-based therapy, gene transfer, etc.) aimed to optimize recovery and increase the number of weaning candidates?
3. Is it possible to facilitate weaning from VADs also in patients with chronic ischemic cardiomyopathy by promoting angiogenesis and myocyte regeneration?
4. Can future research on molecular and cellular level provide data which might allow already before VAD implantation the detection of patients with the potential for cardiac recovery under mechanical unloading?

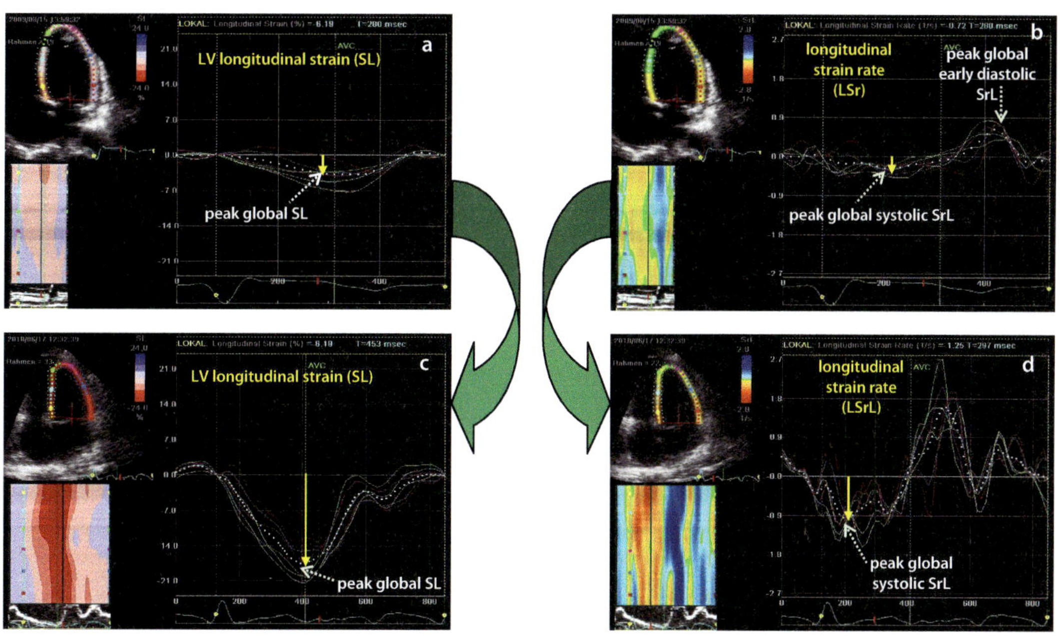

Fig. 12.2 Usefulness of speckle tracking-derived 2D stain imaging for assessment of cardiac improvement after left ventricular assist device (*LVAD*) implantation. The comparison of recordings obtained before LVAD implantation (**a**, **b**) and before LVAD explantation (**c**, **d**) showed striking improvements of systolic global longitudinal strain (myocardial longitudinal shortening) and strain rate (velocity of myocardial longitudinal shortening) which increased during several months of LVAD support from 4% (**a**) and 0.3/s (**b**) to 17.5% (**c**) and 9.6/s (**d**), respectively. The global early diastolic strain rate (early relaxation velocity) also increased from 0.7/s (**b**) to 1.6/s (**d**). Image (**d**) also shows a normalization of early/late diastolic strain rate ratio

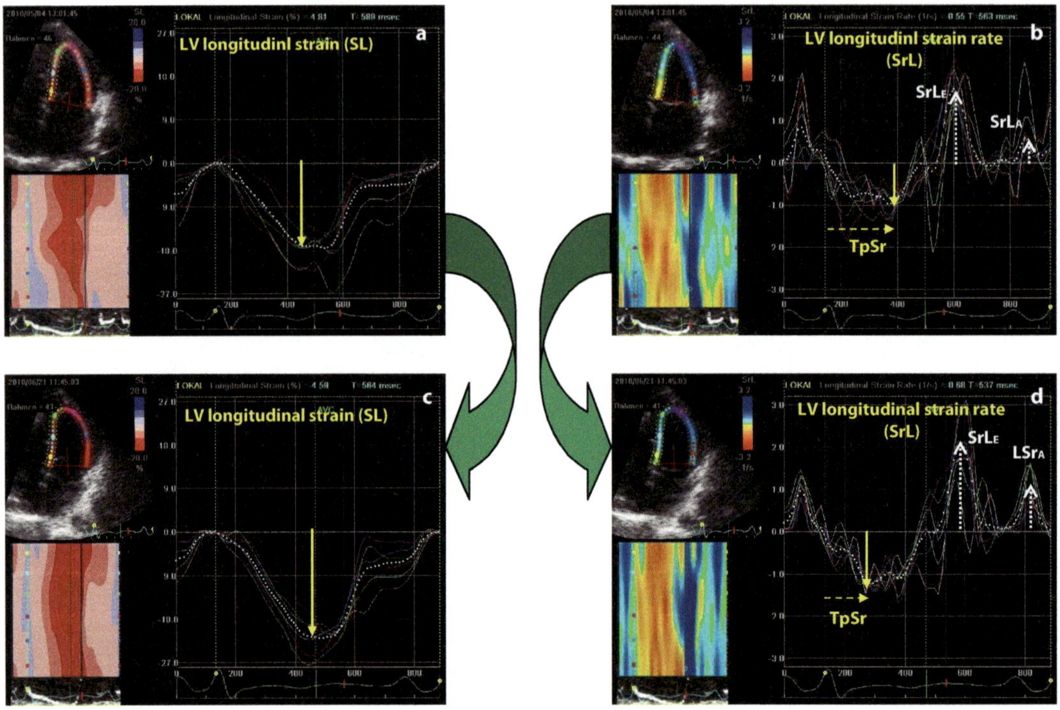

Fig. 12.3 Speckle tracking-derived 2D strain and strain rate off-pump recordings showing further cardiac improvement during left ventricular assist device (*LVAD*) support after off-pump LVEF reached its maximum value of 50%. At the time of maximum LVEF improvement (images **a** and **b**), longitudinal global systolic strain (*SL*) and strain rate (*SrL*) were slightly reduced (17% and 1/s, respectively), and the global early/late diastolic strain rate ratio (SrLE/SrLA) was high. After few weeks of further LVAD support, although the LVEF remained unchanged, both SL and SrL increased, reaching normal values (22% and 1.25/s, respectively), and there was also improvement in intraventricular synchrony of contraction (images **c** and **d**). The 35% shortening of the time to peak strain rate (*TpSr*) additionally indicates improvement of LV systolic function. The early relaxation velocity increase (from 1.7/s to 2.1/s) and the SrLE/SrLA ratio reduction (from 3.5 to 2.1) also indicate an improvement in LV diastolic function

References

1. Müller J, Wallukat G, Weng Y, Dandel M, Spiegelsberger S, Semrau S, Brandes K, Bieda H, Hummel M, Loebe M, Meyer R, Hetzer R (1997) Weaning from mechanical cardiac support in patients with dilated cardiomyopathy. Circulation 96:542–549
2. Hetzer R, Müller J, Weng Y, Wallukat G, Spiegelsberger S, Loebe M (1999) Cardiac recovery in dilated cardiomyopathy by unloading with a left ventricular assist device. Ann Thorac Surg 68:742–749
3. Dandel M, Weng Y, Sinawski H, Potapov E, Lehmkuhl HB, Hetzer R (2005) Long-term results in patients with idiopathic dilated cardiomyopathy after weaning from left ventricular assist devices. Circulation 112:37–45
4. Ferrar DJ, Holmann WR, McBride LR, Kormos RL, Icenogle TB, Hendry PJ, Moore CH, Loisance DY, El-Banayosy A, Frazier H (2002) Long-term follow up of Thoratec ventricular assist device bridge-to-recovery patients successfully removed from support after recovery of ventricular function. J Heart Lung Transplant 21:516–521
5. Mann DL, Barger MP, Burkhoff D (2012) Myocardial recovery and the failing Heart. J Am Coll Cardiol 60(24):2465–2472
6. Hall JL, Fermin DR, Birks EJ, Barton PJ, Slaughter M, Eckman P, Baba HA, Wohlschlaeger J, Miller LW (2011) Clinical, molecular, and genomic changes in response to a left ventricular assist device. J Am Coll Cardiol 57:641–652
7. Dandel M, Knosalla C, Hetzer R (2014) Contribution of ventricular assist devices to the recovery of failing hearts: a review and the Berlin Heart Centert Experience. Eur J Heart Fail 16:248–263
8. Dandel M, Weng Y, Siniawski H, Potapov E, Drews T, Lehmkuhl HB, Knosalla C, Hetzer R (2008) Prediction of cardiac stability after weaning from ventricular assist devices in patients with idiopathic dilated cardiomyopathy. Circulation 118:S94–S105
9. Dandel M, Weng Y, Siniawski H, Potapov E, Krabatsch T, Lehmkuhl HB, Drews T, Knosalla C, Hetzer R (2012) Pre-explant stability of unloading promoted cardiac improvement predicts outcome after weaning from ventricular assist devices. Circulation 126(11):S3–S19
10. Ambardekar AV, Walker JS, Walker LA, Cleveland JC Jr, Lowes BD, Buttrick PM (2011) Incomplete recovery of

myocyte contractile function despite improvement of myocardial architecture with left ventricular assist device support. Circ Heart Fail 4(4):425–432
11. Birks EJ, Hall JL, Barton PJR, Grindle S, Latif N, Hary JP, Rider JE, Banner NR, Khaghani A, Miller LW, Yacoub MH (2005) Gene profiling changes in cytoskeletal proteins during clinical recovery after left ventricular-assist support. Circulation 112(suppl I):I57–I64
12. Akhter SA, D'Souza KM, Malhotra R, Staron ML, Valeroso TB, Fedson SE, Anderson AS, Raman J, Jeevanandam V (2010) Reversal of impaired myocardial beta-adrenergic receptor signaling by continuous-flow left ventricular assist device support. J Heart Lung Transplant 29:603–609
13. Ogletree ML, Sweet WE, Talerico C, Klecka ME, Young JB, Smedira NG, Starling RC, Moravec CS (2010) Duration of left ventricular assist device support: effects on abnormal calcium cycling and functional recovery in the failing human heart. J Heart Lung Transplant 29:554–561
14. Hall JL, Torre-Amione G (2012) Cellular, molecular, genomic and functional changes that occur in the failing heart in response to mechanical circulatory support. In: Kormos RL, Miller LW (eds) Mechanical circulatory support. A companion to braunwald's heart disease. Elsevier, Philadelphia, pp 258–271
15. Baba HA, Grabellus F, August C, Plenz G, Takeda A, Tjan TD, Schmid C, Deng MC (2000) Reversal of metallothionein expression is different throughout the human myocardium after prolonged left-ventricular mechanical support. J Heart Lung Transplant 19(7):668–674
16. Francis GS, Anwar F, Bank AJ, Kubo SH, Jessurun J (1999) Apoptosis, Bcl-2and proliferating cell nuclear antigen in the failing human heart: observation made after implantation of left ventricular assist device. J Card Fail 5:308–315
17. Manginas A, Tsiavou A, Sfyrakis P, Giamouzis G, Tsourelis L, Leontiadis E, Degiannis D, Cokkinos DV, Alivizatos PA (2009) Increased number of circulating progenitor cells after implantation of ventricular assist devices. J Heart Lung Transpl 28(7):710–717
18. Wohlschlaeger J, Levkau B, Brockoff G, Schmitz KJ, von Winterfeld M, Takeda A, Takeda N, Stypmann J, Vahlhaus C, Schmid C, Pomjanski N, Böcking A, Baba HA (2010) Hemodynamic support by left ventricular assist devices reduces cardiomyocyte DNA content in the failing human heart. Circulation 121:989–996
19. Muranaka H, Marui A, Tsukashita M, Wang J, Nakano J, Ikeda T, Sakata R (2010) Prolonged mechanical unloading preserves myocardial contractility but impairs relaxation in rat heart of dilated cardiomyopathy accompanied by myocardial stiffness and apoptosis. J Thorac Cardiovasc Surg 140:916–922
20. Terraciano CMN, Hardy J, Birks EJ, Khaghani A, Banner NR, Yacoub MH (2004) Clinical recovery from end-stage heart failure using left ventricular assist device and pharmacological therapy correlates with increased sarcoplasmic reticulum calcium content but not with regression of cellular hypertrophy. Circulation 109:2263–2265
21. Birks EJ, Tansley PD, Hardy J, George RS, Bowles CT, Burke M, Banner NR, Khagani A, Yacoub MH (2006) Left ventricular assist device and drug therapy for the reversal of heart failure. N Engl J Med 355:1873–1884
22. Dandel M, Weng Y, Siniawski H, Stepanenko A, Krabatsch T, Potapov E, Lehmkuhl HB, Knosalla C, Hetzer R (2011) Heart failure reversal by ventricular unloading in patients with chronic cardio-myopathy: criteria for weaning from ventricular assist devices. Eur Heart J 32:1148–1160
23. Simon MA, Kormos RL, Murali S, Nair P, Heffernan M, Gorcsan J, Winowich S, McNamara DM (2005) Myocardial recovery using ventricular assist devices: prevalence, clinical characteristics, and outcomes. Circulation 112:I32–I36
24. Kirklin JK, Naftel DC, Kormos RL, Stevensen LW, Pagani FD, Miller MM, Baldwin TJ, Joung JB (2013) Fifth INTERMAX annual report: risk factor analysis for more than 6000 mechanical circulatory support patients. J Heart Lung Transplant 32(2):141–156
25. Birks EJ, Miller LW (2012) Myocardial recovery with use of ventricular assist devices. In: Kormos RL, Miller LW (eds) Mechanical circulatory support. A companion to braunwald's heart disease. Elsevier, Philadelphia, pp 258–271
26. Birks EJ, George RS, Firouzi A, Wright G, Bahrami T, Yacoub MH, Khaghani A (2012) Long-term outcomes of patients bridged to recovery versus patients bridged to transplantation. J Thorac Cardiovasc Surg 144:190–196
27. Hetzer R, Müller J, Weng Y, Meyer R, Dandel M (2001) Bridging-to-recovery. Ann Thorac Surg 71: S109–S113
28. Birks EJ, George RS, Hedger M, Bahrami T, Wilton P, Bowles CT, Webb C, Bougard R, Amrani M, Yacoub MH, Dreyfus G, Khaghani A (2011) Reversal of severe heart failure with a continuous-flow left ventricular assist device and pharmacological therapy: a prospective study. Circulation 123(4):381–390
29. Krabatsch T, Schweiger M, Dandel M, Stepanenko A, Drews T, Potapov E, Pasic M, Weng YG, Huebler M, Hetzer R (2011) Is bridge to recovery more likely with pulsatile left ventricular assist devices than with nonpulsatile-flow systems? Ann Thorac Surg 91(5):1335–1340
30. Hetzer R, Potapov EV, Alexi-Meskishvili V, Weng Y, Moera O, Berger F, Hennig E, Hübler M (2011) Single-center experience with treatment of cardiogenic shock in children by pediatric assist devices. J Thorac Cardiovasc Surg 141:616–623
31. Blume ED, Naftel DC, Bastardi HJ, Duncan BW, Kirklin JK, Webber SA (2006) Outcomes of children bridged to heart transplantation with ventricular assist devices. Circulation 113:2213–2319
32. Klotz S, Burkhoff D, Garrelds IM, Boomsma F, Danser AH (2009) The impact of left ventricular assist device induces left ventricular unloading on the myocardial renin-angiotensin-aldosterone system: therapeutic consequences? Eur Heart J 30:805–812
33. Simon MA, Primack BA, Teutenberg J, Kormos RL, Bermudez C, Toyoda Y, Shah H, Gorcsan J 3rd, McNamara DM (2010) Left ventricular remodelling and myocardial recovery on mechanical circulatory support. J Card Fail 16(2):99–105

Mechanical Circulatory Support as Bridge to Candidacy

Maria Frigerio, Manlio Cipriani, and David Feldman

© Springer International Publishing Switzerland 2017
A. Montalto et al. (eds.), *Mechanical Circulatory Support in End-Stage Heart Failure*,
DOI 10.1007/978-3-319-43383-7_13

13.1 Introduction

13.1.1 Definition

Implant of long-term mechanical circulatory support (MCS), ventricular assist device (VAD), or total artificial heart (TAH) in patients who are not yet on the heart transplant (HTX) waiting list, in whom actual or future eligibility for HTX has been neither ascertained nor excluded, is not uncommon in clinical practice. This strategy can be defined as "bridge to candidacy" (BTC); including in this group also are patients with the highest degree of uncertainty, in whom MCS strategy is sometimes classified as "bridge to decision."

13.1.2 Prevalence and Outcome

As per September 2015, in the Interagency Registry for Mechanically Assisted Circulatory Support (INTERMACS), the proportion of patients classified as bridge to transplant (BTT)-likely, BTT-moderate, and BTT-unlikely that all together may be pooled as "BTC" was 40.6% in those enrolled from 2006 to 2009, 36.3% in 2010–2011, and 29.2% since 2012 and thereafter. In the meantime, BTT strategy in patients already listed for HTX decreased from 47.8 to 26.0%, while DT strategy increased from 8.2 to 43.8% of the cases. As a whole, BTC patients represented 1/3 of the entire population (n = 4991/15323) [1]. The Italian Mechanically Assisted Circulatory Support (ITAMACS) Registry, reporting the vast majority of long-term MCS/LVAD/TAH implants in Italy from 2010 to 2013 (n = 289 in adult population), includes 40 patients classified as BTC and 3 as BTD (overall 15%), with the majority of patients implanted with BTT (49%) followed by DT strategy (36%) [2]. In the EUROMACS first published report [3], 312/825 patients (37.8%) who received a device for MCS between January 2011 and December 2013 had been classified as "possible bridge to transplant."

It must be acknowledged that MCS strategy may change over time, as a consequence of improvement, MCS-related complications, or MCS-unrelated adverse events and evolving comorbidities. BTC patients are by definition a dynamic group, in whom decision regarding suitability for HTx has been deferred at the time of the operation. However, initial implant indication maintains an influence on outcomes, being associated with different pre-implant characteristics, different probability to get HTX, and different survival, with or without HTX. A report from patients enrolled in the INTERMACS from 2006 to March 2011 [4, 5] showed that at 2 years, about 40% of BTT and only 6% of DT patients had received HTX, with intermediate percentages in BTC patients, according to the likelihood of becoming BTT as estimated at the time of the operation. Overall 2-year survival, irrespective of HTX, was 77.7% in BTT, 70.1% in BTC, and 60.7% in DT patients. Among BTC patients surviving on support, about 1/3 of those classified as BTT-likely was still on the waiting list at 2 years, while 23% had been switched to DT strategy. A higher proportion of patients initially classified as BTC-moderate or BTC-unlikely (24% and 39%, respectively) had been already switched to DT strategy at 1 year.

13.1.3 MCS as BTC: Clinical Settings and Objectives

The criteria defining need and eligibility for HTX change over time and have been recently updated [6]. Patients receving MCS with BTC strategy are those who are felt in need for HTX, but whose eligibility is under question due to a wide spectrum of reasons, that can be classified as follows.

- Conditions contraindicating HTX, or increasing its risk to unacceptable levels, observed mostly in the setting of known chronic heart failure. Mechanical support may just allow to gain time, as in the case of recent history of treated cancer or severe obesity, or may also contribute directly to remove the obstacle, as in the case of severe, fixed pulmonary hypertension or renal insufficiency. Renal failure is unfrequently the sole or main indication for MCS as BTC, being mostly a feature of refractory low output state, that generally recover quickly on mechanical support. The average weight loss on support in obese LVAD recipients is below 5 Kg [7], leading some groups to suggest to associate bariatric surgery to LVAD implant if obesity is the main obstacle to transplant. Pulmonary hypertension and cancer will be discussed in the following paragraphs.

- Uncertainties or doubts regarding the absence of contraindications or major risk factors, including those related with psychosocial profile, in patients with new onset or new diagnosis of heart failure, presenting with acute, refractory/worsening symptoms, low output state, or cardiogenic shock. In these cases, MCS may serve as a lifesaving, "rescue" therapy and also facilitate myocardial restoration and sometimes recovery. In this setting, initial implant strategy has been also defined as "bridge to decision" (BTD) and in some cases may be classified ex post as "bridge to recovery" (BTR). MCS in the acute heart failure setting, generally corresponding to low INTERMACS profiles, may be implemented initially with short-term circulatory support devices and is discussed in detail in Chaps. 7 and 9; thus, only a brief summary of the decision-making process will be reported here.
- Very low probability to have access to HTX due to hyperimmune status. This condition, called sensitization, is not a true contraindication, but in fact limits the probability to undergo the operation, and mid- to long-term support may be useful to allow desensitization and/or to wait for a compatible donor.

Choices regarding indications for short- or long-term MCSD implant, HTX eligibility, and prioritization on the waiting list may vary according to national regulations, local expertise and practice, donor availability, and individual preferences. Noteworthy, for most conditions, the updated guidelines for HTX candidate selection do not set clear-cut thresholds that define contraindications, but point out the relevance of several risk factors and of their combination [6]. The interplay between MCS and HTX listing and prioritization will be addressed at the end of this chapter.

13.2 Pulmonary Hypertension

It is well known that fixed pulmonary hypertension (PH), unresponsive to acute vasodilator challenge, represents a major risk factor or a contraindication for HTX, being associated with increased probability of early right ventricular failure, multi-organ failure, prolonged mechanical ventilation (with nitric oxide administration), and higher mortality. The recently updated ISHLT guidelines for selection of HTX candidates recommend to evaluate and reevaluate periodically the presence and reversibility of PH with right heart catheterization, considering pulmonary artery systolic pressure ≤50 mmHg and either transpulmonary gradient (TPG) ≤15 mmHg or pulmonary vascular resistance (PVR) ≤3 Wood units (while maintaining a systolic arterial blood pressure > 85 mm Hg) as upper acceptable levels for HTX listing (class I, level of evidence C) [6]. Reversibility may be tested with infusion of sodium nitroprusside or, in case of concomitant severely reduced cardiac output, of an inodilator such as milrinone or enoximone, with an association of an inotropic agent (e.g., dobutamine) and a vasodilator, or after a 24-h infusion of levosimendan. When the patient is severely congested at baseline, it may be better to defer hemodynamic evaluation after volume unloading, with a target right atrial pressure (RAP) <10–12 mmHg, unless hemodynamic monitoring is perceived useful for treating the patient. In most cases, at least partial improvement of the hemodynamic profile may be obtained with pharmacological therapy, but especially when it is accompanied by some renal dysfunction (increased serum creatinine and/or blood urea nitrogen) or the patient is a "frequent flyer," and obviously when the INTERMACS profile is ≤3, LVAD should be considered to maintain patient conditions suitable for HTX regarding both hemodynamics and end-organ function while awaiting. This strategy appears reasonable, also taking into account that several analyses of multicenter cohorts have shown better survival on the waiting list and better overall survival including post-transplant outcome, when patients listed as status 2A are treated with a LVAD with respect to medical therapy alone [8–10]. In cases of resistant, "fixed" PH under pharmacological treatment, LVAD may still be an option, as BTC or for long-term, indefinite treatment. One paper reports that post-HTX outcome after, on average, more than 400 days from LVAD implant may be still dependent on PH reversibility assessed with pharmacological manipulation before LVAD implant, especially when reduction in TPG and/or PVR has been unsatisfactory [10]. However, in this paper the evolution of PH after LVAD implant had not been addressed. After LVAD implant, the immediate hemodynamic change is a dramatic reduction of pulmonary capillary wedge pressure (PCWP). Reduction in pulmonary artery pressure (PAP), TPG, and PVR, which are important for HTX eligibility, is generally also observed over time, but at a slower rate and inferior proportion. Various studies reporting on this point suggest that hemodynamic profiles suitable for HTX are reached in most cases approximately at 3 months after LVAD implant and that in these patients HTX may be performed with good postoperative outcomes [11–18]. Of note, first experiences include patients treated in the 1990s, and various types of pulsatile- and continuous-flow devices had been utilized, providing similar results, suggesting that (1) LV unloading "per se" is the mechanism for secondary PH resolution and (2) this concept has been gradually incorporated into clinical practices. It is prudent to ascertain PH resolution prior to proceed to listing and transplantation and to reassess periodically pulmonary hemodynamics as it is usual in HTX candidates [6]. If reduction in PAP, TPG, or PVR remains unsatisfactory despite LV mechanical unloading, some authors suggest to add medical treatment targeted to pulmonary arterial hypertension, i.e., an endothelin receptor antagonist (bosentan) [19] or a PDE-5 inhibitor (sildenafil) [20]. Observational experiences in a limited number of cases appear to obtain some additional hemodynamic improvement; however, this approach must be considered with caution, taking into account that (1) these studies were not controlled, (2) controlled clinical trials with the same drugs in patients with heart failure and PH secondary to LV dysfunction did not demonstrate any significant benefit, and (3) in patients with "primary" pulmonary hypertension (PPH), clinical benefit appears superior than expected on the basis of the observed, numerically limited hemodynamic changes, suggesting that the mechanisms of PH and of the effects of drugs on clinical and hemodynamic end points are different in the two conditions of PPH and PH secondary to LV disease [21]. An interesting line of research on advanced HF with preserved LVEF, which is characterized by markedly restrictive physiology, pulmonary hypertension, dilated left atrium, and normal LV size, regards the possibility of long-term use of continuous-flow micropumps that drain blood from the left atrium instead of LV, to circumvent surgical and hemodynamic problems that limit the utilization of currently available LVADs in various forms of restrictive or hypertrophic cardiomyopathy [22]. Patients with these diseases are considered as disadvantaged with respect to those with dilated/hypokinetic cardiomyopathy, due to limited resources for both pharmacological and mechanical treatment [6].

13.3 Cancer

Cancer, together with late graft dysfunction and cardiac allograft vasculopathy, is the leading cause of death after HTX [23]. Post-transplant immunosuppression is known to be associated with increased probability to develop malignant disease, in general and especially regarding some malignancies related to viral infections, such as EBV-positive non-Hodgkin lymphoma and HHV8-positive Kaposi's sarcoma [23, 24] Moreover, the course of post-transplant malignant diseases may be very dramatic and aggressive, although in recent years some alternative immunosuppressive regimens, based on antiproliferative mammalian target of rapamycin (M-Tor) inhibitors instead of on calcineurin inhibitors, have been proposed as possibly associated with a reduced risk of developing malignancies and a reduced speed of their progression [25–27]. As a consequence, not only patients with active malignant disease but also those who had been recently treated are considered ineligible for HTX, until there are reasonable motives for considering this disease as definitely "cured" and at very, very low probability of recurrence [6, 25].

After completing treatment, the length of disease-free follow-up time required for eligibility for HTX is variable, in relationship with the site and type of malignancy, individual characteristics and treatments, and the degree of certitude that is felt appropriate. In any case, it may be too long for patients' waiting, especially when INTERMACS profile is 3 and 4; thus, long-term LVAD implant with BTC strategy may be considered [28–30]. Reports regarding outcomes in this specific category of BTC patients are very scant; thus, the strength of pertinent recommendation in the ISHLT guidelines, 2016, is IIb (i.e., possibly recommended, with doubts), and the level of evidence is C (experts' consensus) [6].

It must also be taken into account that a relevant proportion of patients with severe heart failure and treated cancer have received antineoplastic drugs and/or radiotherapy that may have caused heart disease or at least contributed to it. Post-chemotherapy cardiomyopathy is not rarely characterized by biventricular compromise and mildly dilated LV with severe systolic and diastolic dysfunction, leading to restrictive filling pattern, low/very low cardiac index, pulmonary hypertension, high right filling pressure, and reduced tolerability of standard heart failure treatments [28, 31]. Moreover, chest radiotherapy may damage the heart via several mechanisms, including valvular disease, pericardial thickening with tenacious adhesions to the surrounding tissues, diffuse coronary artery stenosis, and myocardial fibrosis, contributing to restrictive physiology and making it difficult the successful implant of a LVAD, for both hemodynamic and surgical reasons [31]. Unfortunately, these conditions are not ideal either for continuing medical therapy alone or for LVAD implant, and a higher rate of postoperative RV failure has been reported in LVAD recipients with post-chemotherapy cardiomyopathy with respect to other etiologies [27, 28, 30, 32].

The availability of mechanical devices for advanced HF may be seen as an opportunity for expanding the cancer patient population that can be treated with contemporary approach, including surgery, pharmacotherapy, and radiotherapy, despite severe heart disease. Some reports showed the feasibility of surgical tumor resection or debulking [33–35], and the safety of radiotherapy without interferences with device functioning [36, 37] when cancer is diagnosed during follow-up after LVAD implantation. However, it does not mean that long-term simultaneous management of LVAD and cancer should be, at present, prospectically planned and practiced in the majority of patients. Such experiences are very few [38]. Malignancies may imply altered – most often increased – thrombogenicity, and pharmacological therapy may cause anemia, leukopenia, pancytopenia, mucositis, gastroenteric disturbances, and increased lung alveolar permeability, all conditions that may alter blood rheology, drug absorption, and hemodynamic and ventilatory requirements and facilitate infections [29, 30]. Moreover, both LVAD and cancer therapy are highly demanding in terms of economic and human resources and also in terms of suffering, expectations, and coping, for the patient and also for the relatives and caregivers. Thus, a situation in which the interests of individuals and of the community could collide, which 10 years ago had been debated as a theoretical case, may be now a real clinical and ethical dilemma [39]. So far, prospective long-term LVAD implant in patients with active serious malignancy should be evaluated very carefully within an expert multidisciplinary team and should represent, in authors' opinion, an exception more than a rule. In any case, expectations and uncertainties should be explained with realism and frankness to the patients and their families.

13.4 Acute/De Novo Heart Failure

Patients presenting with acute, severe/refractory heart failure or cardiogenic shock are a highly heterogenous group in terms of etiology (acute myocardial infarction, post-cardiotomy shock, fulminant myocarditis, peripartum cardiomyopathy), treatment, and probability of recovery [40]. In this setting, implantation of short-term MCS may be the best initial option, leaving room to evaluate further evolution, while transition to long-term LVAD or TAH are critical choices, also because in relatively young patients without relevant comorbidities they imply to consider also HTX listing. Streamlining very acute patients toward HTX is critical because their attitudes and psychological characteristics are not well known, recovery of cardiac function in some cases occurs after several weeks, and multi-organ dysfunction associated with cardiogenic shock represents a risk factor [23]. These aspects are discussed in Chaps. 7 and 9, and the relationship with HTX listing and prioritization is analyzed later, in the last section of this chapter. In the case of post-cardiotomy heart failure or shock, two different conditions must be recognized: the first corresponds to de novo, unexpected HF due to dramatic complications; the second corresponds to difficulties encountered in patients with already known HF/LV dysfunction, undergoing high-risk conservative/reparative surgery. In the latter, rescue strategies in case of surgery failure should have been already discussed, also with the patient, and planned on an individual basis before entering the operating room.

13.5 Sensitization

Hyperimmune status, generally defined as the presence of anti-HLA antibodies against a variety of antigenic profiles that may be encountered in local population (panel-reactive antibody, PRA, >10%), may reduce the probability to get HTX, and when it is performed, post-transplant course may be difficult and survival reduced, due to an immuno-mediated reaction to the graft that may comprise a spectrum from immediate, hyperacute rejection to late graft failure [41]. Hyperacute rejection is a dramatic and lethal event, consisting of immediate aggression to the transplanted heart that happens in the operating room, at reperfusion or early after, due to the cytotoxic effect of pre-existing anti-HLA Class I antibodies. The presence of class II anti-HLA antibodies is associated to an increased probability to experience acute cellular and/or humoral rejection. The burden of cellular rejection has been recognized to facilitate the development and progression of cardiac allograft vasculopathy, while after humoral rejection it is not uncommon to observe a marked acceleration of CAV, with quick development of new, multiple lesions and diffuse arterial narrowing. Although there is an agreement on these general concepts, various criteria, tests, and thresholds for defining sensitization, requiring pre-transplant crossmatch, implementing apheresis at the time of HTX, and pursue desensitization before HTX are used. Desensitization therapies include plasmapheresis, immunoapheresis, immunoadsorption, and administration of high-dose immunoglobulins, cyclophosphamide, and monoclonal antibodies targeted to lymphocyte subpopulations, e.g., rituximab, bortezomib, and others [6, 41]

Thus, sensitized patients have a reduced probability to get HTX unless some prioritization is considered [42, 43] and when hemodynamically unstable may be considered for long-term LVAD therapy. Unfortunately, patients are more prone to produce anti-HLA antibodies after LVAD implant, and regular PRA monitoring and at least "virtual" crossmatch are strongly recommended in LVAD-supported HTX candidates [43–46]. The impact of sensitization on post-transplant overall outcome depends also on patient characteristics, center experience, and donor pool. It must be kept in mind that the sensitized LVAD patients may be challenging HTX recipients [47], with increased risk for both rejection and infection and divergent needs: for example, induction of immunosuppression with polyclonal or monoclonal antibodies is recommended for sensitized patients, but not for HTX candidates with LVAD.

13.6 Considerations on Mechanical Circulatory Support/Left Ventricular Assist Device Therapy and Listing and Prioritization for Heart Transplantation

The setting of MCS with BTC strategy is highly representative of the complex and dynamic interplay between MCS and HTX listing and prioritization, both in terms of general criteria and shared rules and in terms of decision making regarding individuals.

We all agree that the few available donor hearts should be assigned taking into account both the need and the probability of survival after HTX, but when we try to translate these principles into recommendations on eligibility for HTX listing and then into rules for organ allocation and candidate prioritization, there is no universal consensus, also due to geographical differences [48, 49]. Some typical scenarios concerning MCS and HTX will be presented here.

- Short-term MCS. In acute, severe heart failure with (or evolving to) cardiogenic shock (INTERMACS profile 1 and 2), short-term MCS is intended as "rescue therapy," or bridge to decision (BTD), and is by definition a temporary condition. Contemporary trends in the treatment of cardiogenic shock due to acute myocardial infarction appear in favor of MCS with respect to intra-aortic balloon pump [50, 51] and, together with the advanced, aggressive approach to out-of-hospital cardiac arrest [52], may increase in the near future the number of "rescued" patients who do not reach adequate cardiac function for allowing weaning from the device in a few days. Extended support with paracorporeal devices, transition to a long-term device (the so-called bridge to bridge strategy), or fast-track listing for HTX in high-priority status are then the possible choices [40]. Similar options may be considered after high-risk "conservative" surgery or after unexpected complications leading to post-cardiotomy shock requiring short-term MCS. It is well known that temporary circulatory support is one of the major risk factors for early death after HTX [23], but in clinical practice these patients cannot be considered as a homogeneous group. In fact, young patients with de novo heart failure, without relevant comorbidities, and with normal or normalized end-organ function on support may have excellent results after HTX, while patients aged 60 years or more, with prior history of heart failure, diabetes, renal failure, peripheral or cerebral vasculopathy, and/or MCS-related complications such as coagulopathy or limb ischemia, should be considered with much attention when overall medical utility of HTX is also taken into account, besides the efforts to save a single patient. Full – or at least sufficient to get along after weaning – myocardial recovery is not rarely observed in patients with acute myocarditis or peripartum cardiomyopathy, in whom a watchful delay of HTX listing may be justified [40].

- Long-term LVAD without complications. Patients who received LVAD with BTT strategy plus those implanted as BTC who have reached the expected goals for eligibility for HTX are filling in this scenario. Their probability of post-transplant survival is similar to that of the other recipients, but the net benefit conferred by transplantation and the role and weight of specific risk factors remain to be elucidated. The appropriate priority status for organ allocation in these patients is under debate [8, 9, 53, 54], and at present the rules vary from country to country. After LVAD implant, the survival curve shows a constant decline over time, with an acceleration after 2–3 years, mostly due to LVAD-related complications (infections, stroke, aortic insufficiency), system failures (including pump thrombosis), or loss of efficacy (relapsing heart failure, late RV failure) [53]. Thus, some priority for LVAD-supported HTX candidates with respect to other stable outpatients appears to be justified. On the other side, transplanting a stable LVAD patient means to expose this patient to the inherent risks – which are mostly upfront after HTX – and deprive another patient in need who cannot take advantage from long-term MCS. Moreover, the usefulness of an intermediate prioritization of a growing cohort, such as that of LVAD patients, in helping them to actually get a heart is doubtful. In this perspective, LVAD-supported candidates should qualify for priority only if and when they develop some complication. In fact, it seems that even in the USA, where these patients may be classified as status 1A (i.e., highest priority) for 30 days per year, the rate of HTX in BTT patients is getting slower over time, and it is much lower in BTC patients [4, 55, 56].
- Long-term LVAD, complicated. Adverse events and LVAD-related complications – which in many cases may be managed without HTX – are the object of ▶ Chap. 28. HTX may be a lifesaving procedure in some of these patients, and there are optimistic reports regarding post-transplant outcomes in patients deemed "stable" in presence of "controlled" LVAD-related complications. However, deep infections could have a negative impact on post-HTX survival [57], and the additive role and weight of LVAD-specific conditions and complications, besides common risk factors for HTX, has not been analyzed in details so far [58]. Other complications, typically stroke, may cause relevant disability and lead to removal from the waiting list due to loss of functional benefit. In fact, the proportion of patients switched from BTT to DT strategy for any cause is increasing, and the percentage of BTC candidates classified as DT at 2 years is higher that their HTX rate at the same time [4]. Extended use of LVAD therapy in less severe heart failure (non-inotrope-dependent, INTERMACS $\geq$4), now representing less than 20% of the implanted patients, is

currently under evaluation [5, 59, 60]. This approach could further increase the pressure of patients with complicated LVAD on the HTX waiting list in the near future. Since probably not all of them will receive a heart timely, the net benefit of this strategy in patients with advanced – but not end-stage – heart failure could actually result to be smaller than expected.

- In summary:
  1. Long-term LVAD therapy so far appears to be an excellent solution in the mid-term perspective.
  2. Long-term results are not rarely compromised by complications, firstly, infections and stroke and, secondly, pump thrombosis, malfunction, aortic valve insufficiency, or late RV failure.
  3. As a consequence, with extended use of MCS and LVAD therapy, the need for HTX will probably be delayed in individual patient's trajectory, but the number of patients in need will globally increase rather than decrease [60–63].
  4. Dissociating LVAD and HTX at conceptual level, moving away from "bridging" as main objective [5], is theoretically an interesting approach, but will not diminish the competition for the small number of available donor hearts, especially if selection criteria for candidacy are broadened rather than restricted, as in the updated ISHLT guidelines [5, 6, 60].
  5. Possible solutions to this medical and ethical dilemma would come from (a) significant reduction in LVAD-related morbidity in the mid- to long-term perspective; (b) selection of HTX candidates aimed to reduce the number of listed patients, e.g., orienteering older patients toward DT-LVAD whenever possible [63, 64]; (c) reconsideration of priorities in organ allocation, introducing some estimate of the probability of success besides of the urgency of need and taking into account LVAD-specific risk factors and their relationships with demographics and comorbidities. In this perspective, joined analysis of MCS/VAD and HTX registries appears highly advisable [61–64].

References

1. The Data and Clinical Coordinating Center University of Alabama at Birmingham Intermacs (Interagency Registry for Mechanically Assisted Circulatory Support). Quarterly statistical report (2015) Q3 – Implant and event dates: 23 June 2006 to 30 September 2015. Available at ▶ https://www.uab.edu/medicine/intermacs/images/Federal_Quarterly_Report/Statistical_Summaries/Federal_Partners_Report_2015_Q3.pdf. Accessed on 14 Jan 2016
2. Feltrin G, Frigerio M, Martinelli L et al (2015) Preliminary results from ITAMACS, the Italian Multi Center Registry for Mechanically Assisted Circulatory Support. J Heart Lung Transplant 34(Suppl):S11–S12
3. de By TM, Mohacsi P, Gummert J et al (2015) The European Registry for Patients with Mechanical Circulatory Support (EUROMACS): first annual report. Eur J Cardiothorac Surg 47:770–776; (discussion 776–7)
4. Teuteberg JJ, Stewart JC, Jessup M et al (2013) Implant strategies change over time and impact outcomes: insights from the INTERMACS (Interagency Registry for Mechanically Assisted Circulatory Support). JACC Heart Fail 1:369–378
5. Fang JC, Stehlik J (2013) Moving beyond "bridges". JACC Heart Fail 1:379–381
6. Mehra, MR, Canter CE, Hannan MM et al, On Behalf of the International Society for Heart Lung Transplantation (ISHLT) Infectious Diseases, Pediatric and Heart Failure and Transplantation Councils (2016) The 2016 international society for heart lung transplantation listing criteria for heart transplantation: a 10-year update. J Heart Lung Transplant 35:1–23
7. Chaudhry UI, Kanji A, Sai-Sudhakar CB, Higgins RS, Needleman BJ (2015) Laparoscopic sleeve gastrectomy in morbidly obese patients with end-stage heart failure and left ventricular assist adevice: medium-term results. Surg Obes Relat Dis Off J Am Soc Bariatric Surg 11:88–93
8. Singh TP, Milliren CE, Almond CS, Graham D (2014) Survival benefit of transplantation in patients listed for heart transplantation in the United States. J Am Coll Cardiol 63:1169–1178
9. Wever-Pinzon O, Drakos SG, Kfoury AG et al (2013) Morbidity and mortality in heart transplant candidates supported with mechanical circulatory support: is reappraisal of the current United network for organ sharing thoracic organ allocation policy justified? Circulation 127:452–462
10. Wozniak CJ, Stehlik J, Baird BC (2014) Ventricular assist devices or inotropic agents in status 1A patients? Survival analysis of the United Network of Organ Sharing database. Ann Thorac Surg 97(4):1364–71; discussion 1371–2
11. Mikus E, Stepanenko A, Krabatsch T et al (2011) Reversibility of fixed pulmonary hypertension in left ventricular assist device support recipients. Eur J Cardiothorac Surg 40:971–977
12. Kutty RS, Parameshwar J, Lewis C et al (2013) Use of centrifugal left ventricular assist device as a bridge to candidacy in severe heart failure with secondary pulmonary hypertension. Eur J Cardiothorac Surg 43:1237–1242

13. Gupta S, Woldendorp K, Ke M et al (2014) Normalisation of haemodynamics in patients with end-stage heart failure with continuous-flow left ventricular assist device therapy. Heart Lung Circ 23:963–969
14. Atluri P, Fairman AS, MacArthur JW et al (2013) Continuous flow left ventricular assist device implant significantly improves pulmonary hypertension, right ventricular contractility, and tricuspid valve competence. J Card Surg 28:770–775
15. Alba AC, Rao V, Ross HJ et al (2010) Impact of fixed pulmonary hypertension on post-heart transplant outcomes in bridge-to-transplant patients. J Heart Lung Transplant 29:1253–1258
16. Nair PK, Kormos RL, Teuteberg JJ (2010) Pulsatile left ventricular assist device support as a bridge to decision in patients with end-stage heart failure complicated by pulmonary hypertension. J Heart Lung Transplant 29:201–208
17. Liden H, Haraldsson A, Ricksten SE, Kjellman U, Wiklund L (2009) Does pretransplant left ventricular assist device therapy improve results after heart transplantation in patients with elevated pulmonary vascular resistance? Eur J Cardiothorac Surg 35:1029–1034 ; discussion 1034-5
18. Etz CD, Welp HA, Tjan TD et al (2007) Medically refractory pulmonary hypertension: treatment with nonpulsatile left ventricular assist devices. Ann Thorac Surg 83:1697–1705
19. LaRue SJ, Garcia-Cortes R, Nassif ME et al (2015) Treatment of secondary pulmonary hypertension with bosentan after left ventricular assist device implantation. Cardiovasc Ther 33:50–55
20. Tedford RJ, Hemnes AR, Russell SD et al (2008) PDE5A inhibitor treatment of persistent pulmonary hypertension after mechanical circulatory support. Circ Heart Fail 1:213–219
21. Galiè N, Humbert M, Vachiery JL (2016) 2015 ESC/ERS Guidelines for the diagnosis and treatment of pulmonary hypertension: the joint task force for the diagnosis and treatment of pulmonary hypertension of the European Society of Cardiology (ESC) and the European Respiratory Society (ERS): endorsed by: Association for European Paediatric and Congenital Cardiology (AEPC), International Society for Heart and Lung Transplantation (ISHLT). Eur Heart J 37:67–119
22. Burkhoff D, Maurer MS, Joseph SM et al (2015) Left atrial decompression pump for severe heart failure with preserved ejection fraction: theoretical and clinical considerations. JACC Heart Fail 3:275–282
23. Lund LH, Edwards LB, Kucheryavaya AY et al (2015) Registry of the International Society for Heart and Lung Transplantation: thirty-second official adult heart transplantation report—2015; focus theme: early graft failure. J Heart Lung Transplant 34:1244–1254
24. Grulich AE, Vajdic CM (2015) The epidemiology of cancers in human immunodeficiency virus infection and after organ transplantation. Semin Oncol 42: 247–257
25. Mistiaen WP (2015) Heart transplantation in patients with previous malignancy. An overview. Acta Cardiol 70:123–130
26. Rivinius R, Helmschrott M, Ruhparwar A et al (2015) Analysis of malignancies in patients after heart transplantation with subsequent immunosuppressive therapy. Drug Des Devel Ther 9:93–102
27. Doesch AO, Müller S, Konstandin M et al (2010) Malignancies after heart transplantation: incidence, risk factors, and effects of calcineurin inhibitor withdrawal. Transplant Proc 42:3694–3699
28. Shah S, Nohria A (2015) Advanced heart failure due to cancer therapy. Curr Cardiol Rep 17:16
29. Deo SV, Al-Kindi SG, Oliveira GH (2015) Management of advanced heart failure due to cancer therapy: the present role of mechanical circulatory support and cardiac transplantation. Curr Treat Options Cardiovasc Med 17:388
30. Sayin OA, Ozpeker C, Schoenbrodt M (2015) Ventricular assist devices in patients with chemotherapy-induced cardiomyopathy: new modalities. Acta Cardiol 70:430–434
31. Rosa GM, Gigli L, Tagliasacchi MI et al (2016) Update on cardiotoxicity of anti-cancer treatments. Eur J Clin Investig 46:264–284
32. Oliveira GH, Dupont M, Naftel D (2014) Increased need for right ventricular support in patients with chemotherapy-induced cardiomyopathy undergoing mechanical circulatory support: outcomes from the INTERMACS Registry (Interagency Registry for Mechanically Assisted Circulatory Support). J Am Coll Cardiol 63:240–248
33. Smail H, Pfister C, Baste JM et al (2015) A difficult decision: what should we do when malignant tumours are diagnosed in patients supported by left ventricular assist devices? Eur J Cardiothorac Surg 48:e30–e36
34. Loyaga-Rendon RY, Inampudi C, Tallaj JA, Acharya D, Pamboukian SV (2014) Cancer in end-stage heart failure patients supported by left ventricular assist devices. ASAIO J 60:609–612
35. Murakawa T, Murayama T, Nakajima J, Ono M (2011) Lung lobectomy in a patient with an implantable left ventricular assist device. Interact Cardiovasc Thorac Surg 13:676–678
36. Chelikani NM, Masterson K, Down LA et al (2012) Effects of gamma radiation on a ventricular assist device and its percutaneous lead components. ASAIO J 58:19–24
37. Gossman MS, Graham JD, Das IJ (2012) Evaluation of a ventricular assist device system: stability in a proton beam therapy. ASAIO J 58:597–600
38. Netuka I, Stepankova P, Urban M et al (2013) Is severe cardiac dysfunction a contraindication for complex combined oncotherapy of Hodgkin's lymphoma? Not any more. ASAIO J 59:320–321
39. McCarthy PM, Lamm RD, Sade RM (2005) Medical ethics collides with public policy: LVAD for a patient with leukemia. Ann Thorac Surg 80:793–780
40. Teuteberg JJ, Chou JC (2014) Mechanical Circulatory Devices in acute heart failure. Crit Care Clin 30:585–606
41. Cole RM, Kobashigawa JA (2016) Desensitization strategies pre- and post-cardiac transplantation. Curr Treat Options 18:8
42. Chih S, Ross HJ, McDonald MA, Issac DL (2012) Highly sensitized patients in cardiac transplantation: early

outcomes from the Canadian Prioritized Organ Sharing Program. J Heart Lung Transplant 31:780–782
43. Kfoury AG, Kobashigawa JA (2012) Prioritizing sensitized heart transplant candidates: a sensitive affair. J Heart Lung Transplant 31:677–678
44. Urban M, Gazdic T, Slimackova E et al (2012) Alloimmunosensitization in left ventricular assist device recipients and impact on post-transplantation outcome. ASAIO J 58:554–561
45. Arnaoutakis GJ, George TJ, Kilic A et al (2011) Effect of sensitization in US heart transplant recipients bridged with a ventricular assist device: update in a modern cohort. J Thorac Cardiovasc Surg 142:1236–1245
46. Chang D, Kobashigawa JA (2012) The use of calculated panel-reactive antibody and virtual crossmatch in heart transplantation. Curr Opin Organ Transplant 17:423–426
47. Bhimaraj A, Taylor DO (2011) How to deal with presensitized candidates for heart transplantation? Curr Opin Organ Transplant 16:529–535
48. Kobashigawa JA, Johnson M, Rogers J et al (2015) Report from a Forum on US Heart Allocation Policy. Am J Transplant 15:55–63
49. Stehlik J, Stevenson LW, Edwards LB et al (2014) Organ allocation around the world: insights from the ISHLT International Registry for Heart and Lung Transplantation. J Heart Lung Transplant 33:975–984
50. Thiele H, Zeymer U, Neumann FJ et al (2013) Intra-aortic balloon counterpulsation in acute myocardial infarction complicated by cardiogenic shock (IABP-SHOCK II): final 12 month results of a randomised, open-label trial. Lancet 2013(382):1638–1645
51. Khera R, Cram P, Vaughan-Sarrazin M, Horwitz PA, Girotra S (2016) Use of mechanical circulatory support in percutaneous coronary intervention in the United States. Am J Cardiol 117:10–16
52. Link MS, Berkow LC, Kudenchuk PJ et al (2015) Part 7: adult advanced cardiovascular life support: 2015 American Heart Association guidelines update for cardiopulmonary resuscitation and emergency cardiovascular care. Circulation 132(Suppl 2):S444–S464
53. Taghavi S, Jayarajan SN, Komaroff E, Mangi AA (2014) Continuous flow left ventricular assist device technology has influenced wait times and affected donor allocation in cardiac transplantation. J Thorac Cardiovasc Surg 147:1966–1971
54. Meyer DM, Rogers JG, Edwards LB (2015) The future direction of the adult heart allocation system in the United States. Am J Transplant 15:44–54
55. Kirklin JK, Naftel DC, Pagani FD et al (2015) Seventh INTERMACS annual report: 15,000 patients and counting. J Heart Lung Transplant 34:1495–1504
56. Kirklin JK, Naftel DC, Kormos RL et al (2010) Second INTERMACS annual report: more than 1,000 primary left ventricular assist device implants. J Heart Lung Transplant 29:1–10
57. Healy AH, Baird BC, Drakos SG, Stehlik J, Selzman CH (2013) Impact of ventricular assist device complications on posttransplant survival: an analysis of the United network of organ sharing database. Ann Thorac Surg 95:870–875
58. Healy AH, Stehlik J, Edwards LB, McKellar SH, Drakos SG, Selzman CH (2016) Risk of 30-day post-transplant mortality in patients bridged to transplantation with continuous-flow left ventricular assist devices-an analysis of the international society for heart and lung transplantation transplant registry. J Heart Lung Transplant 35:34–39
59. Estep JD, Starling RC, Horstmanshof DA et al (2015) Risk assessment and comparative effectiveness of left ventricular assist device and medical management in ambulatory heart failure patients: results from the ROADMAP Study, for the ROADMAP Study Investigators. J Am Coll Cardiol 66:1747–1761
60. Mancini D, Colombo P (2015) Left ventricular assist devices: a rapidly evolving alternative to transplant. J Am Coll Cardiol 65:2542–2555
61. Smits J, DeUries E, De Pauw M et al (2013) Is it time for a cardiac allocation score? First results from the Eurotransplant pilot on survival benefit based heart allocation. J Heart Lung Transplant 32:873–880
62. Mancini DM, Schulze PC (2014) Heart transplant allocation: in desperate need of revision. J Am Coll Cardiol 63:1179–1181
63. Barr ML, Taylor DO (2015) Changes in donor heart allocation in the United States wfundamental changes in the system: rearranging deck chairs and elephants in the room. Am Journal Transplant 15:7–9
64. Stevenson LW (2013) The urgent priority for transplantation is to trim the waiting list. J Heart Lung Transplant 32:861–867

Intraoperative Tips and Pitfalls

Contents

Engineering and Clinical Considerations in Rotary Blood Pumps

F. Moscato and H. Schima

© Springer International Publishing Switzerland 2017
A. Montalto et al. (eds.), *Mechanical Circulatory Support in End-Stage Heart Failure*,
DOI 10.1007/978-3-319-43383-7_14

In this chapter, general considerations and the operation principle of rotary blood pumps will be first presented with particular focus on the pressure-flow-speed characteristics, on what influences the pump flow rate, and on biocompatibility aspects. Finally current state-of-the-art about hemodynamic monitoring and control of these pumps will be presented.

14.1 General Considerations

Rotary blood pumps are used in the treatment of heart failure. Common indication for the implantation of these devices is end-stage heart failure (NYHA class IV) with expected 50% mortality within 1 year. Typically patients present with a low left ventricular ejection fraction (<25%), elevated pulmonary pressures, reduced cardiac index (<2 $l/min/m^2$), peak-VO_2 <12–14 ml/min/kg, chronic or intermitted inotropic dependence, and secondary progressive hepatic or renal dysfunction [1]. Rotary blood pumps can be used to bridge the patient until heart transplantation becomes possible, or they can even be implanted for lifetime. This latter is described as destination therapy and is considered when there is a contraindication for cardiac transplantation, such as irreversible pulmonary hypertension, active systemic infection, active malignancy or history of malignancy with probability of recurrence, or inability to comply with complex medical regimen. In a few cases, these devices can be used as bridges to recovery, such as in case of acute cardiac failure following cardiac surgery or acute myocarditis infections.

14.2 Working Principle and Classification

Rotary blood pumps are electromagnetically actuated turbodynamic machines [2]. These pumps consist of two main parts: a rotating component (impeller, i.e., a disk/annulus with vanes) and a pump housing. By its rotation, the impeller transfers energy from the electric motor that drives the pump to the blood. As a result of the impeller action, the blood leaves the impeller at a higher pressure and velocity than at its entrance. The impeller is supported within the pump housing by a bearing. In addition, a rotary blood pump assembly comprises inflow and outflow cannulas for its connection to the cardiovascular system and a flexible driveline for connection to electric power supply and to a control unit (◘ Fig. 14.1).

Rotary blood pumps can be classified according to five main factors: geometry, bearing type, implantability, intended duration of use, and intended support function. Concerning the design geometry, one can distinguish three different types according to the flow path through the pump. If the angle between blood inflow and blood outflow is 90° (blood exits the pump in a direction orthogonal to the blood inflow), one speaks of a centrifugal-flow pump. If this angle is 0° (blood enters and leaves the pump along the same axis), one has an axial-flow pump. A pump characterized by angles between these two extreme cases is called a mixed-flow pump. There are three main types of bearing used to support the impeller of a rotary blood pump: mechanical, magnetic, and hydrodynamic bearings. The first bearing type relies on the low friction coefficient of the bearing material (ceramic, ruby), the second on magnetic forces, and the third on hydrodynamic forces to obtain levitation of the impeller and contactless rotation. Concerning implantability, one can distinguish between implantable devices, where the pump housing and cannulas are placed into the body with power supply and driving unit being still extracorporeal, and external devices, where the only implantable components are the pump inflow and outflow cannulas. The duration of use constitutes another factor to distinguish devices: one can have short-term devices that are intended for days or weeks and long-term devices for months or years of implantation. Finally, one can distinguish pumps that support the function of one ventricle (left or right ventricular assist devices, LVAD, RVAD), of both ventricles (BiVAD), or for heart replacement (rotary total artificial heart, rTAH). The focus in the following text will be on rotary pumps used as implantable LVADs, since these are the most commonly developed and used devices.

An implantable LVAD has its inlet cannula typically placed within the left ventricle, but cannulation to the left atrium is sometimes also used. The outlet cannula is commonly sutured to the ascending aorta, but the descending aorta or subclavian cannulation is also used. In ◘ Fig. 14.1, an implantable, axial-flow LVAD with mechanical

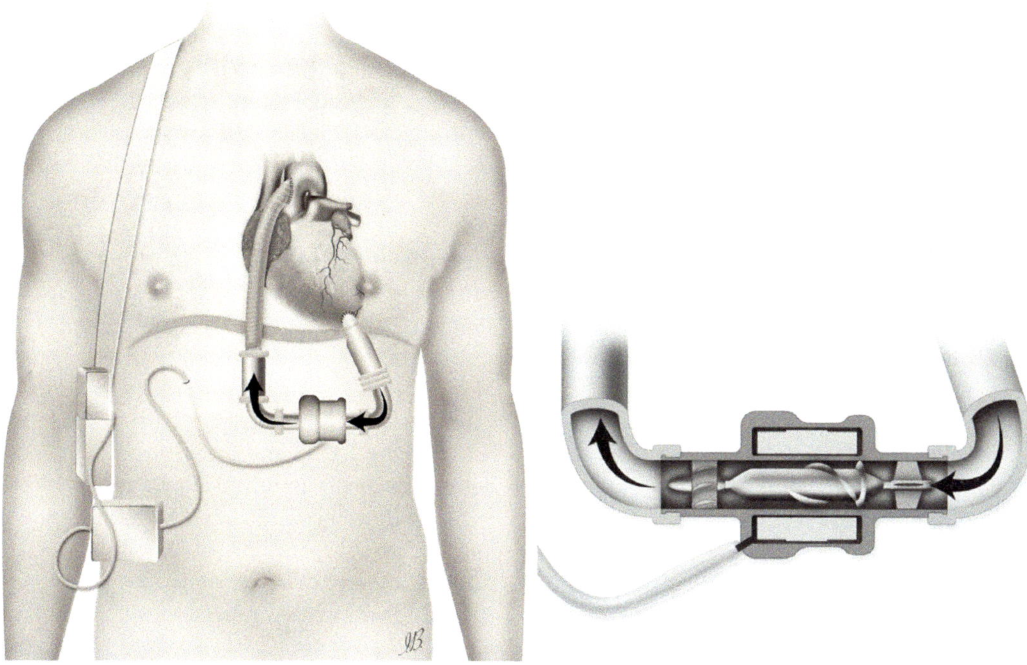

Fig. 14.1 LVAD implanted between the left ventricle and the ascending aorta (*left*); schematic diagram of the different components of an axial-flow pump (*right*) (Illustration by Ilaria Bondi's Peppermint Advertising)

bearings for long-term use is shown. The inflow is cannulated to the left ventricle and outflow to the ascending aorta.

14.3 Functional Requirements

The key functional requirements for rotary blood pumps can be summarized in the following bullet points: They should:

- Generate enough blood flow rate, 5–8 l/min, at physiological arterial pressure (100–150 mmHg for LVADs).
- Adapt to patient hemodynamic requirements (at least have a Starling-like behavior).
- Prevent hemodynamic overload to the right ventricle (in case of LVADs).
- Guarantee right/left flow balance (in case of BiVADs or rTAH).
- Be anatomically compatible with the large variations in patient size (body mass, chest diameter, abdominal girth).
- Be small to reduce surgical trauma and chronic infections at implantation site.
- Be structurally stable in corrosive environments.
- Guarantee continuous operation without maintenance for years (5–10 years).
- Minimize red blood cell damage (hemolysis) and activation of the coagulation cascade.
- Avoid formation of thrombi (all current devices require anticoagulation therapy).
- Be efficient for low power consumption and prolonged battery life.
- Have user-friendly interfaces and deliver unambiguous warnings and alarms.
- Be cost-effective (in terms of device, implantation, usage costs).

Modern rotary blood pumps fulfill most of the abovementioned requirements. They are all powered by a so-called brushless DC motor and have an external power supply: typically two rechargeable batteries or a power cord. The efficiency of these devices allows power consumption up to 10 W and a battery capacity that allows several hours of untethered patient activity. Rotary blood pumps are small in size, which allows minimally invasive implantation. They have with just one moving part (the impeller) and no valves as in the pulsatile counterpart, which increase the durability. This also allows silent operation, which is important for patient quality of life. They suffer however from a lack of adaptation to changing hemodynamics, which leads, for example, to pump flow rate decrease in response to an increasing arterial pressure or to suck-down of the ventricular structures into the inflow cannula in responsed to a decreasing ventricular filling. They require therefore careful monitoring. Thrombus formation, strokes and bleeding still remain an issue with these devices, which although optimized for blood pumping are still challenging for coagulation and hemostasis [3, 4]. Further complications include infections of the percutaneous driveline.

14.4 Pressure-Flow-Speed Characteristics

In the following section, the typical operation of a rotary blood pump used as an LVAD will be presented. Circulatory support by a LVAD depends on the interaction between the residual ventricular function, the overall hemodynamics and the pump speed setting. Generally one distinguishes between partial support and full support. In partial support, the LVAD and the ventricle both eject blood toward the aorta (see ◘ Fig. 14.2, left panel). In case of full support, the LVAD alone pumps the whole cardiac output toward the aorta, and the aortic valve stays permanently closed (see ◘ Fig. 14.2, right panel). In both support types, the flow rate generated by the rotary pump is related to the ventricular and aortic pressures as well as to the pump speed.

In order to understand the interaction between the LVAD and the assisted heart, some definitions will be given first, and then the pressure-flow-speed characteristics will be introduced. The volume of blood pumped in one min by the rotary pump is referred to as the pump capacity or flow rate or even simply named pump flow. It is usually symbolized by the letter

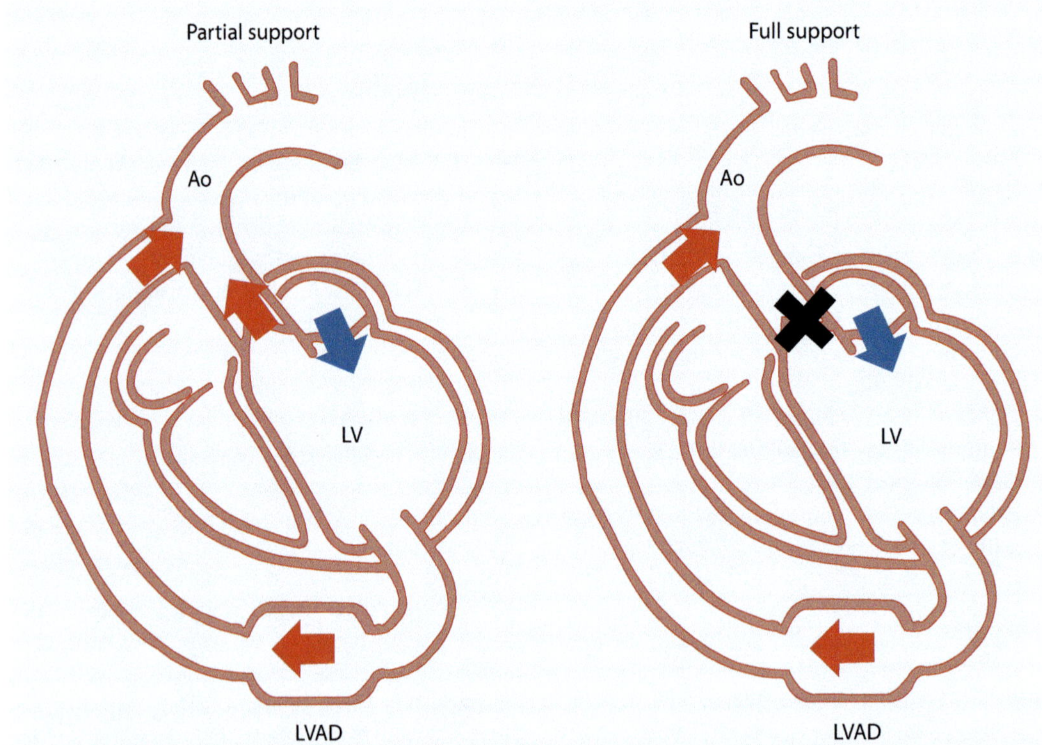

◘ **Fig. 14.2** Partial and full support by a left ventricular assist device (*LVAD*) in ventriculo-aortic cannulation. In case of partial support, the left ventricle (*LV*) and the LVAD pump blood in parallel toward the aorta (*Ao*). In case of full support, the LVAD alone pumps the whole cardiac output toward the Ao, and the aortic valve stays permanently closed (symbolized by *black cross*)

Q, and it is measured in liters per minute (l/min). The pressure difference between pump outlet and inlet is referred to as the head or simply pressure difference (outlet pressure=aortic pressure AoP, inled pressure=left ventricular pressure LVP). This difference is symbolized by the letter *H* or sometimes by ΔP, and it is usually measured in millimeters of mercury (mmHg). The speed at which the impeller rotates is referred to as pump speed. It is symbolized by the letter *N*, and it is measured in revolutions per minute (rpm). A rotary blood pump can be uniquely described by a relationship between these three variables. Specifically, variation of the pressure difference with pump flow at constant speed is called the pump characteristic. Considering the different speeds, one speaks of the pressure-flow-speed characteristics. In ◘ Fig. 14.3, a schematic diagram depicting characteristics for a hypothetical centrifugal-flow pump is shown. For a more technical description of hydraulic characteristics and design concepts of centrifugal- and axial-flow pumps, please refer to [2].

14.5 Pump Flow Rate-Influencing Factors

Pump characteristics are extremely useful to understand how much blood the assist device will pump at a given rotational speed and pressure difference/head between outlet and inlet (H = AoP – LVP). In this paragraph, a simplified and graphical analysis of the influence of these factors on the pump flow rate will be presented.

Due to a residual ventricular contractile function, the LVP (and to some extent the AoP) will pulsate during the cardiac cycle, leading to a periodic change of the pump pressure head (Hs and Hd in ◘ Fig. 14.4a). This pulsating pressure head will lead, via the pump characteristic for a given rotational speed, to a pulsatile pattern of the pump flow rate (Qs and Qd in ◘ Fig. 14.4b, c).

A rotary blood pump provides a continuous unloading of the ventricle since blood is continuously pumped through the heart cycle (the flow rate is >0). The blood flow rate retains a certain pulsatility that depends on the residual

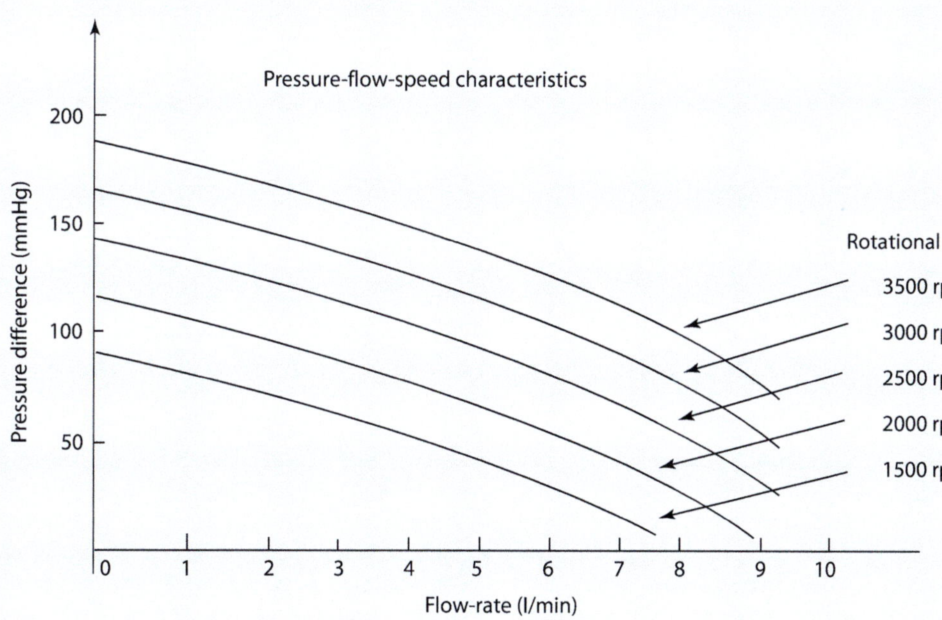

◘ **Fig. 14.3** Schematic drawing of pump characteristics (*solid lines*) of a hypothetical centrifugal-flow pump. For an LVAD connected between the left ventricle and the aorta, the pressure difference across the pump is equal to the aortic pressure minus the left ventricular pressure

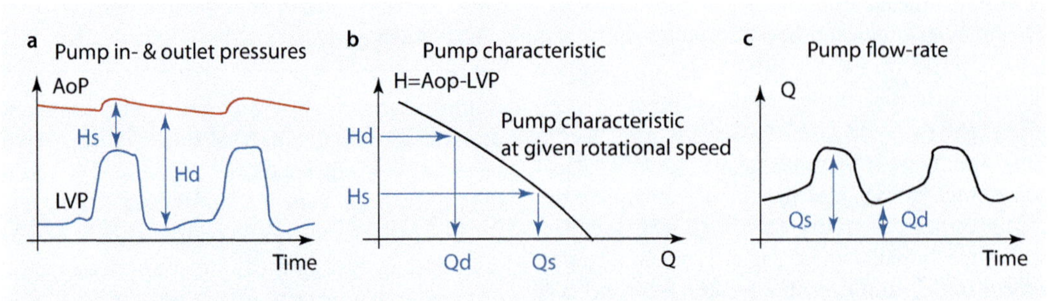

Fig. 14.4 In the leftmost panel (**a**), the time course of pressures at the LVAD outlet and inlet as well as their difference during systole (*Hs*) and diastole (*Hd*) is shown. In the middle panel (**b**), a pump characteristic relating the Hs and Hd to the systolic and diastolic flow rates (*Qs* and *Qd*) is shown. In the rightmost panel (**c**), the time course of the LVAD flow rate is shown

contractile function of the assisted ventricle. It is therefore incorrect to name rotary blood pumps as "nonpulsatile" assist devices. Only in the rare case of ventricular fibrillation (no residual contraction) these devices will deliver a truly nonpulsatile flow rate. It must be however noted that the flow rate pulsatility that these devices are able to provide is often small compared to native pulsatility. This reduced flow pulsatility leads to small arterial pressure pulse, which can be difficult to measure using conventional auscultation or automated cuffs. Instead Doppler ultrasound can be used to detect flow in the radial artery when the cuff pressure becomes lower that the systolic arterial pressure [5].

By means of the simple three diagrams presented in Fig. 14.4, the effect of changes in pump speed, pump preload (LVP), and pump afterload (AoP) can be analyzed. In the following analysis, a condition of full support (see Fig. 14.2, right panel) is considered. An increase in the three abovementioned variables is considered here; when a decrease occurs, the opposite changes will take place.

In Fig. 14.5a, the effect of a pump speed increase at constant pre- and afterload is shown. Because of constant pre- and afterload, the systolic and diastolic pressure head are constant too. The new pump characteristic at a higher speed will lead therefore to an increase in both systolic and diastolic flow rates (Qd' and Qs' in Fig. 14.5a – middle and rightmost panels). This increase in flow rate will lead to circulatory adaptation and consequent later changes in LVP and AoP (mostly by reducing LVP and increasing AoP). The assumption of constant preload and afterload is therefore strictly valid in the short time after the speed change; the later changes can be investigated in a similar manner, however, as it is presented next.

In Fig. 14.5b, the effect of an increased pump preload (LVP) at constant afterload and speed is depicted. Pump preload can increase, for example, due to increased venous return to the LV or increased LV contractility. With a change in venous return or contractility, the systolic LVP will typically increase much more than the diastolic one, leading to a reduction of the Hs and an almost constant Hd (Fig. 14.5b leftmost panel). This new hemodynamic conditions will lead to an increased systolic flow rate (Qs' in Fig. 14.5b middle and rightmost panels) and consequently an increased waveform pulsatility (defined as the difference between systolic and diastolic flow rates Qpuls=Qs-Qd). In this analysis, the pump afterload is considered constant. Also this assumption is strictly valid in the short time after the preload change, and a further analysis can be performed considering afterload effects presented next.

Finally, in Fig. 14.5c the effect of an increased afterload (AoP) at constant preload and speed is shown. The increase of AoP leads to an increase of both Hs and Hd (Fig. 14.5c leftmost panel), that leads, via the pump characteristics, to a decrease in pump flow (Qs' and Qd' Fig. 14.5c middle and rightmost panels). This decrease in pump flow will lead a change in the overall hemodynamics, possibly leading to insufficient ventricular unloading and blood accumulation in the pulmonary circulation.

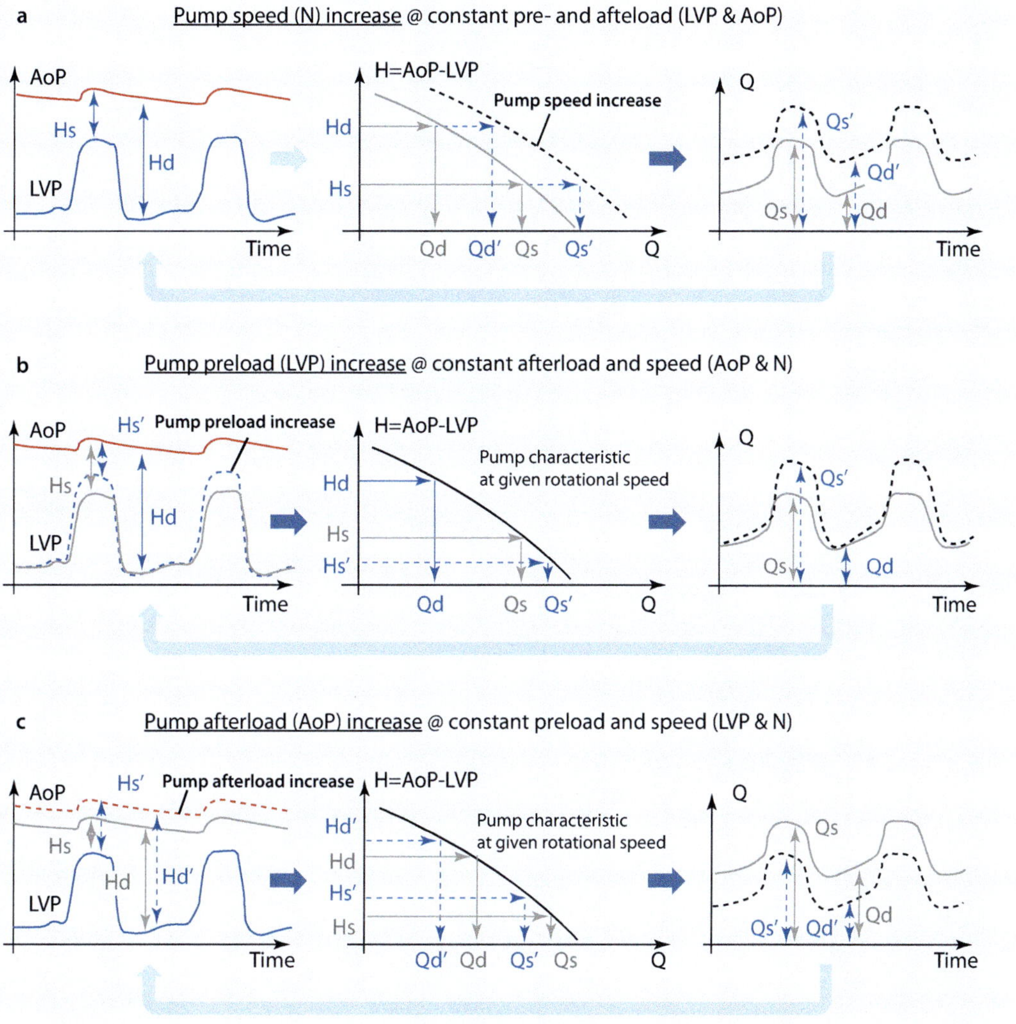

Fig. 14.5 Effect of isolated changes in speed (*panel a*), preload (*panel b*), and afterload (*panel c*) on the pump flow rate. The arrows feeding back from the rightmost to the leftmost panel mean that a change in pump flow will result in a change in the overall hemodynamics, thus a change in LVP and AoP

The condition of partial support was not considered above. The analysis is however similar with just one relevant difference. When the aortic valve opens, the systolic pressure head (AoP-LVP during systole) will be approximately zero (slightly negative), and it remains rather independent on pre- and afterload changes. In this case, the systolic pump flow rate will have a rather constant value that depends only on the speed setting. The systolic flow rate will be indeed the intercept of the pump characteristic with the x-axis (e.g., in Fig. 14.3, $Qs = 9$ l/min for $N = 2000$ rpm).

14.6 Blood Trauma and Thrombogenicity

The probably most crucial aspect in the development of rotary blood pumps is the blood compatibility, both concerning mechanical blood trauma and triggering platelet activation and coagulation of thrombi.

In the early developments, spinning disks were preferably used to avoid high shear stress exposure [6]. It is known since long time that the damage of erythrocytes depends on shear stress value, exposure time, and type of flow [7]. Therefore, an ultrashort exposure to high shear can be preferable to longer exposures to less shear [8], which explains the shape of many of the impellers of rotary pumps, which have different (e.g., straight) vane geometries compared to classic rotary pumps [9, 10]. However, the trauma (far less than one erythrocyte out of 1 mio should be destroyed per passage) is difficult to measure, and short exposure times at well-defined shear would require new test setups, which are not available yet. As a consequence, even after decades of research, numerical models of blood trauma are limited in reliability and accuracy [11].

Thrombogenicity and particularly platelet activation can be caused by local shear stress, hot spots due to bearing/sealing friction, surface roughness, and long residence times in stagnation areas [12]. To provide thrombogenicity tests for pumps and specific blood pathways, several in vitro setups have been developed [13, 14]. Mechanical bearings have been identified as the most critical parts in design, due to their shear gradient, the generated friction heat, and critical location in the center of the rotor in usually low-flow areas. As a potential solution to this issue, pumps with either actively controlled magnetic bearings or combinations of permanent magnets with hydrodynamic bearings have been developed and successfully implemented in commercially available devices.

14.7 Hemodynamic Monitoring and Physiological Control

14.7.1 LVAD Patient Monitoring

A detailed knowledge of the hemodynamic interaction of the pump and the cardiovascular system allows one to predict hemodynamic behavior depending on the pump flow rate waveform and therefore perform patient monitoring using pump data. This is especially important in rotary blood pumps because of their lack of adaptation to hemodynamic changes. Apart from standard clinical diagnostics [5], approaches to monitor the LVAD patient can be divided in those which make use of external sensors and those that rely on assist device motor parameters to estimate hemodynamic variables [15]. Monitoring using an implantable pump flow rate sensor has been reported in patients [16]. Developments of pressure sensors [17, 18] as well as impedance sensors [19] to be embedded in LVAD systems have been reported. In [20] the possibility of utilizing in LVAD patients remote pressure monitoring tools designed for non-LVAD heart failure patients is reviewed. Patient monitoring that relies only on available pump data seems very promising, particularly because additional sensors are often affected by drifts and may be prone to failure. Several hemodynamic indices and methods were developed based on available pump signals: a ventricular contractility index [21], a ventricular relaxation index [22], as well as the discrimination between full and partial assistance (state of the aortic valve opening during support) [23–26]. A method to evaluate heart rate and arrhythmic events (e.g., sustained ventricular tachycardia or atrial fibrillation) as well as heart rate variability [27] and methods to detect conditions of overpumping (i.e., ventricular suction) [28, 29] were also developed. All these methods and indices use either pump flow rate waveform, which can be either measured or estimated from pump motor current and speed [30], or directly the motor current/speed waveforms. In ◘ Fig. 14.6a, graphical overview of hemodynamic features that can be derived from the pump flow rate waveform is shown. These methods take advantage of the pulsatility in the pump flow rate that depends on the residual contractile function of the assisted ventricle (◘ Fig. 14.4).

Pump Physiological Control

Since the first days of clinical application, rotary pumps have been driven at constant speed. In this setting, the pump can be understood as a "turbo discharger" of the ventricle, which – simply speaking – facilitates ventricular output by providing pressure work. If the ventricle has some remaining contractile force or recovers after implant, it can overtake some physiological adaptation by the Starling mechanism still working against a lower output pressure. This explains why most patients can perform their daily activities and some reduced exercise at such constant speed. Only in patients with completely dysfunctional ventricle such adaptation is difficult, with circadian hemodynamic changes that may lead to suction during night and

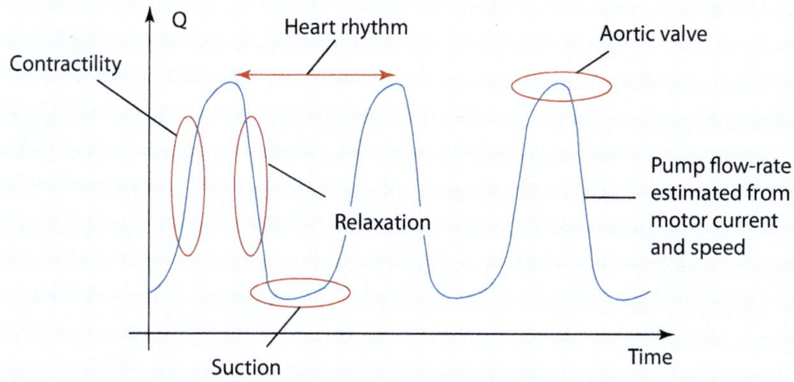

Fig. 14.6 Hemodynamic features that can be derived from an estimation of the pump flow rate waveform

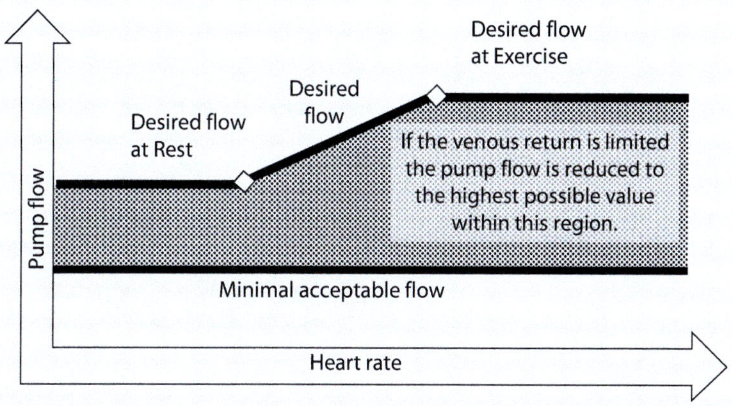

Fig. 14.7 Physiological controller settings and function. A target desired flow depending on heart rate is set by the physician. This is achieved by automatically adjusting pump speed. In case of reduced venous return (suction detected or too low flow pulsatility), the highest possible flow is automatically achieved. If this falls below a minimal acceptable level, set by the physician, a fail-safe mode is activated to avoid further decrease

insufficient supply during the day even at rest [31]. Especially for such weak patients, for early postoperative recovery, and particularly for activity and exercise, a physiologically adaptive speed control would be extremely desirable. The key problem for such algorithms however still is the lack of reliable, drift-free, durable, and biocompatible pressure transducers, which would allow a control based on inflow preload pressure. A control should also fulfil several targets: it should maintain atrial pressure within a physiological range, but at the same time avoid excessive ventricular unloading or suction and provide an overall aortic flow correlated to the demand as in a healthy individual. If a physiological control should allow also intermittent opening of the aortic valve, support pulsatility of aortic pressure, and provide myocardial protection or even myocardial training for recovery, is currently under debate.

To fulfil these requirements, many algorithms have been described and tested in silico and in vitro, but only very few made it into in vivo or even clinical tests. For a review of physiological control strategies for rotary LVADs, please refer to [32, 33]. A physiological control including suction detection and speed based on remaining pulsatility and heart rate has been successfully clinically tested. In Fig. 14.7, a schematic diagram of the controller settings and function is shown. For details about the controller design and the clinical study, please refer to [34, 35].

Although this control algorithm has proven stable in rest, exercise, Valsalva maneuvers, and even during severe arrhythmia, it has not been implemented in commercially available devices yet. Obstacles for an implementation into clinical routine are probably liability challenges and correlated questions of continuous recording of pump control activity ("how to prove the innocence of the control algorithm in case of problems?") and perhaps also the necessity for higher pump flow rates during exercise than current devices can deliver. Currently physicians and patients are satistifed with the basic support provided by LVADs, but this may soon change with increasing patient needs for better life quality related to full participation in life, physical activity, and improved usability of ventricular assist systems.

References

1. Miller LW, Guglin M (2013) Patient selection for ventricular assist devices: a moving target. J Am Coll Cardiol 61(12):1209–1221
2. Stepanoff AJ (1957) Centrifugal and axial flow pumps: theory, design, and application, 2nd edn. John Wiley & Sons, New York, p 462
3. Kirklin JK, Naftel DC, Kormos RL, Stevenson LW, Pagani FD, Miller MA et al (2013) Fifth INTERMACS annual report: risk factor analysis from more than 6,000 mechanical circulatory support patients. J Heart Lung Transplant Off Publ Int Soc Heart Transplant 32(2):141–156
4. Kirklin JK, Naftel DC, Pagani FD, Kormos RL, Stevenson LW, Blume ED et al (2014) Sixth INTERMACS annual report: a 10,000-patient database. J Heart Lung Transplant Off Publ Int Soc Heart Transplant 33(6):555–564
5. Estep JD, Trachtenberg BH, Loza LP, Bruckner BA (2015) Continuous flow left ventricular assist devices: shared care goals of monitoring and treating patients. Methodist Debakey Cardiovasc J 11(1):33–44
6. Bernstein EF, Dorman FD, Blackshear PL, Scott DR (1970) An efficient, compact blood pump for assisted circulation. Surgery 68(1):105–115
7. Schima H, Trubel, W, Muller, MR, Papantonis, D, Salat, A, Schlusche, A et al (1991) Development of a centrifugal blood pump with minimal hemolysis. In: Proceedings of the International Workshop on Rotary Blood Pumps
8. Wampler RK, Moise JC, Frazier OH, Olsen DB (1988) In vivo evaluation of a peripheral vascular access axial flow blood pump. ASAIO Trans Am Soc Artif Intern Organs 34(3):450–454
9. Schima H, Müller MR, Papantonis D, Schlusche C, Huber L, Schmidt C et al (1993) Minimization of hemolysis in centrifugal blood pumps: influence of different geometries. Int J Artif Organs 16(7):521–529
10. Larose JA, Tamez D, Ashenuga M, Reyes C (2010) Design concepts and principle of operation of the HeartWare ventricular assist system. ASAIO J Am Soc Artif Intern Organs 56(4):285–289
11. Hariharan P, D'Souza G, Horner M, Malinauskas RA, Myers MR (2015) Verification benchmarks to assess the implementation of computational fluid dynamics based hemolysis prediction models. J Biomech Eng 137(9): 094501 (10 Pages)
12. Chiu W-C, Girdhar G, Xenos M, Alemu Y, Soares JS, Einav S et al (2014) Thromboresistance comparison of the HeartMate II ventricular assist device with the device thrombogenicity emulation- optimized HeartAssist 5 VAD. J Biomech Eng 136(2):021014
13. Schima H, Siegl H, Mohammad SF, Huber L, Müller MR, Losert U et al (1993) In vitro investigation of thrombogenesis in rotary blood pumps. Artif Organs 17(7):605–608
14. Dimasi A, Rasponi M, Sheriff J, Chiu W-C, Bluestein D, Tran PL et al (2015) Microfluidic emulation of mechanical circulatory support device shear-mediated platelet activation. Biomed Microdevices 17(6):117
15. Bertram CD (2005) Measurement for implantable rotary blood pumps. Physiol Meas 26(4):R99–117
16. Pektok E, Demirozu ZT, Arat N, Yildiz O, Oklu E, Eker D et al (2013) Remote monitoring of left ventricular assist device parameters after HeartAssist-5 implantation. Artif Organs 37(9):820–825
17. Bullister E, Reich S, D'Entremont P, Silverman N, Sluetz J (2001) A blood pressure sensor for long-term implantation. Artif Organs 25(5):376–379
18. Zhou M-D, Yang C, Liu Z, Cysyk JP, Zheng S-Y (2012) An implantable Fabry-Pérot pressure sensor fabricated on left ventricular assist device for heart failure. Biomed Microdevices 14(1):235–245
19. Her K, Ahn CB, Park SM, Choi SW (2015) Heart monitoring using left ventricle impedance and ventricular electrocardiography in left ventricular assist device patients. Biomed Eng Online 14:25
20. Lampert BC, Emani S (2015) Remote hemodynamic monitoring for ambulatory left ventricular assist device patients. J Thorac Dis 7(12):2165–2171
21. Naiyanetr P, Moscato F, Vollkron M, Zimpfer D, Wieselthaler G, Schima H (2010) Continuous assessment of cardiac function during rotary blood pump support: a contractility index derived from pump flow. J Heart Lung Transplant 29(1):37–44
22. Moscato F, Granegger M, Naiyanetr P, Wieselthaler G, Schima H (2012) Evaluation of left ventricular relaxation in rotary blood pump recipients using the pump flow aveform: a simulation study. Artif Organs 36(5):470–478
23. Bishop CJ, Mason NO, Kfoury AG, Lux R, Stoker S, Horton K et al (2010) A novel non-invasive method to assess aortic valve opening in HeartMate II left ventricular assist device patients using a modified Karhunen-Loève transformation. J Heart Lung Transplant Off Publ Int Soc Heart Transplant 29(1):27–31
24. Granegger M, Schima H, Zimpfer D, Moscato F (2014) Assessment of aortic valve opening during rotary blood pump support using pump signals. Artif Organs 38(4):290–297

25. Hayward C, Lim CP, Schima H, Macdonald P, Moscato F, Muthiah K et al (2015) Pump speed waveform analysis to detect aortic valve opening in patients on ventricular assist device support. Artif Organs 39(8):704–709
26. Granegger M, Masetti M, Laohasurayodhin R, Schloglhofer T, Zimpfer D, Schima H et al (2016) Continuous monitoring of aortic valve opening in rotary blood pump patients. IEEE Trans Biomed Eng 63:1201–1207
27. Moscato F, Granegger M, Edelmayer M, Zimpfer D, Schima H (2014) Continuous monitoring of cardiac rhythms in left ventricular assist device patients. Artif Organs 38(3):191–198
28. Vollkron M, Schima H, Huber L, Benkowski R, Morello G, Wieselthaler G (2004) Development of a suction detection system for axial blood pumps. Artif Organs 28(8):709–716
29. Vollkron M, Schima H, Huber L, Benkowski R, Morello G, Wieselthaler G (2006) Advanced suction detection for an axial flow pump. Artif Organs 30(9):665–670
30. Granegger M, Moscato F, Casas F, Wieselthaler G, Schima H (2012) Development of a pump flow estimator for rotary blood pumps to enhance monitoring of ventricular function. Artif Organs 36(8):691–699
31. Wang Y, Koenig SC, Slaughter MS, Giridharan GA (2015) Rotary blood pump control strategy for preventing left ventricular suction. ASAIO J Am Soc Artif Intern Organs 61(1):21–30
32. AlOmari A-HH, Savkin AV, Stevens M, Mason DG, Timms DL, Salamonsen RF et al (2013) Developments in control systems for rotary left ventricular assist devices for heart failure patients: a review. Physiol Meas 34(1):R1–27
33. Pauls JP, Stevens MC, Bartnikowski N, Fraser JF, Gregory SD, Tansley G (2016) Evaluation of physiological control systems for rotary left ventricular assist devices: an in-vitro study. Ann Biomed Eng 44:2377–2387
34. Vollkron M, Schima H, Huber L, Benkowski R, Morello G, Wieselthaler G (2005) Development of a reliable automatic speed control system for rotary blood pumps. J Heart Lung Transplant Off Publ Int Soc Heart Transplant 24(11):1878–1885
35. Schima H, Vollkron M, Jantsch U, Crevenna R, Roethy W, Benkowski R et al (2006) First clinical experience with an automatic control system for rotary blood pumps during ergometry and right-heart catheterization. J Heart Lung Transplant Off Publ Int Soc Heart Transplant. 25(2):167–173

Engineering and Clinical Considerations in Pulsatile Blood Pump

Oliver Voigt and Friedrich Kaufmann

© Springer International Publishing Switzerland 2017
A. Montalto et al. (eds.), *Mechanical Circulatory Support in End-Stage Heart Failure*,
DOI 10.1007/978-3-319-43383-7_15

15.1 Milestones for Clinical Use of Blood Pumps

The development of mechanical circulatory support systems ("MCSS") has been in parallel to donor heart transplantation. In 1966, Michael E. DeBakey did the first successful implant of a partial artificial heart at Methodist Hospital in Houston, USA, by using a paracorporeal blood pump to assist the failing left ventricle of a female patient until her heart has recovered after 10 days [1]. A blood pump connected to the patient's circulatory system to support the pumping function is called ventricular assist device or "VAD." Three years later, in 1969 Denton Cooley implanted the first total artificial heart ("TAH" – a full replacement of the patient's native heart) which was developed by Domingo Liotta into the chest of a 47-year-old patient for 64 h to bridge him for heart transplantation [2]. The first implantations with the aim of permanent life support (so-called destination therapy, "DT") took place 13 years later in 1982 by William DeVries and his team at Utah Medical Center, USA, using the Jarvik-7 TAH developed by Willem Kolff and his team [3]. The first MCSS mimic the layout (anatomy) and function of the natural heart using pulsatile pumping mode of displacement pumps. Nowadays nonpulsatile rotary blood pumps are the first choice for long-term LVAD support. Only for pediatric use and for short- to medium-term support the pulsatile displacement pumps are being used in the clinical arena. The first implantation of an axial flow rotary blood pump was in 1998 at the German Heart Institute Berlin, Germany, performed by Roland Hetzer [4]. In 2012, Martin Strueber reported the first use of two continuous flow centrifugal blood pumps as TAH in a patient after cardioectomy at Hannover Medical School, Germany [5]. Nevertheless, the current TAH systems and those in clinical or preclinical evaluation are all pulsatile pump systems. The pulsatile TAH offers advantages like high physiologic flows in case of biventricular failure.

15.2 General Concept of Pulsatile MCSS

15.2.1 Cannulas (or the Biological-Technical Interface)

Like with all MCSS, the pump itself has to be connected to the circulatory system of the patient using cannulas representing the interface between the biological and technical system. These may be very short with a TAH, where the inflow section is "condensed" into a sewing cuff with some sort of quick connector system. The cannulas may be made of graft prosthesis material like woven polyester fabric (Dacron) and thus are sewn to the vessels like any standard vascular surgery procedure.

In case of para- or extracorporeal systems, at least the external part of the cannula has to be manufactured from some solid material like silicone (Berlin Heart EXCOR) or polyurethane tubing (Thoratec PVAD) to prevent leaking, kinking, and damaging. A sewing ring and some sort of stabilizing metallic structure helps to facilitate a secure and tight anastomosis. Besides the obligatory accuracy providing a dry anastomosis, special attention has to be given to an optimal position of the anastomosis with respect to the direction the cannula will take: the position of the percutaneous exit site in case of extracorporeal systems has to be chosen carefully so that no kinking will occur, neither passively nor by movements of the patient like bending, sitting up, etc. Rules for correct orientation of the inflow cannula have to be followed, e.g., the Berlin Heart apical inflow cannula has an asymmetrical tip; the slope of the opening should point to the mitral valve to prevent obstruction by the lateral wall.

Pulsatile flow requires higher maximal flow velocities (about three times higher flow peaks compared to continuous flow systems) because the blood volume stored in the pump has to be pushed through the cannula in less than 50% of the time, whereas with rotary blood pumps, it will be constantly flowing. Accordingly the pressure loss will be high during peak flow plus the acceleration of the blood column in the long cannula. The required driving energy amounts to high driving pressures especially with extracorporeal devices.

The cannula connection to the pump is a sensitive spot. All transitions are predestined locations for thrombus development because even a small step at the junction is causing disturbances of the laminar flow. Thus, when using the pediatric device, selecting the cannula size should be preferential to the size of the pump, respectively, to the size of the connectors of the chosen pump size, which mainly is dependent on the body weight of the patient. Though adapters are available with the EXCOR system to match small cannulas to the next order of pump size, their use imposes an additional risk for thrombosis because two additional junctions are created. Plastic (usually polycarbonate) connectors, used by various other brands, need a certain material thickness to provide the necessary strength for a safe attachment of a cannula. Thus, the step is big and the risk and incidence of ring thrombi at these plastic connectors is much higher than with the titanium connectors of the EXCOR device, which are almost sharp at the tip.

15.3 Pulsatile Blood Pump

15.3.1 Ventricles

Pulsatile systems consist of displacement pumps. Blood is accumulating in the pump chamber (blood chamber) and then ejected into the arterial vessel connected to the pump. The necessary volume change of the blood chamber is facilitated by an elastic membrane (usually a multiple membrane to provide a high degree of safety as well as flexibility: four layers in the SynCardia ventricle and three layers in the Berlin Heart EXCOR ventricle). Both types use graphite powder as a lubricant between the membranes to prevent abrasion and thus weakening of the membrane in the long run. The Thoratec PVAD and the formerly WorldHeart NOVACOR were both systems of the blood sack type which provides an absolute seamless blood contact surface but can be manufactured only single-layered.

To eject the blood out of the blood chamber, the membrane has to be moved to "squeeze out" the blood volume. Both devices under consideration use pressurized air to achieve this – thus, they are called "pneumatic devices." The pressure pulse is delivered via a tube connected to the air chamber of the pump – adjacent to the blood chamber, separated by the membrane – the so-called driveline. The pressurized air is generated in the pneumatic driver, an external component. In order to move the membrane, the housing itself has to be rigid. This is realized by a much higher wall thickness of the same material used to mold the membranes. The SynCardia ventricle housing is reinforced with a Dacron mesh. However, there will be a small amount of flexibility of the ventricle housing. A tiny fracture of the driving pressurized air pulse will get lost in this small expansion of the housing, which has to be taken into account if the blood flow is derived from the airflow of the driver (▶ see Sect. 15.5).

To prevent any thrombotic material adhering to the surface of the blood chamber, it is manufactured as smoothly as possible. This is realized by a finish of purified polyurethane solution. In addition, the Berlin Heart EXCOR ventricles are coated with heparin according to the Carmeda® process [6]. Deposits adhering to the membrane surface have not been reported in literature; probably they do not develop at this part of the pump because of the constant movement of the membranes. However, thrombus formation at the housing is to be expected if anticoagulation is inappropriate. Most sensitive are regions of poor washout and vortices, as are the housing in between the inflow and outflow connector disturbing the inflow vortex and the attaching line of the membrane to the housing.

One of the big advantages of extracorporeal devices is the opportunity to inspect the pump for any thrombotic deposits developing on the housing of the transparent pump and cannulas. Adapting the anticoagulation therapy or a pump exchange can be initiated before embolization occurs.

15.4 Membranes

One of the most feared complications are ruptures of the membranes, though they are very rare adverse events. Blood leakage or air embolism is almost impossible and never reported because this would imply rupture of all membranes of the multimembrane set. Rupture of the blood membrane or the driving membrane is reported [7]. This would produce a cushion between the two adjacent membranes progressively reducing the stroke volume up to a total loss of pumping capacity. A tiny hole will act as a small valve, trapping blood or air, respectively, pushed into the intermediate space at the end position of the membrane due to a slight stretching. This complication represents a life-threatening complication if not detected in time. A leakage of the blood membrane is easily detected with extracorporeal systems by traces of blood in the intermembrane space visible at the attaching line of the housing. A leak of the outer air or driving membrane can be detected only by correct interpretation of an incomplete end-systolic emptying despite sufficient driving pressures caused by an air cushion between driving membrane layers. For fully implanted ventricles like the SynCardia TAH, membrane ruptures cannot be seen directly, but improper filling volume (alarm) on the external driver could be a hint. The standard operation of SynCardia TAH is "full eject and partial fill." The latter is being achieved by proper heart rate setting (typically around 130 beats per minute). Lowering the heart rate increases the filling volume (per stroke). If the maximum filling volume cannot be reached anymore by a rather low heart rate (assuming the patient has a normal volume status), then echocardiography or CT should be done to check the cross-sectional view of the membrane to look for increased thickness.

15.4.1 Valves

To create a unidirectional flow, valves are required like in the natural heart. Each ventricle has an inflow and an outflow valve. Apart from the former implantable mechanically driven pumps using a pusher plate where biological valves were used in favor of lower anticoagulation levels, the discussed systems use mechanical valves – as of today, SynCardia TAH uses tilting disk Hall valves (in the past MedHall valve and since 2014 the in-house assembled SynHall™ valve, whereas Berlin Heart EXCOR typically used Sorin monoleaflet valves, now Sorin bileaflet mechanical valves "Bicarbon" for the larger size adult ventricles and trileaflet PU valves for the small pediatric ventricles).

Biological valves would not be suitable in an extracorporeal device because the pressure difference in the closed position is too high according to the driving pressures necessary to propel the blood through the long cannulas. Mechanical valves are stable enough to stand the high driving pressures and the high dp/dt of pneumatic drivers. They have a low incidence of thrombotic complications because there is some leakage flow in the closed position, which provides the necessary washout. Disadvantageous are a noisy operation and a more profound "water hammer effect" producing high pressure peaks during valve closure.

The relative closing and leaking volume is increasing with a smaller valve diameter because the circumferential gap to ensure a safe opening cannot be diminished equivalent to downsizing the cross section of the valve. For pediatric pumps, the smallest available mechanical tilting disks would have a combined closing volume plus leakage flow in the range of the stroke volume of the smallest pump size of the Berlin Heart EXCOR pediatric ventricle (10 ml). Thus, no significant effective flow would be produced using mechanical valves for these small ventricles. To overcome this limitation, trileaflet valves cast from the same polyurethane solution used to mold the membranes had to be developed. These are produced from a single mold by dipping into the solution and cut open at the end of the manufacturing process. So the leaflets form a perfect fitting line to effectuate almost no leakage. Advantageous also is a soundless closure. A disadvantage of the tight closure of the leaflets is a higher risk of thrombus formation because of a poor washout, almost stasis during the closed half cycle. Especially at the attaching line of the leaflets at the valve housing, some recirculating vortex causes prolonged residence time of blood in the cusp of the valve. The leaflets always differ a little in thickness. Thus, with increasing flow during systole, they open separately one after the other. With the small pumps, the stroke volume may be not high enough to open all leaflets. While using the smallest (10 ml) pump, it is likely that one leaflet will stay closed all the time. Respectively, thrombus formation preferably will develop in the cusp of this leaflet if at all.

15.5 Pneumatic Drivers

Historically the first drivers used for TAH pumps were pneumatic drivers of the switching type with the big advantage of a very simple design, easy control, almost no necessary maintenance because of only few moving parts, and a low level of noise when operated on a wall air pressure outlet. These switching devices have pressure regulated tanks providing the necessary driving pressure. A small "ventilator" produces the necessary low vacuum to assist venous filling of the pump by removing the air from the air chamber and driveline during the pump diastole. Most advantageous of pneumatic devices is the elasticity of the medium air. No special sensors and high-speed reaction control circuits are required compared to hydraulically operated systems to prevent damage by excessive suction. To enable patient mobility, pressurized air is supplied from exchangeable tanks, which provides only limited time of operation. However, these big devices with very limited mobility were suitable in the beginning when patients were bedridden and restricted to intensive care units anyway. To gain more mobility, energy conversion by electric motor-driven pneumatic compressors was necessary. Various types were realized: membrane compressors loading air pressure tanks and electronically controlled proportional valves regulating the set driving pressure and vacuum offer a wide range of settings of pressure, systolic operation percentage, and matching of left and right pump cycles (synchronous, async., different rates). Switching between pressure and vacuum reservoir produces high dp/dt rates which allow high-frequency rates which are necessary in pediatric systems. On the other hand, these devices are less efficient, thus need a lot of power and are heavy. Battery operating time is short; these devices are designed for in-hospital use and offer therefore only restricted mobility (e.g., Berlin Heart IKUS2000 driver, weight 90 kg, power consumption abt. 400 W, battery operating time abt. 30 min). Also both described principles can be combined to have an effective low-noise operating device utilizing pressurized air from wall outlet during room stay and a membrane compressor kicking in if the wall pressure is disconnected, providing some kind of mobility (SynCardia "Companion 2" driver with 1 h battery operation time, weighting 35 kg including batteries and caddy).

To provide the necessary pneumatic power by a small, low power consuming preferably wearable device, piston compressors are utilized. Two principles are followed in clinically established devices: fixed cylinder capacity (displacement) with adaption to the maximum pressures needed by venting surplus displaced air volume (former Berlin Heart "Heimes" driver, SynCardia "Companion 1") or using reversing high-torque motors moving the exact amount of air volume back and forth to move the respective membrane of the pump (Berlin Heart EXCOR). The latter offer the means to calculate blood flow from air volume displacement taking into account the produced pressures, whereas all other types need airflow measurements usually by measuring the pressure gradient generated, e.g., by a "Fleischsche Düse," which is less accurate. Piston compressor-activated devices have restricted pneumatic capacity because of lower dp/dt but are much more efficient, thus allowing miniaturization to realize portable devices which can be carried in a backpack or on a caddy/trolley. If both ventricles of a BiVAD or a TAH device are driven by one compressor using both sides of the piston, a lot of components, weight, and space can be saved (e.g., Berlin Heart "Heimes" driver). The feasibility of this resulting alternating pump mode concept has been proven by long-term use in a lot of patients. A disadvantage however is the coupling of systole of the LVAD to the diastole of the RVAD and vice versa, limiting the range of useful systolic duration variability. Another principle to reduce volume is the idea to use "staged pistons" driven by one motor making use of the fact that the driving pressures of the pump creating the low pulmonary blood pressures are much lower than those creating systemic pressure and thus need much less displacement volume (e.g., SynCardia "Freedom" driver [8]).

Various principles were realized to offer high system immanent safety: totally redundant motor compressor and pressure regulation units (a third set in the IKUS2000) and in case of biventricular operation the ability to provide both ventricles with pneumatic power from only one unit by alternate mode (emergency mode of the Berlin Heart EXCOR driver) or a redundant motor concept ("Heimes" driver or SynCardia "Freedom" driver with an extra set of motor wires). The hazard by failing components has to be weighed against additional weight and volume.

15.6 Main Principles of Operation

The basic principle for operation of displacement pumps is maximum end-systolic ejection of the blood volume (an "empty" pump). The point of maximum end-systolic position of the membrane can be detected from the air (driving) pressure curve, which shows an abrupt increase by the sudden fixed volume of the air chamber – the end-systolic pressure peak (see ◻ Fig. 15.1. of SynCardia pressure curve).

If this peak is not existent because at the end of the ejection cycle the membrane is still moving, there could be an imbalance. The hazard of right to left mismatch may result in lung edema or low output. The immediate reaction would be to increase systolic driving pressures, and possibly to adjust pump rate upwards or extend the relative systolic operation period. So long as the driving pressures are high enough to overcome the needs to secure an empty pump in the range of expected systolic blood pressures, displacement pumps are afterload independent. Thus, blood pressure shall be controlled to avoid episodes of high blood pressure.

Filling of the pump during diastole is ideally passive. A small vacuum has to be applied to quickly remove the air from the air chamber through the long and narrow drivelines because of their resistance. The necessary pressure difference (vacuum) could be reduced by bigger diameters of the driveline, which on the other hand heightens the necessary pneumatic displacement volume of the driver because a bigger dead volume has to be filled to create the desired systolic driving pressures.

With the extracorporeal VADs, a higher vacuum may be useful to compensate for pressure losses along the long and narrow venous cannulas, especially with the pediatric settings. If the negative pressures in accordance to the available diastolic time, defined by the pumping rate and relative diastolic operation time, are adjusted correctly, this will result in a near total filling of the ventricle (please note that proper operation for SynCardia TAH requires a filling of about 75 percent only). Pneumatic devices are preload respondent. A sudden decrease of the filling volume thus indicates rather a medical problem (hypovolemia, obstruction by tamponade) than an increased need for vacuum.

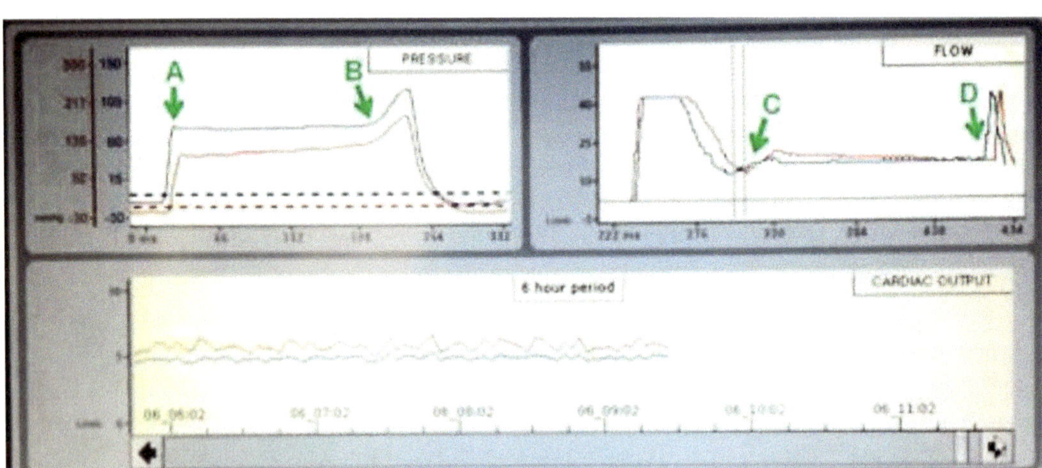

◻ **Fig. 15.1** Pressure curves (*top left*), filling curves (*top right*) and cardiac output curves (*bottom*) displayed on the SynCardia "Companion 2" driver

Box

In ◘ Fig. 15.1, the curves from the screen of the Companion driver can be seen. The red lines represent the left ventricle and the blue lines the right ventricle. The top left curves show the pressure of air inside the ventricles during systole (blood inside the ventricles is being ejected). The top right curves show the velocity of air flow coming outside the ventricles during diastole (ventricle fills with blood). The bottom curves are the cardiac output (in liters per minute) and evolve over time by adding a dot every minute. A reminder: the ventricles of the SynCardia TAH system have no sensors. The system is in balance as long as both ventricles *full eject* and *partial fill*. Full eject can be seen on the pressure curves (top left in ◘ Fig. 15.1). In the beginning, the ventricles are filled with blood. The driver starts to build up air pressure rapidly. When the air pressure gets higher than the arterial blood pressure, the outflow valve opens (at point "*A*" in ◘ Fig. 15.1), and the membrane starts to move pushing out the blood from the ventricle. During the movement of the membrane, the air pressure is not increasing (from "*A*" to "*B*" in ◘ Fig. 15.1). When the membrane reached the end position (at point "*B*"), the blood from the ventricle is fully ejected. The pressure rises up again to reach the programmed maximum driving pressure (e.g., 210 mmHg for left and 110 mmHg for right driving pressure, seen in ◘ Fig. 15.1). This pressure increase at the end of the curve is called the full eject flag. After systole, a valve in the driver opens and relieves the air from the ventricles. The air from the ventricles travels through the drivelines and a flow sensor before exiting the driver. The sensor can be simplified as a wheel spinning when air goes through. The top right curves in ◘ Fig. 15.1 are showing the speed of the wheel spinning during diastole. In the beginning, the ventricles decompress, meaning the high pressure is released to ambient air pressure. The wheel accelerates fast and eventually comes down. When the pressure inside the ventricles is lower than the filling blood pressure, the inflow valve opens (at point "*C*" in ◘ Fig. 15.1). The membrane moves while blood is coming into the ventricles. The air that is displaced by the blood let the wheel spinning at constant speed (indicating a smooth filling). The diastolic phase is stopped before the ventricle is completely filled with blood, so the curves at point "*D*" in ◘ Fig. 15.1 don't touch the zero line. The beginning of the systolic phase is seen at the end of the curves as sharp increase in wheel spin. No further explanation is needed for the cardiac output curves on the bottom of ◘ Fig. 15.1.

References

1. Liotta D (2002) Early clinical application of assisted circulation. Tex Heart Inst J 29(3):229–230
2. Cooley DA (2001) The total artificial heart as a bridge to cardiac transplantation: personal recollections. Tex Heart Inst J 28(3):200–202
3. DeVries WC, Anderson JL, Joyce LD, Anderson FL, Hammond EH, Jarvik RK, Kolff WJ (1984) Clinical use of the total artificial heart. N Engl J Med 310(5):273–278
4. Noon GP, Morley DL, Irwin S, Abdelsayed SV, Benkowski RJ, Lynch BE (2001) Clinical experience with the MicroMed DeBakey ventricular assist device. Ann Thorac Surg 71(3 Suppl):S133–8; discussion S144–6
5. Strueber M, Schmitto J, Kutschka I, Haverich A (2012) Placement of 2 implantable centrifugal pumps to serve as a total artificial heart after cardiectomy. J Thorac Cardiovasc Surg 143(2):507–509
6. Werkkala K, Jokinen JJ, Soininen L, Dellgren G et al (2016) Clinical durability of the CARMEDA® BioActive Surface in EXCOR® VAD pumps. ASAIO J 62:139–142
7. Völz S, Holmberg M, Redfors B, Dellgren G (2014) Acute tamponade of the left paracorporeal pump house due to membrane defect in a patient with a Berlin Heart EXCOR biventricular assist device. Eur J Cardiothorac Surg 46:743–744
8. Jaroszewski DE, Anderson EM, Pierce CN, Arabia FA (2011) The SynCardia freedom driver: a portable driver for discharge home with the total artificial heart. J Heart Lung Transplant 30:844–845

Intraoperative Anesthesiological Monitoring and Management

M. Baiocchi, M. Benedetto, and G. Frascaroli

© Springer International Publishing Switzerland 2017
A. Montalto et al. (eds.), *Mechanical Circulatory Support in End-Stage Heart Failure*,
DOI 10.1007/978-3-319-43383-7_16

16.1 Introduction

Patients undergoing ventricular assist device (VAD) implantation are critically ill, usually receiving multiple inotropic drugs and/or an intra-aortic balloon pump, often showing a no more than 20% mean ejection fraction (EF) [1]. So intraoperative management for VAD surgery may be challenging for cardiac anesthesiologists as this patient cohort is associated with significant comorbidities: pulmonary hypertension, peripheral vascular disease, kidney, hepatobiliary, and central nervous dysfunction. Even minor changes in hemodynamics may dramatically increase morbidity and mortality. In other words, the anesthesiologist should become familiar with the various assist devices; the anesthetic plan must take into account the severity of cardiac dysfunction and the degree of organ dysfunction. The use of diagnostic (transesophageal echocardiography), hemodynamic (MAPs, CVP, SvO2, PAPs), and therapeutic (vasopressors, inotropes) tools is mandatory. Particularly, the diagnosis of right-sided heart failure after implantation of left-ventricular assist devices should be intraoperatively investigated. Patients suffering from severe congestive heart failure (CHF) are typically chronically treated with ß-blockers, intensive diuretic therapy, ACE inhibitors, and/or angiotensin receptor blockers, the latter in order to reduce peripheral vascular resistances, but with the controversy of a theoretical increase in inotrope support requirement [2]. Patient that comes to theater has usually received premedication with benzodiazepine or opioids in order to reduce the sympathetic tone. However, an overtreatment with sedatives may cause hypoventilation and hypoxia, thus increasing pulmonary vascular resistances and acidosis [3].

16.2 Preoperative Standard Monitoring

A standard invasive hemodynamic monitoring should be ensured before inducing general anesthesia for VAD placement (Table 16.1):

- Five-lead electrocardiography (ECG), pulse oximetry, capnography, core and peripheral temperature probes, and an invasive arterial blood pressure monitoring are mandatory.

Table 16.1 Standard monitoring

Device	Measure
PAC	PVR, SvO2
TEE	Right ventricle function, shape of ventricular septum, LV filling, PFO, etc.
NIRS	ScvO2 correlation, adequate tissue perfusion
LAP	LV filling pressure

- A large-bore peripheral venous access (14 gauge) and five-lumen central venous line, vascath, and PA sheet catheters are strongly indicated due to the high risk of massive intra- and postoperative blood loss [4]. An ultrasound scanning and guidance for internal jugular vein catheter positioning is usually preferred than the landmark technique, due to high incidence (10%) of central venous thrombosis in these long-term hospitalized CHF patients [5–7]. When VAD is thought to be the only bridge to heart transplant, it's better to preserve the RIJV in order to facilitate myocardial biopsy posttransplantation to evaluate for cardiac rejection.
- Pulmonary artery catheter (PAC) should be floated through the PA sheet. Although it has not been demonstrated a direct improvement in clinical outcomes for cardiac surgical patients [8, 9], a recent survey of cardiac anesthesiologists shows they still choose to use PAC during VAD implantation [10] in order to monitor pulmonary vascular resistances, right ventricular function, and mixed central venous oxygen saturation [11].
- ICD must be turned off, and external plates should be positioned for eventual shock delivery before and after chest closure.
- TEE probe: TEE is a useful diagnostic and monitoring tool, providing information about the position of the inflow cannula, the ventricular function, and the filling volume status [12–14]. It's the best device to monitor RV function and compliance before and after LVAD insertion and measure pulmonary arterial pressures (PAPs) by using the continuous wave (CW) on the tricuspid valve and applying the Bernoulli's equation. RV

Table 16.2 TEE evaluation during LVAD insertion, check for:

LV thrombus	
RV failure	RVEDD >85 mm RVEDV >20 cm^2
Tricuspid valve	Severe TR reduces LV filling LV septal movement can distort the annulus
PFO	Prior to insertion After LVAD positioning (decompression of LA can unmask PFO) It can be the reason for unexplained hypoxia
Atheromasic disease in the descending aorta	It can increase the risk of stroke

dysfunction occurs in 25–50% of cases after LVAD implantation [15–17]. Echocardiographic predictors are an increased RV to LV diastolic diameter, moderate to severe tricuspid regurgitation, and RV geometry with a decreased long axis to short axis ratio (Table 16.2).

- Neuromonitoring: Continuous measurement of cerebral oxygenation with near-infrared spectroscopy (NIRS) is strongly recommended during the entire perioperative period [18], especially with second-/third-generation VADs providing a continuous less pulsatile flow that may get peripheral pulse oximetry unreliable [19]. Bispectral index (BIS) monitoring is also recommended to assess the depth of anesthesia throughout the intraoperative period.

16.2.1 Anesthetic Drugs

The induction of general anesthesia for congestive heart failure (CHF) patients undergoing VAD placement is crucial due to the risk of myocardial depression, severe hypotension, and multiorgan dysfunction, the latter potentially related to anesthetic drug metabolism. Compared with normal physiology, heart failure also results in a slow circulation and a reduced distribution volume for anesthetic drugs. As a result, when conventional doses are administered, drug concentrations are usually higher among heart failure patients. The anesthesiologist must be mindful of this fact using incremental doses of anesthetic drugs and allowing time to evaluate their effects [20]. Furthermore, in this patients high endogenous catecholamine level supports hemodynamics, and induction of general anesthesia may alter this balance; for this reason, start the induction only when operating room is available and, in critical patients (high inotropic support, very low cardiac performance), perform the induction of GA having ECLS/CPB in "stand-by" support.

- Unawareness: etomidate is usually preferable to propofol due to less risk of negative inotropic effect or vasodilation. The risk of relative adrenal insufficiency as a consequence of single dose of etomidate (20 mg) is well described, but did not result in a higher demand for vasopressors [21]. However, it has been found there is no significant difference in cardiac output changes by using either propofol or etomidate and that propofol does not lead to the induction of myoclonic movements and the inhibition of 11-b-hydroxylase as seen with etomidate [22]. Furthermore, in experimental models, it can induce a relaxation of the pulmonary vessels [23]. Midazolam is a good choice to provide unawareness due to low hemodynamic impact. Ketamine is also a useful sedation drug, increasing heart rate, blood pressure, and cardiac output, mediated through the sympathetic nervous stimulation, with minimal effects on respiratory drive.
- Analgesia: fentanyl seems to be the standard choice for induction of general anesthesia [4, 24]. A choice of continuous infusion of remifentanil (instead of sufentanil, alfentanyl, or fentanyl) has the major advantage – its metabolism is related to plasma esterase and not to liver or kidneys.
- Mioresolution: pancuronium and rocuronium are usually appropriate for VAD patients.

Pancuronium provides hemodynamic stability due to vagolytic and indirect sympathomimetic properties and a longer duration of action. It may result in a prolonged neuromuscular blockade in patients with kidney dysfunction and CHF.

Table 16.3 Practical guide to drug administration during GA for LVAD positioning

Induction	Etomidate 0.3–0.6 mg/kg (not available in all countries) Ketamine 1–2 mg/kg Midazolam 0.05–0.25 mg/kg Propofol 1.5–2 mg/kg (focus on myocardial depression and vasodilation) Conditioning with volatile agents (SEV/DESF) Fentanyl 2–4 mcg/kg or sufentanil 0.15–0.4 mcg/kg Rocuronium 0.6–1 mg/kg or pancuronium 0.08–0.1 mg/kg
Maintenance	Propofol 1–3 mg/kg/h or sevorane/desflurane Remifentanil 0.05–0.1 mcg/kg/min or sufentanil 0.15–0.5 mcg/kg/h

Rocuronium enables fast-track anesthesia, has a rapid onset of effect, and has an antidote.

- Maintenance out of CPB: It has been shown that sevoflurane and desflurane reduce mortality and morbidity in cardiac surgery [25]. Preconditioning (APC) using volatile agents (sevoflurane and desflurane) is known to improve clinical outcomes in cardiac surgery. APC depends on the concentration and the timing of volatile agent delivering [25].
- Maintenance of anesthesia during CPB in most centers is usually achieved by continuous infusion of propofol with significant reduction in cerebral metabolic rate, which can contribute to a decreased incidence of cerebrovascular events [26] (Table 16.3).

16.2.2 Mechanical Ventilation

Patients undergoing LVAD implantation are at particular risk for developing right-sided heart failure. Pulmonary hypertension may impair this situation due to increased RV afterload. Mechanical ventilation must be set in order to avoid hypoxia and hypercapnia that contribute to pulmonary vasoconstriction and subsequent pulmonary hypertension [27, 28]. VAD patients may often undergo medium- to long-term ventilation afterward. A protective ventilations strategy, as for ARDS patients, has been promoted in order to minimize the potential for ventilator-induced lung injury [29]. Positive end-expiratory pressure could be carefully used, though high PEEP has been not shown to systematically influence right-ventricular function [30]. That's why, as a conclusion, a maximum tidal volume of 6–8 mL/kg (ideal body weight) is preferable, and a best PEEP should be set to optimize lung compliance and minimize vascular pulmonary resistance and then RV dysfunction (which can be continuously monitored via transesophageal echocardiography during ventilation setup) (Table 16.4).

Table 16.4 Mechanical ventilation during LVAD positioning

Decrease pulmonary vascular resistances Monitor RV function	Avoid hypoxia and hypercapnia (PaCO2 30–40 mmHg/PaO_2 >70 mmh) Set maximum tidal volume of 6–8 ml/kg ideal body weight Set best PEEP (at least 4–5 cmH_2O)

16.2.3 Fluid Management

Perioperative fluid management during VAD surgery should aim to guarantee adequate intravascular volume and VAD flows but without overloading the right ventricle.

VAD patients usually have a preexisting volume deficiency due to diuretic therapy.

Although there has been a longstanding debate on this topic and the controversy between colloids and crystalloids is still open [31], intravascular volume optimization for VAD implantation is a crucial point. Before and during the induction of anesthesia, the volume deficiency should be replaced. After weaning from CPB, volume management should aim to provide sufficient VAD flows and avoid a collapse of the left ventricle. Transfusion of RBCs is often required to provide adequate tissue oxygenation; the trigger for that must come from a combination of mixed venous oxygen saturation, lactate plasma levels, and hemoglobin plasma levels [32–34]. Hemolysis is an important issue in VAD patients, less in the intracorporeal centrifugal VAD and

Table 16.5 Fluid management LVAD positioning

Intravascular volume optimization	Replace preexisting volume deficiency during anesthesia induction and before starting CPB Ensure adequate VAD flows and avoid LV collapse after weaning from CPB Don't be too liberal: remember to protect the RV function Help yourself with TEE monitoring

axial technology LVAD and more in BVAD support; hemopexin and haptoglobin, in addition to free hemoglobin, can assess erythrocyte damage [35] (Table 16.5).

16.2.4 Inotropes and Vasopressors

Patients suffering from CHF are typically managed preoperatively with inotropes (dopamine, dobutamine, epinephrine) and phosphodiesterase-III (PDE-III) inhibitors (milrinone or enoximone). Vasopressors such as norepinephrine or vasopressin should be available to ensure a sufficient perfusion pressure, since vasoplegia occurs in up to 40% of VAD patients [36–38]. The main causes of the abovementioned vasoplegia are the lack of vasopressin and the increased production of nitric oxide by nitric oxide synthases [39, 40]. Low-dose vasopressin (defined as <0.04 U/min) started before CPB generally decreases the need of postoperative vasopressors [38–41], but not in severe cases of vasoplegia where high doses of multiple vasopressors (norepinephrine, vasopressin, or phenylephrine) are needed. Methylene blue administration can be considered in catecholamine-resistant vasoplegic shock.

Inotropes and PDE inhibitors support the right ventricle during weaning from CPB after LVAD placement. This must be highlighted since the performance of the right ventricle is the most crucial parameter for successful weaning from CPB post-LVAD implantation. Milrinone was preferred as the primary inotropic drug due to lack of blood pressure increase during implantation of continuous flow-generating assist devices in one study [42].

It can be used even in inhalatory manner to reduce pulmonary vascular resistance. The calcium-sensitizing agent Levosimendan and its long-lasting active metabolite OR-1896 bind to troponin C, significantly increase contractility, and reduce peripheral vascular resistances by opening adenosine triphosphate (ATP)-sensitive K channels in vascular smooth muscles [43, 44]. However, the increased myocardial contractility, which lasts at least for 7 days after a 24-h infusion is maintained, is not associated with an increase in myocardial oxygen consumption. At present, levosimendan nonresponders have been identified as high-risk candidates for right ventricular failure. Presurgery levosimendan treatment nonresponse has been identified by elevated N-terminal prohormone brain natriuretic peptide (NT-proBNP) levels and predicted postsurgery RV failure. Levosimendan however did not prevent right-sided heart failure (RHF) [45], and prospective large multicentric studies for its use in LVAD implantation are still lacking. Inotropes are usually not required in biventricular assist device placement. Vasopressors are generally required to provide adequate perfusion pressure for unsupported right ventricle and to treat also hypotension due to systemic inflammatory response coming from CPB and LVAD placement itself [46]. A number of pharmacological approaches have been promoted in order to prevent or attenuate RV dysfunction, especially inhaled nitric oxide in the contest of weaning from CPB after LVAD placement. A reduced RV contractility is revealed intraoperatively when at least three different factors increase RV preload beyond optimal filling status resulting in increased wall tension. Firstly, the increased systemic blood flow from the LVAD fills the RV more efficiently leading to RV dilatation. Too aggressive offloading of the LV with the device may cause a leftward shift in the ventricular septum increasing end diastolic volume of the RV. Thirdly, intraoperative bleeding may be quite severe, thus requiring massive transfusion. These factors may also increase PVR with devastating consequences to the dysfunctional RV. The failure of the RV to offload venous return will increase venous pressures further reducing

Table 16.6 Inotropes/vasoactive: average therapeutic dosage to support hemodynamics and the right ventricle

Drug	Average dosage	Advantages	Side effects
Epinephrine	0.05–0.25 mcg/kg/min	Supported RV overload	Tachycardia, arrhythmias, raised O_2 demand
Norepinephrine	Up to 0.15 mcg/kg/min	Contrasted vasodilation	Increased PVR
Levosimendan	0.05–0.2 mcg/kg/min	Supported RV overload	Vasodilation
Milrinone	0.3–0.75 mcg/kg/min	Supported RV overload	Arrhythmias, raised O_2 demand, vasodilation
Vasopressin	2.5–5 U/h	Contrasted vasodilation	Increased SVR impairs forward flow of LVAD
i-NO	5–20 ppm	Reduced PVR (if not fixed)	
i-Milrinone	5 mg for 15 min	Reduced PVR (if not fixed)	
i-Iloprost	10–20 ng	Reduced PVR (if not fixed)	
Methylene blue	0.5–2 mg/kg	Contrasted vasodilation	

systemic organ perfusion, which ultimately leads to multiorgan failure [47]. It's mandatory to prevent vicious cycle of hypotension and ischemia, maintaining systolic arterial pressure, minimizing right ventricular dilation, and reducing right ventricular afterload (inhaled NO or milrinone). Indeed various case reports, observational studies, and small-scale RCTs have demonstrated beneficial effects of iNO therapy [48–51] in patients who required LVAD insertion. Nearly all of these small studies showed that iNO decreased mean PAPs and RV afterload and resulted in more stable LVAD performance. In 2005 the European expert panel concluded that it was reasonable to consider iNO during LVAD insertion because of the perceived physiological and clinical benefits and the life-threatening impact of RV failure on the overall survival [51]. A practical prospective definition of RV failure in LVAD literature includes high CVP, inotrope requirement, and LVAD flow less than 2 l/min/m^2, and this should guide the start of iNO therapy in theater together with high PAPs, low SvO2, and low ScVo2. However, the threshold of LVAD flows less than 2 l/min/m^2 seems to be too conservative. The most recent scientific statement of the American Heart Association in their recommendations for the Use of Mechanical Circulatory Support concludes that the use of selective pulmonary vasodilators (nitric oxide, prostanoids, or type 5 phosphodiesterase inhibitors) may attenuate the development of early RV failure [52]. The majority of independent consultants agree with the original European recommendations by 92% and support the use of iNO during LVAD implantation. The debate about the real effectiveness of iNO in LVADs is still open since large RCTs are still lacking and most of the small-size ones reveal the need to crossover from double-blind to open-label investigation if patients met RV failure criteria before 15 min of monitoring. This creates several bias and gets the production of systematic review and meta-analysis quite hard (Table 16.6). Inhaled prostacyclin may offer an alternative to nitric oxide in the treatment of pulmonary hypertension [53].

To Resume: Intraoperative Hemodynamic Management During LVAD Positioning – Tip and Tricks for Anesthesiologists

The goal for anesthesiologists during LVAD positioning is to support hemodynamics by managing pulmonary hypertension and avoiding RV failure which is the first cause of poor clinical outcome (Table 16.7). This is achieved by contemporary decreasing mPAPs and RV

Table 16.7 Practice guide to wean from CPB

Sustain SVR and arterial pressure	Norepinephrine Vasopressin
Maintain DO2 level 272 ml/min/m^2	Raise in pump flow Raise Hb level Raise O_2 Sat Decrease body temp
Support RV	Milrinone (0.5 mcg/kg/min) Dobutamine (4–6 mcg/kg/min) Epinephrine (0.05–0.2 mcg/kg/min)
Hb level	10 g/dl
Maintain regular rhythm and A-V synchrony	K+ / Mg+ Sotalol 40–80 mg Amiodarone 150–300 mg Pacing
Pacing with 110–120 bpm	Increase of HR increases CI in LVAD due to continuous drainage of the LV
Reduce PVR	iNO (5–20 ppm) Inhalatory iloprost (10–20 ng) Inhalatory milrinone (5 mg) for 15 min
Slowly reduce CPB flow and start LVAD (careful monitoring CVP, TEE, LAP)	Continue inhalation of iloprost or milrinone for 30 min every hour

afterload, by supporting peripheral vascular resistances, and by avoiding hypoxia and hypercapnia that can further increase the pulmonary vascular resistances, thus affecting the RV function. Inotrope-vasopressor delivery must be guided by the TEE and hemodynamic parameters and may be expressed by the inotropic score (IS) or the more updated vasopressor-inotropic score (VIS), which have been considered an independent marker of poor clinical outcome (Table 16.8). During CPB in VAD implantation, it is recommended to calibrate the DO2, the oxygen delivery on tissue, or the volume of oxygen provided by the pump (flow rate × [Hb] × SatO2) to the metabolic demand of the tissues. The critical level of DO2 is debatable and is proportionate to CPB temperature. Ranucci et al., in a retrospective review, found that a DO2 (indexed to BSA) less than 272 ml/min/m^2 was the single best predictor for renal failure following CPB [54].

Table 16.8 Scores

Inotropic score [53]	
Dopamine (μg/kg/min) + dobutamine (μg/kg/min) +100 × epinephrine (μg/kg/min)	
Vasoactive inotropic score (Modified by Davidson et al. with inclusion of vasoactive medication [54])	
IS + 10 × milrinone (μg/kg/min) + 10 × vasopressin (U/kg/min) + 100 × norepinephrine (μg/kg/min)	
Vasoactive inotropic score plus levosimendan [55]	
VIS + 10 × levosimendan (mcg/kg/min)	
VIS 20–24 (in the first 24 h) + VIS 15–19 (in the subsequent 24 h)	Poor clinical outcome

16.2.5 Mentions of Anesthesia During Off-Pump VAD Positioning

Usually LVAD is being implanted by median sternotomy and cardiopulmonary bypass, but operative risk is high in patient undergoing repeated heart surgery. Left thoracotomy approach without CPB ensures adequate view of the surgical field without the need of heart manipulation in patients with unstable hemodynamics. However, patient selection is important, because right-sided cardiac structures may not be reached when using this technique. The anesthesiologist should be aware about the pathophysiology of patient heart failure, the off-pump procedure, and the type of implanted devices. Many procedures can be performed by single lumen endotracheal tube (ETT), considering that the single lung ventilation is often not tolerated, leading to hypoxia and hemodynamic instability. The drug management follows the same principles of on-pump procedure with the maximum effort to maintain vascular resistance, support the right ventricle, and minimize the pulmonary vascular resistances. The duration of anesthesia, surgery and mechanical ventilation, as well as the transfusion requirements appears to fall in off-pump procedures, but more studies on this topic are needed.

Implantation of LVAD with non-fibrillatory technique has been also described. It consists of administration of an intravenous bolus of adenosine to induce a short bradycardic arrest during off-pump LVAD placement [55]. Decreasing the heartbeats also helps to reduce the blood loss together with a reduction in the volume of blood ejected from the heart during LVAD implantation (reduction in blood pressure). Furthermore, adenosine may mediate pulmonary vasodilatation, thus protecting the RV function.

References

1. Kocabas S et al (2013) Anesthesia for ventricular assist device placement: experience from a single center. Transplantation Proceedings 45:1005–1008
2. Hasija S et al (2010) Prophylactic vasopressin in patients receiving the angiotensin-converting enzyme inhibitor ramipril undergoing coronary artery bypass graft surgery. J Cardiothorac Vasc Anesth 24:230–238
3. Feussner M et al (2012) Best Pract Res Clin Anaesthesiol 26(2):167–177
4. Broussard D et al (2011) Anesthesia for left ventricular assist device insertion: a case series and review. Ochsner J 11:70–77
5. Long DA et al (2006) Effect of heparin-bonded central venous catheters on the incidence of catheter-related thrombosis and infection in children and adults. Anaesth Intensive Care 34:481–484
6. Palepu GB et al (2009) Impact of ultrasonography on central venous catheter insertion in intensive care. Indian J Radiol Imaging 19:191–198
7. Calvert N et al (2003) The effectiveness and cost-effectiveness of ultrasound locating devices for central venous access: a systematic review and economic evaluation. Health Technol Assess 7:1–84
8. Schwann NM et al (2011) Lack of effectiveness of the pulmonary artery catheter in cardiac surgery. Anesth Analg 113:994–1002
9. Cowie BS (2011) Does the pulmonary artery catheter still have a role in the perioperative period? Anaesth Intensive Care 39:345–355
10. Kanchi M (2011) Do we need a pulmonary artery catheter in cardiac anesthesia? – An Indian perspective. Ann Card Anaesth 14:25–29
11. El-Magharbel I (2005) Ventricular assist devices and anesthesia. Semin Cardiothorac Vasc Anesth 9:241–249
12. Chumnanvej S et al (2007) Perioperative echocardiographic examination for ventricular assist device implantation. Anesth Analg 105:583
13. Scalia GM et al (2000) Clinical utility of echocardiography in the management of implantable ventricular assist devices. J Am Soc Echocardiogr 13:754
14. Nicoara A et al (2007) Mal- positioned left ventricular assist device cannula: diagnosis and management with transesophageal echocardiography guidance. Anesth Analg 105:1574
15. Potapov EV et al (2008) Tricuspid incompetence and geometry of the right ventricle as predictors of right ventricular function after implantation of a left ventricular assist device. J Heart Lung Transplant 27:1275–1281
16. Drakos SG et al (2010) Risk factors predictive of right ventricular failure after left ventricular assist device implantation. Am J Cardiol 105:1030–1035
17. Kavarana MN et al (2002) Right ventricular dysfunction and organ failure in left ventricular assist device recipients: a continuing problem. Ann Thorac Surg 73:745–750
18. De Tournay-Jetté E et al (2011) The relationship between cerebral oxygen saturation changes and postoperative cognitive dysfunction in elderly patients after coronary artery bypass graft surgery. J Cardiothorac Vasc Anesth 25:95–104
19. Heringlake M et al (2011) Preoperative cerebral oxygen saturation and clinical outcomes in cardiac surgery. Anesthesiology 114
20. Magner JJ, Royston D (2004) Heart failure. Br J Anaesth 93:74
21. Morel J et al (2011) Haemodynamic consequences of etomidate administration in elective cardiac surgery: a randomized double-blinded study. Br J Anaesth 107:503–509
22. Bendel S et al (2007) Propofol causes more hypotension than etomidate in patients with severe aortic stenosis: a double-blind, randomized study comparing propofol and etomidate. Acta Anaesthesiol Scand 51:284–289
23. Horibe M et al (2000) Propofol attenuates acetylcholine-induced pulmonary vasorelaxation: role of nitric oxide and endothelium-derived hyperpolarizing factors. Anesthesiology 93:447–455
24. Stone ME (2007) Current status of mechanical circulatory assistance. Semin Cardiothorac Vasc Anesth 11:185–204
25. Landoni G, Biondi-Zoccai GG, Zangrillo A et al (2007) Desflurane and sevoflurane in cardiac surgery: a meta-analysis of randomized clinical trials. J Cardiothorac Vasc Anesth 21:502–511
26. Newman MF et al (1995) Cerebral physiologic effects of burst suppression doses of propofol during nonpulsatile cardiopulmonary bypass. CNS subgroup of McSPI. Anesth Analg 81:452–457
27. Aviado DM et al (1957) Effects of anoxia on pulmonary circulation: reflex pulmonary vasoconstriction. Am J Phys 189:253–262
28. Barer GR et al (1971) Pulmonary vasodilator and vasoconstrictor actions of carbon dioxide. J Physiol 213:633–645
29. (2000) Ventilation with lower tidal volumes as compared with traditional tidal volumes for acute lung injury and the acute respiratory distress syndrome. N Engl J Med 342:1301–1308

30. Berglund JE et al (1994) Echocardiographic analysis of cardiac function during high PEEP ventilation. Intensive Care Med 20:174–180
31. Roberts I et al. (2004) Colloids versus crystalloids for fluid resuscitation in critically ill patients. Cochrane Database Syst Rev (2):CD000567
32. Vallet B et al (2010) Venous oxygen saturation as a physiologic transfusion trigger. Crit Care 14:213
33. (2010) Transfusion requirements after cardiac surgery. JAMA 304:1559–1567
34. Reeves BC et al (2008) Increased mortality, morbidity, and cost associated with red blood cell transfusion after cardiac surgery. Curr Opin Cardiol 23:607-612
35. Heilmann C et al (2009) Haemolysis in patients with ventricular assit devices: major differences between systems. Eur J Cardiothorac Surg 36:580–584
36. Lavigne D (2010) Vasopressin and methylene blue: alternate therapies in vasodilatory shock. Semin Cardiothorac Vasc Anesth 14:186–189
37. Levin MA et al (2009) Early on-cardiopulmonary bypass hypotension and other factors associated with vasoplegic syndrome. Circulation 120:1664–1671
38. Riha H et al (2011) Pro: methylene blue as a rescue therapy for vasoplegia after cardiac surgery. J Cardiothorac Vasc Anesth 25:736–738
39. Fischer GW et al (2010) Vasoplegia during cardiac surgery: current concepts and management. Thorac Cardiovasc Surg 22(2):140–144
40. Levy JH et al (2003) Inflammatory response to cardiopulmonary bypass. Ann Thorac Surg 75:S715–S720
41. Papadopoulos G et al (2010) Perioperative infusion of low-dose of vasopressin for prevention and management of vasodilatory vasoplegic syndrome in patients undergoing coronary artery bypass grafting-A double blind randomized study. J Cardiothorac Surg 5:17
42. Nussmeier NA et al (2003) Anesthetic management for implantation of the Jarvik 2000 left ventricular assist system. Anesth Analg 97:964–971
43. Papp Z et al (2005) Pharmacological mechanisms contributing to the clinical efficacy of levosimendan. Cardiovasc Drug Rev 23:71–98
44. Parle NM et al (2008) Repeated infusions of levosimendan: well tolerated and improves functional capacity in decompensated heart failure – a single-centre experience. Heart Lung Circ 17:206–210
45. Sponga S et al (2012) Reversible circumflex coronary artery occlusion during percutaneous transvenous mitral annuloplasty with the viacor system. J Am Coll Cardiol 59:288
46. Van Meter Jr CH (2001) Right heart failure: best treated by avoidance. Ann Thorac Surg 71:S220–S222
47. Kormos RL et al (2010) Right ventricular failure in patients with the HeartMate II continuous-flow left ventricular assist device: incidence, risk factors, and effect on outcomes. J Thorac Cardiovasc Surg 139(5):1316–1324
48. Hare JM et al (1997) Influence of inhaled nitric oxide on systemic flow and ventricular filling pressure in patients receiving mechanical circulatory assistance. Circulation 95(9):2250–2253
49. Argenziano M et al (1998) Randomized, double-blind trial of inhaled nitric oxide in LVAD recipients with pulmonary hypertension. Ann Thorac Surg 65(2):340–345
50. Macdonald PS et al (1998) Adjunctive use of inhaled nitric oxide during implantation of a left ventricular assist device. J Heart Lung Transplant Off Publ Int Soc Heart Transplant 17(3):312–316
51. Benedetto M et al (2015) Inhaled nitric oxide in cardiac surgery: evidence or tradition? Nitric Oxide 49:67–79
52. Peura JL et al (2012) Recommendations for the use of mechanical circulatory support: device strategies and patient selection: a scientific statement from the American Heart Association. Circulation 126(22): 2648–2667
53. Khan A et al (2009) A prospective, randomized, crossover pilot study of inhaled nitric oxide versus inhaled prostacyclin in heart transplant and lung transplant recipients. J Thorac Cardiovasc Surg 138:1417–1424
54. Ranucci M et al (2005) Oxygen delivery during cardiopulmonary bypass and acute renal failure after coronary operations. Ann Thorac Surg 80:2213
55. Awad H, Abd El Dayem M, Heard J et al (2010) Initial experience with off-pump left ventricular assist device implantation in single center: retrospective analysis. J Cardiothorac Surg 5:123

Transesophageal Echocardiography During LVAD Implantation

Marian Kukucka

© Springer International Publishing Switzerland 2017
A. Montalto et al. (eds.), *Mechanical Circulatory Support in End-Stage Heart Failure*,
DOI 10.1007/978-3-319-43383-7_17

Transesophageal echocardiography (TEE) has become a standard diagnostic and monitoring technique during ventricular assist device (VAD) implantation [1]. Morphological and functional information impacts patient management during the pre-, intra-, and post-procedural periods.

17.1 Pre-procedural Period

Despite application of several imaging methods such as transthoracic echocardiography or computer tomography during the preoperative period for diagnosis of end-stage heart failure (HF) and scheduling for VAD implantation, important questions remain to be answered immediately before implantation. Here intraoperative TEE is of advantage due to its actuality and the superior image quality.

17.1.1 Thrombus Exclusion

For exclusion of intracavitary thrombus formation, a comprehensive TEE examination is necessary. Preferred localization of thrombus in patients with end-stage HF is the left ventricular (LV) apex due to the blood flow stasis resulting from the severe reduction of myocardial contractility. This phenomenon is more pronounced following myocardial infarction (ischemic cardiomyopathy) in scaring apical regions of LV (◘ Fig. 17.1). In addition, exclusion of thrombus in the left atrial appendage is essential. Further, yet rare left-sided thrombus localizations are the submitral region of the LV and the wall of the left atrium.

RV function is usually partially retained which would prevent thrombus formation. However, most of the VAD candidates receive electrophysiological therapies (automated implantable cardioverter defibrillator or cardiac resynchronization), and the concomitant intracavitary wires are a predominant localization of thrombus formation (◘ Fig. 17.1).

Thrombus size, its localization, and degree of flotation have to be discussed with the surgeon and may impact the surgical strategy (with/without CPB, thrombectomy, left atrial appendage occlusion). Not all kinds of thrombus (wide wall adhesion) require therapy, but have to be exactly described in TEE reports.

17.1.2 Patent Foramen Ovale (PFO)

In patients with end-stage HF, left atrial pressure exceeds right atrial pressure, and echocardiographic identification of left to right shunting is performed with colored Doppler after adjusting velocity range to 30–40 cm/s using bicaval view (midesophageal, rotation 90°, ◘ Fig. 17.2). Contrast echocardiography is obsolete in this indication. Because of the profound hemodynamic changes following LVAD implantation with right atrial pressure now exceeding left atrial pressure, determination of shunting volume at this time does not support decision making. Postoperative risks in patients with PFO include

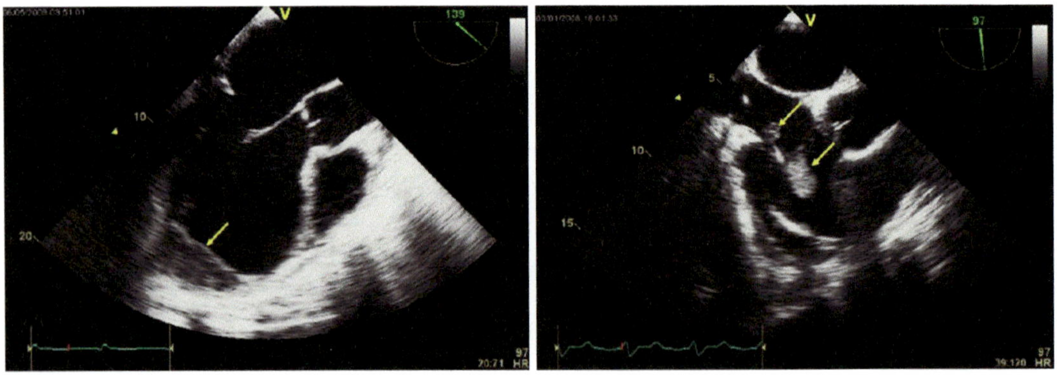

◘ **Fig. 17.1** Left apical thrombus in ischemic cardiomyopathy (*left panel*), multiple floated thrombi in the right atrium, and ventricle with adhesion to AICD wire (*right panel*)

right to left shunting with consequent decrease of arterial oxygen saturation and, in the long term, systemic embolization via PFO. In VAD surgery, direct closure (in case of bicaval cannulation) or interventional closure with an occluder (in case of VAD implantation via minimal approach without CPB) has to be considered.

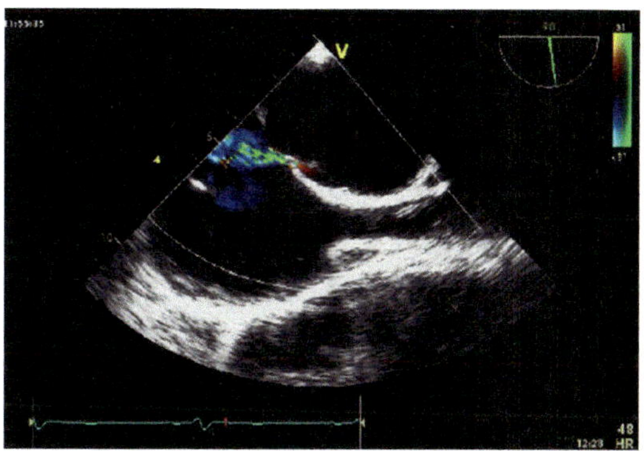

Fig. 17.2 Patent foramen ovale with left to right shunt imaged using color Doppler echocardiography

17.1.3 Aortic Regurgitation

In the case of aortic regurgitation (AR) following LVAD implantation, efficiency of mechanical support decreases, LV unloading is inadequate, and patients clinically present with limited exercise tolerance due to increased pulmonary pressures and subsequent right ventricular failure.

Careful quantification of AR is important. Due to increased left ventricular diastolic pressure in patients with end-stage HF, assessment by color Doppler may underestimate the degree of regurgitation. Therefore, quantification of AR has to be repeated while on cardiopulmonary bypass when hemodynamics are similar to the situation after LVAD implantation. Thus, it is possible to estimate the degree of AR following LVAD implantation.

Using the long axis aortic view (midesophageal, 120°) in color Doppler modus, the width of the regurgitant jet (1 cm below its origin) relative to the width of the left ventricular outflow tract is calculated, and a value above 25% identifies moderate to severe regurgitation (Fig. 17.3).

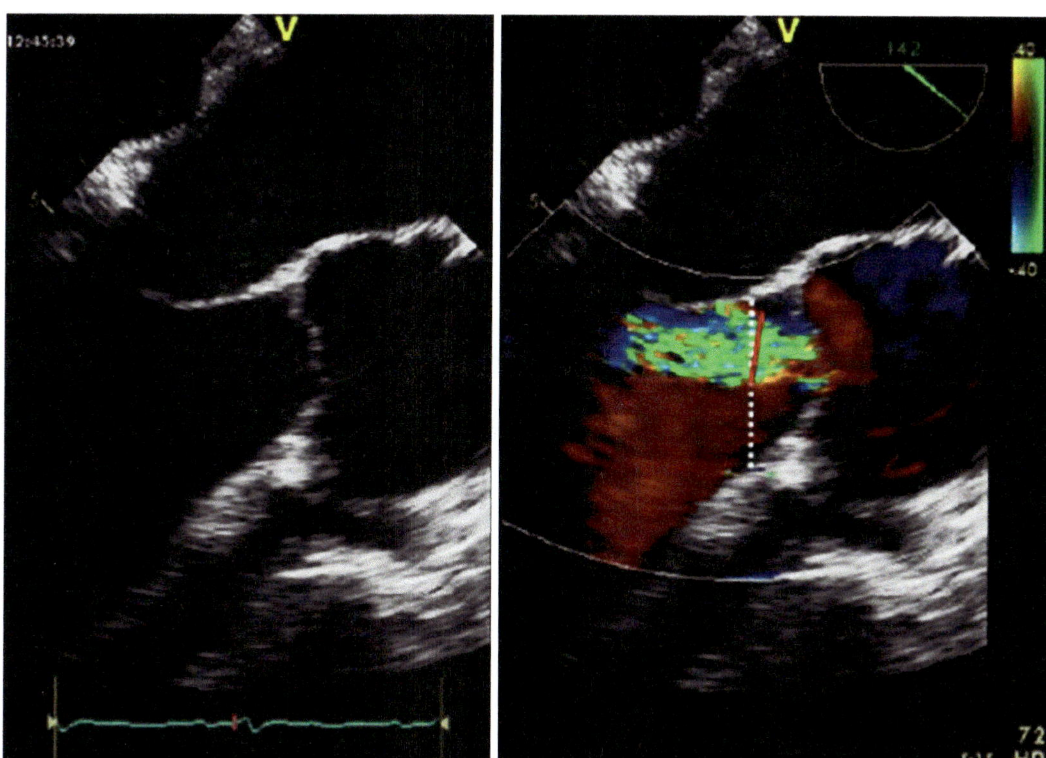

Fig. 17.3 Aortic regurgitation on CPB, left ventricular outflow tract measurement (*dot line*), and measurement of regurgitant jet width (*red line*)

It is generally accepted that AR of moderate or higher degree presents an indication for concomitant aortic valve surgery [2].

17.1.4 Assessment of RV Function

Following LVAD implantation, the right ventricle (RV) receives systemic venous blood and generates transpulmonary flow and adequate loading of the left ventricle and consequently of the LVAD. Right ventricular failure (RVF) is a well-known and frequent complication during the early post-procedural period. In high-volume centers, incidence of RVF decreases below 10%, probably due to exact pre- procedural risk stratification and therapy adjustment [3, 4].

TEE provides valuable information about RV morphology and function. To assess RV inflow tract and apex, acquisition of the midesophageal 4-chamber view (ME 4C) is necessary. Turning the probe to the right until the tricuspid valve comes into the center of the display and adjustment of probe depth to visualize the RV apex help to optimize image acquisition. To quantify RV geometry, annular (RVEDD 1), midcavity (RVEDD 2), and maximal (RVEDD max) short axis diameters at end-diastole are measured (◘ Fig. 17.4a). For assessment of RV function, the RV fractional area change using end-diastolic and end-systolic areas measured in the ME 4C view is calculated. Additional assessment of the RV systolic function includes measurement of tricuspid annular systolic plane excursion (TAPSE) from the ME 4C view

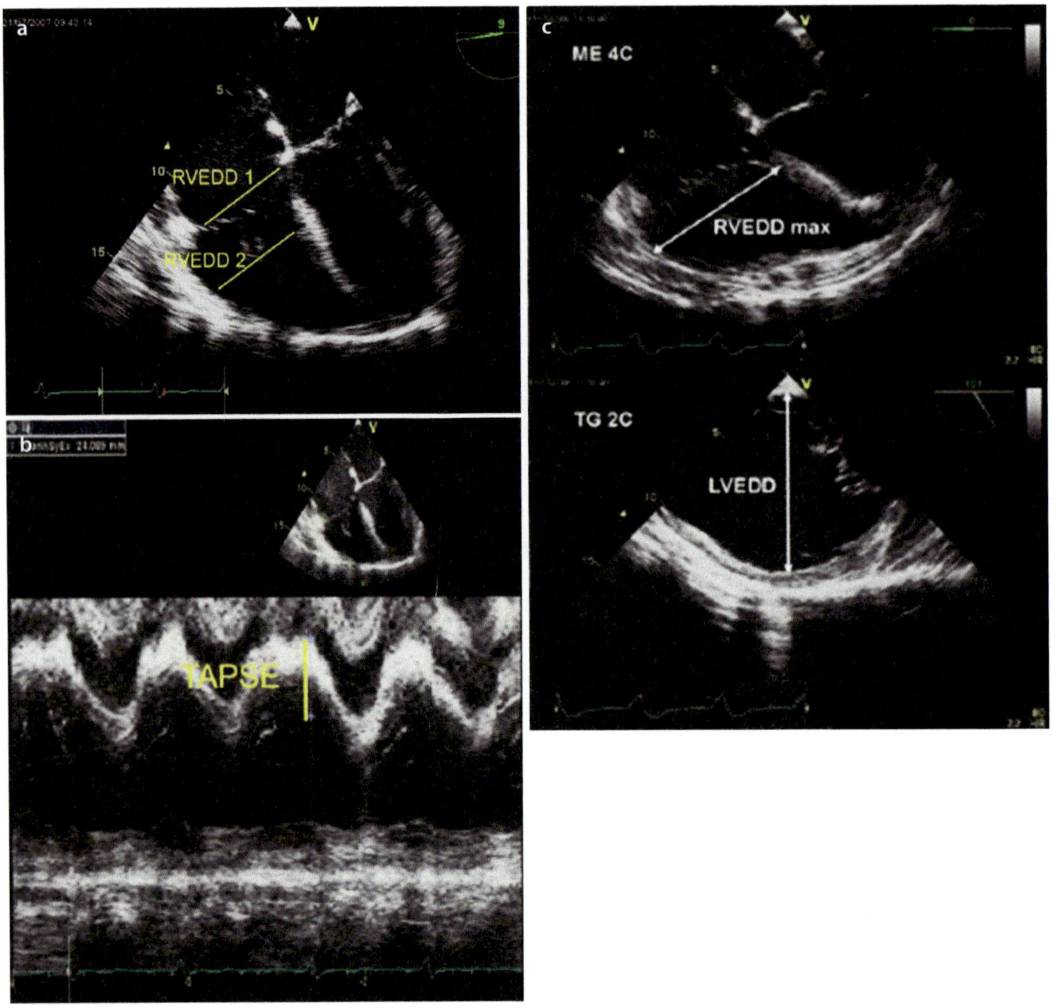

◘ **Fig. 17.4** RV geometrical measurements **a**, TAPSE measurement using anatomical M-Mode **b**, measurements for R/L ratio calculation **c**

using anatomical M-mode (◘ Fig. 17.4b). In patients scheduled for VAD implantations, critical values for these echocardiographic parameters are RVEDD >40 mm, RV FAC <20%, and TAPSE <10 mm [5].

Assessment of tricuspid regurgitation completes the TEE examination of the RV. 2D echocardiography allows for the discrimination between functional TR, frequently associated with secondary pulmonary hypertension in patients with end-stage HF, and structural TR with direct changes of the valvular apparatus (rare as complication of RV wires) which usually requires concomitant surgery. Using color Doppler imaging of vena contracta (VC) and its width measurement add to TR severity quantification (VC< 3 mm, mild; VC >7 mm, severe). Measurement of TR jet velocity with continuous-wave Doppler renders possible the calculation of RV pressure according to Bernoulli's equation (RV systolic pressure = 4 × Vmax2 + central venous pressure). Indication for concomitant tricuspid valve surgery in functional TR and annular dilatation is not definitely resolved. It has been suggested that patients with severe annular dilatation (RVEDD 1 > 43 mm) could later develop RVF [6].

Diverse scoring systems using clinical, hemodynamic, and echocardiographic parameters have been devised to predict RVF after isolated LVAD implantation. Most of these use complex calculations and are not reproducible in different patient cohorts [4].

In the course of the disease, RVF will also develop in many patients with predominant LV failure, with consecutive deterioration of LV preload and stroke volume and development of right-sided congestion and dilatation. Our group hypothesized that the severity of secondary RV dysfunction in patients with primary LV disease may be predicted by the easily determined preoperative RV-to-LV end-diastolic diameter ratio (R/L ratio, ◘ Fig. 17.4). In our study, a R/L ratio >0.72 predicted RVF after isolated LVAD implantation [7]. Importantly, Vivo et al. [8] compared our R/L ratio with different hemodynamic and surgical parameters in their patients' cohort and confirmed a R/L ratio >0.75 as a strong predictor of RVF following LVAD. Clinically, the R/L ratio supports risk stratification during LVAD, decision for the specific surgical approach, and guiding of pharmacological therapy. 3D echocardiography and the respective quantification software (e.g., TomTec Imaging Systems, Unterschleissheim, Germany) allow for direct end-diastolic and end-systolic RV volume measurements and quantification of ejection fraction. These 3D parameters may add important information for description of RV function during LVAD implantation in the near future.

17.2 Intraprocedural Period

17.2.1 Apex Cannula Position

Optimal position of apex (inflow) cannula of LVAD is required to enable unimpeded LV unloading and generation of LVAD flow. Target position is in parallel with the LV long axis toward the mitral valve. To find the optimal insertion spot, palpation of the LV apex under echocardiographic imaging is performed (◘ Fig. 17.5a). Best visualization to avoid positioning toward the myocardial wall is achieved in triplane/biplane 2D imaging (three or two views at the same time). Following insertion, the position is verified in triplane or biplane modus (◘ Fig. 17.5b).

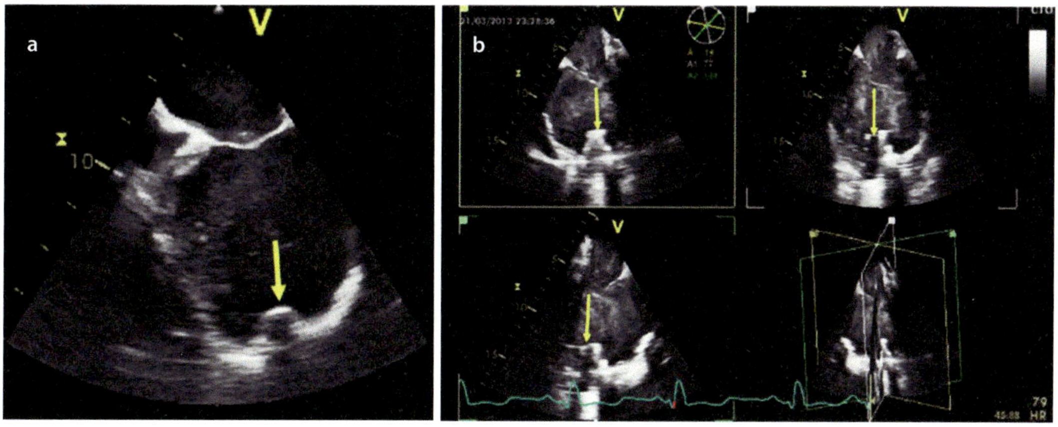

◘ **Fig. 17.5** Palpation of LV apex **a**, Apex cannula position in triplane imaging (four chamber, two chamber and long axis views) **b**

17.2.2 Ascending Aorta Anastomosis

Imaging of the LVAD outflow tract anastomosis is possible in the midesophageal view of the ascending aorta in short and long axis or biplane views. In case of a left lateral approach, the anastomosis with the descending aorta may also be visualized. Outflow from the LVAD may be visualized using color Doppler or quantified using continuous-wave Doppler. Usual velocities range between 1.5 and 2.5 m/s. Extremely low velocities indicate low flow caused by LVAD thrombosis, high velocities signify stenosis of outflow anastomosis on aorta.

17.3 Early Post-procedural Period

17.3.1 Therapy Guiding

Pre-procedurally measured RV echocardiographic parameters support post-procedural pharmacological therapy guiding. Patients with high risk for RVF have to be weaned from cardiopulmonary bypass (CPB) with pharmacological support of myocardial contractility (epinephrine, milrinone) and additional reduction of pulmonary vascular resistance (inhaled nitric oxide, iloprost).

17.3.2 Interventricular Septum Position

Echocardiographic target of pharmacological support during weaning from CPB, i.e., while reducing CPB flow and increasing LVAD performance, is a middle position of the interventricular septum (IVS) as imaged in 4CH view (◘ Fig. 17.6). Bulging of the IVS to the left and complete unloading of the left atrium and the LV indicate either excess performance (rotational speed) of the LVAD or RVF (◘ Fig. 17.6). Reduction of LVAD performance and increase of pharmacological RV support are the logical consequences. When IVS is still bulging to the left despite pharmacological therapy at its upper limit and LVAD flow at or below target, early temporary mechanical support for the RV is inevitable.

In the case of temporary RVAD target, balanced position of IVS optimizes the ratio between RVAD and LVAD flow.

For continuous post-procedural monitoring, echocardiography is not appropriate. Therefore, additional monitoring of left atrial pressure is recommended in critical patients. The ratio of right to left atrial pressure reflects the IVS position in echocardiography. Empirical knowledge identifies a right to left atrial pressure difference of more than 8 mmHg or left atrial pressure near zero as early hemodynamic signs of RV dysfunction.

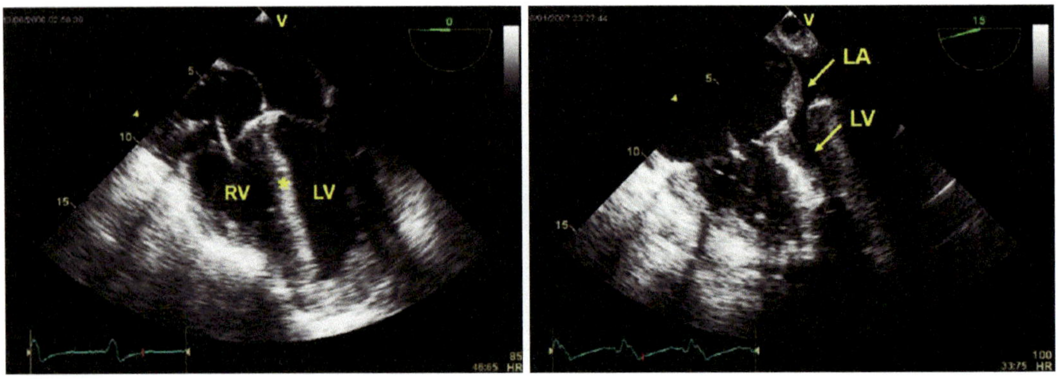

◘ **Fig. 17.6** Balance position of interventricular septum (*) following CPB weaning (*left panel*), completely empty left atrium and ventricle (*arrows*) in patient with right ventricular failure

References

1. Estep JD, Stainback RF, Little SH, Torre G, Zoghbi WA (2010) The role of echocardiography and other imaging modalities in patients with left ventricular assist devices. JACC Cardiovasc Imaging 3:1049–1064
2. Slaughter MS, Pagani FD, Rogers JG, Miller LW, Sun B, Russell SD, Starling RC, Chen L, Boyle AJ, Chillcott S, Adamson RM, Blood MS, Camacho MT, Idrissi KA, Petty M, Sobieski M, Wright S, Myers TJ, Farrar DJ (2010) Clinical management of continuous-flow left ventricular assist devices in advanced heart failure. J Heart Lung Transplant 29:S1–39
3. Meineri M, Van Rensburg AE, Vegas A (2012) Right ventricular failure after lvad implantation: Prevention and treatment. Best Pract Res Clin Anaesthesiol 26:217–229
4. Rich JD (2012) Right ventricular failure in patients with left ventricular assist devices. Cardiol Clin 30:291–302
5. Lang RM, Badano LP, Mor-Avi V, Afilalo J, Armstrong A, Ernande L, Flachskampf FA, Foster E, Goldstein SA, Kuznetsova T, Lancellotti P, Muraru D, Picard MH, Rietzschel ER, Rudski L, Spencer KT, Tsang W, Voigt JU (2015) Recommendations for cardiac chamber quantification by echocardiography in adults: an update from the american society of echocardiography and the european association of cardiovascular imaging. Eur Heart J Cardiovasc Imaging 16:233–270
6. Kukucka M, Stepanenko A, Potapov E, Krabatsch T, Kuppe H, Habazettl H (2012) Impact of tricuspid valve annulus dilation on mid-term survival after implantation of a left ventricular assist device. J Heart Lung Transplant. 31:967–971
7. Kukucka M, Stepanenko A, Potapov E, Krabatsch T, Redlin M, Mladenow A, Kuppe H, Hetzer R, Habazettl H Right-to-left ventricular end-diastolic diameter ratio and prediction of right ventricular failure with continuous-flow left ventricular assist devices. J Heart Lung Transplant 30:64–69
8. Vivo RP, Cordero-Reyes AM, Qamar U, Garikipati S, Trevino AR, Aldeiri M, Loebe M, Bruckner BA, Torre-Amione G, Bhimaraj A, Trachtenberg BH, Estep JD (2013) Increased right-to-left ventricle diameter ratio is a strong predictor of right ventricular failure after left ventricular assist device. J Heart Lung Transplant 32:792–799

Intraoperative Anticoagulation and Coagulation Management

Andreas Koster and Federico Pappalardo

© Springer International Publishing Switzerland 2017
A. Montalto et al. (eds.), *Mechanical Circulatory Support in End-Stage Heart Failure*,
DOI 10.1007/978-3-319-43383-7_18

18.1 General Aspects

Patients undergoing VAD implantation are at an increased risk for excessive perioperative hemorrhage. Therefore, blood conservation strategies should be implemented during VAD implantation. The surgical trauma and the patient's critical preoperative status are the most relevant risk factors. Alternative surgical routes for implantation to minimize surgical trauma, especially in reoperations, should be taken into account. Additionally, the use of completely closed and biocompatible "minimal extracorporeal circulation/perfusion systems", to minimize blood trauma, the degree of systemic anticoagulation needed and attenuate inflammatory response should be considered whenever possible [1].

18.2 Antifibrinolytic Therapy

As aprotinin has been suspended from the market by the Canadian Health and the European Medicines Agency, the lysine analogues tranexamic acid (TXA) and epsilon-aminocaproic acid remain the drugs of choice. Although TXA has been associated with an increase in convulsive seizures, it is the most commonly used antifibrinolytic agent in Europe and the USA. The dosing of TXA varies considerably [2]. Viewing its potential side effects, a *modified low-dose protocol of TXA*, with a 1 g bolus for the patient, 0.5 g in the CPB prime, and 1 g over 8 h as continuous infusion, may be suggested.

18.3 Heparin/Protamine Management

Heparin and protamine management during VAD implantation follows the institutional standards with respect to the dosing and target activated clotting times (ACTs). If the patient is on ECMO, the operation might be performed without switching to an open CPB system, and therefore a lower ACT might be considered.

18.3.1 Heparin Resistance

Heparin resistance (HR) is defined as a condition where excessive dosages (>600 IU/kg) of heparin are needed to achieve the target ACT value of >400 seconds to safely initiate CPB [3]. In most cases of HR, a critical decrease of the antithrombin concentration following prolonged therapy with heparin is the underlying cause. Administration of antithrombin concentrates (1000–2000 IU), to achieve a target concentration of >70%, usually is the most effective treatment strategy. Other causes of HR are massive thrombocytosis or hyperfibrinogenemia. Unfortunately, there is limited literature describing successful management of these conditions: according to our experience, in line with concepts used for management of heparin-induced thrombocytopenia during CPB (see below), an anticoagulation concept of "platelet anesthesia," achieved by the additional (to heparin) administration of short-acting platelet antagonists such as iloprost, might be an effective strategy (see ◘ Table 18.1).

◘ **Table 18.1** Dosing of heparin and target ACT values[a] for different systems and procedures

Procedure/system	Heparin [IU/Kg][a]	Target ACT [s][b]
Open CPB circuit	400	400–480
MECC system (complete heparin coating)	150–300	300–400
ECLS (complete biocompatible coating)	50–100	160–180[c]
ECLS (noncoated)	100–150	180–220[c]
"Off-pump"	100–150	180–300

CPB cardiopulmonary bypass, *MECC* minimal extracorporeal circulation system, *ECLS* extracorporeal life support system, *ACT* activated clotting time
[a]Response will vary rather individually
[b]Please follow suggestions of manufacturer
[c]Periods of stasis in the ventricles or VAD system should be as short as possible

18.4 Heparin-Induced Thrombocytopenia

18.4.1 Pathophysiology, Diagnosis, and Incidence

Heparin-induced thrombocytopenia (HIT) is an immune-mediated disease where antibodies against a neo-antigen of heparin bound to a plasma protein (mostly platelet factor 4 (PF4)) are generated. The antigen/antibody complexes bind to the Fc receptor of platelets thus causing platelet activation, with further release of PF4, and massive thrombin generation. The clinical correlate of this self-amplifying cascade is a rapid decrease of the platelet count, which in some patients is associated with massive thromboembolic events: thrombotic HIT (T) [4].

Typically, HIT antibodies generate after a prolonged therapy with heparins (5–14 days) and disappear 40–100 days after stop of heparin therapy. In case of re-exposure to heparin (even a single bolus), it usually takes 5–7 days until new HIT antibodies are generated.

Clinical scoring systems, such as the *"4 T Score,"* are helpful to assess the probability of HIT [4, 5]. However, the diagnosis is finally confirmed using a specific ELISA test which detects the HIT/PF4 IgG antibodies or by a platelet activation test in which patient serum and defined amounts of heparin lead to the aggregation of washed donor platelets [5].

If HIT is diagnosed or even suspected, heparin must be stopped and therapeutic anticoagulation started with an alternative anticoagulant [5]. Argatroban, a direct thrombin inhibitor, is approved for therapy and prophylaxis of HIT in the USA and most countries in Europe.

The incidence of HIT varies largely among different patient populations. While in standard cardiac surgical patients the incidence of HIT is 0.5–1%, in MCS patients a rate of approximately 10% has been described [6, 7]. If HIT occurs in this special patient population, the rate of thromboembolic complications is high and patient outcome worse, if alternative anticoagulation strategies are not initiated immediately [6, 7].

Management of a patient with HIT during cardiac surgery, particularly when CPB must be used, is difficult as no alternative anticoagulation strategies are approved. However, the actual 9th ACCP Guidelines provide useful information for management of this complex condition [5].

18.4.2 The 9th ACCP Guidelines and Choice of the Anticoagulation Procedure

The highest premise in the management of a patient diagnosed with HIT(T) is that the underlying risks of the alternative anticoagulation procedure should not exceed the HIT-associated risks, which, however, is hard to be defined prospectively. The risk of the alternative anticoagulation approach should be clearly defined in the light of the status of the patient, the issues of the planned surgery, and the experience of the team involved with the use of such strategies. In select cases, it should be discussed if modification of the surgical strategy may help to reduce the intraoperative risk. For example, the implantation of a LVAD on ECLS and interventional implantation of a closure device may be preferred to implantation of the LVAD and surgical closure of a persistent foramen ovale with use of CPB. Only after such a process of "risk stratification" the optimal case-sensitive decision can be made.

18.4.3 Patients Without Acute HIT Antibodies

The HIT antibodies are transient, and after re-exposure to heparin, it takes days until new antibodies are generated. Therefore, when a negative HIT antibody status is proven by laboratory assays, surgery can be safely performed using heparin anticoagulation. However, special care must be taken that any further exposure to heparin in the pre- and postoperative period is strictly avoided [5].

18.4.4 Delay of Surgery

In line with this recommendation, surgery in patients with a positive HIT antibody status should be postponed whenever possible until antibodies have been proven to have disappeared [5]. Although this strategy might not be applicable for most of the urgent candidates for VAD implantation, it might be useful in selected patients which can be recompensated by further medical therapy.

18.4.5 Patients with Acute HIT Antibodies Needing Urgent Surgery

In patients with acute HIT who need urgent surgery, bivalirudin anticoagulation should be preferred to other alternative agents or strategies using heparin and a short-acting antiplatelet agent [5].

18.4.6 Bivalirudin Anticoagulation

Bivalirudin, a short-acting (elimination half-life approximately 25 min) direct thrombin inhibitor, is the only agent which has been prospectively studied in cardiac surgical patients with and without HIT. Bivalirudin binds bivalent to thrombin and thereby inhibits its anticoagulant action. However, the bonded bivalirudin molecule is cleaved by thrombin itself, so that the thrombin molecule achieves its anticoagulant action again. While approximately 80% of the elimination of bivalirudin is performed via this enzymatic mechanism, only 20% are eliminated via the renal pathway. An antidote is not available. The administration of bivalirudin usually follows a strict protocol with an initial bolus and a defined constant infusion to maintain drug concentrations [5] (◘ Table 18.2). As hemofiltration impacts bivalirudin concentrations, this procedure is not recommended during the course of CPB, particularly as the ACT is not a specific assay for monitoring bivalirudin concentrations.

The fact that bivalirudin has a short elimination half-life and an elimination mechanism largely independent of the function of special organ systems makes it an optimal agent for short and effective anticoagulation. However, what at the first sight appears promising, particularly when a VAD implantation is performed, turns out to increase the complexity of the procedure. In spaces where there is no flow and blood stagnation and therapeutic bivalirudin concentrations cannot be maintained by continuous systemic infusion, "clot formation" will occur. Under the special condition of VAD implantation using CPB, this will occur in the pericardial and pleural space, the CPB reservoir, and flushed grafts, cannulas, or the chamber of flushed devices. Therefore, cardiotomy suction should be replaced by cell salvage and flow in reservoirs maintained by using shunting lines and continuous stirring of the volume. When a VAD system is implanted, modification of the surgical strategy may be necessary to reduce the risk of "clot formation." Grafts and cannulas of a VAD system should remain clamped or periodically flushed until all anastomoses are performed. Only after having completed this the chamber of the device can be deaired, and the action of the VAD should be started immediately. Successful use of bivalirudin anticoagulation for total artificial heart and LVAD implantation on CPB and LVAD implantation on an ECLS, using a lower-dose bivalirudin protocol, has been described [8–10].

18.4.7 Argatroban

A case series using argatroban anticoagulation during ECLS support has been published recently [11]. After having experienced massive

◘ **Table 18.2** Dosing and precautions when using bivalirudin or iloprost and heparin during extracorporeal circulation

	Bolus patient	Bolus CPB	Infusion	Precautions
Bivalirudin: CPB	1 mg/Kg	50 mg	2.5 mg/Kg/h	Avoid cardiotomy suction Avoid hemofiltration Avoid stasis in reservoirs, cannulas, and device chamber
Bivalirudin: ECLS	0.5 mg/Kg		0.5 mg/Kg/h	Dose reduced by 50% when preoperative argatroban anticoagulation and baseline ACT>160 sec
Iloprost + Heparin: CPB/ECLS			≥10 ng/Kg/min	Required dose may be higher in patients with HITT or high HIT antibody titers Slowly increase infusion rate to target Counterbalance vasodilatory effect by administration of vasoconstrictors Early postoperative start of DTI

CPB cardiopulmonary bypass, system, *ECLS* extracorporeal life support, *ACT* activated clotting time, *HIT(T)* heparin-induced thrombocytopenia (with thrombosis), *DTI* direct thrombin inhibitor intraventricular thrombus formation in one patient, changing the implantation strategy, and increasing argatroban dosing (target activated partial thromboplastin time 70–80 s), four of six patients needed re-exploration due to bleeding complications. Therefore, argatroban may not be recommended in this indication.

18.4.8 Heparin and Antiplatelet Agents

Anticoagulation with bivalirudin increases the complexity of the procedure and particularly in patients with multiorgan failure; the administration of an anticoagulant which cannot be reversed by an antidote may cause excessive bleeding.

The combination of the established "safe" anticoagulation with unfractionated heparins (UFHs), ACT monitoring, and protamine reversal, with a short-acting antiplatelet agent to inhibit the HIT reaction, is another option [12]. Iloprost is a short-acting (elimination half-life of 30–40 min) prostaglandin which is eliminated via hepatic biotransformation. Lower dosages of 0.5–2 ng/kg/min of iloprost are clinically used to reduce pulmonary artery vascular resistance, while higher concentrations effectively inhibit platelet aggregation. Palatianos et al. assayed individual concentrations of iloprost, which were able to inhibit HIT-induced platelet aggregation in vitro preoperatively and thereafter administered intraoperatively [12]. The individual dosages to inhibit HIT-induced platelet aggregation varied largely between 6 and 24 ng/kg/min, largely dependent on the magnitude of the HIT antibody status [12]. However, in most of the patients, a dose between 10 and 12 ng/kg/min was effective [12]. The strong systemic vasodilatory effect of iloprost may induce or further increase vasoplegia and thus require the administration of high dosages of potent vasoconstrictors. However, limitations of such a concept are evident: platelet aggregation tests for HIT are technically demanding, time consuming, and not available in every institution. It remains unclear if iloprost completely inhibits or only attenuates the in vivo HIT reaction. Currently, there are no data with regard to the elimination half-life of the HIT antigen/antibody complexes. Therefore, it is not known, what happens after termination of CPB when platelet function recovers, platelet concentrates are transfused or when rebound of cell bonded heparin might occur.

Authors' Suggestion

In patients with HITT or a high antibody status, UFH should be avoided whenever possible. The implantation of an LVAD on ECLS using bivalirudin anticoagulation is the strategy of choice. The HVAD® system (HeartWare Inc., Miami Lakes, Florida USA) appears to be preferable for this approach, as the quick ventriculotomy with the "punch" reduces the risk of excessive blood loss and entry of air when inserting the device into the left ventricular apex. However, when use of CPB is necessary, bivalirudin may also be the preferred option under these conditions. In case of increased bleeding, the chest may be closed secondarily.

The use of iloprost and UFH may be restricted to patients with nonthrombotic HIT, patients with a low HIT antibody titer, and patients who are in multiorgan failure and have to undergo complex surgical procedures. In such cases, the risk of excessive perioperative hemorrhage following bivalirudin anticoagulation may outweigh the risk of a perioperative HIT(T) reaction when using iloprost and heparin.

In order to reduce the risk of HIT, a "heparin-free" approach is suggested in the preoperative period: this turns into a systematic administration of an alternative anticoagulant to all patients who are deemed potential candidates for LVAD implantation. Apart from its potential beneficial role on outcomes, this approach obviates for any preoperative diagnostic procedure in case thrombocytopenia ensues and allows for safe use of heparin/protamine anticoagulation during CPB [13, 14]. In the authors' perspective, the administration of a direct thrombin inhibitor after the implant until INR is in the target range takes HIT out of the field for potential urgent-emergent surgeries with CPB (heart transplantation, pump exchange removal) [15].

18.5 Intraoperative Coagulation Management

18.5.1 Impact of Preoperative Anticoagulation

Preoperative anticoagulation strategies vary significantly among different institutions. Additionally, national and international guidelines referring to "bridging strategies" of current anticoagulants and antiplatelet agents are discrepant. Viewing the increased risk of severe bleeding in patients undergoing VAD implantation, we deem it to be of upmost importance that plasma concentrations of nonreversible agents are in subtherapeutic concentrations. Particularly in patients with chronic heart failure and impairment of multiple organ systems, pharmacokinetics of drugs might be altered significantly due to an impaired metabolism/elimination or redistribution phenomena. Therefore, special emphasis should be taken that not only "standard" intervals for discontinuation of these agents are obeyed but specific laboratory assays performed, to confirm that drug levels are markedly below therapeutic concentrations before surgery is started.

▣ Table 18.3 summarizes information about the most relevant anticoagulants and antiplatelet agents.

18.5.2 Restoration of the Plasmatic Procoagulants

There is an ongoing intensive debate if the transfusion of coagulation factor concentrates is superior to the transfusion of fresh frozen plasma (FFP). However, as most of the patients undergoing VAD implantation are under actual vitamin K antagonist therapy or present an elevated INR due to impairment of hepatic function, large amounts of FFP must be quickly transfused to adequately replace the coagulation factors. The concentration of coagulation factors in 1 ml of FFP is approximately 0.8 units. Therefore, in an attempt to replace approximately 2000 units of coagulation factors, approximately 2.5 l of FFP must be administered. As particularly in patients undergoing LVAD implantation the "volume tolerance" of the patients is restricted by RV function, there are obvious limits in this regard. Therefore, in this special patient population, the transfusion of prothrombin complex concentrates (PCCs) and fibrinogen concentrates (FGC) appears to be attractive. However, once coagulation factors are restored by the quick transfusion of concentrates, the transfusion of FFP may be helpful in maintaining the status.

> In patients with HIT who undergo VAD implantation with bivalirudin anticoagulation, care must be taken when PCCs are transfused. Most PCCs contain heparin. Therefore, only heparin-free PCC should be transfused, for example, "Cofact®" (Biotest AG, Dreieich, Germany). Additionally, we recommend waiting for approx. 60 min after stop of the continuous bivalirudin infusion before the PCC is given. Otherwise, the high bivalirudin concentrations will rapidly "cleave" the generated thrombin and bleeding persists.

18.5.3 Transfusion of Platelet Concentrates

In contrast to the restoration of procoagulants, the indications for the transfusion of platelet concentrates (PC) are more homogeneous. In patients with preoperative antiplatelet therapy, in vitro inhibition of platelet aggregation, and clinical signs of microvascular bleeding, PCs are transfused. In patients without preoperative antiplatelet therapy and clinical signs of microvascular bleeding, PCs are usually transfused when the platelet count is below 100.000 × 109/L.

Table 18.3 Current anticoagulants/antiplatelet agents

Agent	Action	Approx. elimination ½ life/duration of effect	Monitoring	Reversal agent/ procedure	Preoperative discontinuation
Warfarin	Vitamin K antagonist	48 h	INR	PCC	5 days
Apixaban	Anti-Xa	10–14 h	Modified thrombin time	Hemofiltration/ dialysis, Idarucizumab as antidote under FDA approval	2–4 days
Rivaroxaban	Anti-Xa	10–12 h	Calibrated anti-Xa activity	No	2–4 days
Enoxaparin	Anti-Xa	4–8 h	Calibrated anti-Xa activity	Protamine (only partially)	24 h
Unfractionated heparin	Antithrombin	4 h	aPTT, ACT	Protamine	No discontinuation
Bivalirudin	DTI	25 min	aPTT, calibrated ECT	Hemofiltration	2–6 h
Argatroban	DTI	40 min	aPTT, calibrated ECT	No	4–12 h
Aspirin	Irreversible inhibition of platelet Thromboxane A2 synthesis	8–10 days	Arachidonic acid-induced platelet aggregation	PRP-PC	No discontinuation
Clopidogrel/ prasugrel	Irreversible inhibition of platelet ADP – P2Y12 receptor	8–10 days	ADP-induced platelet aggregation	PRP-PC	5–7 days
Ticagrelor	Irreversible inhibition of platelet ADP – P2Y12 receptor	1–3 days	ADP-induced platelet aggregation	PRP-PC	3 days

PCC prothrombin complex concentrate, *DTI* direct thrombin inhibitor, *PRP-PC* platelet-rich plasma platelet concentrate, *ECT* ecarin clotting time

Authors' Suggestion

In patients with preoperative antiplatelet therapy, therapy should be stopped 5 days before surgery if the timeline of LVAD implantation allows; alternatives to these molecules, such as short-acting GpIIb–IIIa antagonists, can be used as bridging therapy, if they are part of an institutional practice. Moreover, preoperatively "platelet aggregation testing" can be performed to assess if the patient responded to the antiplatelet therapy. In patients who are responders and present clinical signs of microvascular bleeding, PCs are transfused regardless of the platelet count. Approximately 20 minutes before weaning from CPB or administration of protamine, thromboelastometry using the EXTEM and FIBTEM test of the ROTEM® device (Tem International GmbH, Munich, Germany) is performed (■ Fig. 18.1). These assays are not susceptible to approximately <4 IU/Heparin/ml, so that the sample can be obtained even during CPB and the results be evaluated after approximately 20 min. Although the coagulation time (CT) in the EXTEM test does not correlate with the INR or prothrombin time, to our experience, a prolongation of the CT (normal value 35–80 s) appears to signal massive deficiency of plasmatic coagulation factors. Therefore, in patients with an EXTEM CT of <80 s, approximately 4 units of FFP are transfused. In patients with a CT of 80–120 s, approximately 20 U/kg PCCs are given, and in patients with an EXTEM CT of >120 s, approximately 50 U/kg of PCCs are transfused. The maximal clot firmness (MCF) of the EXTEM test provides a good correlation to the platelet count. However, the effect of antiplatelet therapy cannot be assessed by this method. Therefore, an impaired MCF in this assay is helpful to guide PC transfusions only in patients without preoperative antiplatelet therapy. In case the EXTEM shows an increased fibrinolysis, an additional bolus of 1 g of TXA is given, and the infusion continued until 12 h postoperatively. A maximal clot firmness of <8 mm in the FIBTEM test (normal value 9–22 mm) helps to guide the transfusion of 2–4 g FGC in case of persistent bleeding. Once PCs and PCC/FGC are transfused, FFP is given to maintain the status. If diffuse bleeding persists despite these efforts, 0.3 µg/kg of desmopressin is given as a bolus infusion over approximately 30 min, to augment the release of von Willebrand factor from the endothelial stores. If diffuse bleeding further persists, it is discussed with the surgeon to packing the thorax and to leave the chest temporarily open. Due to the potential thromboembolic risks, the administration of recombinant factor VIIa is restricted to patients with excessive microvascular bleeding which prevents the surgeon even to transfer the patient with an open chest to the ICU.

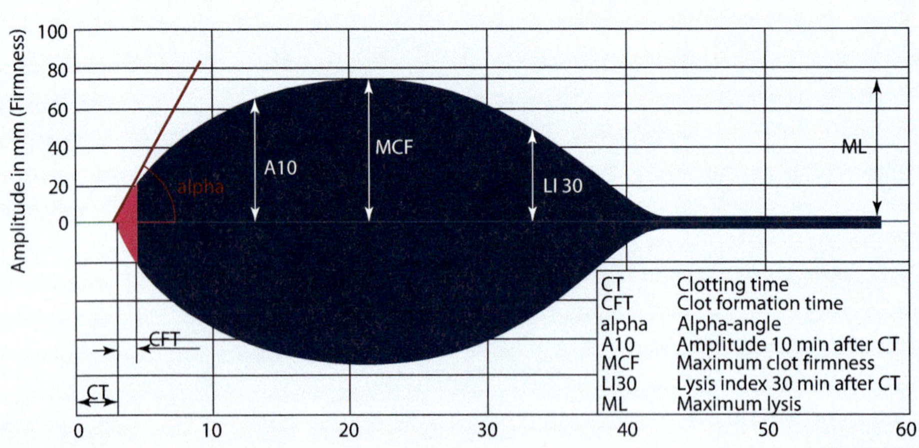

■ **Fig. 18.1** Parameters of ROTEM® Thromboelastometry

Disclosure None.

References

1. Haneya A, Philipp A, Puehler T, Ried M, Hilker M, Zink W et al (2012) Ventricular assist device implantation in patients on percutaneous extracorporeal life support without switching to conventional cardiopulmonary bypass system. Eur J Cardiothorac Surg 41:1366–1370
2. Koster A, Faraoni D, Levy JH (2015) Antifibrinolytic therapy for cardiac surgery: an update. Anesthesiology 123:214–221
3. Finley A, Greenberg C (2013) Review article. Heparin sensitivity and resistance: management during cardiopulmonary bypass. Anesth Analg 116:1210–1222
4. Greinacher A (2015) Heparin-induced thrombocy topenia. N Engl J Med 373:252–261
5. Linkins LA, Dans AL, Moores LK, Bona R, Davidson BL, Schulmann S, Crowther M (2012) Treatment and prevention of Heparin-induced thrombocytopenia: antithrombotic therapy and prevention of thrombosis, 9th ed: American College of Chest Physicians Evidence-Based Clinical Practice Guidelines. Chest 141:e495S–e530S
6. Schenk S, El-Banayosy A, Prohaska W, Arusoglu L, Morshuis M, Koester-Eiserfunke W et al (2006) Heparin-induced thrombocytopenia in patients receiving mechanical circulatory support. J Thorac Cardiovasc Surg 131:1373–1381
7. Koster A, Huebler S, Potapov E, Meyer O, Jurmann M, Weng Y et al (2007) Impact of heparin-induced thrombocytopenia on outcome in patients with ventricular assist device support: single-institution experience in 258 consecutive patients. Ann Thorac Surg 83:72–76
8. Morshuis M, Boergermann J, Gummert J, Koster A (2013) A modified technique for implantation of the HeartWare™ left ventricular assist device when using bivalirudin anticoagulation in patients with acute heparin-induced thrombocytopenia. Interact Cardiovasc Thorac Surg 17:225–226
9. Federmann M, Dragomer D, Grant S, Reemtsen B, Biniwale R (2014) Use of bivalirudin for anticoagulation during implantation of total artificial heart. J Extra Corpor Technol 46:170–172
10. Awad H, Bryant R, Malik O, Dimitrova G, Sai-Sudhakar C (2013) Thrombosis during off pump LVAD placement in a patient with heparin induced thrombocytopenia using bivalirudin. J Cardiothorac Surg 8:115
11. Hillebrand J, Sindermann J, Schmidt C, Mesters R, Martens S, Scherer M Implantation of left ventricular assist device under extracorporeal life support in patients with heparin-induced thrombocytopenia. J Artif Organs. doi:10.1007/s10047-015-0846-9
12. Palatianos G, Michalis A, Alivizatos P, Lacoumenda S, Geroulanos S, Karabinis A et al (2015) Perioperative use of iloprost in cardiac surgery patients diagnosed with heparin-induced thrombocytopenia-reactive antibodies or with true HIT (HIT-reactive antibodies plus thrombocytopenia): an 11-year experience. Am J Hematol 90:608–617
13. Pappalardo F, Agracheva N, Covello RD, Pieri M, De Bonis M, Calabrò MG, Koster A, Zangrillo A (2014) Anticoagulation for critically ill cardiac surgery patients: is primary bivalirudin the next step? J Cardiothorac Vasc Anesth. 28(4):1025–1029
14. Pappalardo F, Scandroglio AM, Potapov E, Stepanenko A, Maj G, Krabatsch T, Zangrillo A, Koster A, Hetzer R (2012) Argatroban anticoagulation for heparin induced thrombocytopenia in patients with ventricular assist devices. Minerva Anestesiol. 78(3): 330–335
15. Pieri M, Agracheva N, Di Prima AL, Nisi T, De Bonis M, Isella F, Zangrillo A, Pappalardo F (2014) Primary anticoagulation with bivalirudin for patients with implantable ventricular assist devices. Artif Organs 38(4):342–346

Intraoperative Right Ventricular Failure Management

Matteo Attisani, Paolo Centofanti, and Mauro Rinaldi

© Springer International Publishing Switzerland 2017

A. Montalto et al. (eds.), *Mechanical Circulatory Support in End-Stage Heart Failure*,
DOI 10.1007/978-3-319-43383-7_19

19.1 Introduction

Left ventricular assist devices are currently implanted using three different techniques [1]:

- Median sternotomy with cardiopulmonary bypass (CPB).
- Left posterolateral thoracotomy with the outflow graft connected to the descending aorta with or without CPB. This approach is more frequently used in case of reoperations to avoid re-sternotomy.
- Minimally invasive left mini-thoracotomy (with or without CPB).

According to the estimated risk of right ventricular failure (RVF) post-LVAD, a different surgical strategy of implantation can be preferred although in elective patients (INTERMACS level 3 or more).

LVAD implantation through median sternotomy is the most used and in this setting CPB is always necessary. CPB is associated with activation of inflammatory mediators, increased pulmonary vascular resistance, platelet activation, coagulopathy, and impaired renal function, increasing also the risk of bleeding and vasoplegia (clinical status defined as *post-perfusion syndrome*) [2].

Endotoxin and pro-inflammatory cytokines can also negatively affect RV function on several levels [3–5].

Minimally invasive approaches allow to avoid the use of CPB in selected patients minimizing surgical trauma, risk of bleeding, and transfusions.

In case of a preplanned right ventricular assist device implantation or concomitant valves, surgery CPB and central approach with sternotomy is mandatory [5].

19.2 Intraoperative Management of Cardiopulmonary Bypass (CPB)

Patency of foramen ovale (PFO) should be verified with transesophageal echocardiogram before the institution of CPB. Any intracardiac shunt should be closed before LVAD implantation [6].

Cardiopulmonary bypass is routinely established between right atrium and ascending aorta. In case of concomitant surgery on the tricuspid valve, mitral valve, or interatrial septum, bicaval cannulation is mandatory.

When LVAD is implanted as bridge to transplant, the ascending aorta should be cannulated more proximally, and the outflow-graft anastomosis should be performed just behind the sinotubular junction. This configuration leaves more native aorta available for the anastomosis at the time of transplantation.

Left ventricular venting through the right superior pulmonary vein is highly encouraged. An accurate unloading of the left ventricle during the inflow cannula position is mandatory to perform visual inspection inside the left ventricle to remove thrombi and potential obstructing trabeculae [7].

A careful volume management in order to reduce hypervolemia and hemodilution during CPB time is recommended, maintaining urinary output over 1 ml/kg/h also during the implantation.

The optimization of preload contractility and afterload perioperatively is the target for right ventricular failure (RVF) prevention, especially in patients with preoperative RV dysfunction [5, 8].

19.2.1 Mini Extracorporeal Circulation (MECC) LVAD Implantation

The use of minimal extracorporeal circulation circuit (MECC) in the setting of LVAD implantation can provide optimal perfusion throughout while attenuating the adverse effects of conventional CPB.

MECC system is connected directly to the atrial line avoiding the interposition of an open reservoir and the use of a cardiotomy suction. The system comprises a closed heparin-coated circuit requiring less heparin (maintain ACT from 250 to 350 s). The closed reservoir eliminates the interaction between air and blood, reducing the activation of humoral cascades. The lower dose of protamine required at the end of the procedure reduces the amount of complement activation by the classical pathway [1, 9].

MECC minimizes hemodilution and requires a lower priming volume (<500 ml). Sometimes hemodilution can be completely avoided using retrograde autologous perfusion (RAP) technique. In this case priming fluid is completely removed by filling the circuit in a retrograde fashion with autologous blood [9].

19.2.2 Off-Pump LVAD Implantation

LVAD implantation is safe and feasible also without CPB. In this case any type of extracorporeal circulation is not used, avoiding the danger of hemodilution, of systemic inflammatory response syndrome, and of coagulopathy. In condition of severe hemodynamic decompensation in critically ill patients, this approach can be dangerous, since no safety net is provided. Therefore the utility of off-pump implantation in INTERMACS levels 1 and 2 patients is highly debated.

Through a left mini-thoracotomy, the apex of the heart is exposed without any need for cardiac displacement as compared to midline access. In case of reoperation, this approach can be particularly favored to avoid tedious dissection. If there are dense pericardial adhesions, the pump can be also implanted transpericardially. Heparin is administered (10,000 U). No activate clotting time control is needed. Two guidewires in the femoral vein and artery are inserted percutaneously in case of emergency CPB institution is needed. In alternative surgical exposure of the femoral vessels is possible.

After performing the end-to-side anastomosis of the outflow conduit to the mid-descending aorta, the epicardial apical cuff is sutured to the apex. Pacing wires are implanted in the left ventricle, and rapid ventricular pacing is instituted at 180 beats/min before opening the left ventricular apex using the coring knife. Once the apical opening is created, bleeding is controlled by finger pressure. During a second rapid ventricular pacing, the pump is rapidly inserted.

New pump technologies and miniaturization of the devices are well suited for minimally invasive approach without the use of CPB.

The presence of a perfusion team, a cell-saving suction, and a backup CPB circuit is mandatory because severe heart failure patients may become unstable in anytime or may not recover after rapid ventricular pacing.

19.2.3 Venoarterial Extracorporeal Circulation (VA ECMO)-Assisted Implantation

Venoarterial extracorporeal membrane oxygenator (VA ECMO) prior to LVAD implantation has recently been reported to significantly worsen survival rates. ECMO is also associated with systemic inflammatory response syndrome [10].

The implantation could be performed on VA ECMO without converting the circuit to a standard CPB and avoiding complications related to an additional anticoagulation and to an increased hemodilution.

No additional heparin is required during implantation.

In these cases ECMO prolongation is suggested by some authors [10] to support RV function after LVAD implantation, allowing a progressive loading of the RV without prolonging surgery.

After LVAD implantation, VA ECMO flow is gradually reduced to the level of 2.5–3.0 l/min. Pump speed and flow are adjusted to obtain an adequate unloading of the LV avoiding the leftward shift of the septum as assessed by echo [10].

It is very important to check the adequacy of the outflows (LVAD+ VA ECMO) by a continuous determination of appropriate perfusion parameters such as lactates, creatinine, and diuresis. In this setting, the intraoperative insertion of a transseptal left atrial pressure (LAP) line can help to assist the weaning from VA ECMO in the intensive care unit during the following days. Sometimes VA ECMO can be converted to a temporary RV support by removing the oxygenator.

19.2.4 On-Pump Versus Off-Pump Implantation: Impact on Right Ventricular Function

Minimally invasive off-pump LVAD implantation avoids the deleterious effects of CPB and limits the surgical trauma reducing the risk of post-implant RV failure. In patients with INTERMACS level 3 or more with a lower risk of hemodynamic instability during the implantation and in the presence of preoperative risk factors for RV failure, minimally invasive off-pump implantation is encouraged.

This approach is not clearly recommended when the patient is unstable (INTERMACS level 1 and 2) or on ECMO support. In these recipients preoperative RV function and pathophysiology of the pulmonary circulation are not adequately known.

Table 19.1 Major advantages and disadvantages of LVADs implantation with CPB, MECC, venoarterial ECMO, Off-pump

LVAD implantation advantages/disadvantages	Total CPB	MECC	Off-pump	VA ECMO
Hemodilution – priming	+++	+	–	++
Heparin and anticoagulation level	+++	++	+	++
Inflammatory response syndrome	+++	+	–	++
Reactive vasoplegia	++	+	–	++
Increased PVR	++	+	–	+
Platelets activation	++	+	–	++
Impaired renal function	++	+	–	++
Feasibility of concomitant open-heart procedures	Yes	Yes	No	No
Feasibility in middle sternotomy	Yes	Yes	No	Yes
Risk of intraprocedural hemodynamic instabilization	No	No	Yes	No
Risk of postoperative bleeding	++	+	–	+++
Risk of blood transfusion	++	+	–	+++
Accurate visual inspection of LV cavity	+++	+	–	+

CPB cardiopulmonary bypass, *MECC* mini extracorporeal circulation, *VA ECMO* venoarterial extracorporeal circulation

Table 19.1 summarizes the main biological effects and major advantages and disadvantages of the LVAD implantation with CPB, MECC, venoarterial ECMO, or off-pump.

19.2.5 De-airing Procedure

De-airing of the LVAD and the native ventricle is crucial before weaning from the CPB. It prevents air embolism, reducing the risk of RV transitory dysfunction. The most common locations for air embolism are the right coronary artery and the innominate artery. This may produce RV dysfunction or contribute to postoperative neurocognitive impairment [11, 12].

Initially, the components of the LVAD are flushed with saline and prepared for implantation at the temperature of 37°. The left ventricular vent has to be clamped and removed just after the inflow cannula insertion and before starting the LVAD pump. This cannula is removed underwater to avoid potential entry of air.

After positioning the inflow cannula, the clamp occluding the outflow graft is rapidly removed in order to avoid the increase of the LV filling pressure and air embolization across the opening aortic valve. Additional de-airing is accomplished by passively filling the heart and pump and elevating the apex and gently shaking the ventricle while lungs are ventilated.

In case of left mini-thoracotomy LVAD implantation, CO_2 flooding of the operative field is mandatory, since with this approach the elevation and shaking of left ventricular apex is almost impossible.

After outflow-graft anastomosis, additional needles can be placed into the graft between the cross clamp and the aorta. The patient is then placed in the Trendelenburg position and ventilation is resumed.

The ascending aortic vent should remain open until all visible air is removed. A sufficient quantity of air entering the right coronary artery causes RV ischemia and manifest as RV dysfunction. The treatment consists of further de-airing, an adequate coronary perfusion pressure, assisting the heart on CPB until RV contractility recovers.

19.3 Weaning from CPB

Low-dose inotrope infusion should be started to support the RV function at least 10 min before the weaning from CPB.

Norepinephrine may therefore be beneficial in patients with hypotension and tachycardia who do not tolerate dobutamine, but it must be carefully used in case of pulmonary hypertension and acute RVF without significant hypotension or vasoplegia.

Adrenaline and IABP should be considered only in case of severe RV failure.

Inhalatory nitric oxide (iNO) has not been clearly showed to be effective despite it is frequently used in many center at this stage. Levosimendan also plays a debated role in this crucial phase.

Ventilation should be started as soon as possible after de-airing to decrease pulmonary vascular resistances. Higher tidal volume (VT) and positive end-expiratory pressure may increase pulmonary artery pressure and right atrial pressure, worsen tricuspid regurgitation, and increase RV afterload [16].

The lowest VT, plateau pressure, and positive end-expiratory pressure needed to provide adequate ventilation and oxygenation should be used [16, 17].

Hypoxic pulmonary vasoconstriction should be avoided. During CPB alveolar nutritive flow relies solely on bronchial circulation which is less than 10% of total pulmonary flow [18].

Reperfusion and restoration of pulmonary flow at the end of CPB contributes to ischemia-reperfusion injury. CPB is also associated with interstitial edema, disruption of gas-capillary exchange, decreased compliance, and increased pulmonary vascular resistance. These effects could impact on the RV function during the weaning from CPB [18, 19].

Recent reports suggest to maintain continuous pulmonary ventilation and perfusion through the main pulmonary artery during CPB thus reducing ischemia-reperfusion injury and minimizing the risk of post-implant RV failure [19].

19.3.1 Pump Speed

Cardiopulmonary bypass (CPB) flow should be gradually reduced to allow filling of the left ventricle. Prior to start LVAD pump the LV should be full. After reducing CPB flow to 2 l per minute, the cross clamp is removed, and the pump started at the minimum speed (HVAD at 1800 rpm; HM II at 6000 rpm; Jarvik 2000 at 8000 rpm; Incor I at 5000 rpm).

RV function is greatly affected by pump speed. It is important to avoid setting the pump speed so high that it causes an abnormal RV geometry, which can adversely affect RV function. Pump speed has to be increased slowly to avoid suction events. Suction events can lead to the ingestion of tissue/clot from inside the LV and may also lead to episodes of ectopy and arrhythmias such as atrial fibrillation or ventricular fibrillation.

Pump speed should be maintained as low as possible at the same flow rate delivered. The pump flow is not exactly the cardiac output which is influenced by the combination of the device flow and the stroke volume of the heart.

When adjusting pump speed, the aortic valve should open every second or third beat. This low pump speed policy reduces the risk of aortic valve thrombosis, and it assures that the LV is reasonably loaded. In some cases even at low pump speed, the aortic valve will not open due to poor LV function.

19.3.2 Ventricular Interdependence: Changes in LVAD Setting

LVAD decompresses the LV and reduces LV end-diastolic pressure and pulmonary artery pressure, and it may improve right ventricular (RV) function. However the increased LVAD output increases venous return to the RV and can potentially worsen pre-existing RVF.

An aggressive LV unloading can cause an excessive leftward shift of the septum decreasing septal contribution to RV contraction.

LV unloading frequently reduces tricuspid regurgitation (TR) reducing RV afterload. However increased RV volume and tethering of valve leaflets to a leftward shifted septum can increase TR. Prolonged CPB and cardioplegic arrest are significant risk factors for early postoperative RV failure.

19.3.3 Intraoperative Transesophageal Echocardiographic Findings

Immediately after CPB, the positions of the inflow and outflow conduit, the blood flow velocity and direction are assessed using color and spectral Doppler. LVAD should have a consistent phasic, slightly pulsatile, low-velocity inflow and outflow patterns [20].

LV decompression and septum position should be monitored. A neutral position of the interventricular septum indicates adequate LV filling (◘ Fig. 19.1). If the LV is not adequately decompressed, a rightward septum shift can be seen (◘ Fig. 19.2). A leftward septal shift may indicate excessive decompression due to high pump speed or RV dysfunction (◘ Fig. 19.3). An

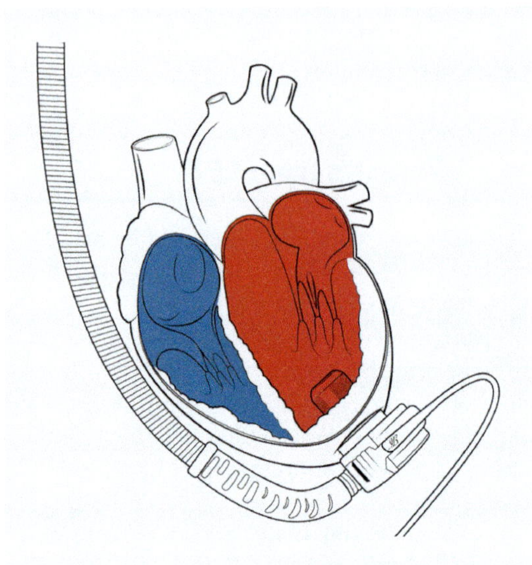

◘ **Fig. 19.2** Rightward shift of interventricular septum indicates non-adequate LV unloading (Illustration by Ilaria Bondi's Peppermint Advertising)

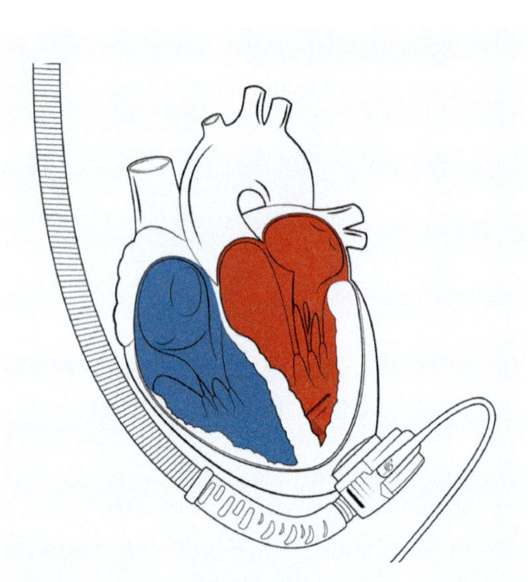

◘ **Fig. 19.1** Neutral position of the interventricular septum indicates adequate LV filling (Illustration by Ilaria Bondi's Peppermint Advertising)

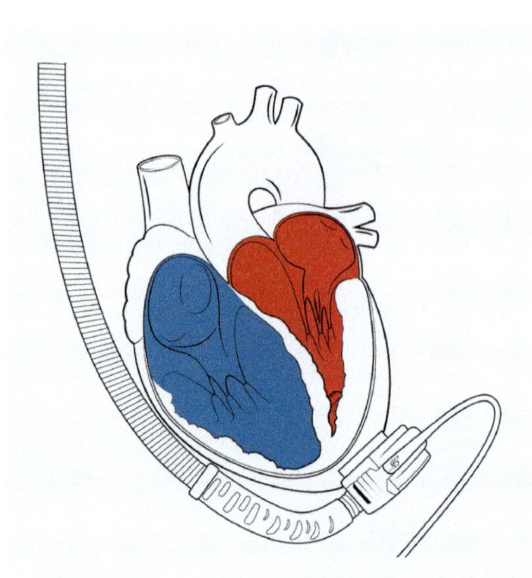

◘ **Fig. 19.3** Leftward shift of interventricular septum is associated to an excessive LV unloading for high pump speed or right ventricular failure (Illustration by Ilaria Bondi's Peppermint Advertising)

increase in RV size, a reduction in RV systolic function, and the presence of significant TR may be demonstrated on TEE [21].

Mitral regurgitation should be less than moderate.

19.3.4 Intraoperative Hemodynamic Monitoring

Hemodynamic monitoring with Swan-Ganz catheter is highly recommended during weaning from CPB in all patients with these preoperative criteria [22, 23]:

- Severe pulmonary hypertension (pulmonary vascular resistance >2 Wood units)
- Preoperative RV dysfunction (CVP >15 mmHg; CVP/Wedge pressure ≤0.66, or echocardiographic evidence of a severe RV dysfunction)
- Preoperative Matthews score >5 points
- Preoperative VA ECMO support

RVF after LVAD implantation is diagnosed if any of the following [24]:

- Inability to wean from CPB
- Or any two of the following (sustained for 15 min after complete withdrawal from CPB):
  - Left ventricular flow rate index ≤2.0 l/min/m2
  - Administration of ≥20 inotropic equivalents (IE):
    - 10 mcg/kg/min dopamine, dobutamine, enoximone, and amrinone are equivalent to 10 IE.
    - 0.1 mcg/kg/min adrenaline or noradrenaline are equivalent to 10 IE.
    - 1 mcg/kg/min milrinone is equivalent to 15 IE.
    - 0.1 U/min vasopressin is equivalent to 10 IE.
  - Mean arterial pressure (MAP) ≤55 mmHg
  - Central venous pressure (CVP) ≥16 mmHg
  - Mixed venous saturation (SvO2) ≤55%

In case of RVF, insertion of a transseptal catheter for continuous monitoring of the left atrial pressure (LAP) is mandatory. During LAP line placement, extreme caution should be used to avoid sucking air into the LA through the insertion site and to avoid flushing air into the LA directly through the LA catheter.

General principle to successfully wean patients from CPB can be summarized as follows:

- CVP should be maintained below 14 mmHg.
- LAP should be in the range between 8 and 14 mmHg in order to avoid suction and overloading of the LV.
- CVP and LAP need to be balanced and kept at similar values.
- In case CVP exceeds LAP more than 4 mmHg, pump speed needs to be reduced and inotropic support to be increased and the use of iNO to reduce RV afterload can be considered. Diuretics should be administered, and in case of severe renal dysfunction, hemofiltration and dialysis should be considered.
- A certain degree of arterial trace pulsatility should be pursued with an intermittent aortic valve opening with a mean arterial pressure over 60 mmHg. Cardiac index needs to be around 2.2 l/min with a mixed venous saturation of more than 60%.

Echocardiographic, hemodynamic, and biochemical targets for weaning from CPB are summarized in Table 19.2.

19.4 Intraoperative Bleeding

Excessive bleeding and blood transfusion can precipitate RV failure [13].

Preoperative coagulopathy must be corrected in advance since it predisposes to bleeding and increases the need for blood transfusion. Studies on first-generation LVADs have validated the administration of vitamin K preoperatively or aprotinin intra-operatively to reduce bleeding [13, 14].

Table 19.2 Targets for the weaning of CPB

TEE parameters
Neutral septal position
TR less than moderate
MR less than moderate
Opening aortic valve
Hemodynamic parameters
CVP ≤ 14 mmHg
8 mmHg ≤ LAP ≤ 14 mmHg
LAP – CVP ≤ ± 4 mmHg
CI >2.2 l/min/m^2
SVO$_2$ >60%
MAP >60 mmHg
Pulsatile arterial line
Pump speed
Minimum speed at the same flow delivered
Biochemical markers
Normal lactates
Diuresis >1 ml/Kg/h
Ventilatory parameters
PaO$_2$/FiO$_2$ fraction >200
Low positive end expiratory pressure
Normocapnia

TEE transesophageal echocardiogram, *MR* mitral regurgitation, *TR* tricuspid regurgitation, *CVP* central venous pressure, *LAP* left atrial pressure, *CI* cardiac Index, *MAP* mean arterial pressure, *SVO$_2$* oxygen venous saturation

A normal preoperative hepatic function (total bilirubin <2.5 mg/dL; AST and ALT <2 times normal) and an accurate nutritional state (albumin >3 g/dL; pre-albumin >15 mg/dL; transferrin >250 mg/dL) significantly reduce the risk of bleeding [14, 15].

A complete antagonization of heparin with protamine is necessary at the end of CPB. Protamine should be given slowly only when patient is hemodynamically stable. Activate clotting time (ACT) should be lower than 140 s [13].

For the assessment of platelet function, the maximal amplitude (MA) at thromboelastography (TEG) is the most useful parameter to tailor therapy to individual patient. MA in the 50–75 range has been used as an appropriate target range for platelet activity. Avoid plasma and platelets transfusion.

Minimally invasive approaches allow to avoid the use of CPB in selected patients minimizing the surgical trauma and the risk of blood loss.

19.5 Arrhythmias and Right Ventricular Failure

Tachyarrhythmias contribute to RVF (25). Atrial arrhythmia occurs in more than 20% of LVAD recipient.

In this group of patients, the risk of RVF seems to be double compared to standard patients.

As the RV is extremely susceptible to alterations in cardiac rhythm and ventricular synchrony, restoration of sinus rhythm and/or atrioventricular synchrony plays an important role [3, 25].

19.6 The Role of Intact Pericardium

The pericardium is the external support of the RV. It plays an active role during the systolic shortening of the free wall-septum dimension of the ventricle, the so-called bellow action [26].

RV long-axis function is known to be depressed after cardiac surgery. A rapid loss in RV systolic velocity occurs as early as 3 min after pericardial opening. It has been clearly shown that RV long-axis reduction during coronary bypass surgery is not caused by CPB or cross clamp, but rather by pericardial incision [26].

The reason of this long-lasting reduction remains unclear. The pericardium contributes much more to the preservation of peak RV myocardial annular velocities than previous supposed, and it probably plays an important role of mechanical support of the free wall of the right ventricle preventing diastolic dilatation.

Minimally invasive implantation, minimizing the opening of the pericardium at the level of the LV apex, could preserve the RV geometry and function after LVAD implantation.

The miniaturization of the devices and the development of intravascular or transcatheter devices in the future could give the chance to implant LVADs leaving the pericardium fully intact.

In case of sternotomy, a RV protective strategy could be implemented with a very limited opening of pericardium before starting CPB, thus avoiding over-dilatation of the RV before LVAD implantation.

19.7 Conclusions

A careful weaning from CPB and optimization of the preimplantation clinical conditions reduce the risk of RV failure post-LVAD. LAP insertion is highly advised in the management of intraoperative RVF in addition to transesophageal echocardiographic monitoring.

Minimally invasive and off-pump LVAD implantation seems to have a protective effect on the right ventricle, and it is encouraged in selected patients with a significant preoperative risk of post-implant RVF.

A minimally invasive approach should be also considered as option in order to avoid future re-sternotomy in bridge-to-transplant patients.

Efficacy and advantages of this technique in critical patients (INTERMACS level 1 and 2) remain to be determined due to the risk of sudden hemodynamic deterioration. One of the main limitations of this approach is the difficult access to the right heart in case of temporary RVAD need. It is not indicated in case of already planned biventricular support.

References

1. Krabatsch T et al (2014) Different strategies for implantation of continuous-flow VADs- experience from Deutsches Herzzentrum Berlin. Ann Cardiothorac Surg 3(5):472–474
2. Levy JH, Tanaka KA (2003) Inflammatory response to cardiopulmonary bypass. Ann Thorac Surg 75: 715–720
3. Lahm T et al (2010) Medical and surgical treatment of acute right ventricular failure. Am Coll Cardiol 56(18):1435–1446
4. Chen JM et al (2000) Management of perioperative right-sided circulatory failure. Cardiac Assist Devices 83-101
5. Kormos RL et al (2010) Right ventricular failure in patients with the HeartMate II continuous-flow left ventricular assist device: incidence, risk factors, and effect on outcomes. J Thorac Cardiovasc Surg 139: 1316–1324
6. Shapiro GC et al (1995) Diagnosis of patent foramen ovale with transesophageal echocardiography in a patient supported with a left ventricular assist device. J Heart Lung Transplant 14:594–597
7. Benk C et al (2013) Effect of cannula position in the thoracic aorta with continuous left ventricular support: four-dimensional flow-sensitive magnetic resonance imaging in an in vitro model. Eur J Cardiothorac Surg 44(3):551–558
8. Kato TS et al (2012) Usefulness of two-dimensional echocardiographic parameters of the left side of the heart to predict right ventricular failure after left ventricular assist device implantation. Am J Cardiol 109:246–251
9. Anastasiadis K et al (2011) Use of minimal extracorporeal circulation circuit for left ventricular assist device implantation. ASAIO J 57(6):547–549
10. Lebretone G et al (2011) Implantation of left ventricular support under extracorporeal membrane oxygenation. Eur J Cardiothorac Surg 40:e165–e167
11. Leyvi G et al (2005) Transient right ventricular failure and transient weakness: a TEE diagnosis. J Cardiothorac Vasc Anesth 19:406–408
12. Tingleff J et al (1995) Intraoperative echocardiographic study of air embolism during cardiac operations. Ann Thorac Surg 60:673–677
13. Meineri M et al (2012) Right ventricular failure after LVAD implantation: prevention and treatment. Best Pract Res Clin Anaesthesiol 26:217–229
14. Holdy K et al (2005) Nutrition assessment and management of left ventricular assist device patients. J Heart Lung Transplant 24(10):1690–1696
15. Kaplon RJ et al (1999) Vitamin K reduces bleeding in left ventricular assist device recipients. J Heart Lung Transplant 18:346–350
16. Jardin F et al (2003) Right ventricular function and positive pressure ventilation in clinical practice: from hemodynamic subsets to respirator settings. Intensive Care Med 29:1426–1434
17. The Acute Respiratory Distress Syndrome Network (2000) Ventilation with lower tidal volumes as compared with traditional tidal volumes for acute lung injury and the acute respiratory distress syndrome. N Engl J Med 342:1301–1308
18. Apostolakis E et al (2010) Strategies to prevent intraoperative lung injury during cardiopulmonary bypass. J Cardiothorac Surg 5:1–9
19. Francisco I, Macedo B et al (2013) Lung perfusion and ventilation during implantation of left ventricular assist device as a strategy to avoid postoperative pulmonary complications and right ventricular failure. Interact Cardiovasc Thorac Surg 17:764–766
20. Estep JD et al (2010) The role of echocardiography and other imaging modalities in patients with left ventricular assist devices. JACC Cardiovasc Imaging 3:1049–1064
21. Maeder MT et al (2009) Changes in right ventricular function during continuous-flow left ventricular assist device support corrected. J Heart Lung Transplant 28:360–366

22. Haneya A et al (2012) Temporary percutaneous right ventricular support using a centrifugal pump in patients with postoperative acute refractory right ventricular failure after left ventricular assist device implantation. Eur J Cardiothorac Surg 41:219–223
23. Matthews JC et al (2008) The right ventricular failure risk score a pre-operative tool for assessing the risk of right ventricular failure in left ventricular assist device candidates. J Am Coll Cardiol 51(22):2163–2172
24. Potapov E et al (2011) Inhaled nitric oxide after left ventricular assist device implantation: a prospective, randomized, doubleblind, multicenter, placebo-controlled trial. J Heart Lung Transplant 30:870–878
25. Garan AR et al (2015) Early post-operative ventricular arrhythmias in patients with continuous-flow left ventricular assist devices. J Heart Lung Transplant 34(12):1611–1616
26. Sakuma M et al (2002) Right ventricular ejection function assessed by cineangiography – Importance of bellows action. Circ J 66(6):605–609

Tricuspid Valve Regurgitation and Right Ventricular Dysfunction During Left Ventricular Assist Device Implantation

Paul C. Tang, Alina Nicoara, and Carmelo A. Milano

© Springer International Publishing Switzerland 2017
A. Montalto et al. (eds.), *Mechanical Circulatory Support in End-Stage Heart Failure*,
DOI 10.1007/978-3-319-43383-7_20

20.1 Introduction

Significant right ventricular dysfunction occurs in approximately 22% of patients undergoing left ventricular assist device (LVAD) implantation and is a predictor of early and late mortality [1, 2]. Despite previously described predictors of RV failure such as right ventricular stroke work index (RVSWI) and central venous pressure to pulmonary capillary wedge pressure (CVP/PCWP) ratio [1], reliable identification of patients who will require mechanical RV support has been challenging. Early failure of right ventricular (RV) output in the operating room may be evidenced by an elevated central venous pressure (CVP) >16 mmHg, poor RV performance parameters (e.g., tricuspid annular plane systolic excursion (TAPSE) <16 mm), reduced mixed venous oxygen saturation (SVO2 <55%), and cardiac index <2 L/min/m^2, in the presence of low pulmonary capillary wedge pressures (PCWP) as assessed by invasive monitoring [3]. Resultant insufficient delivery of volume to the left heart leads to low LVAD pump output. Delayed RV failure in the intensive care or step down unit can manifest as LVAD suction events with insufficient forward flow, hypotension, as well as elevated CVP with secondary renal or hepatic dysfunction. Potential treatment options include the use of pulmonary vasodilators and intravenous inotropic therapy with potential escalation to right-sided mechanical support.

Tricuspid regurgitation (TR) is well recognized as a manifestation of RV dysfunction that may improve with RV pressure and volume unloading with subsequent decrease in RV dimensions [4]. Tricuspid annulus dilation is the primary mediator of functional TR. While the amount of regurgitation resulting from tricuspid annular dilatation may be improved with inotropic support, pulmonary vasodilatation, and LVAD unloading, a part of annular dilatation resulting from chronic remodeling of the cardiac skeleton is unlikely to be improved with conservative measures. Dilatation tends to occur at the mural annulus along the right ventricle free wall, while the septal annulus is relatively stable [6, 7]. This fixed increase in annular diameter represents a chronic outward remodeling of the failing RV and tricuspid fibrous skeleton. Therefore, tricuspid annulus dilation is the main target for surgical correction with the goal of decreasing tricuspid annulus circumference and increasing leaflet coaptation. A preoperative tricuspid annular diameter of >43 mm was associated with decreased survival at 36 months after LVAD implantation [8]. An increasing body of literature from patients with significant TR undergoing left-heart surgery has shown that the downsizing a dilated tricuspid annulus irrespective of TR may lead to better functional capacity and to improvement in RV function by acutely reducing RV volume and promoting reverse remodeling of the RV in the longer term. A tricuspid annular diameter of >40 mm is suggested as a criterion for surgical intervention [9, 10]. We found that immediately after LVAD implantation alone, TR severity remained unchanged despite adequate unloading of the left heart. Late evaluation at 5–6 months demonstrated improvement with the incidence of moderate or severe TR decreasing from 57 to 32%. However, this still left a large proportion of patients with significant TR which correlated with decreased survival (◘ Fig. 20.1) [5]. Therefore persistent moderate to severe TR

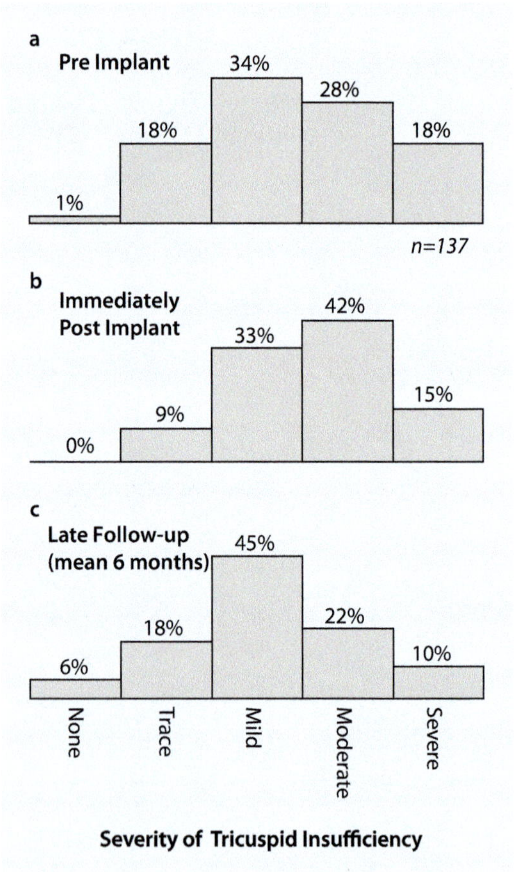

◘ **Fig. 20.1** Tricuspid regurgitation severity frequency distribution for 137 patients who did not receive a concurrent tricuspid valve procedure during LVAD implantation [5]. Figure demonstrates tricuspid valve regurgitation severity; (**a**) pre-implant, (**b**) immediately post-implant, (**c**) on late follow up as evidenced by hepatic vein flow reversal in pre-implant LVAD patients may be an indication for concurrent tricuspid repair [11, 12].

20.2 Echocardiographic Assessment of the Tricuspid Valve

Tricuspid annular dimension is commonly assessed via transthoracic or transesophageal echocardiogram. It is important to appreciate that TV regurgitation is dynamic and may have some variability between echocardiographic assessments. Therefore, the operator should make a summative evaluation of regurgitation severity based on both preoperative and intraoperative studies. Detection and quantitation of TR is performed through a combination of two-dimensional echocardiography, color flow Doppler, and spectral Doppler. The tricuspid valve can be evaluated intraoperatively by transesophageal echocardiography (TEE) in several views at the mid-esophageal (ME) level: four-chamber view, right ventricular inflow-outflow view, and modified bicaval. When performing the TEE, a four-chamber mid-esophageal view is obtained, and the probe is turned to the right to optimize visualization of the TV and annulus [8]. Color flow Doppler can facilitate assessment of TR by measuring the width of the vena contracta of the regurgitant jet as well as area of the regurgitant jet in the right atrium. A vena contracta width greater than 0.7 cm and a jet area greater than 10 cm^2 are criteria for the grade of severe TR. However, despite its simplicity, color flow Doppler is limited by technical and hemodynamic factors such as color gain, frame rate, and decrease in preload and afterload that occur under general anesthesia. Spectral Doppler can provide additional clues regarding the severity of tricuspid regurgitation. A dense, triangular-shaped, early peaking Doppler envelope of the regurgitant jet by continuous wave Doppler is consistent with severe TR. Hepatic vein flow systolic reversal by pulsed-wave Doppler of the hepatic veins is specific but relatively insensitive for the presence of severe TR. Tricuspid annulus diameter can be measured by TEE in the ME four-chamber view or the ME right ventricular inflow-outflow view or by transthoracic in the apical four-chamber or the parasternal short axis view. Given the complex anatomy of the TV and the tricuspid annulus, the geometric assumptions of the regurgitant orifice, and the limitations of each technique, no parameter should be used in isolation, but rather a comprehensive evaluation should be performed. Semiquantitative characterization of TR is determined by measuring the distance of the regurgitate jet from the tricuspid orifice toward the posterior wall. The severity scale is none (grade 0), mild (grade I), moderate (grade II), and severe (grade III/IV) [13].

20.3 Tricuspid Valve Surgery Technique

Appropriate vascular access and monitoring (e.g., pulmonary artery catheter) are obtained in the intubated patient in the operating room after induction of general anesthesia. A careful intraoperative transesophageal echocardiographic assessment for valvular abnormalities, atrial septal defect, and right ventricular function is obtained. TV intervention is planned if moderate or severe TR is confirmed. TV repair during LVAD implantation necessitates a median sternotomy approach with bicaval venous cannulation. Umbilical tapes may be placed around the SVC and IVC. However, vacuum-assisted venous drainage may obviate the need for caval snares. Following full cardiopulmonary bypass, the right atrium is opened. Notably, cardioplegic arrest and aortic cross clamping is not required in most cases. Care is taken to avoid injury to permanent pacer leads, which may be present in the right atrium. The pulmonary artery catheter tip is extracted from the right atrium and moved out of the immediate surgical field. The tricuspid valve is exposed, and assessment of annulus size, leaflet pathology, and position of any leads is performed. TV competence is tested by injecting saline into the RV. It is important to confirm that the RV shocking lead does not tether or perforate any of the leaflets. If the lead perforates any leaflet, this must be rectified in addition to the annuloplasty.

After confirming significant TR, if the findings suggest a dilated annulus without significant leaflet disease, an annuloplasty using a semi-rigid partial ring is most commonly performed [11]. This usually consists of 7–9 annular stitches using a 2-0 braided suture that spares the conduction system in the septal area. A 26 or 28 mm semi-rigid annuloplasty ring generally achieves significant downsizing of the annulus. Others have had success using suture annuloplasty techniques.

The De Vega suture annuloplasty is performed using 3-0 polypropylene suture in mattress technique supported by pericardial or felt pledgets [12]. The Kay (bicuspidization) annuloplasty is performed by plication of the posterior leaflet annulus using pledgeted 4-0 polypropylene horizontal mattress sutures [10, 14].

Primary leaflet pathology or damage (e.g., perforation, tethering, subvalvular chordal fusion), often from pacer/defibrillator leads traversing the tricuspid valve (TV), may preclude an adequate repair with annuloplasty alone. If there is leaflet pathology not amenable to a simple repair strategy such as the closure of a cleft or patching a perforation, TV replacement with a bioprosthesis is recommended. We do not recommend a mechanical prosthesis for the TV position due to the elevated risks of thrombosis, while a bioprosthesis tends to have a durable course with an 89% freedom from reoperation at 10 years [15–19].

Following completion of the tricuspid intervention, the pulmonary artery catheter is maneuvered back into the pulmonary artery manually, and the right atrium is closed in two layers using 4-0 Prolene suture. We then proceed with the LVAD implant portion of the operation. Lifting of the left ventricular apex anteriorly for exposure to place the LVAD inflow cannula has not caused disruption of the tricuspid repair or replacement in our experience. After weaning off cardiopulmonary bypass, the TV is again assessed on TEE, and we would accept mild or less TR as a reasonable result.

20.3.1 Outcome of Tricuspid Valve Interventions

Reports in the literature vary regarding the clinical benefits for concurrent tricuspid repair during LVAD implantation. In a small group of patients, we reported reduced need for inotropes, reduced length of postoperative hospitalization, and improved renal function for patients undergoing LVAD implantation with significant TR who received concurrent TV procedures versus a similar cohort who did not receive the surgical correction of the tricuspid insufficiency [11, 20, 21]. Furthermore, in a multicenter trials, LVAD patients who received concurrent tricuspid valvular procedures experienced equivalent survival outcomes relative to the cohort which underwent LVAD implantation alone [22, 23] (◘ Fig. 20.2). This suggests that the addition of these procedures to the LVAD implant does not greatly increase procedural morbidity/mortality. Finally, in one multicenter experience, late right heart failure appeared to be decreased among patients receiving the tricuspid procedure versus those with significant TR who did not receive the concurrent procedure [22] (◘ Fig. 20.2). Analysis of the STS database by Silvestry et al. however, failed to demonstrate these potential clinical benefits for concurrent tricuspid procedures [24]. Some of the discrepancy may arise from the fact that all studies on this topic have poorly defined control groups. Ultimately, a prospective randomized study would help define the benefits of concurrent tricuspid repair at the time of LVAD for patients with significant tricuspid insufficiency.

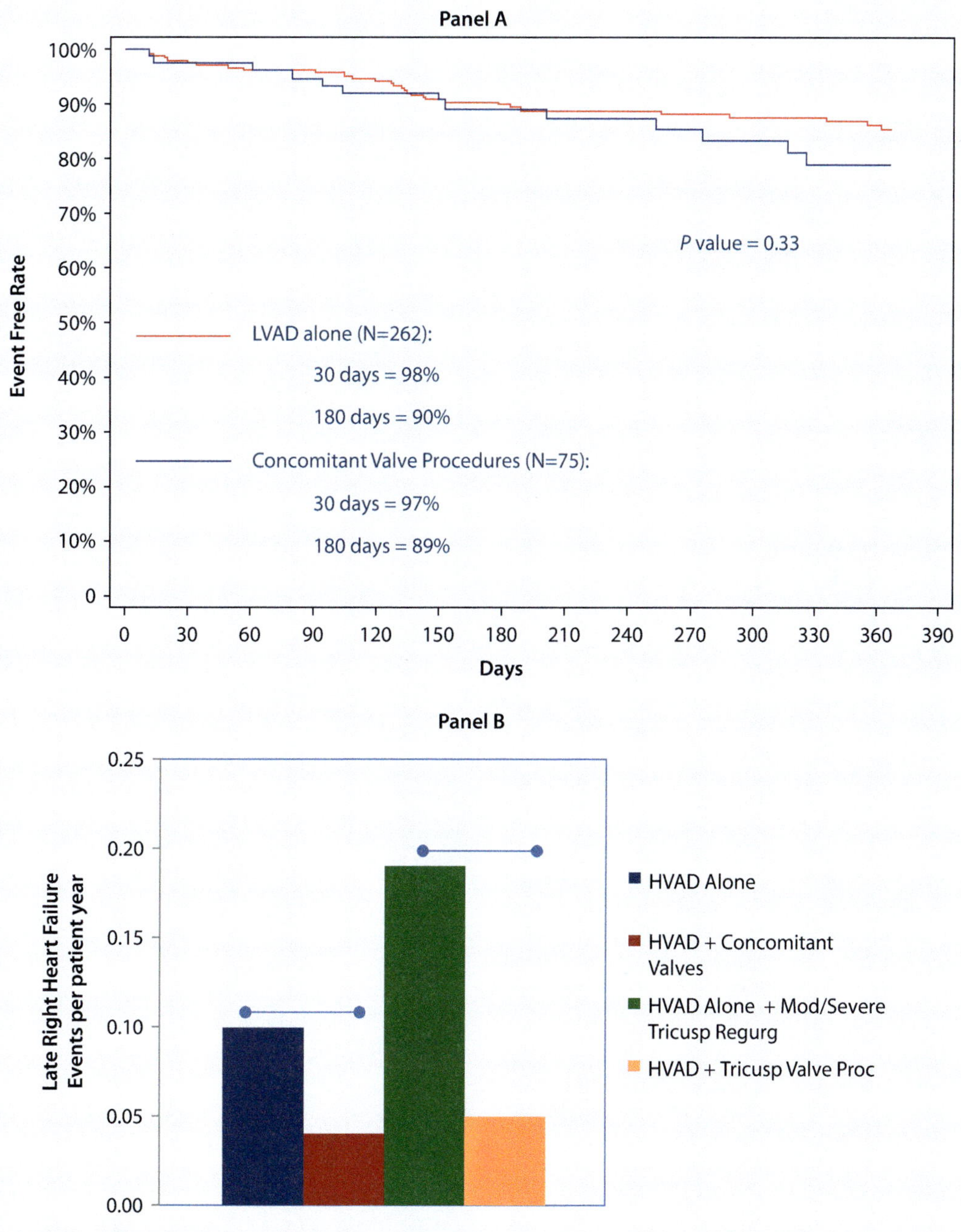

Fig. 20.2 Data from the ADVANCE HeartWare bridge-to-transplant trial are shown. Concurrent valve procedures were not associated with reduced survival outcomes relative to LVAD implantation alone; see *Panel A*. Late right heart failure was an important adverse event. Concurrent tricuspid procedures were associated with reduced late right heart failure compared to patients with significant TR who underwent LVAD alone [22]

References

1. Kormos RL et al (2010) Right ventricular failure in patients with the HeartMate II continuous-flow left ventricular assist device: incidence, risk factors, and effect on outcomes. J Thorac Cardiovasc Surg 139(5):1316–1324
2. Fujita T et al (2014) Right heart failure and benefits of adjuvant tricuspid valve repair in patients undergoing left ventricular assist device implantation. Eur J Cardiothorac Surg 46(5):802–807
3. Kukucka M et al (2011) Right-to-left ventricular end-diastolic diameter ratio and prediction of right ventricular failure with continuous-flow left ventricular assist devices. J Heart Lung Transplant 30(1):64–69
4. Atluri P et al (2013) Continuous flow left ventricular assist device implant significantly improves pulmonary hypertension, right ventricular contractility, and tricuspid valve competence. J Card Surg 28(6):770–775
5. Piacentino V et al (2011) Impact of tricuspid valve regurgitation in patients treated with implantable left ventricular assist devices. Ann Thorac Surg 91(5):1342–1346 ; discussion 1346-7
6. Frater R (2001) Tricuspid insufficiency. J Thorac Cardiovasc Surg 122(3):427–429
7. Foale R et al (1986) Echocardiographic measurement of the normal adult right ventricle. Br Heart J 56(1):33–44
8. Kukucka M et al (2012) Impact of tricuspid valve annulus dilation on mid-term survival after implantation of a left ventricular assist device. J Heart Lung Transplant 31(9):967–971
9. Dreyfus GD et al (2005) Secondary tricuspid regurgitation or dilatation: which should be the criteria for surgical repair? Ann Thorac Surg 79(1):127–132
10. Maltais S et al (2012) Surgical treatment of tricuspid valve insufficiency promotes early reverse remodeling in patients with axial-flow left ventricular assist devices. J Thorac Cardiovasc Surg 143(6):1370–1376
11. Piacentino V et al (2012) Utility of concomitant tricuspid valve procedures for patients undergoing implantation of a continuous-flow left ventricular device. J Thorac Cardiovasc Surg 144(5):1217–1221
12. Akhter SA et al (2014) Durability of De Vega tricuspid valve annuloplasty for severe tricuspid regurgitation during left ventricular assist device implantation. Ann Thorac Surg 98(1):81–83
13. Miyatake K et al (1982) Evaluation of tricuspid regurgitation by pulsed Doppler and two-dimensional echocardiography. Circulation 66(4):777–784
14. Navia JL et al (2010) Surgical management of secondary tricuspid valve regurgitation: annulus, commissure, or leaflet procedure? J Thorac Cardiovasc Surg 139(6):1473–1482.e5
15. Emery RW et al (2008) Anticoagulation for mechanical heart valves: a role for patient based therapy. J Thromb Thrombolysis 25(1):18–25
16. Dalrymple-Hay MJ et al (1999) Tricuspid valve replacement: bioprostheses are preferable. J Heart Valve Dis 8(6):644–648
17. Deo SV et al (2012) Concomitant tricuspid valve repair or replacement during left ventricular assist device implant demonstrates comparable outcomes in the long term. J Card Surg 27(6):760–766
18. McCarthy PM et al (2004) Tricuspid valve repair: durability and risk factors for failure. J Thorac Cardiovasc Surg 127(3):674–685
19. Krishan K et al (2012) Liberal use of tricuspid-valve annuloplasty during left-ventricular assist device implantation. Eur J Cardiothorac Surg 41(1):213–217
20. Piacentino V et al (2011) Clinical impact of concomitant tricuspid valve procedures during left ventricular assist device implantation. Ann Thorac Surg 92(4):1414–1418 ; discussion 1418-9
21. Brewer RJ et al (2014) Relationship of tricuspid repair at the time of left ventricular assist device implantation and survival. Int J Artif Organs 37(11):834–838
22. Milano C et al (2014) Clinical outcomes after implantation of a centrifugal flow left ventricular assist device and concurrent cardiac valve procedures. Circulation 130(11 Suppl 1):S3–11
23. Pal JD et al (2009) Low operative mortality with implantation of a continuous-flow left ventricular assist device and impact of concurrent cardiac procedures. Circulation 120(11 Suppl):S215–S219
24. Silvestry SC et al (2014) Concomitant tricuspid valve surgery during implantation of continuous-flow left ventricular assist devices: a society of thoracic surgeons database analysis. J Heart Lung Transplant 33(6):609–617

Role of Inotropes, Pulmonary Vasodilators, and Other Pharmacologic Interventions for Right Ventricular Dysfunction

Diyar Saeed

© Springer International Publishing Switzerland 2017
A. Montalto et al. (eds.), *Mechanical Circulatory Support in End-Stage Heart Failure*,
DOI 10.1007/978-3-319-43383-7_21

21.1 Introduction

Left ventricular assist device (LVAD) is currently a vital therapy option for patients with end-stage heart failure. Some degree of right ventricular dysfunction can be observed in the majority of patients with advanced heart failure assed for LVAD implantation. It has been reported that right ventricular failure (RVF) complicates 10–40% of patients after LVAD implantation [1–5]. Severe RVF is described by INTERMACS as the need for prolonged post-implant inotropes, inhaled nitric oxide or intravenous vasodilators, or requirement for right ventricular (RV) mechanical support. Severe right ventricular failure after LVAD implantation is associated with increased perioperative mortality, prolonged length of stay, and worse survival [6, 7].

Multiple mechanisms can combine to cause RVF after LVAD implantation. Increased venous return to RV due to higher cardiac output from the LVAD may potentially worsen preexisting RVF [8]. Excessive leftward shift of the interventricular septum with continuous-flow (cf) LVADs may also decrease septal contribution to RV contraction, leading to RVF [9]. Excessive perioperative volume resuscitation may also exacerbate RV dilation and causes tricuspid valve incompetence and RVF [10]. Finally atrial and ventricular tachyarrhythmias may also contribute to RVF. Atrial arrhythmias occur in more than 20% of LVAD patients and double the risk of RVF [11]. In addition, ventricular fibrillation may cause more than a 30% decrease in LVAD flow [12].

21.2 Managing RVF in Patients with LVAD

21.2.1 Preoperative

Prevention of RVF after LVAD implantation usually starts prior to the LVAD surgery. Due to difficulty reliably predicting RVF, it is basically recommended to implant LVAD before developing RVF. However, as many patients are still referred late for LVAD therapy, many of these patients have some forms of RV dysfunction and need prior hospitalization to optimize the RV prior to LVAD implant. Several strategies have evolved to optimize RV function that focus on modifying the hemodynamic and/or laboratory abnormalities associated with RVF [7, 13]. Based on increasing clinical experience with continuous-flow LVADs, many clinicians report positive outcome in correlation with RV optimization prior to LVAD surgery.

Preoperative RV optimization therapies include aggressive diuresis or ultrafiltration if diuresis is ineffective, targeting a lower central venous pressure (CVP) [13]. The optimal CVP is basically unknown, but CVP > 15 mm Hg may be associated with RVF [2], and it has been recommended to target as low as possible CVP prior to LVAD surgery [13].

Using preoperative oral phosphodiesterase-5 inhibitors, such as sildenafil, has been reported to decrease pulmonary artery pressure (PAP) after LVAD implantation, but whether their preoperative use decreases postoperative RVF is unknown [14]. If inotropes are necessary, milrinone may be more useful than dobutamine due to its more pronounced vasodilatory effects [7]. Although preoperative use of intra-aortic balloon pump (IABP) is considered a risk factor for RHF post implantation, some authors suggest using it, if left ventricular function cannot be adequately supported by pharmacological therapy. Imamura et al. reported a positive single center experience using prophylactic IABP support in heart failure patients with worsening hemodynamics prior to LVAD implantation [15]. In their study, the post LVAD clinical course was improved. However, many centers, including ours, rarely use prophylactic IABP prior to LVAD implantation.

Another important preoperative therapy option to precondition the RV is the use of calcium sensitizer levosimendan. Extensive literature search revealed two retrospective studies that reported levosimendan use prior to LVAD implantation [16, 17]. In the first study from Sponga et al., the effect of preoperative levosimendan treatment in LVAD patients with moderate RV dysfunction was investigated [16]. The study included 21 patients, who received levosimendan infusion (0.1–0.2 mg/kg/min) for 48 h prior to LVAD surgery. During levosimendan treatment, all patients demonstrated a significant improvement in cardiac index, pulmonary pressure, and CVP. The NT-proBNP level was significantly higher in patients who died because of RVF after 24 h of levosimendan treatment. During levosimendan treatment, the median NT-proBNP value in patients who survived decreased by 39%, whereas in patients who died, there was an increase of 3% ($p = 0.008$) at 72 h. The authors conclude that Levosimendan treatment improves preimplant hemodynamic performance and may predict patients who will develop RVF [16]. Meanwhile, Theiss et al. evaluated in another retrospective study the impact of preconditioning of the RV with the calcium sensitizer levosimendan immediately before LVAD implantation on outcome and survival [17]. The study included 9 patients with echocardiographic and invasive evidence of right heart insufficiency who were treated with levosimendan (0.1 μg/kg body weight/min) for 24 h before implantation of LVAD. Administration of levosimendan was safe, and no relevant side effects were observed. Merely, two temporary extracorporeal membrane-oxygenation implantations were necessary due to intraoperative RVF. Based on superior outcome after LVAD implantation in this small cohort of patients, the authors conclude that levosimendan might improve clinical outcome and survival when used as pretreatment in patients with right heart insufficiency prior to LVAD implantation. In summary, only two small retrospective studies reported the positive impact of levosimendan on outcome after LVAD implantation. Randomized controlled studies are necessary to confirm the possible advantage of this therapy option in lowering postoperative RVF in LVAD patients. Nevertheless, it is policy of our center to use levosimendan (0.1 μg/kg body weight/min) in every patient considered for LVAD implantation 2–3 days prior to LVAD surgery. Except for vasodilatory effect and increasing need for vasoconstrictive agents after administration, no relevant side effects were observed at our institution.

Apart from the abovementioned hemodynamic managements and optimization agents, other preoperative optimization includes therapy of coagulopathies prior to VAD surgery. Many patients have a spontaneous high INR value due to liver congestion secondary to RVF [18]. Preoperative coagulopathy predisposes to increased intraoperative bleeding. Intraoperative blood transfusions in this setting are particularly detrimental since these risk RV volume overload, increase PVR, and worsen SIRS. Preoperative administration of vitamin K [19] and intraoperative use of aprotinin are common practices to reduce bleeding that are validated by studies on first-generation LVADs [20]. With these measures, intra- and postoperative bleeding and transfusion risks are minimized, and risks of transfusion-related RVF are reduced [21].

Finally, when all above measures have been considered prior to LVAD implantation and the patient is still high risk for RVF despite hemodynamic optimization, a planned biventricular support or a total artificial heart (TAH) need to be considered. This is particularly important in patients with VA-ECMO prior to LVAD implantation [22]. Assessing RV in these patients with VA-ECMO is challenging, the incidence of RVF is higher than elective LVAD patients, and sometimes RVF may occur after LVAD implantation despite preoperative hemodynamic optimization [22].

21.2.2 Intraoperative

Since higher PVR results in increased RV afterload and increased work for RV, some of the general intraoperative principles used in the management of patients with pulmonary hypertension can be applied to the management of RVF after LVAD implantation. Appropriate ventilator setting is required to avoid hypoxia as alveolar hypoxia results in local vasoconstriction and increased pulmonary hypertension. It is also important to avoid acidosis as this can exacerbate RV ischemic injury [23]. Meticulous surgical hemostasis, using minimal invasive approaches; reducing cardiopulmonary bypass time; performing off-pump VAD implantation; minimizing blood product use, optimal pump flow, and speed management; and pharmacological RV support are important measures to prevent RV failure [7, 24]. Other important intraoperative management strategies include maintaining the heart rate at 80–100 bpm. This can be achieved by using cardioversion, $MgSO_4$, or digoxin if >100 bpm and DDD pacing, adrenaline, or isoproterenol if heart rate is slow. Normal sinus rhythm can be maintained/restored by using $MgSO_4$, cardioversion, and/or amiodarone or lidocaine [25]. ◘ Figure 21.1 summarizes the most important management strategies for perioperative RVF.

A study from our group and another recent review of 2196 patients in The Society of Thoracic Surgeons National Database found that tricuspid valve (TV) procedures in LVAD patients with moderate to severe tricuspid valve regurgitation failed to reduce early mortality or the need for an

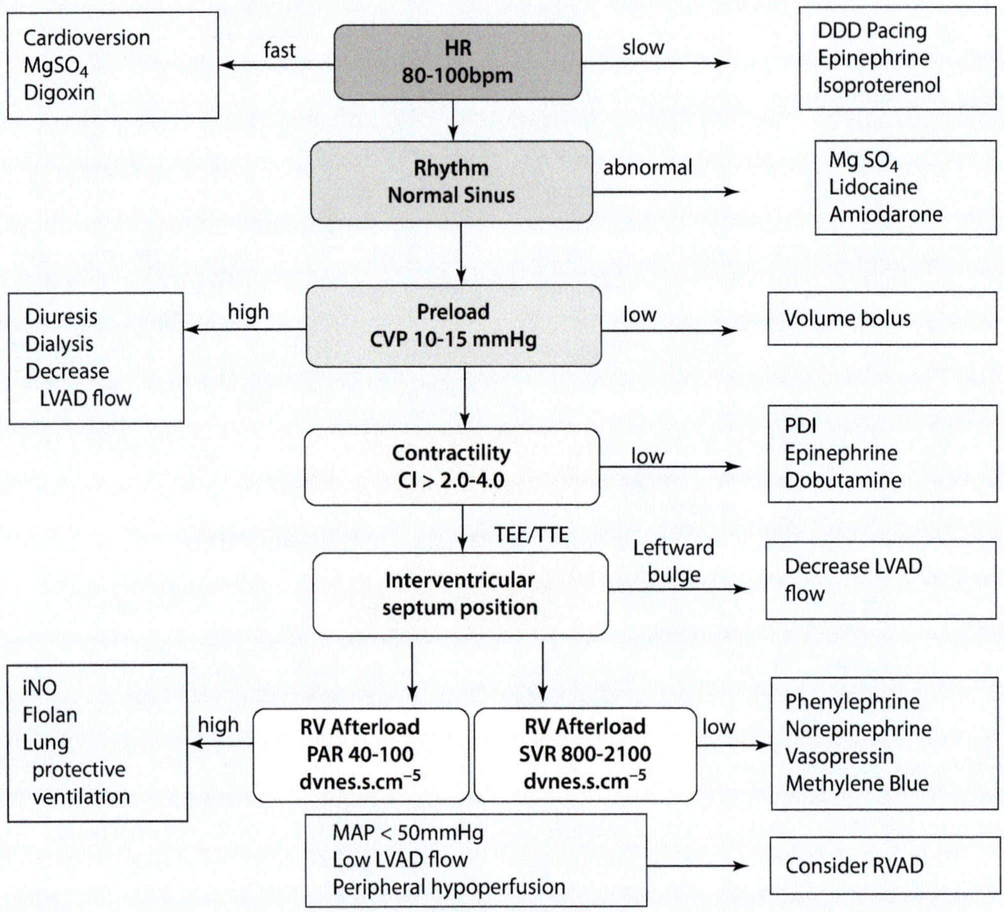

CI, cardiac index; CVP, central venous pressure; HR, heart rate; iNo, nitric oxide; LVAD, left ventricular assist device; MAP, mean arterial pressure; Mg SO_4, magnesium sulphate; PDI, phosphodiesterase inhibitor; RVAD, right ventricular assist device; TEE, transesoephageal echocardiography

Fig. 21.1 Management algorithm for perioperative right ventricular management (Ref. [31])

RV assist device (RVAD) but was associated with more postoperative renal failure and prolonged intensive care unit and hospital lengths of stay [10, 26]. Therefore, we don't consider TV repair procedures at the time of LVAD surgery. As previously described in the preoperative management, aggressive diuresis is among important preoperative measures to prevent postoperative RVF. Our experience and experience of several other groups have shown that tricuspid valve regurgitation can be significantly reduced with aggressive diuresis prior to LVAD implantation.

Pharmacological therapies of RV dysfunction include inhalative and intravenous agents. The role of pulmonary vasodilators (inhaled nitric oxide (NO) or prostacyclin) or a phosphodiesterase inhibitor such as sildenafil is still the subject of current investigation. Current evidence suggests that pulmonary hemodynamics may be improved in some patients with LVAD therapy receiving inhaled NO. In the study by Argenziano et al. including 11 patients with LVAD and pulmonary hypertension were randomized to receive either inhaled NO at 20 ppm ($n = 6$) or nitrogen ($n = 5$). In that study, the use of inhaled NO was associated with a decrease in mean PAP and improvement in LVAD flow compared with the placebo group [27]. However, Kukucka et al. investigated in a randomized trial the effects of inhaled nitric oxide on the hemodynamics of LVAD patients with PVR above 200 dyne s/cm^5 [28]. In their study, no significant difference in hemodynamics was found between groups, although hemodynamics improved after LVAD implantation in both groups. In another small study including seven patients with RV dysfunction after LVAD insertion, inotropes, inhaled NO (10 ppm), and iloprost (10 g) in repeated doses were evaluated [29]. The authors conclude that inhaled vasodilators mainly affected the pulmonary vasculature. Furthermore, combination treatment with inhaled NO and iloprost sufficiently decreased PVR and mean PAP on the basis of an additive effect, improved RV function, and avoided the need for RVAD.

The effect of inhaled milrinone was prospectively evaluated in ten postoperative LVAD patients with a mean INTERMACS profile of 2.5 ± 0.8 [30]. Inhaled milrinone was delivered into a ventilator circuit for 24 hours. Tolerability, efficacy, pharmacokinetics, and cost data were evaluated. Invasive mean PAP from baseline to during milrinone therapy was improved. The authors conclude that inhaled milrinone delivery after cf-LVAD implantation was well tolerated and feasible and demonstrated favorable hemodynamic, pharmacokinetic, and cost profiles.

Considering inotropic agents for RV support, it is important to consider supporting the RV with inotropes that allow some pulmonary vasodilatation (dobutamine or milrinone) while maintaining adequate systolic blood pressure (epinephrine) for coronary perfusion. Ideally, inotropic support can be withdrawn in the first few days after surgery as volume status is optimized and RV function recovers. The most commonly used inotropes are milrinone, dobutamine, and epinephrine depending on center preference. Milrinone is a phosphodiesterase- 3 inhibitor that has inotropic and vasodilatory effects. Dobutamine directly stimulates β1-adrenergic receptors resulting in increased contractility. While dobutamine provides some peripheral vasodilation, its systemic hypotensive effects are substantially less pronounced compared to milrinone. Therefore, dobutamine may be the inotrope of choice in a patient with systemic hypotension and/or postoperative vasoplegic syndrome. In addition, milrinone has a half-life of more than 2 h in patients with normal renal function but substantially longer in patients with renal dysfunction. The longer half-life of milrinone compared with dobutamine (which has a half-life of minutes) may be an advantage when inotropes are being slowly weaned, but may be a disadvantage in patients with significant renal dysfunction [23]. Epinephrine and dopamine do have inotropic effects, but they produce dose-dependent increases in PVR (epinephrine at doses of >0.05 μg/kg/min and dopamine at doses of >5 μg/kg/min). Therefore, these agents are usually used as adjuncts when systemic vasopressor support is needed to maintain coronary perfusion [23, 31].

21.2.3 Postoperative

It is crucial to the importance of early weaning from ventilator and extubation after LVAD implantation. The advantages of early extubation include reducing sedative agents (e.g., propofol) that lowers vascular resistance and has negative inotropic effect. Moreover, extubation lowers the negative impact of the ventilator on respiratory pressures and RV allowing early RV recovery after VAD implantation.

Considering pharmacological agents, it is important to reduce the inotropic agents gradually after LVAD implantation.

Considering pharmacological agents , Tedford et al. investigated the effects of sildenafil (average dose 51.9 mg) in 26 LVAD patients with persistently elevated PVR [14]. In their study, the treatment group had a significant decrease in PVR with the use of sildenafil. Moreover, Klodell et al. also investigated the effects of sildenafil in a small group of 10 LVAD patients with persistent pulmonary hypertension. A dose of 25–50 mg was given to the patients orally [32]. In those patients, there was a significant reduction in pulmonary artery systolic pressure as early as 90 min of oral administration.

La Rau et al. evaluated the safety and clinical course of patients treated with bosentan, an endothelin receptor antagonist, after the implantation of a LVAD in a single center [33]. The study included 50 consecutive patients with mean PAP >25 mmHg that were treated with bosentan after LVAD implantation for a mean duration of 15.7 months. Comparison of baseline to 6-month follow-up data revealed laboratory evidence for decongestion with a decrease in bilirubin and an improvement in pulmonary hemodynamics with echocardiographically calculated mean pulmonary vascular resistance decreasing 1.4 woods units. Therefore, the authors concluded that the tolerability of bosentan in LVAD-supported patients with secondary PH is comparable to prior experience in patients with heart failure.

Apart from the above measures, it is important to emphasize the importance of keeping all LVAD outpatients on known oral medications for heart failure (beta-blockers, ACE inhibitors, diuretics, Aldactone, and digoxin), as tolerated. With these medications, the incidence of post LVAD chronic RVF and repeated hospital admissions may be significantly reduced.

21.3 Summary and Conclusion

Some degree of right ventricular dysfunction can be observed in the majority of patients with advanced heart failure assed for LVAD implantation. Due to difficulty reliably predicting RVF, it is basically recommended to implant LVAD before developing RVF. Several pre-, intra-, and postoperative strategies have evolved to optimize RV function that focus on modifying the hemodynamic and/or laboratory abnormalities associated with RVF. Using the above measures, the risk of RVF may be minimized. However, despite aggressive risk stratification and medical management, some patients still develop RVF requiring RVAD support. The need for an RVAD is associated with worse outcomes. However, it has been reported that elective RVAD implantation correlates with better long-term survival than an emergency implantation. Therefore, a planned biventricular support or a TAH needs to be considered in these high-risk patients.

References

1. Dang NC et al (2006) Right heart failure after left ventricular assist device implantation in patients with chronic congestive heart failure. J Heart Lung Transplant 25(1):1–6
2. Kormos RL et al (2010) Right ventricular failure in patients with the HeartMate II continuous-flow left ventricular assist device: incidence, risk factors, and effect on outcomes. J Thorac Cardiovasc Surg 139(5):1316–1324
3. Matthews JC et al (2008) The right ventricular failure risk score a pre-operative tool for assessing the risk of right ventricular failure in left ventricular assist device candidates. J Am Coll Cardiol 51(22):2163–2172
4. Patel ND et al (2008) Right heart dysfunction after left ventricular assist device implantation: a comparison of the pulsatile HeartMate I and axial-flow HeartMate II devices. Ann Thorac Surg 86(3):832–840 ; discussion 832-40
5. Saeed D et al (2015) Alternative right ventricular assist device implantation technique for patients with perioperative right ventricular failure. J Thorac Cardiovasc Surg 149(3):927–932
6. Baumwol J et al (2011) Right heart failure and "failure to thrive" after left ventricular assist device: clinical predictors and outcomes. J Heart Lung Transplant 30(8):888–895
7. Lampert BC, Teuteberg JJ (2015) Right ventricular failure after left ventricular assist devices. J Heart Lung Transplant 34(9):1123–1130
8. Farrar DJ et al (1985) Right heart interaction with the mechanically assisted left heart. World J Surg 9(1):89–102
9. Moon MR et al (1997) Septal function during left ventricular unloading. Circulation 95(5):1320–1327
10. Saeed D et al (2011) Tricuspid valve repair with left ventricular assist device implantation: is it warranted? J Heart Lung Transplant 30(5):530–535
11. Brisco MA et al (2014) Incidence, risk, and consequences of atrial arrhythmias in patients with continuous-flow left ventricular assist devices. J Card Surg 29(4):572–580
12. Cantillon DJ et al (2014) Low cardiac output associated with ventricular tachyarrhythmias in continuous-flow LVAD recipients with a concomitant ICD (LoCo VT Study). J Heart Lung Transplant 33(3):318–320
13. Feldman D et al (2013) The 2013 International Society for Heart and Lung Transplantation Guidelines for mechanical circulatory support: executive summary. J Heart Lung Transplant 32(2):157–187
14. Tedford RJ et al (2008) PDE5A inhibitor treatment of persistent pulmonary hypertension after mechanical circulatory support. Circ Heart Fail 1(4):213–219
15. Imamura T et al (2015) Prophylactic intra-aortic balloon pump before ventricular assist device implantation reduces perioperative medical expenses and improves postoperative clinical course in INTERMACS profile 2 patients. Circ J 79(9):1963–1969
16. Sponga S et al (2012) Preoperative treatment with levosimendan in candidates for mechanical circulatory support. ASAIO J 58(1):6–11
17. Theiss HD et al (2014) Preconditioning with levosimendan before implantation of left ventricular assist devices. Artif Organs 38(3):231–234
18. Woolley JR et al (2015) Preoperative liver dysfunction influences blood product administration and alterations in circulating haemostatic markers following ventricular assist device implantation. Eur J Cardiothorac Surg 47(3):497–504
19. Kaplon RJ et al (1999) Vitamin K reduces bleeding in left ventricular assist device recipients. J Heart Lung Transplant 18(4):346–350
20. Goldstein DJ et al (1995) Use of aprotinin in LVAD recipients reduces blood loss, blood use, and perioperative mortality. Ann Thorac Surg 59(5):1063–1067 ; discussion 1068

21. Goldstein DJ, Beauford RB (2003) Left ventricular assist devices and bleeding: adding insult to injury. Ann Thorac Surg 75(6 Suppl):S42–S47
22. Maxhera B et al (2014) Survival predictors in ventricular assist device patients with prior extracorporeal life support: selecting appropriate candidates. Artif Organs 38(9):727–732
23. Marzec LN, Ambardekar AV (2013) Preoperative evaluation and perioperative management of right ventricular failure after left ventricular assist device implantation. Semin Cardiothorac Vasc Anesth 17(4):249–261
24. Haberl T et al (2014) Viennese approach to minimize the invasiveness of ventricular assist device implantationdagger. Eur J Cardiothorac Surg 46(6):991–996; discussion 996
25. Argiriou M et al (2014) Right heart failure post left ventricular assist device implantation. J Thorac Dis 6(Suppl 1):S52–S59
26. Robertson JO et al (2014) Concomitant tricuspid valve surgery during implantation of continuous-flow left ventricular assist devices: a Society of Thoracic Surgeons database analysis. J Heart Lung Transplant 33(6):609–617
27. Argenziano M et al (1998) Randomized, double-blind trial of inhaled nitric oxide in LVAD recipients with pulmonary hypertension. Ann Thorac Surg 65(2):340–345
28. Kukucka M et al (2011) Acute impact of left ventricular unloading by left ventricular assist device on the right ventricle geometry and function: effect of nitric oxide inhalation. J Thorac Cardiovasc Surg 141(4):1009–1014
29. Antoniou T et al (2012) Inhaled nitric oxide plus iloprost in the setting of post-left assist device right heart dysfunction. Ann Thorac Surg 94(3):792–798
30. Haglund NA et al (2015) Inhaled milrinone after left ventricular assist device implantation. J Card Fail 21(10):792–797
31. Meineri M, Van Rensburg AE, Vegas A (2012) Right ventricular failure after LVAD implantation: prevention and treatment. Best Pract Res Clin Anaesthesiol 26(2):217–229
32. Klodell CT Jr et al (2007) Effect of sildenafil on pulmonary artery pressure, systemic pressure, and nitric oxide utilization in patients with left ventricular assist devices. Ann Thorac Surg 83(1):68–71; discussion 71
33. LaRue SJ et al (2015) Treatment of secondary pulmonary hypertension with bosentan after left ventricular assist device implantation. Cardiovasc Ther 33(2):50–55

Temporary RVAD

Alexander Stepanenko

© Springer International Publishing Switzerland 2017
A. Montalto et al. (eds.), *Mechanical Circulatory Support in End-Stage Heart Failure*,
DOI 10.1007/978-3-319-43383-7_22

22.1 Introduction

Right ventricular failure (RVF) is a major cause of morbidity and early postoperative mortality in patients suffering from end-stage heart failure who have undergone placement of a left ventricular assist device (LVAD) [1]. Poor LVAD output with prolonged shock in the case of RV failure may lead to deterioration in the function of pre-damaged end organs. Right ventricular assist device (RVAD) insertion in this case is a valid therapy option.

22.2 Indication for RVAD

There are several definitions of RV failure. However, most of them are retrospective (2 weeks on inotropes, need for RVAD, etc.) and fail to help form bedside decision, if LVAD support seems to be ineffective due to RVF [2].

In our center, we use modified RV failure criteria worked out by multicenter, double-blind, randomized studies of the effect of inhaled nitric oxide on RV failure after LVAD implantation (iNOT-41; iNO Therapeutics, Clinton, NJ). These criteria are bedside applicable for all LVAD recipients during support [1, 3, 4].

Intraoperative indications to RVAD insertion were defined as any of the following:

Inability to wean from CPB or any two of the following (sustained for 15 min after complete withdrawal from CPB or LVAD initiation in case of surgical technique used with CPB standby):

- Cardiac index ≤ 2.0 l/min/m^2, calculated as LVAD flow divided by body surface area or evaluated by placing of Swan-Ganz catheter
- Administration of ≥ 20 inotropic equivalents (IE):
  - 10 μg/kg/min dopamine, dobutamine, enoximone, or amrinone is equivalent to 10 IE
  - 0.1 μg/kg/min epinephrine or norepinephrine is equivalent to 10 IE
  - 1 μg/kg/min milrinone is equivalent to 15 IE
  - 0.1 U/min vasopressin is equivalent to 10 IE
- MAP ≤ 55 mmHg
- CVP ≥ 16 mmHg
- SvO2 $\leq$ 55%

Last five criteria persistent for over 15 min in absence of cardiac tamponade may be used as criteria need for temporary RVAD support in LVAD recipients.

22.3 Devices

Several devices are reported efficiently used as temporary RVAD such as CentriMag (Thoratec, Pleasanton), Rotaflow (Maquet, Hirrlingen, Germany), TandemHeart (CardiacAssist Inc., Pittsburgh, PA), Abiomed AB 5000 (Abiomed, Danvers, MA), percutaneous RVAD Impella RP (Abiomed), or modified peripheral VA ECMO circuit [5–8].

RVAD circuit may be coated (heparin, bioline, etc.) or uncoated. In case of postoperative HIT, onset heparin-coated circuit is still a subject of debate.

Few reports show RVAD cannula sizing. Appropriate size of inflow and outflow cannula should be used to maintain adequate venous drainage and support RVAD flow of up to 7–8 l/min by "full" support. "Partial" support devices cannulas (Impella, VA ECMO) are chosen according to patient's vessel characteristic to allow correct device placement and functioning without complication at cannulation site.

■ Inflow Cannulation

In our series of 49 RVADs implanted since 2008, we used predominantly 32F EDWARDS cannula for direct RA drainage. In case of femoral vein use, 28F EDWARDS cannula had been placed.

■ Outflow Cannulation

In all our RVAD recipients disregard surgical technique used 22F EOPA cannula had been inserted.

22.4 Approaches to RVAD Circuit Connection

22.4.1 Conventional Insertion RA-PA via Sternotomy

The RVAD inflow and outflow cannulas were placed in the right atrium and main pulmonary artery and secured by double purse-string sutures. In all our cases, a 32F single-stage venous drainage cannula for the inflow and a 22F arterial cannula for the outflow line were introduced through separate skin incisions in the right upper abdominal quadrant. Explantation requires re-sternotomy (see ◘ Fig. 22.1).

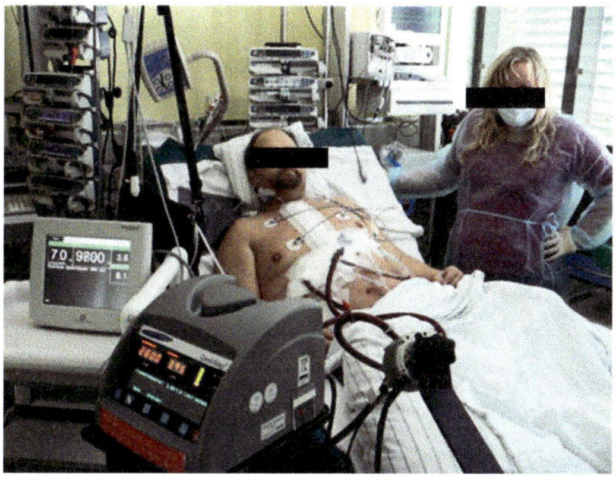

■ **Fig. 22.1** RV Failure after LVAD implantation via MS (direct cannulation of RA and PA), explantation via re-sternotomy

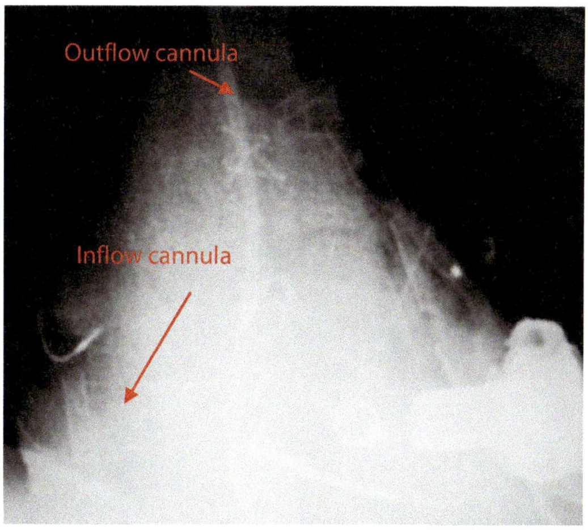

■ **Fig. 22.2** RV failure after LVAD insertion via left lateral thoracotomy

22.4.2 Minimally Invasive Placement/Withdrawal

Several reports have shown the feasibility of minimally invasive RVAD insertion using different approaches. Cohn et al. described RVAD insertion through vessel grafts with bedside removal [9].

Strauch et al. suggested a modified technique for RVAD insertion via sternotomy [10].

Minami et al. described cannulation of the outflow graft through the right pulmonary artery between the ascending aorta and the superior vena cava using Seldinger technique, to avoid excessive adhesion dissection in cases of reoperation [11].

22.4.3 After LVAD Placement Through Left Lateral or Bilateral Minithoracotomy

- Transpericardial outflow cannulation of main PA by Seldinger technique.

After localization of the main pulmonary artery with needle under TEE monitoring, two additional purse string sutures (5–0 polypropylene) were placed at the pericardium to protect the left lateral aspect of the artery. Pressure measurement and blood gas analysis confirmed correct position of the needle in the lumen of the main pulmonary artery. The venous cannula of RVAD was advanced through the inferior vena cava into the cavum of the right atrium using the Seldinger technique. The location and hemostasis were secured by purse string sutures and cutaneous fixation. After that the wound was provisionally closed and the skin adapted with metal clamps (see ■ Fig. 22.2).

Venous cannulation via a femoral vein and transpericardial outflow cannulation of the main pulmonary artery by Seldinger technique RVAD

Our approach is limited if there are severe adhesions after left lung decortication or previous thoracic surgery or lack of TEE to localize the main pulmonary artery transpericardially. Using self-expanding smart venous cannulas may minimize the risk of venous thrombosis and maintain sufficient perfusion of the leg if RV recovery is expected to be prolonged [12]:

- PA cannulation via RV apex (Personal communication Dr. Woo, Dr. Loebe, Berlin MCS Meeting 2009) and femoral vein for drainage
- Peripheral VA ECMO

Peripheral venoarterial ECMO for maintaining systemic circulation may be of value. However, the ECMO flow in this approach is limited to 2–4 l/min and may carry an additional thromboembolic and bleeding risk for the patient:

- Impella RP (Abiomed).
- Son et al. presented an animal and cadaver feasibility study to show possible means of VAD implantation via right thoracotomy [13].

RVAD Flow Reduction
Weaning patients, n=27

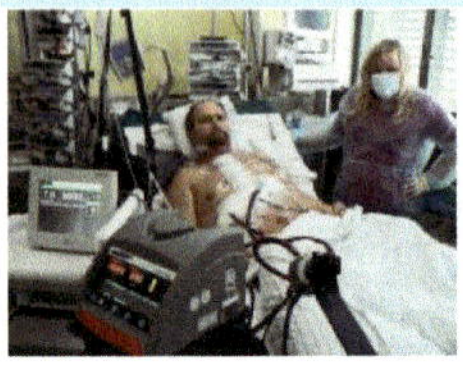

Median RVAD support duration, days	20 (3-65)
RVAD duration <14 days, n=6	9 (3-11)
RVAD duration 14-30 days, n=15	20 (15-27)
RVAD duration >30 days, n=6	34 (30-65)

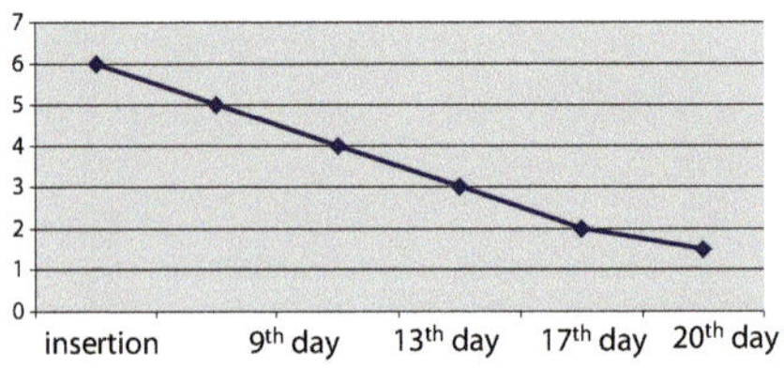

Fig. 22.3 Temporary RVAD between January 2008 and October 2013

22.5 Management and RVAD Weaning

22.5.1 Weaning

Potential for right ventricular myocardial recovery induced by mechanical assistance and exact guidelines for right ventricular assist device weaning are still challenging. Most of publication did not provide exact criteria for weaning start.

Most of the groups suggest first echocardiographic weaning study in the intensive care unit after 24–72 h of support. Low-dose inotropic support with milrinone (0.25 g/kg/min), dopamine (3.0 g/kg/min), or epinephrine (0.05 g/kg/min) was initiated before attempting to wean the device. Signs consistent with RV recovery included increased amplitude of the pulmonary arterial waveform, no need for escalation of inotropic support, maintenance of a low central venous pressure (CVP), and improved RV systolic function on echocardiography [5, 14].

In our experience between January 2008 and October 2013, 49 of total 584 LVAD recipients required implantation of a temporary RVAD (Thoratec® CentriMag®) for treatment of RV failure after the initiation of LVAD support. Thirty-three patients on RVAD reached candidacy for weaning after a median of 6 (range 1–36) days of full RVAD support. Four of them were nonweanable and bridged to the heart of sepsis and late tamponade (both died on RVAD after 25 and 39 days). Weaning patients (n = 27) required a median support duration of 20 (range 3–65) days (see Fig. 22.3) [14].

Based on this center experience, we introduced RVAD weaning protocol. Briefly, after RVAD insertion, full flow (5–7 l/min) of VAD, minimization, or freedom from catecholamines, euvolemia, and support of end-organ function is targeted.

Important is to maintain a balance between RVAD and LVAD flow – maximal flow without lung congestion confirmed by echocardiography and lung function. In any case of lung suggestion, RVAD overflow has to be ruled out first. Membrane oxygenation included into RVAD circuit may be a therapy option in case of refractory lung failure.

After 3–4 days of support, first echocardiographic assessment of RV function is performed, ruling out significant pericardial effusion, high degree of tricuspid insufficiency, interventricular septum position, and RV systolic function.

Criteria for start to reduce RVAD flow in absence of cardiac tamponade are:

- SR or absence of arrhythmias
  - Freedom from or low-dose vasopressors
  - Stable pulmonary function
  - Euvolemia
  - Recovered liver and kidney function
  - Controlled infection status

If pts met these criteria, RVAD flow reduction is performed 0.5/l per day with attention on CVP/LVAD flow/end-organ function. Daily echocardiographic assessment is performed. Pulmonary afterload reduction may be of value (iloprost, sildenafil).

Criteria for weaning discontinuation are drop-off of LVAD flow more than 25%, hypotonia with MAP < 60 mmHg, and signs of hypoperfusion (calculated CI less than 2 l/min/m^2, mixed or central venous saturation less than 60%). RVAD flow is restarted as full again. After recompensation, repeated weaning attempt may be of value. In case of failing recovery of RV, selected pts are then screened for heart transplantation or insertion of long-term implantable RVAD [15, 16].

Once RVAD flow has reached 2 l/min, echocardiographic rump test under increased (blousing) anticoagulation is performed. Stable tricuspid annulus dimension, absence of severe tricuspid regurgitation, stable TAPSE > 15 mm, stable RV geometry and LV feeling (LVEDD), absence of LVAD suction events, stable arterial pressure over 60 mmHg, CVP below 12 mmHg, and stable rhythmus are decision criteria for RVAD explantation.

Device explantation may be performed in OR or bedside in ICU (if minimal invasive implantation via grafts used) after clamping of RVAD cannula and RVAD circuit recirculation under TEE monitoring.

22.5.2 Anticoagulation

The infusion of unfractionated heparin or argatroban was started 12–24 h after CentriMag placement or at the point that chest tube drainage was less than 50 mL/h; the infusion was therefore titrated to an aPTT of 50–60 s for 24 h and to an aPTT target of 60–80 s for the duration of support. During phases of flow reduction, the aPTT target was increased to above 80 s, with bolusing in selected cases (echocardiographic examination with RVAD pump stop).

22.5.3 RV Function After RVAD Removal

After RVAD removal, several groups report stable RV function in LVAD outpatients. In our group of temporary RVAD LVAD outpatients (n = 19, 13.2 ± 5.3 months, cumulative support 25 patient/years), all showed stable right ventricular function after previous weaning from temporary RVAD.

22.6 Conclusion

In general, the outcomes of patients who require implantation of a temporary RVAD after LVAD insertion are still unsatisfactory. Sequelae of preoperative shock or delayed RVAD insertion together with surgical revisions for bleeding and following sepsis currently limits the clinical success of temporary RVAD therapy.

Several devices used for RVAD circuit showed good flow profile for full and partial support options.

In our experience, after reaching weaning candidacy, the overall procedural success rate is rising up to 90% with RV myocardial recovery allowing weaning of over 80%.

Weaned patients achieve acceptable functional status and stable RV function and LVAD flow in outpatient studies.

References

1. Potapov EV, Stepanenko A, Dandel M, Kukucka M, Lehmkuhl HB, Weng Y et al (2008) Tricuspid incompetence and geometry of the right ventricle as predictors of right ventricular function after implantation of a left ventricular assist device. J Heart Lung Transplant 27(12):1275–1281
2. Lampert BC, Teuteberg JJ (2015) Right ventricular failure after left ventricular assist devices. J Heart Lung Transplant 34(9):1123–1130
3. Kukucka M, Potapov E, Stepanenko A, Weller K, Mladenow A, Kuppe H et al (2011) Acute impact of left ventricular unloading by left ventricular assist device on the right ventricle geometry and function: effect of nitric oxide inhalation. J Thorac Cardiovasc Surg 141(4):1009–1014
4. Potapov E, Meyer D, Swaminathan M, Ramsay M, El Banayosy A, Diehl C et al (2011) Inhaled nitric oxide after left ventricular assist device implantation: a prospective, randomized, double-blind, multicenter, placebo-controlled trial. J Heart Lung Transplant 30(8):870–878
5. Bhama JK, Kormos RL, Toyoda Y, Teuteberg JJ, McCurry KR, Siegenthaler MP (2009) Clinical experience using the Levitronix CentriMag system for temporary right ventricular mechanical circulatory support. J Heart Lung Transplant 28(9):971–976
6. Khani-Hanjani A, Loor G, Chamogeorgakis T, Shafii A, Mountis M, Hanna M et al (2013) Case series using the ROTAFLOW system as a temporary right ventricular

assist device after HeartMate II implantation. ASAIO J 59(4):456–460
7. Haneya A, Philipp A, Diez C, Metterlein T, Puehler T, Hilker M et al (2011) Successful use of temporary right ventricular support to avoid implantation of biventricular long-term assist device: a transcutaneous approach. ASAIO J 57(4):274–277
8. Takeda K, Naka Y, Yang JA, Uriel N, Colombo PC, Jorde UP et al (2013) Timing of temporary right ventricular assist device insertion for severe right heart failure after left ventricular assist device implantation. ASAIO J 59(6):564–569
9. Cohn WE, Gregoric ID, La Francesca S, Frazier OH (2007 Apr) Bedside right ventricular assist device removal in the conscious patient. Ann Thorac Surg 83(4): 1556–1557
10. Strauch JT, Franke UF, Madershahian N, Wahlers T (2004 Dec) Right ventricular assist device implantation – A new transcutaneous approach. Thorac Cardiovasc Surg 52(6):378–379
11. Minami K, Bonkohara Y, Arusoglu L, El-Banayosy A, Korfer R (1999) New technique for the outflow cannulation of right ventricular assist device. Ann Thorac Surg 68(3):1092–1093
12. Stepanenko A, Potapov EV, Krabatsch T, Hetzer R (2011) Simple implantation of a temporary right ventricular device for right ventricular failure after left ventricular device implantation via a left lateral thoracotomy. ASAIO J 57(1):17–18
13. Son HS, Sun K, Hwang CM, Fang YH, Lim CH, Lee HW et al (2006) Ventricular assist device implantation using a right thoracotomy. ASAIO J 52(4):386–390
14. Stepanenko A, Dandel M, Kukucka M, Vierecke J, Jurmann B, Maroto Perez L, Chavez T, Gromann T, Pasic M, Wenig Y et al (2015). Right ventricular recovery induced by temporary right ventricular assist device support. Zeitschrift Thoracic Cardiovascular Surgeon 63(Suppl 1):S88. (this has to be inserted into references)
15. Saito S, Sakaguchi T, Miyagawa S, Nishi H, Yoshikawa Y, Fukushima S et al (2012) Recovery of right heart function with temporary right ventricular assist using a centrifugal pump in patients with severe biventricular failure. J Heart Lung Transplant 31(8):858–864
16. Krabatsch T, Potapov E, Stepanenko A, Schweiger M, Kukucka M, Huebler M et al (2011) Biventricular circulatory support with two miniaturized implantable assist devices. Circulation 124(11 Suppl):S179–S186

Which Approach? Traditional Versus MICS

Sebastian V. Rojas, Jasmin S. Hanke, Ezin Deniz, Christina Feldmann, Axel Haverich, Thomas Krabatsch, Evgenij Potapov, Daniel Zimpfer, Simon Maltais, and Jan D. Schmitto

© Springer International Publishing Switzerland 2017
A. Montalto et al. (eds.), *Mechanical Circulatory Support in End-Stage Heart Failure*,
DOI 10.1007/978-3-319-43383-7_23

23.1 Introduction

Cardiac transplantation has been the only therapy providing a definite solution for congestive heart failure during the past decades [1]. Nevertheless, especially in Europe and the USA, the new century has brought important changes to this field leading to a growing gap between the number of heart failure patients and the number of performed heart transplantations. As cardiac transplantation is no longer capable to provide a solution for an increasing incidence of heart failure patients, ventricular assist device (VAD) therapy has developed from its beginnings as bridge-to-transplant (BTT) strategy to more recently destination therapy (DT) [1]. Thus, devices that were originally designed to work for only some months have shown considerable durability surpassing the 10-year mark [2–4]. Moreover, during the past 15 years of LVAD-therapy, 2-year survival rates have dramatically improved from 30% to almost 80%. This is remarkable and it seems difficult to find another therapy, even in other medical areas that has shown such important improvements in such a brief period of time. Even if cardiac transplantation is still considered as gold standard for heart failure treatment, the worldwide number of yearly implanted VADs has already surpassed the number of cardiac transplantation [5]. Thus, VAD therapy has become indispensable in the treatment of terminal congestive heart failure. However, along with larger application of VAD, therapy patient collective has changed: (1) especially with a growing number of DT patients, mean age of patients at time of implantation has raised [5], (2) severity of illness has worsened due to increased comorbidities, and (3) the number of patients receiving LVAD as redo surgery has grown. All these factors contribute to a more critical risk profile of LVAD candidates. Therefore, there is a need of alternative surgical strategies to deal with these challenges. With the venue of miniaturized latest generation VADs, less invasive procedures became possible. What started as single center case reports is now being applied in most important VAD centers worldwide and has revolutionized this surgical field [6–8]. Next to the implantation itself [9], device explantation [10] and exchange [11] can now be performed through LIS techniques.

The aim of less invasive procedures is to reduce mortality and morbidity by minimizing surgical trauma, avoiding myocardial ischemia, and reducing the immunological trauma. In addition to less invasive surgery, there is also a need for optimized patient management including preoperative conditioning, during anesthesia and while being at the intensive care unit. Thus, a faster convalescence and rehabilitation of VAD patients is accomplished. From another perspective, LIS procedures also contribute to economical resource optimization by means of shorter ICU and total hospital stays. It has also been shown that minimally invasive LVAD implantation can be performed without the need for blood transfusion. This is beneficial not only for all heart failure patients, but also for special cases such as during treatment of patients with various religious backgrounds (eg. Jehovah's witness patients) [35].

While it remains unclear until which point the miniaturization of LVADs will continue in future, it is already clear that less invasive techniques will be used for most implantations in the future. In this book chapter, we will first summarize and describe important surgical advances of past years with a special focus on less invasive state-of-the-art surgical techniques. Moreover, we will give a stepwise description of less invasive LVAD implantation, including optimized perioperative patient management.

23.2 Standard Approach

The standard implantation approach for common LVAD systems involves a full sternotomy with right-atrial and aortic cannulation for the heart-lung machine (see ◘ Fig. 23.1).

A key advantage of this approach is that it provides the best overview of the heart and all major vessels (see ◘ Figs. 23.2, 23.3, and 23.4). This is especially beneficial in combined surgery. Most common concomitant procedures to LVAD surgery are aortic valve replacement, tricuspid valve repair/replacement, closure of patent foramen ovale/atrial septal defects, ligation/appendectomy of the left atrium, and placement of epicardial pacing wires. While aortic valve replacement can be performed safely by LIS techniques, all the other procedures are not performed routinely by

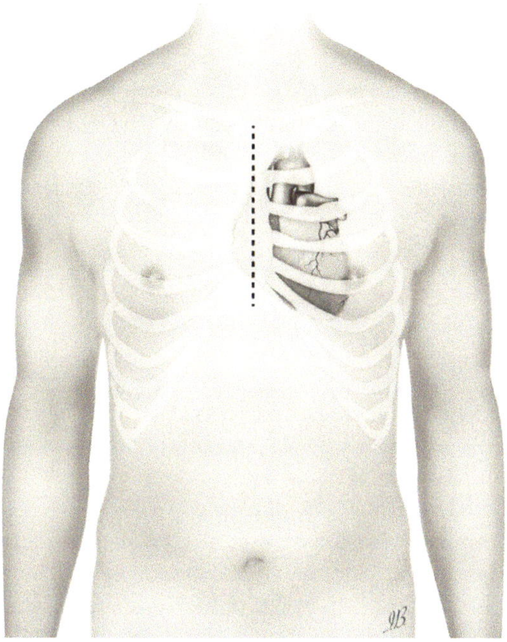

■ **Fig. 23.1** Conventional implantation technique: full sternotomy (Illustration by Ilaria Bondi's Peppermint Advertising)

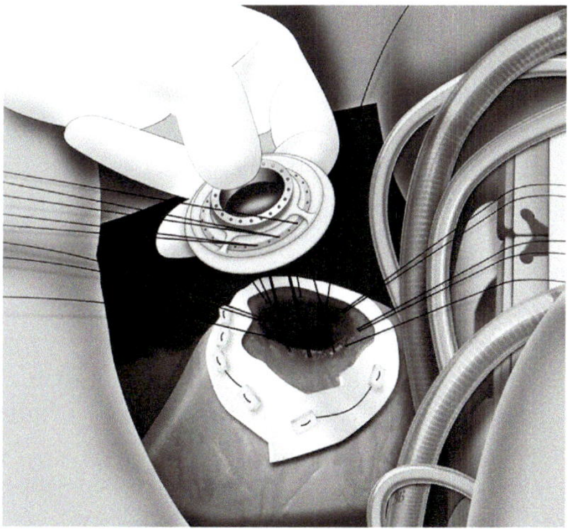

■ **Fig. 23.2** 2–0 Tevdek sutures are placed in a full-thickness fashion through the myocardial core and passed through the felt portion of the sewing cuff or ring. According to the surgeon, a Teflon strip is used to reinforce the outer wall of the myocardium and provide better hemostasis (Illustration by Ilaria Bondi's Peppermint Advertising)

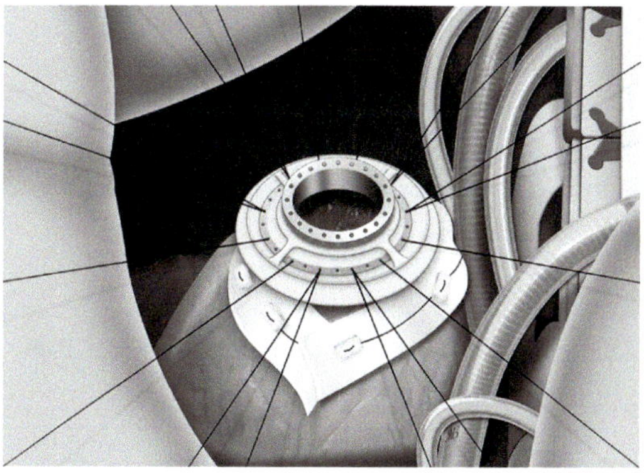

■ **Fig. 23.3** These sutures are then tied down carefully to secure the sewing cuff or ring to the apical opening (Illustration by Ilaria Bondi's Peppermint Advertising)

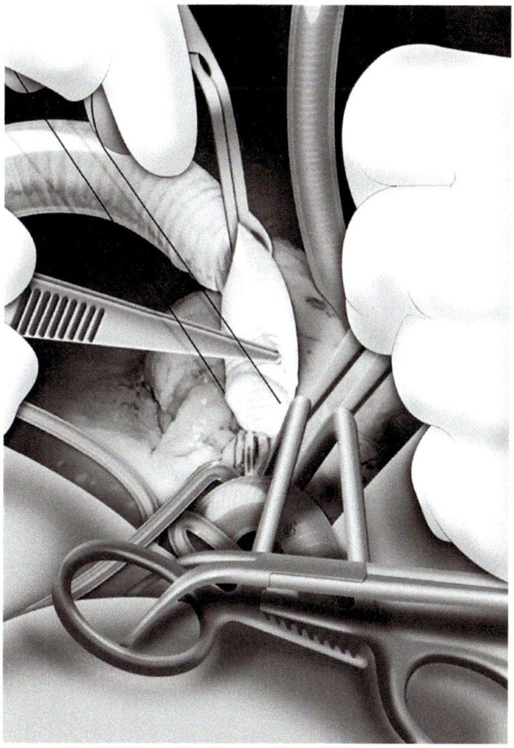

■ **Fig. 23.4** Anastomosis of outflow graft to ascending aorta during a conventional full sternotomy approach (Illustration by Ilaria Bondi's Peppermint Advertising)

smaller incisions. Disadvantages of this approach are increased surgical trauma with higher incidence of postoperative bleeding, full opening of the pericardium with risk of RV dilatation/RV failure, and higher risk of sternal instability and wound infections.

23.3 Development of Less Invasive LVAD Surgery

Initial approaches for less invasive LVAD surgery were hampered by large devices which even required external or abdominal pump placement [7, 12, 13]. Hill et al. introduced the concept of less invasive implantation in three patients receiving the paracorporeal Thoratec LVAD (Thoratec Corporation, USA) [12]. They advocated a combination of a right minithoracotomy and a left subcostal incision. Of 3 LVAD patients with dilated cardiomyopathy, 2 experienced postoperative bleeding and needed drainage (by chest tubes) and blood transfusions. One patient died (for technically unrelated reasons), but the other 2 were able to safely undergo a heart transplant. After those early results reported by Hill et al., the new minimally invasive technique was applied by other groups using new-generation devices, with significant improvements. Gregoric et al. described a less invasive approach for implanting the Heartmate II LVAD (Thoratec Corporation, USA) [13]. They advocated a subcostal incision, followed by separating the interfering muscles (stopping extraperitoneally above the transverse muscle fascia). Then the pleura should be opened, in order to allow access to the pericardium and the left ventricular apex below. Before LVAD placement, a pocket must be created subcostally for the pump housing. A parasternal minithoracotomy on the third right intercostal space is done in order to perform the aortic anastomosis of the outflow graft [38]. Overall, Gregoric et al. performed the procedure successfully in three patients [14].

More recently, Anyanwu et al. also successfully applied this sternotomy-avoiding technique with minor modifications [15]. Samuels et al. used a less invasive approach including an upper hemisternotomy, a left-sided lateral thoracotomy, and a partial midline upper abdominal pre-peritoneal laparotomy; the upper pre-peritoneal incision created the LVAD pocket in the subrectus muscle plane, while 2 lateral dissections connected to both inflow and outflow pathways [16]. An alternative approach was described by Riebandt et al. from Vienna: in the setting of severe thoracic aortic calcification, they anastomosed the outflow graft to the right subclavian artery [17].

23.4 Less Invasive LVAD Implantation

The first pump to be completely placed inside the pericardium by less invasive surgery was the HVAD (HeartWare Inc., Framingham, MA, USA) [9, 18–20, 36–37]. Before surgery we recommend to assess each patient by using preoperative and intraoperative checklists (▫ Tables 23.1 and 23.2). In order to perform the implant by LIS, two independent surgical steps have to be performed: (1) access to the apex of the left ventricle and (2) access to the upper mediastinum. While the first step is routinely performed by a left-sided thoracotomy (see ▫ Fig. 23.5), there are two different approaches to gain access to the ascending aorta: upper hemisternotomy or right-sided thoracotomy [9, 18]. Even though the sternum is preserved entirely, the right-sided thoracotomy can be associated with more pain, and also the access to the ascending aorta might be more challenging, too. Since surgical access to the ascending aorta is superior, the hemisternotomy is better suited for redo LVAD cases and concomitant procedures. This is important because a growing number of LVAD candidates already received prior surgical treatment such as coronary artery bypass grafting, valvular repairs, or replacements [21].

After checking the perioperative checklist, the procedure starts by placing the wire for venous cannulation through the right femoral vein into the right atrium. This should be performed under TEE control. In redo cases, it makes sense to place an additional wire or an arterial sheath into the right femoral artery previous to sternotomy. Afterward, the access to the ascending aorta is achieved either by hemisternotomy or right-sided thoracotomy with opening of the aorta-covering pericardium. Once the

Table 23.1 Preoperative patient assessment

Item	Purpose
Blood analysis	Hemogram (exclude anemia/leukocytosis) Coagulation assessment (normalize INR) HF markers (NT-proBNP) Liver enzymes (ALT, AST, LDH, Bilirubine) (acute backward failure vs. chronic liver dysfunction) Kidney function (creatinine, urea, GFR) Infection (CRP, procalcitonin) (exclude acute infection) Capillary blood gas analysis (oxygenation/decarboxylation)
Chest x-ray	Thoracic assessment (calcified aorta, pulmonary congestion, pleural effusion)
Spirometry	Lung function tests (FVC, FEV) Only viable in INTERMACS IV+ patients
Carotid Doppler	Exclude carotid stenosis
Pacemaker follow-up	Assessment of ICD or pacemaker function (exclude dysfunction/low power supply)
Transthoracic echocardiography	Assessment of the left ventricle LV-EF (Simpson), LVEDD, exclude LV aneurysm/thrombus, aortic valve function (exclude regurgitation), mitral valve function (exclude stenosis), LA diameter Assessment of the right ventricle TAPSE, tricuspid valve function (evaluate grade of regurgitation), Tissue doppler TV annulus (PW vs. CW), PASP, RVD1, RVD2, RVD3, RVOT prox, RVOT dist, 3D RV-EF (More detailed: [33])
Right heart catheterization	Assessment of cardiac output, RV function and PHT RA (sys/dia/mean), RV (sys/dia/mean), PA (sys/dia/mean), PCWP (sys/dia/mean), cardiac output*, cardiac index*, PA SO_2 *Fick's technique is most accurate in low output states and considered gold standard (More detailed assessment of RV failure risk: [34])
CT scan	Thoracic assessment in redo cases Distance heart/major vessels/sternum (exclude calcified aorta)

pericardial holding stitches are in place, aortic purse strings should be positioned. Ensure that there is enough space for later partial aortic clamping in order to perform outflow-graft anastomosis to the aorta. According to surgeon's preference, arterial cannulas especially designed for MIC surgery can help to save space. By these steps, initiation of extracorporeal circulation can be achieved fast and safely in case of unexpected instability. Next the thoracotomy is performed after echo-controlled marking of the incision and thoracic projection of the apex. This is of importance as the position of the apex varies from case to case. Usually it is found in the sixth intercostal space within the intersection of the left midclavicular line. After dissection of the pectoralis muscle, the pleura is opened, and the rip spreaders (usually two) are inserted. Even if the skin incision is kept as minimal as possible, it is important to thoroughly dissect the intracostal muscles to the left midaxillary line to avoid rip fracture. After performing the thoracotomy, the apex surrounding pericardium is opened, and the epicardial HVAD sewing ring is sutured to the left ventricular apex off-pump (see Fig. 23.6).

This step can still be performed without full heparinization, reducing apical-associated bleeding. The sewing ring is primarily fixed by 12 pledget-armed epicardial sutures. Consequently, a running suture with 4-0 prolene is performed to

Table 23.2 Intraoperative management

Item	Purpose
Swan-Ganz-Catheter	Assess RV function and continuous CO monitoring during surgery Should be placed during anaesthetization, avoid bedding the patient in a fully horizontal supine position (RV overload)
Respirator	NO application during surgery Nitric oxide should be used routinely in all LVAD implants
Transesophageal echocardiography	Perioperative assessment of cardiac function/venous cannula placement/inflow cannula placement Exclude PFO, ASD, thrombotic material in the LV/LAA The TEE transducer should be placer during anesthetization
Transthoracic echocardiography	Localization of the LV apex Once the patient is bedded inside the OR, the surgeon should seek for the 4-chamber view in order to find the projection of the LV apex to minimize the anterolateral thoracic incision
External defibrillator electrodes	The electrodes have to be placed on the backside (right shoulder and left torso) of the patient in all LIS procedures
Pacemaker/ICD	Deactivate defibrillator function during surgery by placing a magnet or direct deactivation
Skin disinfection	Disinfection should be performed according to hospital's standard covering thorax (the left side until posterior axillary line), abdomen, thighs, and genital area. When placing the drapes, keep umbilicus (landmark for driveline placement) and both inguinal regions (cannulation) free
Preparation for CPB	Cannula selection In LIS procedures, venous cannulation is usually performed by the right femoral vein (control cannula placement by TEE, vacuum-assisted drain is mandatory), and arterial cannula placement can be performed to the ascending aorta (consider using an elongated cannula) or to femoral artery In case of full sternotomy access, consider venting the LV in case the sewing ring is attached before LV coring Evaluation of CO_2 flooding
Antibiotic management	Perioperative prophylaxis should be more aggressive than in common cardiac surgery. It should be adapted according to previous microbiological tests and local guidelines but always include agents against gram-positive and gram-negative bacteria. In addition you should include a bloodstream active agent. A possible combination would be 1 g oxacillin, 1 g meropenem, 1 g vancomycin
Hemostasis	Blood products should be reserved: 6 units of packed red blood cells, 6 units of fresh frozen plasma, 2 units of thrombocytes Coagulation factors for LIS: 2 g fibrinogen Coagulation factors for sternotomy: 4 g fibrinogen + 2000 units PPSB (factors II, VII, IX, and X) + 2500 units (factor XIII)

seal the space between epicardium and sewing ring. In addition surgical glue can be used as sealant too. Next, cardiopulmonary bypass is performed targeting a mean pulmonary artery pressure of 12 mmHg. The myocardium is cored throughout the ring with the specialized tool. After coring, a careful inspection of the LV cavity should be performed in order to resect trabecular tissue that has the potential to occlude the inflow cannula. Now the HVAD pump is placed through the sewing ring into the left ventricular apex. Once the pump is placed and the apex inspected for eventual bleeding, it might be useful to vent the outflow graft for deairing LVAD and LV. Now the driveline has to be tunneled to the exit site and connected to the controller. The outflow graft is

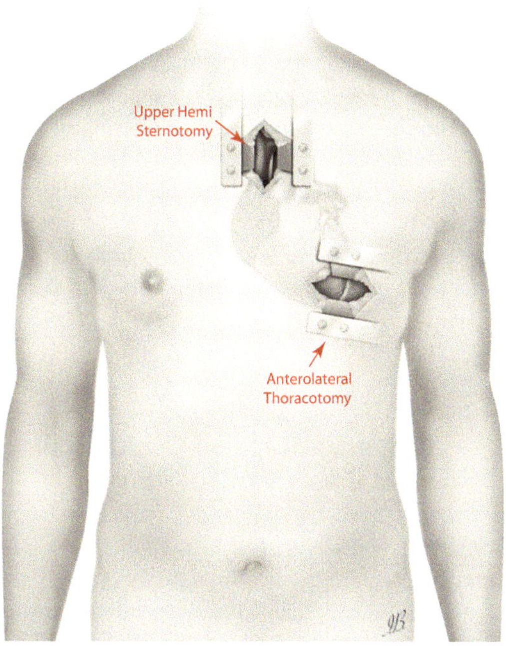

Fig. 23.5 Minimally invasive LVAD implantation, the "Hannover Approach" (Illustration by Ilaria Bondi's Peppermint Advertising)

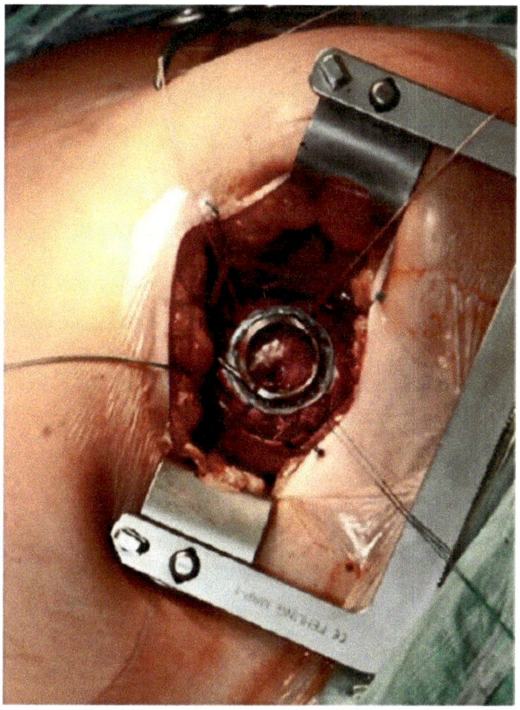

Fig. 23.6 HVAD sewing ring sutured to the apex of left ventricle by thoracotomy

then tunneled through the pericardium and then anastomosed end to side to the ascending aorta through the upper hemisternotomy. Before securing the suture by knots, it is possible to start the LVAD at minimum speed to further deair the system through the opened anastomosis. Deairing process should be controlled by transesophageal echocardiography before opening the partial clamp. Once the anastomosis is finished and the system deaired, it is time for LVAD onset and decrease of extracorporeal circulation. For this purpose, NO application and continuous application of epinephrine support RV function during and after LVAD onset. The transition from full extracorporeal circulation to full LVAD support should be performed stepwise by surgeon, anesthesiologist, and perfusionist. In this context, a key benefit of the LIS approach is that the part of pericardium that surrounds the right ventricle remains mainly closed, preserving the natural right ventricular delimitations and thereby avoiding right ventricular dilatation. In addition, the heart remains within its original position (more or less "no-touch-technique"), which avoids the RV from failing, too. Thus, right ventricular function remains passively sustained [9].

23.5 Less Invasive LVAD Exchange and Explantation

As the number of implanted LVADs is growing, the number of patients requiring a pump exchange is growing too [22]. Most important indications of LVAD exchange are extended driveline infection, LVAD thrombus, or technical fault [23]. LVAD exchange through full sternotomy implies a high-risk procedure because of tissue adhesions with increased bleeding risk [24]. Thus, in cases where the outflow graft can be preserved, it is possible to perform the LVAD exchange through left-sided thoracotomy [11]. To assess exact LVAD localization and to plan the incision, it is helpful to perform a CT scan with 3D reconstruction of the ribcage, the VDA housing, and the outflow graft prosthesis. In addition, in cases of LVAD infection, a PET-CT scan can be helpful to assess extent of infection [25]. Especially in cases of severe tissue adhesions, partial costal resection must be performed in order to gain access to the LVAD. The next step consists of identifying the outflow graft and to gain enough space for clamping it and for the later anastomosis. In LVAD exchange without thrombus formation, it is possible to perform the exchange without application of cardiopulmonary bypass. If extracorporeal circulation is required, peripheral cannulation of femoral vessels is recommended. Once everything is prepared for VAD-exchange, the LVAD must be turned off previous to outflow-graft clamping and transection. Now, the screw of the sewing ring has to be unscrewed for explanting the LVAD. In order to avoid exsanguination, the hemodynamic management is crucial at this point. Therefore, the mean arterial blood pressure and heart must be kept as low as possible. Then, the new HVAD pump has to be placed immediately through the old sewing ring into the left ventricular apex. To ensure good backward flow, retrograde flushing of the old outflow graft has to be performed before the anastomosis. Now, the outflow-graft anastomosis is performed end-to-end to the former outflow graft. The new driveline should be on to the opposite side of the old exit site. Following careful deairing of the device, the new pump can be started in situ. After closure of the left anterior-lateral thoracotomy, the old driveline of the old pump has to be fully explanted. In cases of driveline infection, the old exit site and surround infected tissue should be thoroughly excised and drained.

Despite the fact that recovery of myocardial function during LVAD support is lower than expected, considering the total number of implanted patients, the cases of successful LVAD weaning are growing too [26]. However, especially in patients without LVAD-related complications, the weighing up of operative risks and potential benefits of performing a complete LVAD explantation with ventriculoplasty might argue against surgery. Nevertheless with the development of less invasive LVAD surgery, explantation surgery can now be performed with lower risks. There are two options for less invasive LVAD explantation [10].

23.6 Option A: Ventriculoplasty with Sewing Ring Removal

The left-sided thoracotomy should be performed according the same routine as in LVAD exchange surgery. In this case, the application of cardiopulmonary bypass is mandatory. After the patient is put on extracorporeal circulation, ventricular fibrillation is electrically induced and the HVAD pump removed. The outflow graft should be closed by multiple ligations. Afterward, the sewing ring has to be detached from its sutures and the ventricle inspected for eventual LV thrombus. Finally, the ventricle has to be closed with surgical sutures and stabilized by pledgets. Following defibrillation, the patient can be weaned from extracorporeal circulation.

23.7 Option B: Sewing Ring Preservation and Occlusion with a Mechanical Plug

The surgical procedure is similar to the previously described technique, however in this case as the sewing ring is kept in place and occluded bleeding risk is considerably lower than in option A. Thus, this procedure can be performed without extracorporeal circulation. After HVAD pump removal, a specially designed mechanical plug is inserted and fixed by the sewing ring screw. As previously described, the remaining outflow graft is sutured distally and remained in situ [10].

23.8 Discussion

The surgical treatment of terminal heart failure has been experiencing a paradigm change through the past years. While cardiac transplantation has been considered as the gold standard of treatment for patients with terminal heart failure, the continuously growing gap between the number of donor hearts and the number of candidates has led to an increased mortality rate on the waiting list. Even in countries with traditional high donor rates like Spain, cardiac transplantation has decreased, leading to the circumstance that cardiac transplantation is increasingly performed on patients fulfilling high-urgency criteria [27]. Thus, LVAD implantation has become a serious alternative for patients with terminal heart failure, being often considered as first choice before putting patients on the transplant list. Continuous technical improvements, enhanced patient selection, and perioperative management have improved operative outcomes reaching 90% of 6-month survival [36]. These short-term results are comparable to those of heart transplant recipients. Despite these major advances, some hurdles like perioperative bleeding, right ventricular failure, driveline infections, and thrombus formation remain unsolved. From another perspective, rising implantation number have also provoked higher hospitalization costs. As conventional LVAD procedures have been associated with major incisions, high complication rates, and poor outcomes, less invasive LVAD surgery represents a paradigm shift especially in view of abovementioned challenges. The introduction of minimally invasive techniques is changing the entire field with promising expectations [9, 12, 14, 28]: minimally invasive procedures not only mean smaller incisions with less operative trauma or blood loss but also imply shorter hospital stays with lower hospitalization costs [29, 30]. Less invasive LVAD implantation has also changed the organization standard in the operation room: traditionally with only one incision (i.e., full sternotomy), only one surgeon was capable to operate. Now, with the two-folded approach (hemisternotomy and lateral thoracotomy), two surgeons can work parallel together in a time-sparing joint venture. Furthermore, Khalpey et al. developed a robotic technique for LVAD implantation (r-VAD) that enables total endoscopic anastomosis of the aortic outflow graft [31, 32]. Although less invasive LVAD surgery is generating much well-deserved enthusiasm among surgical community, the need for caution cannot be overemphasized – particularly since comparative studies with mid-term and long-term results are still missing. Another limitation of less invasive LVAD surgery is the realization of concomitant procedures. While aortic valve replacement can be performed routinely by upper hemisternotomy [30], surgery of the tricuspid valve, patent foramen ovale (PFO) closure, or left atrial appendectomy are currently not being performed routinely as concomitant procedures in LVAD surgery by less invasive techniques. Especially in cases of moderate tricuspid regurgitation, minor aortic valve regurgitation, or small PFO, there is presently no consensus if patients take benefit of concomitant surgery in addition to LVAD implantation. As patient selection and management for LVAD surgery are complex, the heart team has to take individual decisions for each patient being diligent in evaluating the risk benefit ratio. In the future, experience with larger patient numbers of long-term VAD support (>5 years) will help to elucidate the impact of atrial fibrillation, aortic insufficiency, tricuspid regurgitation, or mitral valve regurgitation during long-term LVAD support. In some institutions, all patients that are enrolled for HVAD implantation will already undergo less invasive surgery unless concomitant procedures are planned. Thus, most of the patients can be included for less invasive LVAD implantation. In this context, the incidence of conversion to sternotomy in HVAD implantations is neglectable. Still, a potential cause of conversion to full sternotomy is uncontrolled apical bleeding after LVAD placement.

In contrast to other cardiothoracic procedures, less invasive LVAD surgery has been introduced only recently. Therefore, no comparative studies showing mid-term or long-term results have been published. However, with several ongoing studies, it is expected that several prospective studies about this subject will be published during the next year.

Another important discussion point in less invasive LVAD surgery is the application of cardiopulmonary bypass. The avoidance of cardiopulmonary bypass has two important benefits: it shortens the surgical time and decreases activation of the inflammatory and coagulation cascade decreasing the incidence of vasoplegia and coagulopathy which often occur following LVAD surgery [18]. However, LVAD candidates with terminal heart failure might decompensate due to cardiac manipulations during implantation. In these cases, on-pump surgery is a much safer alternative. Even with future LVAD studies in the pipeline investigating these topics, implantation strategies are always patient specific, and surgeons adopting minimally invasive techniques must be diligent in evaluating their results to ensure the highest quality of LVAD implantations. Regarding the impact of new devices hitting field, the Heartmate 3 (St. Jude Medical) showed excellent results in the CE mark trial. Survival rates after 6 months were over 90%, and none of the patients suffered from pump thrombosis and hemolytic events or required pump exchange. On the other hand, the MVAD is designed to become the first full-support LVAD system for less invasive implantation. It is considerably decreased in its size with enhanced positioning capabilities.

23.9 Conclusion

Given all these benefits and having the perspective of more and more LVAD implantations worldwide, we are convinced that the future of LVAD surgery will be marked by novel technical features as well as by less invasive implantation techniques.

References

1. Lund LH, Edwards LB, Kucheryavaya AY, Benden C, Dipchand AI, Goldfarb S, Levvey BJ, Meiser B, Rossano JW, Yusen RD, Stehlik J (2015) The registry of the international society for heart and lung transplantation: thirty-second official adult heart transplantation report – 2015; focus theme: early graft failure. J Heart Lung Transplant 34:1244–1254. doi:10.1016/j.healun.2015.08.003
2. Rose EA, Gelijns AC, Moskowitz AJ, Heitjan DF, Stevenson LW, Dembitsky W, Long JW, Ascheim DD, Tierney AR, Levitan RG, Watson JT, Meier P, Ronan NS, Shapiro PA, Lazar RM, Miller LW, Gupta L, Frazier OH, Desvigne-Nickens P, Oz MC, Poirier VL, Randomized Evaluation of Mechanical Assistance for the Treatment of Congestive Heart Failure (REMATCH) Study Group (2001) Long-term use of a left ventricular assist device for end-stage heart failure. N Engl J Med 345:1435–1443. doi:10.1056/NEJMoa012175
3. Slaughter MS, Rogers JG, Milano CA, Russell SD, Conte JV, Feldman D, Sun B, Tatooles AJ, Delgado RM, Long JW, Wozniak TC, Ghumman W, Farrar DJ, Frazier OH, HeartMate II Investigators (2009) Advanced heart failure treated with continuous-flow left ventricular assist device. N Engl J Med 361:2241–2251. doi:10.1056/NEJMoa0909938
4. Strueber M, O'Driscoll G, Jansz P, Khaghani A, Levy WC, Wieselthaler GM, Investigators HW (2011) Multicenter evaluation of an intrapericardial left ventricular assist system. J Am Coll Cardiol 57:1375–1382. doi:10.1016/j.jacc.2010.10.040
5. Kirklin JK, Naftel DC, Pagani FD, Kormos RL, Stevenson LW, Blume ED, Myers SL, Miller MA, Baldwin JT, Young JB (2015) Seventh INTERMACS annual report: 15,000 patients and counting. J Heart Lung Transplant 34:1495–1504. doi:10.1016/j.healun.2015.10.003
6. Rojas SV, Avsar M, Hanke JS, Khalpey Z, Maltais S, Haverich A, Schmitto JD (2015) Minimally invasive ventricular assist device surgery. Artif Organs 39:473–479. doi:10.1111/aor.12422
7. Rojas SV, Avsar M, Uribarri A, Hanke JS, Haverich A, Schmitto JD (2015) A new era of ventricular assist device surgery: less invasive procedures. Minerva Chir 70:63–68
8. Pedemonte O, Vera A, Schmitto JD, Rojas SV, Haverich A, Merello L, Novajas M, Aranda F, Ibarra J, Muñoz JA, Albuquerque J, Diaz R, Aranguiz-Santander E (2014) Asistencia ventricular intracorpórea en falla cardiaca terminal. Rev Med Chil 142:914–918
9. Schmitto JD, Molitoris U, Haverich A, Strueber M (2012) Implantation of a centrifugal pump as a left ventricular assist device through a novel, minimized approach: upper hemisternotomy combined with anterolateral thoracotomy. J Thorac Cardiovasc Surg 143:511–513. doi:10.1016/j.jtcvs.2011.07.046
10. Schmitto JD, Rojas SV, Hanke JS, Avsar M, Haverich A (2014) Minimally invasive left ventricular assist device explantation after cardiac recovery: surgical technical considerations. Artif Organs 38:507–510. doi:10.1111/aor.12201
11. Rojas SV, Avsar M, Khalpey Z, Hanke JS, Haverich A, Schmitto JD (2014) Minimally invasive off-pump left ventricular assist device exchange: anterolateral thoracotomy. Artif Organs 38:539–542. doi:10.1111/aor.12226
12. Hill JD, Avery GJ, Egrie G, Turley K, Reichenbach S (2000) Less invasive Thoratec LVAD insertion: a surgical technique. Heart Surg Forum 3:218–223
13. Gregoric ID, La Francesca S, Myers T, Cohn W, Loyalka P, Kar B, Gemmato C, Frazier OH (2008) A less invasive approach to axial flow pump insertion. J Heart Lung Transplant 27:423–426. doi:10.1016/j.healun.2008.01.002
14. Gregoric ID, Bruckner BA, Jacob L, Kar B, Cohn WE, La Francesca S, Frazier OH (2008) Clinical experience with sternotomy versus subcostal approach for exchange of the heartMate XVE to the HeartMate II ventricular assist device. Ann Thorac Surg 85:1646–1649. doi:10.1016/j.athoracsur.2008.01.020
15. Anyanwu AC (2011) Technique for less invasive implantation of Heartmate II left ventricular assist device without median sternotomy. Semin Thorac Cardiovasc Surg 23:241–244. doi:10.1053/j.semtcvs.2011.10.002
16. Samuels LE, Casanova-Ghosh E, Rodriguez R, Droogan C (2012) Left ventricular assist device implantation in high risk destination therapy patients: an alternative surgical approach. J Cardiothorac Surg 7:21. doi:10.1186/1749-8090-7-21
17. Riebandt J, Sandner S, Mahr S, Haberl T, Rajek A, Laufer G, Schima H, Zimpfer D (2013) Minimally invasive thoratec Heartmate II implantation in the setting of severe thoracic aortic calcification. Ann Thorac Surg 96:1094–1096. doi:10.1016/j.athoracsur.2013.04.114
18. Cheung A, Lamarche Y, Kaan A, Munt B, Doyle A, Bashir J, Janz P (2011) Off-pump implantation of the HeartWare HVAD left ventricular assist device through minimally invasive incisions. Ann Thorac Surg 91:1294–1296. doi:10.1016/j.athoracsur.2010.08.031
19. Popov AF, Hosseini MT, Zych B, Simon AR, Bahrami T (2012) HeartWare left ventricular assist device implantation through bilateral anterior thoracotomy. Ann Thorac Surg 93:674–676. doi:10.1016/j.athoracsur.2011.09.055
20. Maltais S, Davis ME, Haglund N (2014) Minimally invasive and alternative approaches for long-term LVAD

placement: the Vanderbilt strategy. Ann Cardiothorac Surg 3:563–569. doi:10.3978/j.issn.2225-319X.2014.10.02

21. Kirklin JK, Naftel DC, Pagani FD, Kormos RL, Stevenson LW, Blume ED, Miller MA, Baldwin JT, Young JB (2014) Sixth INTERMACS annual report: a 10,000-patient database. J Heart Lung Transplant 33:555–564. doi:10.1016/j.healun.2014.04.010
22. Moazami N, Milano CA, John R, Sun B, Adamson RM, Pagani FD, Smedira N, Slaughter MS, Farrar DJ, Frazier OH, HeartMate II Investigators (2012) Pump replacement for left ventricular assist device failure can be done safely and is associated with low mortality. Ann Thorac Surg 95:500–505. doi:10.1016/j.athoracsur.2012.09.011
23. Stulak JM, Cowger J, Haft JW, Romano MA, Aaronson KD, Pagani FD (2012) Device exchange after primary left ventricular assist device implantation: indications and outcomes. Ann Thorac Surg 95:1262–1268. doi:10.1016/j.athoracsur.2012.08.031
24. Gregoric ID (2008) Exchange techniques for implantable ventricular assist devices. ASAIO J 54:14–19. doi:10.1097/MAT.0b013e318161d705
25. Kim J, Feller ED, Chen W, Dilsizian V (2014) FDG PET/CT imaging for LVAD associated infections. JACC Cardiovasc Imaging 7:839–842. doi:10.1016/j.jcmg.2014.04.013
26. Dandel M, Weng Y, Siniawski H, Potapov E, Lehmkuhl HB, Hetzer R (2005) Long-term results in patients with idiopathic dilated cardiomyopathy after weaning from left ventricular assist devices. Circulation 112:I37–I45. doi:10.1161/CIRCULATIONAHA.104.525352
27. González-Vílchez F, Gómez-Bueno M, Almenar L, Crespo-Leiro MG, Arizón JM, Palomo J, Delgado J, Roig E, Lage E, Manito N (2014) Registro Español de Trasplante Cardiaco. XXV Informe Oficial de la Sección de Insuficiencia Cardiaca y Trasplante Cardiaco de la Sociedad Española de Cardiología (1984-2013). Rev Esp Cardiol 67:1039–1051. doi:10.1016/j.recesp.2014.09.004
28. Schmitto JD, Ortmann P, Akdis M, Alekuzei H, Steinke K, Kolat P, Popov AF, Liakopoulos OJ, Waldmann-Beushausen R, Mirzaie M, Grossmann M, Seipelt R, Schöndube FA (2008) Miniaturized HIA microdiagonal pump as left ventricular assist device in a sheep model. ASAIO J 54:233–236. doi:10.1097/MAT.0b013e318175258e
29. Schmitto JD, Mokashi SA, Cohn LH (2010) Minimally-invasive valve surgery. J Am Coll Cardiol 56:455–462. doi:10.1016/j.jacc.2010.03.053
30. Rojas SV, Haverich A (2013) Minimally invasive cardiac surgery: a safe alternative for aortic valve replacement? Rev Esp Cardiol (Engl Ed) 66:685–686. doi:10.1016/j.rec.2013.05.010
31. Khalpey Z, Riaz IB, Marsh KM, Ansari MZA, Bilal J, Cooper A, Paidy S, Schmitto JD, Smith R, Friedman M, Slepian MJ, Poston R (2015) Robotic left ventricular assist device (LVAD) implantation using left thoracotomy approach in patients with previous sternotomies. ASAIO J 61:e44–e46. doi:10.1097/MAT.0000000000000251
32. Khalpey Z, Sydow N, Paidy S, Slepian MJ, Friedman M, Cooper A, Marsh KM, Schmitto JD, Poston R (2014) Robotic-assisted implantation of ventricular assist device after sternectomy and pectoralis muscle flap. ASAIO J 60(6):742–743
33. Rudski LG, Lai WW, Afilalo J, Hua L, Handschumacher MD, Chandrasekaran K, Solomon SD, Louie EK, Schiller NB (2010) Guidelines for the echocardiographic assessment of the right heart in adults: a report from the American Society of Echocardiography endorsed by the European Association of Echocardiography, a registered branch of the European Society of Cardiology, and the Canadian Society of Echocardiography. J Am Soc Echocardiogr 23:685–713. doi:10.1016/j.echo.2010.05.010quiz 786–8
34. Dandel M, Potapov E, Krabatsch T, Stepanenko A, Löw A, Vierecke J, Knosalla C, Hetzer R (2013) Load dependency of right ventricular performance is a major factor to be considered in decision making before ventricular assist device implantation. Circulation 128:S14–S23. doi:10.1161/CIRCULATIONAHA.112.000335
35. Hanke JS, Avsar M, Haverich A, Schmitto JD (2015) Heart-Failing Jehovah's Witness Patient Successfully Treated by Minimally Invasive LVAD Implantation without Any Blood Transfusions. Thorac Cardiovasc Surg Rep 4(1):21–4
36. Hanke JS, Rojas SV, Avsar M, Bara C, Ismail I, Haverich A, et al. (2016) HeartWare left ventricular assist device for the treatment of advanced heart failure. Future Cardiol. 12(1):17–26
37. Hanke JS, Rojas SV, Avsar M, Haverich A, Schmitto JD (2015) Minimally-invasive LVAD Implantation: State of the Art. Curr Cardiol Rev 11(3):246–51
38. Hanke JS, Rojas SV, Martens A, Schmitto JD (2015) Minimally invasive left ventricular assist device implantation with outflow graft anastomosis to the innominate artery. J Thorac Cardiovasc Surg 149(4):e69–70

Minimal Invasive: Padua's Approach and Technique

Tomaso Bottio, Jonida Bejko, Vincenzo Tarzia, and Gino Gerosa

© Springer International Publishing Switzerland 2017
A. Montalto et al. (eds.), *Mechanical Circulatory Support in End-Stage Heart Failure*,
DOI 10.1007/978-3-319-43383-7_24

24.1 Introduction

Heart transplantation is the most effective method of enhancing quality of life and survival in end-stage heart failure (HF) patients. Unfortunately, the Achilles' heel of this excellent treatment is the severe shortage of donor organs. Consequent to this mismatch between supply and demand, of particular importance has become the application of the ventricular assist devices (VADs) [1–9]. The field of circulatory support has matured dramatically in recent years, thanks to the advent of smaller, rotary pumps and new surgical and anesthetic solutions. These improvements have changed the face of advanced heart failure care [10, 11]. New management strategies associated to new pump technology over the years modified the mechanical circulatory support (MCS) candidate selection and risk stratification. In the next future, familiarity with newer pump devices and patient management strategies should accelerate the timing and improve the referral for MCS evaluation.

Therefore, MCS device use in severe heart failure, opened to discussion decades ago, is now well established, either for temporary support such as bridge to transplantation or destination therapy [4]. Consequently, left ventricular assist devices (LVADs) have become nowadays the principle alternative treatment for end-stage heart failure unresponsive to optimal medical therapy.

The typical VAD candidate is commonly very compromised and may not have sufficient resources to tolerate major surgical insults and trauma. Therefore, device implantation through smaller, less traumatic incisions is a desirable goal. The median sternotomy decreases lung volumes and reduces thoracic motion with significant decrease in functional residual capacity and total lung capacity months later [12]. Minimally invasive cardiac surgery via mini-thoracotomy was devised to reduce morbidity because of potentially less inflammatory response and reduce transfusion requirements and scarring, with consequent rapid rehabilitation to normal life activity [13]. Additionally, avoiding the cardiopulmonary circulatory support (CPB) even for short period of time might reduce the release of inflammatory cytokines and their consequences, as most CPB-related damage happens within the first few minutes [14, 15].

Different approaches are described for implantation of VADs, including off-pump [16], subcostal [11], or mini upper sternotomy implantation [17]. In this chapter, we describe the minimally invasive techniques used for the implantation of an LVAD that involve three distinct professional figures within the operating room: the surgeon, the anesthesiologist, and the perfusion technician [18–24].

24.2 Why Should It Be Considered a Minimally Invasive LVAD Implantation Technique

Off-pump implantation: Avoiding CPB reduces the release of inflammatory cascade and its consequences [8, 11, 13]. The reduced heparin dose necessary for the off-pump implantation favors a reduction in intraoperative and postoperative bleeding and thus a decreased blood unit transfusion and immunization, particularly important for patient's bridge to transplantation.

Minimally invasive surgical approach: There is a growing trend toward the use of non-sternotomy incisions and/or mini-thoracotomy in all fields of cardiac surgery [14, 15]. Although full-median sternotomy provides the best access to the heart and the adjacent structures, it can be replaced by smaller incisions in most of the cases. The choice for minimally invasive approaches was powered by the possibility of a preserved good exposure of the great vessels (through upper mini-sternotomy or II intercostal space mini-thoracotomy) and the minimal displacement of the heart for left ventricle apex exposure (through mini-thoracotomy), with decreased rate of arrhythmias and hemodynamic instability related to the heart manipulation, mandatory when in full sternotomy. Additionally, less-extensive mediastinal dissection reduces the risk and the degree of postoperative bleeding.

Paravertebral analgesia and mild general anesthesia: The hemodynamic fragility of these patients is well reported, and renal insufficiency, pulmonary hypertension, as well as COPD stand out as risk factors. Furthermore, when a prolonged mechanical ventilation is required, the cerebral perfusion and oxygenation are compromised [12, 25–33]. In order to improve the patient management, paravertebral analgesia has been suggested in association to a mild general anesthesia. Many authors [12, 25–33] have confirmed the advantages and efficacy of continuous paravertebral block (PVB) for analgesic treatment of thoracotomies when compared to epidural analgesia with lower complication rate (pulmonary, renal, gastrointestinal, and hemodynamic). Additionally, PVB provides safe, effective analgesia, diminishes the early reduction of postoperative pulmonary function, and restores respiratory mechanics more rapidly, with consequent facilitated extubation. The local anesthetics migrate from this injection site, both caudally and rostrally, and produce unilateral somatic and sympathetic nerve blockade. The risk of wrong positioning the PVB catheter in the epidural or spinal space with subsequent risk of epidural hematoma is considered low when the preoperative coagulation tests are normal and when lower doses of heparin are administrated. Same low risk was considered when PVB catheter is removed 48 h after surgery. This analgesia does not influence the hemodynamic stability and permits a mild general anesthesia approach.

24.3 Padua Experience

From December 2008 to January 2016, 96 patients with HF refractory to medical therapy were implanted with the last-generation LVAD: 53 % with Jarvik 2000 (Jarvik 2000 (Jarvik Heart Inc., New York, NY)) and 44 % with HeartWare HVAD (HeartWare Inc., Framingham, MA). Three additional patients (3 %) received HeartMate II (Thoratec, Pleasanton, California) (two patients) and HeartMate III VAD (Thoratec Corp, Pleasanton, CA) (one patient). Mainly male patients (83.1 %) with dilated cardiomyopathy prevalent (58.5 %), followed by ischemic (33.7 %) and fewer different cardiomyopathies such as peripartum, myocarditis, amyloidosis, and arrhythmogenic, came to our attention in very compromised hemodynamic conditions (INTERMACS I and II 92.3 %). Initially, the policy of our center was the implantation of Jarvik 2000 as destination therapy (DT) and HeartWare HVAD as bridge to transplantation (BTT). Recently, we focus on the expected duration of assistance (short or long time), right ventricle performance, pulmonary artery pressure, BSA, technical considerations, pathology, residency, behavior of the coagulation system, and INTERMACS class.

Hereunder are described the different procedures adopted for the implantation of different models of VAD. Afterward, a step-by-step description of the evolution of minimally invasive implantation techniques, for each model of VAD used at the Cardiac Surgery Unit of Padua, is described, with also a discussion of the tricks and traps of the surgical and anesthetic aspect for each evolution of the minimally invasive procedures.

24.4 Anesthesia: Paravertebral Block

In the operating room, after light sedation (IV 1 mg midazolam), thoracic paravertebral block (PVB) is performed in the awake patient placed in lateral or sitting position by skillful anesthesiologist. After local anesthetic infiltration of the skin and muscular plane (5 ml lidocaine 2 %), a Tuohy 17-gauge needle is inserted at level of T4-T5, 3 cm on the left side of the spinous process of the T4 dorsalis vertebra. Identification of the paravertebral space is done by *loss-of-resistance* technique, without ultrasound or nerve stimulator, first identifying T4 transversus process with a recently reviewed technique [33]. According to the surgical approach (mono- or bithoracotomic), asymmetric mono- and/or bilateral PVB analgesia is performed. The left block is set by a catheter inserted 3 cm on the left side of the spinous process of T4 dorsalis vertebra, between fourth and fifth inter-transverse process, and the right PVB is established by a catheter inserted 3 cm on the right of the spinous process of T2 dorsalis vertebra, between third and fourth inter-transverse process.

When paravertebral space is reached, an epidural catheter (19 gauge) is inserted and left at 2 cm beyond the tip of the needle. A subcutaneous tunnel is made for avoiding accidental catheter removal. A cumulative dose of 20 ml of 0.5 % ropivacaine (100 mg) is done for intraoperative analgesia (10 ml at left mini-thoracotomy closure). Induction of general anesthesia is performed with doses of sodium thiopental (4 mg/kg), fentanyl (200 mcg total dose), and rocuronium (0.6 mg/kg). A single lumen tube (monolateral approach) or a bi-lumen endotracheal tube (bilateral approach) is inserted for endotracheal intubation and mechanical ventilation performed with a protective strategy (tidal volume 8 ml/kg, respiratory rate 10 b/min, PEEP: 4 cmH2O). Anesthesia is maintained by propofol (3–5 mg/kg/h) and remifentanil infusions (0.05–0.1 mcg/kg/min). At the end of the surgical procedure, remifentanil and propofol infusion are suspended, and extubation is performed if possible in short time in OR, in order to guarantee afterload reduction of the right ventricle. The patients are transferred to the ICU. Postoperative pain control is assured by 0.2 % ropivacaine continuous infusion at speed of 5 ml/h by paravertebral route, intravenous continuous infusion (elastomeric device) at 3 mcg/h of sufentanil, and intravenous analgesics upon patient request. PVB catheter is maintained for 48 hrs and afterward removed.

24.5 General Anesthesia

As premedication, flunitrazepam, 2 mg, is administered orally 90 mins before surgery. On arrival in the operating room, a large-bore peripheral venous catheter and a radial artery catheter are inserted. After baseline monitoring, intravenous (IV) anesthesia is induced, following preoxygenation, over a period of 10 mins with thiopental, 1.5 mg/kg; fentanyl, 5 mcg/kg; and rocuronium, 0.6 mg/kg. Endotracheal intubation is performed 5 mins after administration of rocuronium, and controlled ventilation with oxygen/air (FIO_2 = 0.6) is instituted to normocapnia (end-tidal PCO_2 35–40 mmHg). Endotracheal intubation is performed with single or double lumen tube, with possibility to exclude right or left lung when necessary. After induction of anesthesia, a central venous catheter is inserted in the right internal jugular vein. The central venous catheter (CVC) is positioned on the left jugular vein for not cluttering the pedestal implant procedure (in case of Jarvik 2000 implantation). In this phase, anesthesia is maintained with continuous inhalation of sevoflurane (0.9 %) and sufentanil (0.1 mcg/kg/h). Before thoracotomy and mini-sternotomy, IV continuous infusion of propofol at a rate of 4–6 mg/kg/h is started. During and after the incisions, both groups are supplemented with intermittent boluses (5 mcg/kg) of fentanyl (up to a total maintenance dose of 30 mcg/kg) received prophylactically to blunt brief but intense periods of pain and autonomic stimulation (sternal splitting and spread, aortic mobilization, clamping and de-clamping, and sternal thoracotomy closure). Each patient receives 0.025 mg/kg of pancuronium every hour for muscle relaxation and mechanical ventilation during surgery. Propofol infusion is stopped at the end of surgery, and extubation is performed if possible in the operating room (OR). Postoperative pain control is assured by intravenous continuous infusion (elastomeric device) at 3 mcg/h of sufentanil at the first 48 postoperative hours and intravenous analgesics upon patient request.

24.6 Common Anesthetist Strategies

In both modalities, anesthesia is monitored by the bispectral index of the EEG (BIS) [BIS® monitor; Aspect MS, Newton, MA-USA]. A Swan-Ganz catheter and a transesophageal echocardiography probe are inserted for monitoring right and left ventricular function and LVAD inflow cannula orientation. The visual analog scale (VAS) is used to assess the quality of analgesia, and data are collected at 1, 6, 24, and 48 h postoperatively [18–24].

24.7 Surgical Technique Evolution at Padua University

Initially the routine technique was the left thoracotomy (17 pts.; 17.8 %). It currently is used only in cases of reoperation or impossibility to approach the ascending aorta. Subsequently, we experienced full sternotomy for only 13 cases (13.5 %). Almost immediately, the technique evolved toward a less invasive approach with the combination of the anterior left mini-thoracotomy (LMT) to high mini-sternotomy (28 pts.; 29.2 %). Nowadays, the approach of choice is the association of anterior LMT in fifth intercostal space with anterior right mini-thoracotomy (RMT) in II intercostal space (32 pts.; 33.4 %) or left axillary artery (6 pts.; 6.1 %).

24.8 Implant Procedure

▪▪ **LMT associated to mini-midline upper sternotomy:**

(off-pump implantation and thoracic monolateral PVB analgesia)

- **Surgical times:**

First step: LVAD implantation requires LV apex isolation, for inflow cannula insertion. In minimally invasive approaches, the isolation of the cardiac apex is obtained through a 5–8 cm LMT. The patient is placed in supine position, as usually in cardiac surgery for a sternotomy access. The skin incision is performed in correspondence of the first intercostal space below the left areola in men and in correspondence of the submammary sulcus in women. The intercostal space target depends on the location of the heart apex and is detected by physical palpation or with the aid of echocardiography. In most of the cases, it matches with the fifth intercostal space. After incision of the intercostal muscles and the pleural space, a soft tissue retractor is used for exposure and a rib retractor is positioned. The left lung is at this phase excluded from the ventilation, providing a good exposure of the apical pericardium, that once opened is fixed to the skin, so as to displace out the cardiac apex and also to reduce interference with the left lung. The insertion site of LVAD is marked on the LV by echocardiographic assessment using a finger on the apex for mimicking the inflow cannula. At this stage, we are ready to prepare the apical sewing cuff to which to anchor the VAD. This is the single action during minimally invasive VAD implantation, which is equal for all the available devices and for all the different procedures (◘ Fig. 24.1).

Second step: When we decide to proceed toward mini-sternotomy, we can saw the manubrium and/or the manubrium and part of the body, up to the third–fourth intercostal space. The outflow vascular graft is tunneled and stretched underneath the left mini-thoracotomy to the high mini-sternotomy, in order to measure

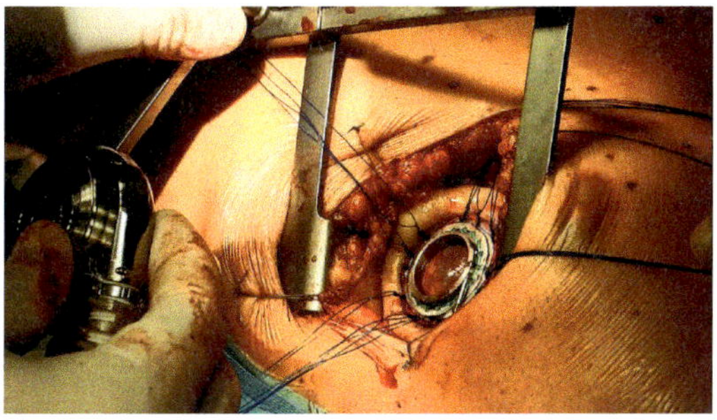

◘ **Fig. 24.1** Left mini-thoracotomy for HVAD implantation

and next cut the right length of the graft without kinking or overstretching it. According to the extension of the mini-sternotomy, a different section of the ascending aorta is exposed. When mini-sternotomy up to the fourth intercostal space is performed, the outflow graft anastomosis will match with the anterior face of the aorta, in its portion near the sino-tubular junction. Otherwise, when the sternum is split up to the third intercostal space, the anastomosis will be performed in correspondence of the frontal face of the ascending aorta in an intermediate position between the sino-tubular junction and the trunk anonymous emergency. Finally, if the sole sternal manubrium is interrupted, the anastomosis will be in the front position of the aorta, close to the emergence of anonymous arterial trunk. In all cases, the outflow graft anastomosis is performed with the aid of a side clamp on the ascending aorta.

Third step: The timing and methods for the driveline management are different depending on the device.

For the HVAD, the technique is simple and rapid: the driveline is tunneled subcutaneously from LMT to the exit point at left lower abdominal quadrant and thereafter re-tunneled to exit its tip contralaterally at right lower abdominal quadrant.

For the Jarvik 2000, the driveline positioning is more complex and time-consuming: the power cable is tunneled through the LMT underneath the pericardium following the profile, by using a blunt-tip instrument, and stretched to the upper mini-sternotomy. The pedestal is then secured to the parietal bone behind and slightly above, indifferently the right or left ear. A C-shaped incision is performed around the ear, and a full-thickness flap is raised down to the periosteum. Recently we changed the incision shape versus a straight line incision, to preserve the vascularization of the flap. The periosteum is elevated beneath the skin flap, and a template is used to define the position of the bone screws. Any skull irregularity is burred-off to give a flat surface. The three-pin connector is tunneled from the jugular space, through the neck, to the behind-the-ear connector position, and then inserted in the titanium pedestal. To convey the three-pin connector and power cable to the skull pedestal site, the incision is made on the neck, almost 2 cm under the basis of the ear. The tunneling is achieved by inserting the three-pin connector within the end of an intercostal drain. The drain is withdrawn out of the chest and through the neck to the scalp. The three-pin connector is then inserted through the titanium pedestal. This is then implanted firmly onto the external table by using 7 or 8 mm bone screws. The postauricular skin flap is repositioned with the percutaneous pedestal through the punched-out defect. The scalp and skin incisions are then closed securely. The external power cable is attached to the skull pedestal, and with the Jarvik 2000 LVAD outside the ventricle, the power is switched on to test the device in a basket filled with saline solution.

Fourth step: The VAD sewing ring is secured by using interrupted 2–0 polypropylene-pledgeted sutures and sealing the suture line applying BioGlue (CryoLife, Kennesaw, GA). Once 5000 UI of heparin is administered, VAD inflow cannula is off-pump inserted into LV through the apex. The correct housing position of the cannula is echocardiographically monitored and then tightened the sewing ring (■ Fig. 24.2).

Fifth step: A side clamp is placed on the ascending aorta and the outflow graft anastomosed, by using a 4-0 RBII polypropylene suture, and then reinforced with BioGlue surgical adhesive. After complete deairing, the outflow graft cross clamp is released and gradually increased pump speed to achieve the desired flow.

Sixth step: Once suspended remifentanil and propofol infusions, the patient is extubated when possible, in short time in OR, in order to guarantee self-inotropic support and afterload reduction to right ventricle. The patient is then transferred in the ICU.

Seventh step: Postoperative pain control is assured by continuous infusions of 0.2 % paravertebral ropivacaine at 5 ml/h speed when PVB is performed, in addition to 3 mcg/h in elastomeric device of sufentanil and paracetamol boluses (1 g/6 h). The visual analog scale is used to assess the quality of analgesia with a target between 2 and 3. PVB catheter is maintained for almost 48 hrs and removed when the patient is discharged from ICU.

LMT associated to right mini-thoracotomy:
(off-pump implantation and bilateral-thoracic PVB analgesia)

Surgical times:
First step: *(See First step of the previous paragraph.)*

Second step: The procedure continues through an incision in the second right intercostal space (RMT). The medial edge of the surgical incision should correspond 1.1–1.5 cm lateral to the right margin of the sternal bone and the course of the right internal mammary artery. The lateral edge is extended for 4–5 cm along the intercostal space without rib resection (■ Fig. 24.3). Once dissected the subcutaneous tissue, the fascia and the intercostal muscle, the pleural space is opened and the right lung is gently pushed down with moist gauze. The right lung is at this time excluded from the ventilation. The internal thoracic artery and vein are isolated and interrupted by applying two clips. The space is better exposed by using a soft tissue retractor and rib retractor. The anterolateral mediastinal fat tissue and thymic remnants are dissected and coagulated for better hemostasis. Particular attention should be paid to hemostasis of fat tissue, because this maneuver would become very complicated if delayed at the end of the procedure. Once opened the pericardium longitudinally, and fixed it to the skin (medial edge of the pericardium), in the foreground appears the

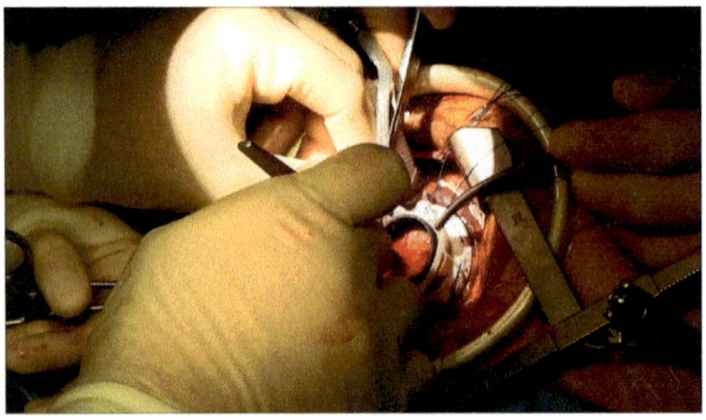

■ **Fig. 24.2** Left mini-thoracotomy for Jarvik 2000 implantation

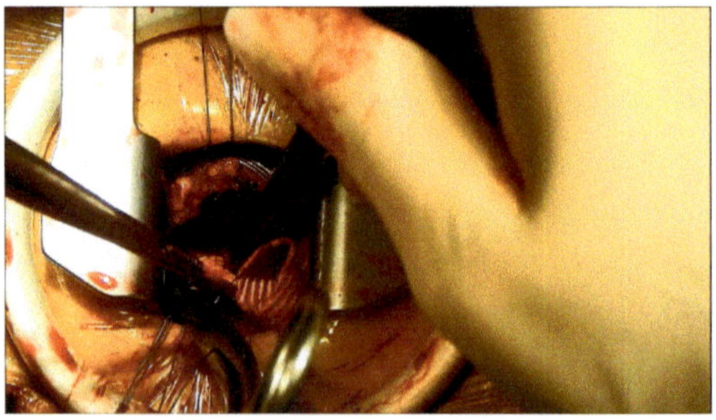

■ **Fig. 24.3** Right mini-thoracotomy for ascending aorta exposure during Jarvik 2000 implantation

ascending aorta, on a lower level the superior vena cava, while the right atrial appendage in a few cases overhangs the ascending aorta. The pulmonary artery on the contrary lies much deeper in the chest, and the best maneuver to manage it is to release the pericardium (medial edge) and to pull on the pericardium (distal edge) in order to cause a twisting of the great vessel axis, shifting the pulmonary artery in a higher plane than the aorta. The outflow graft is then tunneled through the LMT underneath the pericardium following the profile, by using a blunt-tip instrument, and stretched to the RMT.

Third step: The timing and methods for the driveline management are different depending on the device.

The HVAD driveline positioning is the same already described in the previous chapter (LMT associated to mini-sternotomy).

The Jarvik 2000 power cable supply is more tough and time-consuming: the power cable is tunneled through the LMT underneath the pericardium following the profile, by using a blunt-tip instrument, and stretched to the upper mini-thoracotomy.

The pedestal is then secured to the parietal bone behind and slightly above the right ear *(see third step of the previous procedure)*. The choice of positioning the pedestal on the right side is detected by major facility of tunneling the power cable from the second right intercostal space than tunneling it from the fifth intercostal LMT. The three-pin connector is tunneled from the RMT, through the neck, to the behind-the-ear connector position, and then inserted in the titanium pedestal. To convey the three-pin connector and power cable to the skull pedestal site, the incisions are made at the first 1 cm under the clavicle bone and the other on the neck, almost 2 cm under the basis of the ear. In case we want to avoid the subclavicular incision, the driveline can be tunnelized with a single incision along the neck. The tunneling is achieved by inserting the three-pin connector within the end of an intercostal drain. The drain is withdrawn out of the chest and through the neck to the scalp. The three-pin connector is then inserted through the titanium pedestal and is implanted firmly onto the external table by using 7 or 8 mm bone screws. The postauricular skin flap and scalp are sutured back with the percutaneous pedestal through the punched-out defect. The external power cable is attached to the skull pedestal, and the LVAD switched on and tested in a basket filled with saline solution.

Fourth step: Heparin is administered (5.000 UI). The activated clotting time target is between 180 and 200 s. The sewing ring is sutured to the myocardium using 8–10 interrupted pledgeted, double-armed 3-0 polypropylene sutures. The sutures are tied to secure the sewing ring. The coring knife is inserted through a cruciate incision. As the coring knife is removed, the LVAD simultaneously is off-pump inserted into the LV cavity. The correct housing of the cannula is echocardiographically monitored and then secured to the ring by screwing the connecting ring. In case of Jarvik 2000 implantation, once inserted, it is secured to the ring by tightening the connecting strings. Immediate venting of the air bubbles detected into the LV by TEE is performed by releasing the clamp on the outflow vascular prosthesis, paying attention to hold it high over the heart level, so that the blood pumping out from the ventricle deairs through the graft.

Fifth step: Measurement of the right length and position of the outflow graft is echocardiography monitored, in order that no encumbrances on the right ventricle (RV) are detected. A side-biting clamp is placed on the ascending aorta. The prosthesis is cut and anastomosed to the aorta using a continuous 4-0 polypropylene suture and then reinforced with BioGlue surgical adhesive. Air removal is accomplished using a needle inserted into the outflow graft and activating the pump at low speed. Once no air bubbles are detected into the LV by TEE, the side-biting clamp is released and the LVAD is fully activated. Two drainage tubes and a catheter for continuous flushing with saline and antibiotic solution for each access are positioned.

Sixth step: Immediately after skin suturing, the mild GA with remifentanil and propofol infusions is suspended. Attempt to rapidly wean and extubation of the patients in OR is done in order to guarantee self-inotropic support and afterload reduction to RV.

Eighth step: PVB catheters are maintained for almost 48 hrs and removed when the patients are discharged from ICU. The patients are usually transferred in ward 3–5 postoperative days later. In almost 2 weeks, they become autonomous for their daily activities and VAD management and are discharged from the hospital to the rehabilitation unit.

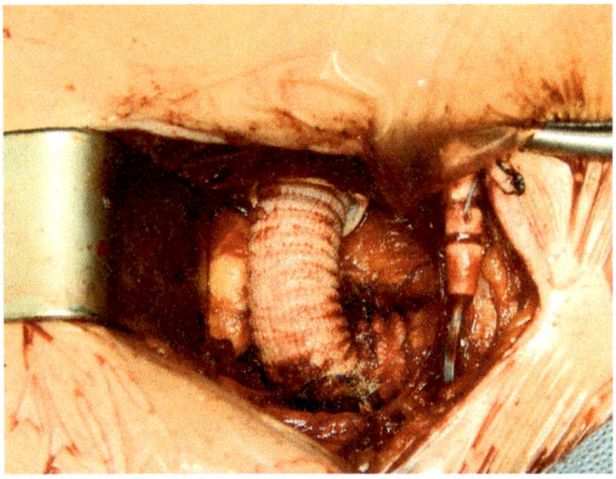

■ **Fig. 24.4** Left axillary artery access for HVAD implantation

■ ■ LMT associated to left axillary artery isolation:

(off-pump implantation and monolateral-thoracic PVB analgesia)

This approach, for now, is limited to a single device available on the market: HVAD. This is due to its vascular outflow 10 mm diameter. Other devices are provided of larger vascular prosthesis sizes, therefore not compatible with the size of the common axillary arteries.

The surgical times and steps are different when we decide to anastomose the outflow graft to the left axillary artery.

First step: (See First step of the mini upper sternotomy-associated procedure.)

Second step: Axillary artery isolation (■ Fig. 24.4). There are different possibilities:

1. Subclavicular incision
2. Deltopectoral incision

■ Subclavicular incision

Through a 6–8 cm incision below and parallel to the lateral two thirds of the clavicle, the axillary artery can be exposed. The incision proceeds deep to the muscle pectoralis major, which is divided in the direction of its fibers. The clavipectoral fascia is incised secondly, exposing the pectoralis minor, which may be divided or retracted laterally. By using a Beckman retractor, the axillary vein is identified in its ascending course and once circled is isolated and caudally mobilized. The axillary artery is located just below the vein and once circled can easily externally mobilized. The artery is thereafter dissected from the surrounding tissue. Particular attention should be paid not to injure the brachial plexus. After administration of 5000 UI of heparin, proximal and distal control of the axillary artery is obtained with two different vascular clamps.

■ Deltopectoral incision

A further approach to axillary artery, of relative simplicity, is the so-called deltopectoral approach that allows access to the second portion of the vessel or to its median portion. The reason why usually we prefer a more peripheral surgical approach to the axillary artery is due to steric hindrance with the defibrillator and associated leads in the subclavicular position. Once the patient is placed in the supine position and with the arm in slight abduction and external rotation, skin incision of approximately 5–6 cm is performed along the deltopectoral groove, along a line that connects the anterior midclavicular line with the intersection point of the anterior border of the deltoid with the lateral margin of the biceps. Once dissected skin and subcutaneous tissue, Beckman retractor is placed to better expose. By blunt dissection, we move medially the pectoralis major muscle and laterally the deltoid muscle: the maneuver involves the cephalic vein that is easily identified in the sulcus between the two muscles and accompanies the pectoralis major. The underlying groove is then completely dissected with the tip of the scissors, to the medial margin of coracobrachialis muscle (satellite muscle of the axillary artery). Immediately below, the clavipectoral-axillary fascia is recognized and incised. This leads to exposure of the vascular-nervous structures, covered by soft tissue, which must be thoroughly removed. The median nerve is formed in the axilla by two roots from the medial and lateral cords of brachial plexus. Generally, the medial root joins with the lateral root after crossing the front of the third part of the axillary artery and descends anteriorly. While the vein remains anteromedial, the axillary artery can be exposed by inferiorly displacing the nervous block. Nerve structures must always be preserved during both artery dissection and vascular clamp placement. After administration of 5000 UI of heparin, proximal and distal control of the axillary artery is obtained with two different vascular clamps.

24.9 Axillary Artery Management

Generally the axillary artery identified is less than 8 mm in caliber. The vascular prosthesis of the HVAD, the smallest on the market, is of 10 mm diameter. If the axillary artery is larger than 8 mm, we recommend the first technique (a); contrary, in case of axillary diameter less than 8 mm, we recommend the second technique (b):

(a) After positioning the vascular clamp proximally and distally, the artery is interrupted crosswise. The proximal portion of the axillary artery is then anastomosed to the HVAD vascular prosthesis of 10 mm, in end-to-end fashion, by using a 5-0 polypropylene RBII suture. Once anastomosed, the vascular prosthesis is gently forced to enter into the thorax through the first intercostal space just below the muscle pectoralis major. Afterward the distal portion of the axillary artery is anastomosed, in end-to-lateral fashion, to the vascular prosthesis. A restrictive anastomosis is performed with the aim to avoid arm indwelling caused by blood overflow. In addition, in order to create a preferential centripetal flow, the selected site where to perform the distal anastomosis is the convexity of the curve designed by the vascular prosthesis.

(b) Different is the approach in case of size of the axillary artery less than 8 mm: in all these cases, we prefer to interpose a vascular prosthesis of 8 mm in diameter and almost 2 cm long, like a Dacron bridge along the course of the axillary artery. After positioning the proximal and distal clamps, the axillary artery is interrupted. The 8 mm vascular prosthesis is anastomosed proximally and distally in end-to-end fashion, by using a 5-0 RBII polypropylene suture. After checking the hemostasis of these two sutures through the release of the clamps, we proceed, after vessel re-clamp, with an incision of the vascular prosthesis just interposed, along the long axis of the vessel. The rhyme of the incision on the vascular prosthesis is enlarged by removing some Dacron tissue, with the aim to enhance as much as possible the perimeter of the anastomosis. At this point, we proceed with the suture of the 10 mm vascular graft (HVAD prosthesis), in end-to-side fashion, to the vascular prosthesis interposed along the course of the axillary artery (T-anastomosis), using the same polypropylene suture. A restrictive suture armed with two pledgets is then placed on the distal portion of the vessel to avoid axillary overflow. This is then tightened once started the LVAD assistance, with contemporary monitoring of the arterial pressure in both the radial arteries.

24.10 LVAD Outflow Vascular Graft Management

Once the vascular prosthesis is anastomosed to the axillary artery, it must be tunnelized within the chest through the first intercostal space. Therefore, with the aid of a retractor for the soft tissues, we kindly displace the muscle pectoralis major and thus expose the first intercostal space. After exclusion and collapse of the ipsilateral lung, a 2 cm intercostal space dissection is performed with particular attention to hemostasis. Through this access, we introduce a string as a guide that should be retrieved, from the LMT. It will help to guide and tunnel an armed GORE-TEX vascular prosthesis, from LMT toward the ipsilateral first intercostal space. Another string guide is tied to the outflow graft prosthesis and is slipped from the first intercostal space, through the armed vascular prosthesis, out to the fifth intercostal space LMT, where the Dacron prosthesis is connected to the LVAD. The armed GORE-TEX prosthesis is helpful as an anticollapse protection to the outflow graft along the intrathoracic pathway and in the way out through the first intercostal space.

Third step: The driveline is tunneled subcutaneously to the exit point at the left lower abdominal quadrant and thereafter re-tunneled to exit its tip contralaterally at the right lower abdominal quadrant.

Fourth step: *(See the Fourth step of the previous procedure.)*

Fifth step: Air removal is accomplished using a proximal axillary artery clamping and activating the pump at low speed. Once no air bubbles are detected into the LV by TEE, the clamp is released and the LVAD is fully activated. Two drainage tubes and a catheter for continuous flushing with saline and antibiotic solution for LMT access are positioned.

Sixth step: Immediately after skin suturing, the mild GA with remifentanil and propofol infusions is suspended. The patients are rapidly weaned from the mechanical ventilation and extubated in the OR when possible, in order to guarantee self-inotropic support and afterload reduction to RV.

Eighth step: *(See the Eighth step of the previous procedure.)*

24.11 Comment

Given the shortage of valid organs available, an increasing number of patients refractory to maximum medical therapy are treated with mechanical circulatory assistance, frequently requiring support in short time. Additionally, these patients often present very poor general condition that frequently leads to a challenging emergent heart transplant, when an organ is available, because of high risk of acute graft failure or to waiting list exclusion. For these reasons, the LVAD has become increasingly the main solution for such unstable patients [34]. Data confirming that the VAD therapy leads to pathology remission and clinical condition normalization are already published [35–37]. On the other hand, given the frailty of these patients, an impairment of hemodynamic, pulmonary, and renal function is frequently observed [35–37]. Therefore, the rapid recovery after LVAD implantation is very important, mostly in order to achieve a patient with the best possible conditions when scheduled to receive a new organ. Key therapeutic intervention for frailty is exercise training [38–41], because it decreases hospitalizations and it is also deemed to improve the clinically evident features of declining muscle mass strength [42–44]. As a matter of fact, the entrapment to bed would lead to inevitable consequent loss of muscle mass, which compromises respiratory mechanics and prolonged wound healing. Additionally, several factors related to both the operative phase (duration of surgery, prolonged intubation) and postoperative phase (red blood cell transfusion, delayed mobilization, and postoperative complications) in cardiac surgery may compromise the postoperative course [41, 42]. In order to fulfill these results, both procedures, surgical and anesthetic, must ensure the fastest recovery possible, with the least possible impairment.

We described LVAD implantation with a "less invasive technique": first the off-pump implantation, second the minimally invasive surgical approach, and third the paravertebral analgesia associated to a mild general anesthesia.

Performing the procedure using an off-pump technique might reduce the release of inflammatory cascade and its consequences. Additionally, the reduced need for heparin infusion favors a limited intraoperative and postoperative bleeding and thus a decreased need for blood unit transfusions.

As far as the mini-surgical access concerns, there is a growing trend toward the use of non-sternotomy incisions and/or mini-thoracotomy in all fields of cardiac surgery. Although full-median sternotomy provides the best access to the heart and the adjacent structures, it could be replaced by smaller incisions in most cases. The choice of our approaches is directed by the possibility of a good exposure of the great vessels while maintaining facility on an eventual implantation of a paracorporeal right ventricular assistance in case of right ventricle failure, and the heart no-touch technique for left ventricle apex exposure (mini-thoracotomy), with decreased rate of arrhythmias and hemodynamic instability related to the heart manipulation, mandatory when in full sternotomy. Additionally, the surgical risk of a redo surgery, like transplantation, is limited since the vascular graft at re-intervention is protected by the pericardium. Finally, less extensive mediastinal dissection reduces the risk and the degree of postoperative bleeding.

On the other hand, the hemodynamic fragility of these patients is well reported, and renal insufficiency, pulmonary hypertension, as well as COPD stand out as risk factors. Furthermore, when prolonged mechanical ventilation is required, the cerebral perfusion and oxygenation are compromised. In order to improve the patient management, paravertebral analgesia has been used in addition to a mild general anesthesia. Many authors have confirmed the utility and efficacy of continuous PVB for analgesic control during thoracotomy and thoracic surgery when compared to epidural analgesia techniques, but with more advantages, i.e., lower complication rate (pulmonary, renal, gastrointestinal, and hemodynamic). This analgesia does not influence the hemodynamic stability and permits a mild general anesthesia approach.

These maneuvers allow an entire low blood transfusion entity procedure, an important issue considering patients' bridge to transplantation, and therefore an eventual immunization should be avoided.

Additionally, avoiding full sternotomy and CPB can significantly reduce the alterations to respiratory mechanism. Furthermore, the optimal thoracotomy pain control offered by the continuous PVB analgesia enables early extubation and right ventricle unloading.

In conclusion, our considerations led credence to the notion that minimally invasive surgical technique associated to PVB analgesia is a safe and reproducible technique, and it enables early extubation with optimal pain control.

References

1. Kanter KR, McBride LR, Pennington DG, Swartz MT, Ruzevich SA, Miller LW et al (1988) Bridging to cardiac transplantation with pulsatile ventricular assist devices. Ann Thorac Surg 46:134–140
2. Argenziano M, Catanese KA, Moazami N, Gardocki MT, Weinberg AD, Clavenna MW et al (1997) The influence of infection on survival and successful transplantation in patients with left ventricular assist devices. J Heart Lung Transplant 16:822–831
3. Toda K, Fujita T, Kobayashi J, Shimahara Y, Kitamura S, Seguchi O et al (2012) Impact of preoperative percutaneous cardiopulmonary support on outcome following left ventricular assist device implantation. Circulation 76:88–95
4. Rose EA, Gelijns AC, Moskowitz AJ, Heitjan DF, Stevenson LW, Dembitsky W et al (2001) Long-term use of a left ventricular assist device for end-stage heart failure. N Engl J Med 345:1435–1443
5. Worku B, Naka Y, Pak SW et al (2011) Predictors of mortality after short-term ventricular assist device placement. Ann Thorac Surg 92:1608–1612
6. Sun BC, Firstenberg MS, Louis LB et al (2008) Placement of long-term implantable ventricular assist devices without the use of cardiopulmonary bypass. J Heart Lung Transplant 27:718–721
7. McLoughlin MP, Chapman JR, Gordon SV, Ledwich M, Macdonald G, Mohacsi P (1991) "Go on — say yes": a publicity campaign to increase commitment to organ donation on the driver's license in New South Wales. Transplant Proc 23:2693
8. Goldstein DJ, Oz MC, Rose EA (1998) Implantable left ventricular assist devices. N Engl J Med 339(21): 1522–1533
9. Casarotto D, Bottio T, Gambino A, Testolin L, Gerosa G (2003) The last to die is hope: prolonged mechanical circulatory support with a Novacor left ventricular assist device as a bridge to transplantation. J Thorac Cardiovasc Surg 125:417–418
10. Krabatsch T, Potapov E, Stepanenko A et al (2011) Biventricular circulatory support with two miniaturized implantable assist devices. Circulation 124:S179–S186
11. Gregoric ID, La Francesca S, Myers T, Cohn W, Loyalka P, Kar B et al (2008) A less invasive approach to axial flow pump insertion. J Heart Lung Transplant 27:423–426
12. Kristjánsdóttir A, Ragnarsdóttir M, Hannesson P, Beck HJ, Torfason B (2004) Respiratory movements are altered three months and one year following cardiac surgery. Scand Cardiovasc J 38:98–103
13. Puskas JD, Williams WH, Duke PG, Staples JR, Glas KE, Marshall JJ et al (2003) Off-pump coronary artery bypass grafting provides complete revascularization with reduced myocardial injury, transfusion requirements, and length of stay: a prospective randomized comparison of two hundred unselected patients undergoing off-pump versus conventional coronary artery bypass grafting. J Thorac Cardiovasc Surg 125:797–808
14. Gilmanov D, Bevilacqua S, Murzi M, Cerillo AG, Gasbarri T, Kallushi E et al (2013) Minimally invasive and conventional aortic valve replacement: a propensity score analysis. Ann Thorac Surg 96:837–843
15. Cheng DC, Martin J, Lal A, Diegeler A, Folliguet TA, Nifong LW, Perier P et al (2011) Minimally invasive versus conventional open mitral valve surgery: a meta-analysis and systematic review. Innovations (Phila) 6:84–103
16. Anyanwu AC, Fischer GW, Plotkina I, Pinney S, Adams DH (2007) Off-pump implant of the Jarvik 2000 ventricular assist device through median sternotomy. Ann Thorac Surg 84:1405–1407
17. Gerosa G, Gallo M, Tarzia V, Di Gregorio G, Zanella F, Bottio T (2013) Less invasive surgical and perfusion technique for implantation of the Jarvik 2000 left ventricular assist device. Ann Thorac Surg 96:712–714
18. Bortolussi G, Lika A, Bejko J, Gallo M, Tarzia V, Gerosa G, Bottio T (2015) Left ventricular assist device end-to-end connection to the left subclavian artery: an alternative technique. Ann Thorac Surg 100:e93–e95
19. Bejko J, Bortolussi G, Tarzia V, Gerosa G, Bottio T (2015) Pulmonary embolism and LVAD: is there compatibility? Int J Artif Organs 38:468–470
20. Bejko J, Guariento A, Bortolussi G, Tarzia V, Gerosa G, Bottio T (2015) Minimally invasive surgical Jarvik 2000 off-pump implantation. Multimed Man Cardiothorac Surg 25;2015. pii: mmv020. doi: 10.1093/mmcts/mmv020.
21. Bottio T, Bejko J, Guariento A, Tarzia V, Pittarello D, Gerosa G (2016) Bilateral mini-thoracotomy off-pump Jarvik 2000 implantation in regional asymmetric paravertebral analgesia. J Cardiovasc Med (Hagerstown) 17:160–164
22. Bottio T, Bejko J, Tarzia V, Gerosa G (2014) HeartWare LVAD implantation in a patient with a rare ARVD: carvajal syndrome. Int J Artif Organs 37:563–566

23. Bottio T, Bejko J, Gallo M, Bortolussi G, Gerosa G (2014) Less invasive implantation of HeartWare left ventricular assist device. Multimed Man Cardiothorac Surg 11;2014. pii: mmu008. doi: 10.1093/mmcts/mmu008
24. Bottio T, Bejko J, Falasco G, Bortolussi G, Gallo M, Tarzia V, Gerosa G (2014) Less-invasive off-pump ventricular assist device implantation in regional paravertebral analgesia. J Artif Organs 17:275–277
25. Baidya DK, Khanna P, Maitra S (2014) Analgesic efficacy and safety of thoracic paravertebral and epidural analgesia for thoracic surgery: a systematic review and meta-analysis. Interact Cardiovasc Thorac Surg 18:626–635
26. Ragnarsdóttir M, KristjAnsdóttir A, Ingvarsdóttir I, Hannesson P, Torfason B, Cahalin L (2004) Short-term changes in pulmonary function and respiratory movements after cardiac surgery via median sternotomy. Scand Cardiovasc J 38:46–52
27. Westerdahl E, Lindmark B, Bryngelsson I, Tenling A (2003) Pulmonary function 4 months after coronary artery bypass graft surgery. Respir Med 97:317–322
28. Carmona P, Llagunes J, Cánovas S, de Andrés J, Marqués I (2011) The role of continuous thoracic paravertebral block for fast-track anesthesia after cardiac surgery via thoracotomy. J Cardiothorac Vasc Anesth 25:205–206
29. Mehta Y, Arora D, Sharma KK, Mishra Y, Wasir H, Trehan N (2008) Comparison of continuous thoracic epidural and paravertebral block for postoperative analgesia after robotic assisted coronary artery bypass surgery. Ann Card Anaesth 11:91–96
30. Bottio T, Bisleri G, Piccoli P, Negri A, Manzato A, Muneretto C (2007) Heart valve surgery in a very high-risk population: a preliminary experience in awake patients. J Heart Valve Dis 16:187–194
31. Davies RG, Myles PS, Graham JM (2006) A comparison of the analgesic efficacy and side-effects of paravertebral vs epidural blockade for thoracotomy. A systematic review and meta-analysis of randomized trials. Br J Anaesth 96:418–426
32. Casati A, Alessandrini P, Nuzzi M et al (2006) A prospective, randomized, blinded comparison between continuous thoracic paravertebral and epidural infusion of 0.2% ropivacaine after lung resection surgery. Eur J Anaesthesiol 23:999–1004
33. Boezaart AP, Lucas SD, Elliott CE (2009) Paravertebral block: cervical, thoracic, lumbar, and sacral. Curr Opin Anaesthesiol 22:637–643
34. Afilalo J, Karunananthan S, Eisenberg MJ, Alexander KP, Bergman H (2009) Role of frailty in patients with cardiovascular disease. Am J Cardiol 103:1616–1621
35. Patel AM, Adeseun GA, Ahmed I, Mitter N, Rame JE, Rudnick MR et al (2013) Renal failure in patients with left ventricular assist devices. Clin J Am Soc Nephrol 8:484–496
36. Hasin T, Topilsky Y, Schirger JA, Li Z, Zhao Y, Boilson BA et al (2012) Changes in renal function after implantation of continuous-flow left ventricular assist devices. J Am Coll Cardiol 59:26–36
37. Sato T, Seguchi O, Morikawa N, Hieda M, Watanabe T, Sunami H et al (2013) A heart transplant candidate with severe pulmonary hypertension and extremely high pulmonary vascular resistance. J Artif Organs 16:253–257
38. Theou O, Stathokostas L, Roland KP, Jakobi JM, Patterson C, Vandervoort AA et al (2011) The effectiveness of exercise interventions for the management of frailty: a systematic review. J Aging Res 2011:569194
39. von Haehling S, Anker SD, Doehner W, Morley JE, Vellas B (2013) Frailty and heart disease. Int J Cardiol 13:S0167–S5273
40. Fülster S, Tacke M, Sandek A, Ebner N, Tschöpe C, Doehner W et al (2013) Muscle wasting in patients with chronic heart failure: results from the studies investigating co-morbidities aggravating heart failure (SICA-HF). Eur Heart J 34:512–519
41. Newman MF, Kirchner JL, Phillips-Bute B, Gaver V, Grocott H, Jones RH et al (2001) Longitudinal assessment of neurocognitive function after coronary-artery bypass surgery. N Engl J Med 344:395–402
42. Van Dijk D, Jansen EW, Hijman R, Nierich AP, Diephuis JC, Moons KG et al (2002) Cognitive outcome after off-pump and on-pump coronary artery by-pass graft surgery: a randomized trial. JAMA 287:1405–1412
43. Lazar RM, Shapiro PA, Jaski BE, Parides MK, Bourge RC, Watson JT et al (2004) Neurological events during long-term mechanical circulatory support for heart failure: the Randomized Evaluation of Mechanical Assistance for the Treatment of Congestive Heart Failure (REMATCH) experience. Circulation 109:2423–2427
44. Ballantyne JC, Carr DB, de Ferranti S, Suarez T, Lau J, Chalmers TC (1998) The comparative effects of postoperative analgesic therapies on pulmonary outcome: cumulative meta-analyses of randomized, controlled trials. Anesth Analg 86:598–612

To Pump or Not to Pump: The Role of CPB or ECMO

Daniel Zimpfer

© Springer International Publishing Switzerland 2017
A. Montalto et al. (eds.), *Mechanical Circulatory Support in End-Stage Heart Failure*,
DOI 10.1007/978-3-319-43383-7_25

25.1 Introduction

Left ventricular assist device (LVAD) implantation is routinely performed with cardiopulmonary bypass (CPB) support [1]. The main advantages of CPB are hemodynamic and respiratory stabilization and the ability to open the left ventricular apex allowing for thorough inspection of the left ventricular cavity and eventual resection of ventricular trabeculations and left ventricular thrombus formation during LVAD implantation [1]. Furthermore, CPB allows for concomitant procedures to the aortic, tricuspid, or mitral valve as well as closure of intracardiac shunts [1]. However, CPB causes a severe cascade of adverse events that ultimately result in a systemic inflammatory response syndrome, coagulation disorders, and end-organ injury [2]. Moreover, avoiding CPB and replacing it by ECMO or off-pump strategies has been shown to be associated with improved results in patients undergoing lung transplantation and high-risk coronary artery bypass cases [3]. Therefore, several programs have successfully replaced CPB with ECMO support or off-pump approaches at the time of LVAD implantation in an attempt to reduce the overall invasiveness of the procedure [4, 5]. Especially if combined with a sternotomy-sparing approach, off-pump LVAD implantation is probably the least invasive approach for LVAD implantation today [6]. Obviously, especially multimorbid LVAD candidates with impaired end-organ function might have the biggest benefit from avoiding CPB.

In this chapter, we review surgical technique as well as current evidence for replacing CPB by ECMO or off-pump approaches.

25.2 LVAD Implantation with ECMO Support

LVAD implantation with ECMO support initially has been described in a series of INTERMACS level 1 patients that underwent LVAD implantation after stabilization of end-organ function without switching to CPB [4, 5]. Based on this initial "feasibility" experience, several groups have replaced CPB by ECMO for isolated LVAD implantation. Depending on the initial situation, the patient is either transported to the OR on ECMO support, or ECMO support is initiated in the OR [4, 5]. For a standard procedure, LVAD implantation will be performed via a median sternotomy. After opening of the pericardium and placement of stay sutures, the patient will be fully heparinized and the outflow graft anastomosis performed to the side-clamped ascending aorta after measuring the required outflow graft length. Depending on the used device, a pump pocket has to be dissected before [4]. Thereafter, the left ventricular apex is exposed. Despite the fact that hemodynamic stability will be ensured by ECMO support, exposure of the LV apex can be more demanding as ECMO only provides minimal right and left ventricular decompression. During exposure of the LV apex, distortion or compression of the RCA has to be meticulously avoided as this may result in right ventricular dysfunction. In our experience, tactical placement of deep pericardial sutures similar to LAD exposure for off-pump CABG can be extremely helpful for LV apex exposure in this situation. Depending on surgeons preference, the apical sewing ring is then attached to the apex either in a running or interrupted suture technique. Before incising the LV apex, the driveline should then be tunneled according to surgeons preference and institutional standard. To minimize blood loss during coring, it is advisable to then place temporary ventricular wires and incise the apex during rapid pacing. Alternatively, temporary cardiac arrest can be achieved by adenosine administration. After LV coring, the left ventricular cavity can then be inspected with the aid of a cell saver that should allow for rapid blood reinfusion via the ECMO circuit. However, the ability to suck empty the LV cavity is limited and extensive procedures such as removal of large thrombus formations is impossible. Connection of the assist device to the apical sewing ring is the performed according to the manufacturers recommendations. The described technique is feasible with the HeartMate II and III as well as the HeartWare HVAD system [4, 5]. Depending on the patients general state and RV function, the ECMO is primarily explanted in the OR which or left in place for additional hemodynamic stabilization. The latter is a common approach in those patients previously supported with ECMO as a short-term assist device [4, 5].

25.3 Off-Pump LVAD Implantation

Off-pump LVAD implantation has successfully been performed with the HeartMate II via a sternotomy approach and with the HeartWare HVAD via a thoratomy approach with the outflow graft either to the ascending aorta or left subclavian artery [6–9].

25.3.1 HeartMate II

For HeartMate II off-pump implantation, the patient is prepared in a routine fashion including insertion of a transesophageal echo probe as well as a Swan-Ganz catheter [8, 9]. Cardiopulmonary bypass has to be available and primed in the OR. Any patients with valve pathologies necessitating surgical correction at the time of LVAD implantation have to be excluded from an off-pump approach. Before commencing surgery, a thorough echocardiographic workup of the heart is performed with special emphasis on LV thrombus formation. After opening the pericardium, a pump pocket is prepared and the driveline is tunneled. Thereafter, the patient is heparinized with a target ACT above 300 s, and the outflow graft anastomosis is performed to the side-clamped ascending aorta in a regular fashion after estimating the necessary length of the outflow graft. Thereafter, pericardial stay sutures are placed, and the apex is exposed similar to off-pump CABG cases. To improve exposure, the patient is placed in the Trendelenburg position and rotated toward the surgeon. A large silk stich is then placed into the center of the LV apex, and the apical cuff is sewn to the LV apex using the surgeon's technique of choice (either interrupted or continuous sutures). Before coring of the LV apex, the inflow elbow of the LVAD is occluded with a Foley catheter. For coring, a second Foley catheter is inserted into the LV apex via a small stab incision in the middle of the apical cuff. The apex is then cored with the HeartMate II coring knife. Great care is taken not to destroy the Foley catheter during this procedure. After completion of the apical coring, the LVAD inflow cannula is attached to the apical cuff and connected to the HeartMate II system. To minimize blood loss while coring, adenosine is administrated to achieve a short cardiac arrest or rapid pacing using temporary epicardial wires is performed to minimize cardiac output. The HeartMate II system is then started and routine deairing maneuvers are performed. The rest of the procedure compares to standard HeartMate II implantation.

25.3.2 HeartWare HVAD

For HeartWare HVAD off-pump implantation, the patient is prepared in a routine fashion including insertion of a transesophageal echo probe as well as a Swan-Ganz catheter [5, 7]. We find it extremely useful to use a 3D TEE probe in order to optimize the position of coring as well as ruling out LV thrombus. Cardiopulmonary bypass has to be available and primed in the OR. Any patients with valve pathologies necessitating surgical correction at the time of LVAD implantation have to be excluded from an off-pump approach. The apex is usually approached via a left thoracotomy (◘ Fig. 25.1., ► see also chapter on less invasive approaches for LVAD implantation). The pericardium is then opened, and the apical sewing cuff is attached to the LV apex using an interrupted or running suture technique. To optimize the position of the apical cuff, we routinely insert a needle into the LV and visualize it using TEE. The patient is then heparinized in order to achieve an ACT of at least 300 s. Coring and attaching the HVAD to the apical sewing ring is performed in a two-step procedure that usually ensures perfect hemodynamic stability even in critical cases. First adenosine administration or rapid pacing initiates a short period of low output or cardiac arrest. Then

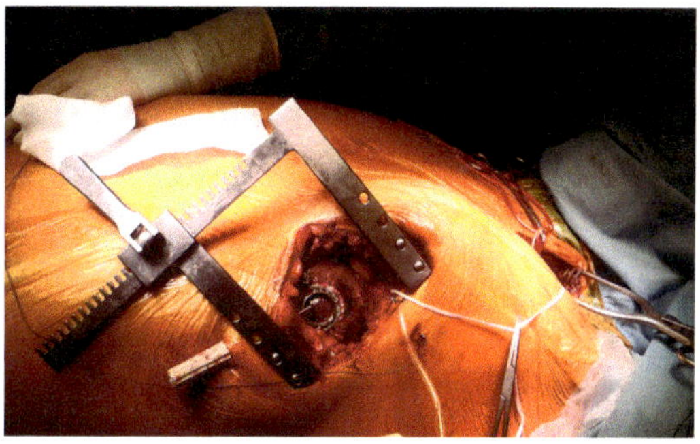

◘ **Fig. 25.1** Thoracotomy access to LV apex. In addition, the left subclavian artery has been exposed via a subclavicular incision and will later on become the site of outflow graft anastomosis. The umbilical tape on display will serve as a pulley for the outflow graft

a cruciate incision is performed and then coring knife is inserted into the LV. This completely seals the LV and rapid pacing is stopped. In case of adenosine administration, the heart will meanwhile regain normal function. After complete hemodynamic stabilization, the procedure is repeated; this time the apex is cored, and the HVAD is connected to the apical sewing ring. For deairing, approximately 100 ml of blood is allowed to exit via the outflow graft before clamping it. The procedure is concluded by performing the outflow graft anastomosis, either to the ascending aorta or left subclavian artery and tunneling the driveline. Additional deairing can be performed via a small needle inserted into the outflow graft after initiation of LVAD support.

25.4 Discussion

Off-pump and ECMO support LVAD implantation have been developed to reduce the overall invasiveness of LVAD implantation. Especially multimorbid patients in terminal heart failure with chronically injured end organs could benefit from these approaches. Despite the obvious advantages, the main concerns with off-pump and ECMO support LVAD implantation are the inability to visualize the LV cavity during surgery to rule out LV thrombus and obstructing trabeculations. Missing LV thrombus formation could lead to devastating thrombus dislodgement or suction into the LVAD, and obstructing trabeculations can limit LVAD flow and LV unloading.

While off-pump LVAD implantation developed as a discrete procedure, ECMO support LVAD implantation was first described in bridge-to-decision patients [4, 5]. In this distinct population, switching to cardiopulmonary bypass can thereby be avoided [4, 5]. Combining the ECMO circuit with a cell saver system also allows for expeditious blood re-transfusion; the overall procedure is very much straightforward, and surgeons do not have to leave the comfort zone provided by the ECMO as a hemodynamic safety net. Results with this approach have to be assessed in light of a high percentage of INTERMACS I patients operated with this approach. Technical success rates of 100% without conversions to cardiopulmonary bypass have been reported in both major series [4, 5]. In-hospital survival of 90–95% and 1 year survival of 86% underline the safety of the procedure [4, 5]. Of note, no thrombus dislodgements or embolization has been reported and the observed stroke rates compare to standard LVAD implantation with cardiopulmonary bypass [4, 5]. So far, no reports on elective ECMO LVAD implantation have been published. Therefore, it can only be speculated that exchanging cardiopulmonary bypass by ECMO might be beneficial. Some evidence supporting this assumption might be derived from lung transplantation [10].

Off-pump LVAD implantation developed as a distinct surgical approach, and many of us have used this approach for experimental VAD implantation in the animal lab [6–9]. In contrast to ECMO support LVAD implantation, off-pump LVA implantation requires the surgeon and the entire surgical team to leave the comfort zone provided by cardiopulmonary bypass and close interactions between all team members become necessary, similar to off-pump CABG [6–9]. However, as soon as the entire team gets comfortable with this approach, it is a perfectly standardized, reproducible, teachable, and safe procedure that truly minimizes the insult of LVAD implantation. Besides technical success and survival rates, off-pump LVAD implantation especially has to be assessed with regard to thromboembolic complications. The three major series on off-pump LVAD implantation report technical success rates of 100% without any conversions to cardiopulmonary bypass [6–9]. Of note, two publications only address HeartWare HVAD off-pump implantation, which is probably best explained by the fact that the HVAD apical sewing ring and coring device allow for a staged procedure and maximal intraoperative hemodynamic stability [5, 7]. Survival rate with off-pump LVAD implantation are excellent and reach up to 90% at 6 months and 85% at 1 year [6–9]. So far no long-term survival rates have been published [6–9]. Importantly, off-pump LVAD implantation was not associated with any intraoperative thromboembolic events in all published series and the overall thromboembolic event rates compare to those reported after standard LVAD implantation [6–9].

Summarizing, off-pump and ECMO support LVAD implantation are reasonable alternatives to standard LVAD implantation with cardiopulmonary bypass. Especially off-pump LVAD implantation will become increasingly adapted as soon as apical connection and coring systems developed specifically for this procedure become commercially available.

References

1. Feldman D, Pamboukian SV, Teuteberg JJ et al (2013) The 2013 International Society for Heart and Lung Transplantation Guidelines for mechanical circulatory support: executive summary. J Heart Lung Transplant Off Publ of Int Soc Heart Transplant 32(2):157–187
2. Edmunds LH Jr (1995) Why cardiopulmonary bypass makes patients sick: strategies to control the blood-synthetic surface interface. Adv Card Surg 6:131–167
3. Kowalewski M, Pawliszak W, Malvindi PG et al (2016) Off-pump coronary artery bypass grafting improves short-term outcomes in high-risk patients compared with on-pump coronary artery bypass grafting: meta-analysis. J Thorac Cardiovasc Surg 151(1):60–77 e61-58
4. Lebreton G, Nicolescu M, Leger P, Leprince P (2011) Implantation of left ventricular support under extracorporeal membrane oxygenation. Eur J Cardiothorac Surg Off J Eur Assoc Cardiothorac Surg 40(5): e165–e167
5. Riebandt J, Haberl T, Mahr S et al (2014) Preoperative patient optimization using extracorporeal life support improves outcomes of INTERMACS Level I patients receiving a permanent ventricular assist device. Eur J Cardiothorac Surg Off J Eur Assoc Cardiothorac Surg 46(3):486–492 discussion 492
6. Moayedifar R, Riebandt J, Haberl T et al (2016) Off-pump heartware HVAD left ventricular assist device implantation. J Heart Lung Transplant 35(4):S319–S320
7. Strueber M, Meyer AL, Feussner M, Ender J, Correia JC, Mohr FW (2014) A minimally invasive off-pump implantation technique for continuous-flow left ventricular assist devices: early experience. J Heart Lung Transplant Off Publ Int Soc Heart Transplant 33(8):851–856
8. Sun BC, Firstenberg MS, Louis LB et al (2008) Placement of long-term implantable ventricular assist devices without the use of cardiopulmonary bypass. J Heart Lung Transplant Off Publ Int Soc Heart Transplant 27(7):718–721
9. Awad H, Abd E, Dayem M, Heard J, Dimitrova G, Yu L, Sun BC (2010) Initial experience with off-pump left ventricular assist device implantation in single center: retrospective analysis. J Cardiothorac Surg 5:123
10. Aigner C, Wisser W, Taghavi S et al (2007) Institutional experience with extracorporeal membrane oxygenation in lung transplantation. Eur J Cardiothorac Surg Off J Eur Assoc Cardiothorac Surg 31(3):468–473 ; discussion 473–464

Techniques for Inflow Cannula Placement

Nicolas A. Brozzi, Antonio Loforte, and Matthias Loebe

© Springer International Publishing Switzerland 2017
A. Montalto et al. (eds.), *Mechanical Circulatory Support in End-Stage Heart Failure*,
DOI 10.1007/978-3-319-43383-7_26

26.1 Introduction

An adequate surgical technique is paramount for the outcome of any surgical procedure. Implantation of left ventricular assist devices (LVADs) presents a series of technical challenges for the appropriate placement and long-term function of the device. The proper positioning of the inflow cannula is possibly the most important technical aspect of LVAD implantation. This chapter is intended to highlight pitfalls related to placement of the inflow cannula during implantation of LVAD.

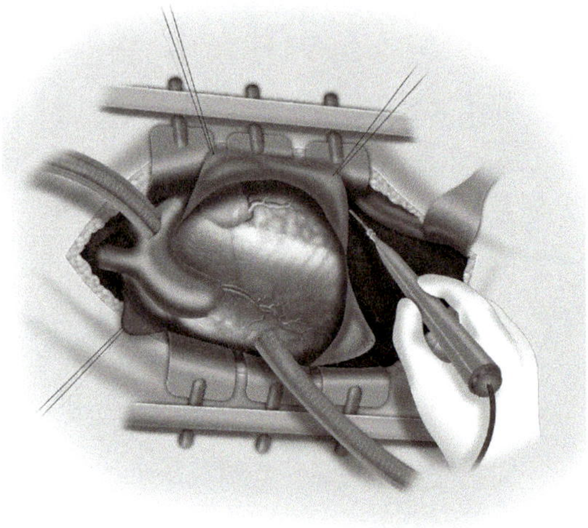

■ **Fig. 26.1** Creation of an adequately sized pump pocket is essential to optimize inflow cannula position. For the HM II LVAD, the exposed part of the diaphragm is cauterized as far as possible laterally. In addition, dividing the pericardial reflection laterally beyond the left ventricular (LV) apex is also necessary (this maneuver alone is sufficient for the HeartWare LVAD, which is placed in an intrapericardial position) (Illustration by Ilaria Bondi's Peppermint Advertising)

26.2 Implantation of Continuous-Flow LVAD

The standard implantation of LVAD through a median sternotomy, with cardiopulmonary bypass, will present the heart decompressed at time of placement of the inflow cannula.

The first step to provide an appropriate placement of the inflow cannula is the division of the pericardium parallel to the diaphragm toward the left hemithorax beyond the apex of the heart. Attention should be placed when opening the pericardium to identify and avoid transection of the left phrenic nerve, which descends vertically and anterior to the lung pedicle.

Creating an adequate-size pump pocket requires division of the muscular fibers of the diaphragm from their insertion in the posterior aspect of the rib cage on the left hemithorax (■ Fig. 26.1). Division of the diaphragm provides access to the pre-peritoneal space, where the tissues can be dissected to create a deep pocket that will accommodate the LVAD pump in the required position. The pump pocket for insertion of LVAD on a small heart will require division of more anterior fibers of the left hemidiaphragm, while patients with larger hearts might require more lateral division of the muscle fibers of the diaphragm extending well under the costal arch into the left pleural space [1].

Patients with prior cardiac surgeries may pose particular challenges related to dissection and exposure of the apex of the heart and creation of the pump pocket. Attention should be placed on preserving patent grafts in patient with prior coronary surgery and to preserve the left phrenic nerve intact during the dissection of the lateral wall of the heart. Exposure and midline retraction of the apex of the heart can become more challenging in patients with prior mitral valve replacement.

26.3 Placement of the Inflow Cannula

The conventional surgical technique for placement of the inflow cannula requires the patient to be on cardiopulmonary bypass to provide hemodynamic stability, while the heart is decompressed to facilitate medial displacement and exposure of the apex of the left ventricle.

Position of arterial cannula and number and position of venous cannulas to establish cardiopulmonary bypass will be determined by the condition of the patient, prior cardiac surgeries, or need to perform additional procedures during the implantation of LVAD. While standard technique is done with single venous cannula, alternative bicaval cannulation will be used if patient requires simultaneous closure of a patent foramen ovale or repair of the tricuspid valve.

Intraoperative transesophageal echocardiogram provides thorough assessment of cardiac anatomy and function, and it is important to determine if patient presents cardiac pathologies that require concomitant surgical repair at time of LVAD implantation, including moderate-severe aortic insufficiency, patent foramen ovale or atrial septal defect, and tricuspid regurgitation. These pathologies are treated before the implantation of LVAD and most of the time can be surgically repaired. Occasionally, patients with severe aortic insufficiency related to a thickened and retracted leaflets will require aortic valve, and we favor implantation of bioprosthesis. While most surgeons will not perform repair for severe mitral valve insufficiency, some authors advocate plication of the central aspect of both leaflets (Alfieri stitch) from the ventricular aspect of the valve after coring the apex of the heart.

Implantation of the inflow cannula of the LVAD continues after any concomitant procedure has been performed. The initial step is the creation of a circular incision in the wall of the left ventricle. The ideal position is usually 1–2 cm anterolateral to the apical dimple, which is an easily palpable location of thinner myocardial wall. A full-thickness piece of myocardial core is removed, and the opening is inspected closely for thrombi or adjacent trabeculae, both of which are carefully removed to create an unobstructed funnel to harbor the inflow cannula (◘ Fig. 26.2). Chronic thrombus that is well embedded to the left ventricular wall and not protruding in the funnel can be left alone. For patients presenting severe mitral regurgitation, some authors favor repair of severe mitral regurgitation with an edge-edge stitch that can be placed from the ventricular core opening at this stage of the procedure.

By choosing the correct position on the LV apex, the ideal orientation of the inflow cannula pointing toward the mitral valve and parallel to the ventricular septum can be achieved. Creating adequate space for the pump pocket is important to prevent inadvertent malposition of the inflow cannula when the heart is returned to the anatomic position.

Next, 2-0 Tevdek sutures supported with 3 x 8 mm Teflon pledgets are placed in a full-thickness fashion through the myocardial core and passed

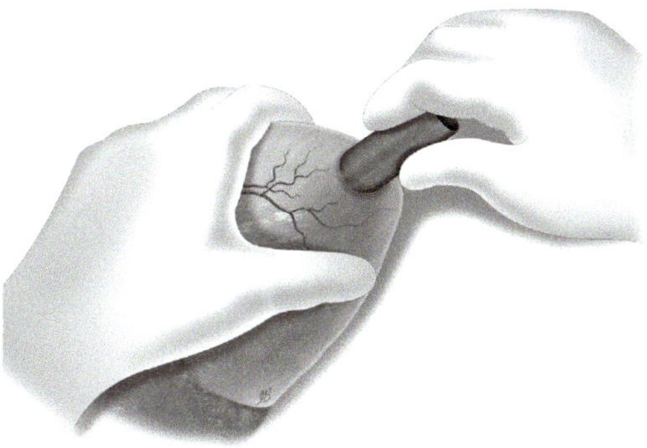

◘ Fig. 26.2 Placement of LVAD inflow cannula. A circular incision to accommodate the inflow cannula of the LVAD is created toward the apex of the heart, lateral to the dimple, and away from the left anterior descending coronary artery. When using a coring knife, it must be directed toward the mitral valve to facilitate proper orientation of the inflow cannula (Illustration by Ilaria Bondi's Peppermint Advertising)

through the felt portion of the sewing cuff or ring. A variety of techniques can be utilized to place this stitches so that they provide adequate support to the inflow cannula. Our preference is to place a total of twelve stitches along the circumference of the LV opening. Four initial stitches are placed in the cardinal points, while the other eight are equally distributed along the circumference with two on each quadrant. We have found that placing each stitch from outside-in about 1 cm from the edge and coming back out 3–5 mm from the edge of the core incision provides very good support and hemostasis.

Alternative techniques include the reinforcement of the sawing ring with a segment of Teflon felt patch or autologous pericardium fashioned as a donut that matches the coring incision on the wall of the left ventricle. These reinforcement strategies may be particularly useful in patients with recent myocardial infarction.

26.4 Alternative Techniques for Implantation of LVAD Inflow Cannula

A couple of alternative techniques have been described to decrease the impact of the surgery on patients receiving LVAD, who are often times debilitated and fragile, and facilitate postoperative recovery. Minimally invasive approaches were proposed to decrease the trauma created by surgery, and techniques that avoid use of cardiopulmonary bypass machine aim to attenuate the inflammatory response of patients triggered by extracorporeal circulation.

Both approaches warrant some specific considerations related to the implantation of the inflow cannula, and more complete discussion of other technical aspects is discussed in detail in other sections of this book.

Of note, cardiopulmonary bypass can be instituted though central or peripheral cannulation, and concomitant structural heart procedures could be performed although the exposure is limited and can add complexity to the procedures [2, 3].

26.5 Minimally Invasive Approaches

Minimally invasive techniques require an 8 cm left thoracotomy through the fifth intercostal space for HeartWare HVAD (HeartWare Inc., Framingham, MA), with subsequent access to the pericardium and direct exposure of the LV apex. Prior cardiac surgery has not been considered a contraindication to this approach, and insertion of the inflow cannula using the support of the adherent pericardium has been described. In these cases, the insertion of a needle in the apex of the heart under TEE guidance can be used to confirm the appropriate location to implant the inflow cannula.

When implanting a HeartMate II (Thoratec Inc., Pleasanton, CA) through a minimally invasive approach, a 10–12 cm left subcostal incision is performed about 2 cm lateral to the xiphoid process, and it is deepened though the subcutaneous tissue, anterior rectus sheath, and rectus muscle, to create a pocket anterior to the posterior rectus sheath [4]. The diaphragm is divided to provide access to the left pleural space and open the pericardium anterior to the left phrenic nerve. Prior cardiac surgery or dense adhesions are considered a contraindication to this approach (◘ Fig. 26.3).

With either of the two approaches, the exposure of the apex of the heart is limited, but sufficient to proceed with implantation of the inflow cannula of either LVAD device.

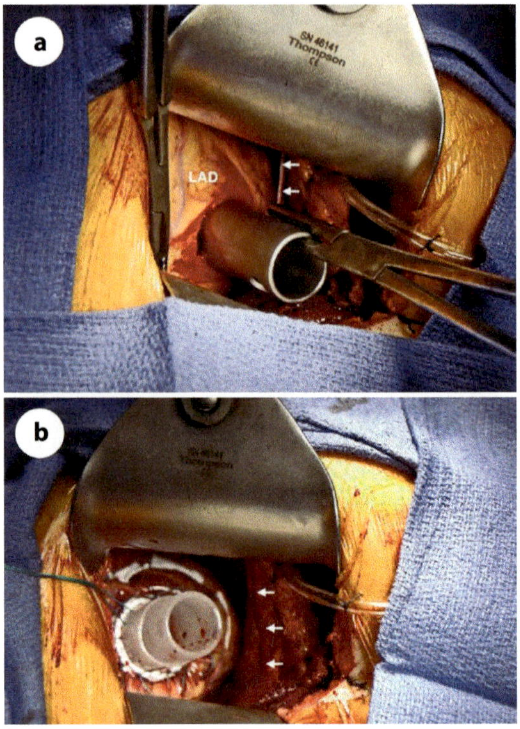

◘ **Fig. 26.3** Minimally invasive placement of LVAD inflow cannula. Exposure of cardiac apex via the subcostal incision. **a** Apex is being cored with a coring knife. **b** Apical sewing ring has been implanted. *LAD* left anterior descending artery. *Arrows* denote left lateral pericardial edge

26.6 Hemodynamic Considerations

The location and direction of the inflow cannula is critical for both early- and long-term pump performance, to facilitate draining blood from the left ventricle, prevent suction events, and possibly formation of clots.

One of the key benefits of LVAD implantation is the ability to unload the left ventricle and decompress the pulmonary vasculature, decreasing pulmonary vascular resistance and intrapulmonary pressures. Patients with optimally placed inflow cannulas and pump pockets have been reported to have up to 20% decrease in left ventricular end-diastolic diameter, which has been related to improved hemodynamics with greater decrease of mean pulmonary artery pressure and central venous pressure.

Meticulous surgical technique with adequate direction of the inflow cannula at the time of operation has also been proposed as an important strategy to reduce the risk of pump thrombosis [2].

26.7 Current Devices and Potential Consequent Alternative Approaches

Several of the newer LVADs that are currently under development use magnetic or hydrodynamic bearings, or both, for frictionless rotation of the pump impeller. These small pumps can provide reliable long-term circulatory support for a wide range of patients with heart failure. Two such devices, the HeartWare HVAD (HeartWare Inc., Framingham, MA) and the HeartMate III (Thoratec Inc., Pleasanton, CA), have an integrated inflow cannula. This compact design allows the device to fit within the pericardial space. Pericardial placement of the pump avoids the need to create a subdiaphragmatic pump pocket, thereby simplifying the implant procedure and eliminating LVAD-related abdominal complications [5, 6].

Correct placement of the integrated inflow cannula of these recent centrifugal pumps is essential for maintaining proper device performance. Ideally, the pump should be positioned so that the cannula resides in the central portion of the LV, away from obstructive surfaces and oriented toward the mitral valve. Usually, HVAD and HeartMate III implantation involves inserting the inflow cannula near the LV apex. If the pump is positioned too far laterally, however, the cannula may abut the interventricular septum after chest closure, thus compromising pump inflow; conversely, if the pump is positioned too far medially, the cannula may abut the lateral LV wall, with resultant impairment of inflow. In addition, apical insertion of the HVAD or HeartMate III necessitates an anterior course for the outflow graft, which may present a hazard on reopening the sternum. Apical cannulation is particularly suboptimal in patients with small lateral thoracic dimensions, an unusually enlarged heart, or both. Additionally apical cannulation may be not feasible in case of postinfarction LV apical aneurysm since a patch placement for Dor procedure makes the LVAD placement difficult and risky [7, 8].

To avoid these complications, some authors recommend an approach in which the inflow cannula is placed posterior to the apex, through the diaphragmatic aspect of the LV ("Frazier's point") (◘ Fig. 26.4). This allows the pump to reside on the left hemidiaphragm, with the inflow cannula directed cephalad and parallel to the short axis of the ventricle, and the outflow graft to lie laterally to the right atrium, far from the retrosternal area (◘ Fig. 26.5). As in the standard technique, this approach eliminates the need for an abdominal pocket.

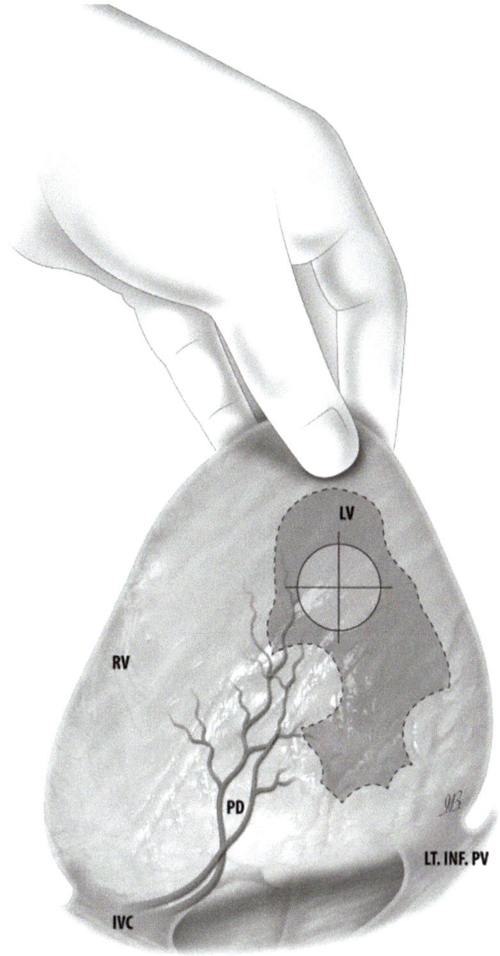

◘ **Fig. 26.4** The heart is reflected in a cephalad direction to expose the diaphragmatic surface of the left ventricle (LV). The dotted line delineates the LV cavity and the posteromedial and anterolateral papillary muscles. The crosshair indicates "Frazier's point," preferred location for inlet cannula insertion during diaphragmatic implantation of a LV assist device. *IVC* inferior vena cava, *Lt. Inf. PV* left inferior pulmonary vein, *PD* posterior descending artery, *RV* right ventricle (Picture by Ilaria Bondi's Peppermint Adertising)

Houston' team experience with HVAD has confirmed that this placement results in the optimal left ventricular position, with orientation of the inlet cannula parallel to the short axis of the left ventricle and anterior to the papillary muscle

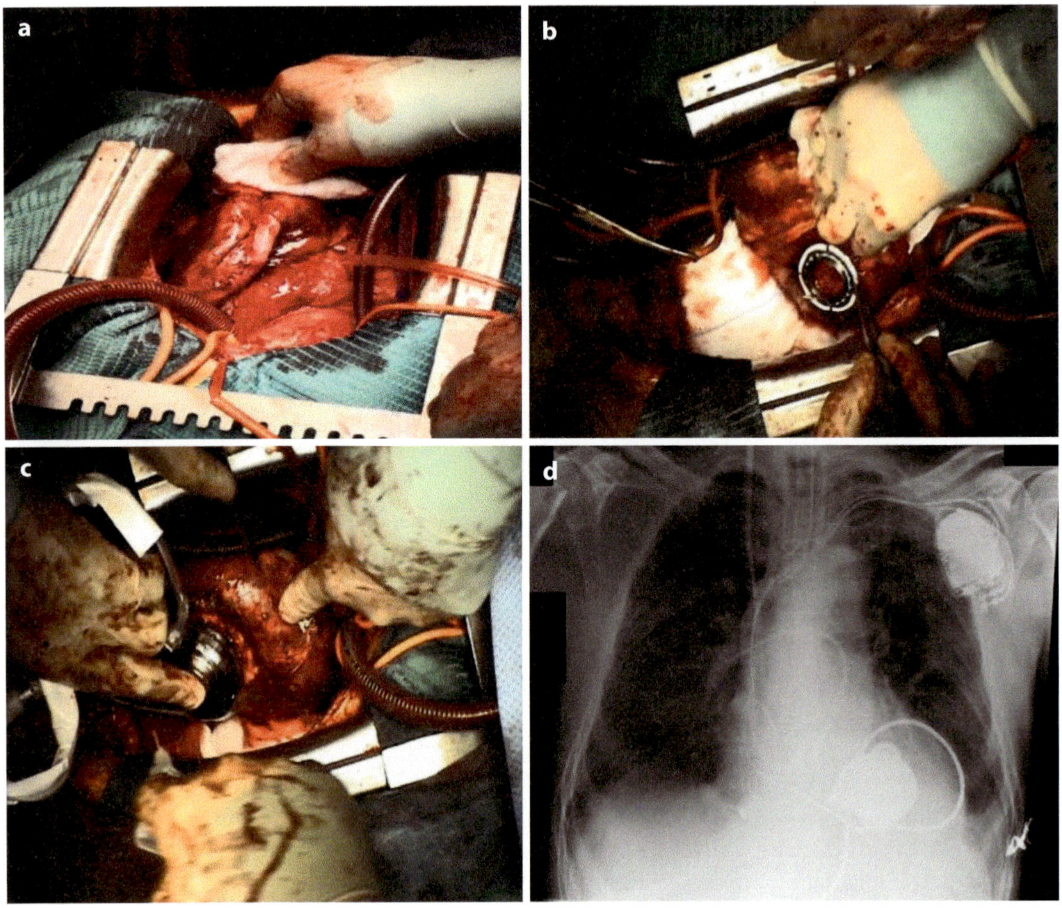

Fig. 26.5 **a** Surgical approach to HVAD implantation. **b** The ring for HVAD is placed posterior to the apex of LV. **c** The pump is inserted and fixed. **d** Postoperative chest radiography showing the pump placed through the diaphragmatic aspect of the LV

insertion. This approach should protect against inflow obstruction and endocardial contact, with resulting arrhythmias. In addition, this position results in lateral placement of the outflow graft, avoiding the anterior and retrosternal surface of the right ventricle.

However, the data are insufficient to demonstrate the superiority of one technique over the other, and further investigations are necessary.

References

1. John R. Implantation of continuous-flow ventricular assist devices: technical considerations. Operative techniques in Thoracic and Cardiovascular Surgery. http://dx.doi.org/10.1053/j.optechstcvs.2012.05.004
2. Taghavi S, Ward C, Jayarajan SN et al (2013) Surgical technique influences Heart Mate II left ventricular assist device thrombosis. Ann Thorac Surg 96: 1259–1265
3. Hall JL, Dr F, Birks EJ et al (2011) Clinical, molecular, and genomic changes in response to a left ventricular assist device. J Am Coll Cardiol 57:641–652
4. Anyanwu AC (2011) Technique for less invasive implantation of Heart mate II left ventricular assist device without median sternotomy. Semin Thorac Cardiovasc Surg 23:241–244
5. Cheung A, Lamarch Y, Kaan A et al (2011) Off-pump implantation of the HeatWare HVAD left ventricular assist device through minimally invasive incisions. Ann Thorac Surg 91(4):1294–1296
6. Gregoric ID, Cohn WE, Frazier OH (2011) Diaphragmatic implantation of the HeartWare ventricular assist device. J Heart Lung Transplant 30:467–470
7. Garbade J, Bittner HB, Barten MJ, Rastan A, Lehmann S, Mohr FW et al (2011) Combined surgical left ventricular reconstruction and left ventricular assist device implantation for destination therapy in end-stage heart failure. Circ Heart Fail 4(4):e14–e15
8. Patil NP, Popov AF, Simon AR (2015) Left ventricular assist device implantation with dor procedure via bilateral limited thoracotomy. Artif Organs 39(7): 641–642

Techniques for Outflow Cannula Placement

Antonio Loforte and Arnt E. Fiane

© Springer International Publishing Switzerland 2017
A. Montalto et al. (eds.), *Mechanical Circulatory Support in End-Stage Heart Failure*,
DOI 10.1007/978-3-319-43383-7_27

With the exception of percuneously placed VADs and the CentriMag device (Thoratec Inc., Pleasanton, CA), each VAD system uses a specific outflow graft and arterial cannula [1–6]. The diameter of these grafts range from 10 to 20 mm. Some are porous, and others are collagen-coated to reduce porosity. To minimize bleeding, non-coated porous grafts require preclotting with the patient's blood or other materials, such as albumin or a surgical adhesive (e.g., BioGlue, CryoLife, Kennesaw, GA). Each VAD system manufacturer has specific, required procedures for preparing the graft before implantation. Currently, last generation of VADs [1–6] has pre-coated Dacron outflow grafts such as HVAD (HeartWare Inc., Miami, FLA) and HeartMate III (Thoratec Inc., Pleasanton, CA) or the silicon material does not need pre-coating such as INCOR (Berlin Heart GmbH, Berlin, Germany).

Before the outflow is anastomosed, its tip should be beveled for the direction of the cannula; both of these procedures are necessary to avoid kinking. Grafts that are too long or too short may cause excessive tension on the anastomosis after they are attached to the pump. Grafts that are too short often lie just below the sternum, creating the risk of being cut during a re-sternotomy. Because the graft stretches after it is pressurized with blood, it should be stretched manually when estimating the proper length. The aortic graft should be beveled at approximately 30 degrees; the pulmonary artery graft bevel, in case of RVAD or BVAD implantation, should be greater. In case of continuous-flow implantable BVAD placement, an adequate narrowing of the graft for pulmonary artery should be done to reduce the risk of pulmonary overflow according to preoperative basal postcapillary pulmonary pressure.

The outflow is anastomosed to the ascending aorta for LVAD support and the main pulmonary artery for right ventricular assist device support. The anterolateral portion of the ascending aorta is the preferred location for the LVAD outflow, but location may vary depending on the presence of coronary artery grafts. With a partial occlusion clamp on the target vessel, a longitudinal aortotomy according to the length of the graft diameter is made, and the graft is anastomosed with a polypropylene suture. The integrity of the anastomosis is carefully inspected by releasing the partial occlusion clamp (◘ Fig. 27.1), allowing blood to fill the graft and expel air. After the graft fills with blood, a cross clamp is placed. If necessary, the anastomotic site can be reinforced by placing pledgeted, buttressed sutures or a felt strip around the site.

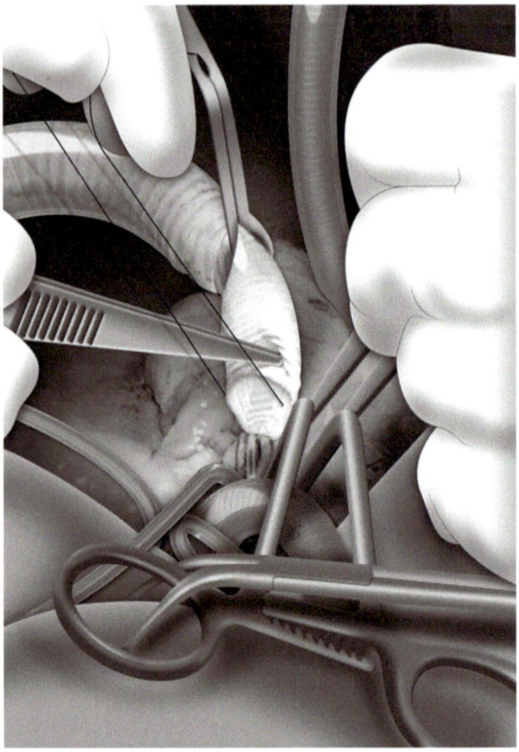

◘ **Fig. 27.1** HeartMate 3 outflow-graft anastomosis on the ascending aorta by adoption of a side clamp (Illustration by Ilaria Bondi's Peppermint Advertising)

Additionally, the outflow may be anastomosed to the descending aorta through a left thoracotomy (◘ Fig. 27.2) as suggested by such manufactures as Jarvik Inc. (Jarvik Heart, NY) for Jarvik 2000 LVAD placement [7, 8]. Or alternatively the descending aorta may be the site for any other LVAD outflow-graft anastomosis in case of redo operation implantation or in case of bridge-to-heart transplantation (Htx) intention to avoid any eventual risky sternal reentry and provide a technically easier surgery.

Outflow-graft protection is of major interest in the bridge-to-transplant therapy with left ventricular assist devices (LVADs). Avoiding adhesions of the outflow graft to the sternum prevents possible graft damages and bleeding events while performing re-thoracotomy for Htx or pump exchange. Furthermore, it reduces the time used for preparation of the anatomical structures before Htx.

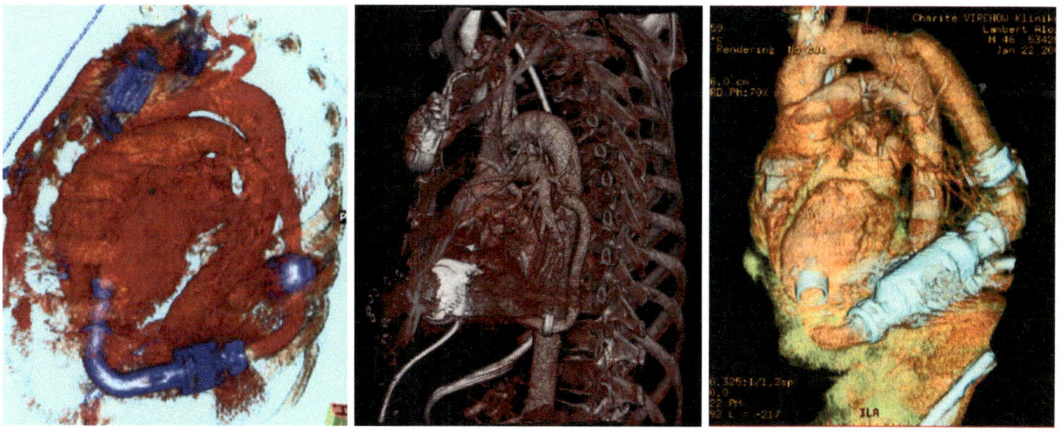

Fig. 27.2 Descending aorta outflow-graft placement by 3D computed tomography (CT) scan reconstruction

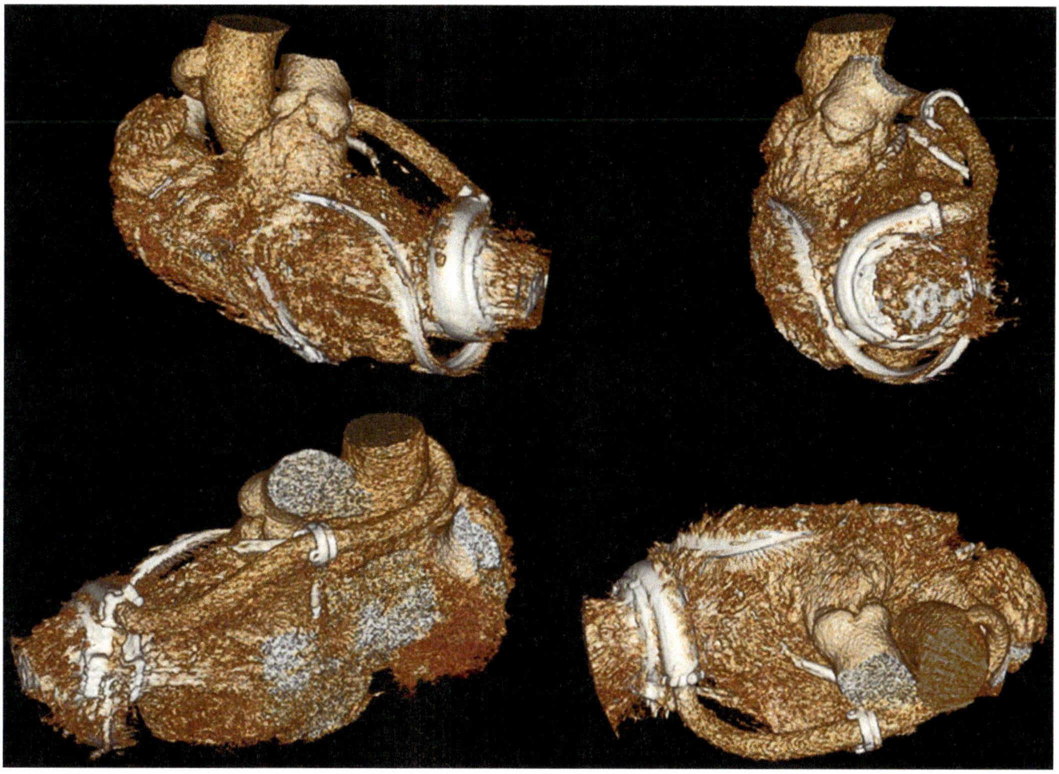

Fig. 27.3 HVAD outflow graft tunneling through the transverse sinus by 3D computed tomography (CT) scan reconstruction

A novel surgical approach for outflow LVAD placement may be its positioning through the transverse sinus (Fig. 27.3), thus performing the anastomosis, after its adequate trimming and orientation, on the right posterolateral side of the ascending aorta [9]. The positioning of the outflow graft plays an important role in the long-term outcome of the patient. False positioning leads to turbulences in the blood flow, resulting in a high risk of outflow-graft thrombosis or kinking. The flow in the outflow graft seems not to be affected by tunneling the outflow graft through the transverse sinus. Due to the augmented physiological angle of the anastomosis of the outflow graft to the aorta, the accelerated blood flow in the ascending aorta is physiological and aortic insufficiency might be

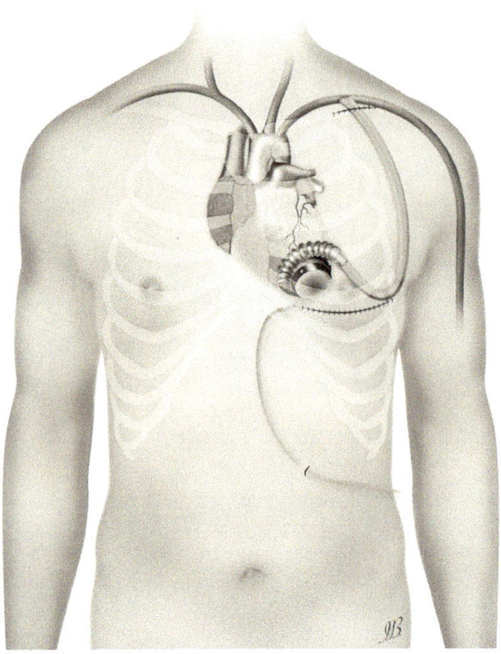

Fig. 27.4 Axillary artery HVAD outflow-graft placement (Illustration by Ilaria Bondi's Peppermint Advertising)

decreased. Preparing the transverse sinus for outflow-graft tunneling is not time-consuming, and, with surgical training, the additional amount of time used for this technique compared to the standard procedure is reduced to a minimal difference.

Moreover, in case of redo scenarios and severely calcified aorta, the outflow may be sutured on the axillary artery [10] (Fig. 27.4). The left ventricular apex is accessed through a left mini-thoracotomy. The outflow graft is tunneled through a small incision in the fourth intercostal space and then subcutaneously to the subclavian region. In order to avoid any outflow-graft kinking and compression at the passage between the ribs, a covering vascular prosthesis with a ring-reinforced Gore-Tex graft may be adopted. After division of the left axillary artery, an end-to-end anastomosis is performed to the proximal part, and the distal vessel is connected end-to-side through a fenestration in the outflow graft. This technique may achieve a more direct blood flow into the aorta and reduces cerebrovascular events while avoiding excessive flow to the arm. Other authors [10] suggest simply a single end-to-side anastomosis between the outflow graft and axillary artery. A distal banding of subclavian artery may be considered to avoid hyperflow and postoperative edema in left arm. The only significant potential adverse event may be compression of outflow graft between under the clavicle, particularly when the left arm is elevated > 90°.

However all these recently introduced challenging techniques need further investigations to be considered extensively well accepted.

References

1. Slaughter MS, Pagani FD, Rogers JG et al (2010) Clinical management of continuous-flow left ventricular assist devices in advanced heart failure. J Heart Lung Transplant 29:S1–S39
2. Thoratec Ventricular Assist Device (VAD) system instructions for use (2009) Thoratec, Pleasanton, CA, www.thoratec.com
3. Thoratec Implantable Ventricular Assist Device (IVAD) system instructions for use (2008) Thoratec, Pleasanton, CA
4. HeartWare Ventricular Assist System HVAD pump surgical implant (2009) HeartWare, Miami Lakes, FL. www.heartware.com.
5. LaRose JA, Tamez D, Ashenuga M, Reyes C (2010) Design concepts and principle of operation of the HeartWare ventricular assist system. ASAIO J 56: 285–289
6. Netuka I, Sood P, Pya Y et al (2015) Fully magnetically levitated left ventricular assist system for treating advanced HF: a multicenter study. J Am Coll Cardiol 66(23):2579–2589
7. Hetzer R, Potapov EV, Weng Y, Sinawski H, Knollmann F, Komoda T et al (2004) Implantation of MicroMed DeBakey VAD through left thoracotomy after previous median sternotomy operations. Ann Thorac Surg 77:347–350
8. Umakanthan R, Haglund NA, Stulak JM, Joyce LD, Ahmad R, Keebler ME et al (2013) Left thoracotomy HeartWare implantation with outflow graft anastomosis to the descending aorta: a simplified bridge for patients with multiple previous sternotomies. ASAIO J 59:664–667
9. Loforte A, Pilato E, Marinelli G (2016) Outflow Graft tunneling through the transverse sinus for left ventricular assist device placement. Artif Organs 2016;40(12):E305-E306.
10. Bortolussi G, Lika A, Bejko J, Gallo M, Tarzia V, Gerosa G, Bottio T (2015) Left ventricular assist device end-to-end connection to the left subclavian artery: an alternative technique. Ann Thorac Surg 100:e93–e95

Techniques for Driveline Positioning

Christina Feldmann, Jasmin S. Hanke, Günes Dogan, Ezin Deniz, Axel Haverich, Thomas Krabatsch, and Jan D. Schmitto

© Springer International Publishing Switzerland 2017
A. Montalto et al. (eds.), *Mechanical Circulatory Support in End-Stage Heart Failure*,
DOI 10.1007/978-3-319-43383-7_28

28.1 Introduction

In addition to the improvements in implantation procedure of the pump itself [1], there are other parts of the LVAD system, which are crucial to the process of LVAD therapy such as graft anastomosis, controller and battery management, and driveline. An optimal driveline position is one variable for a positive outcome of LVAD therapy. As one of the main complications next to bleeding and thromboembolic events, driveline infections influence LVAD implantation outcome as well as survival of patients after heart transplantation [2]. Another important issue in driveline-related complications is the case of fractured fractures of drivelines leading to connectivity problems and consequently to pump stoppage. Besides reducing the incidence of these important risk factors for continuous pump operation, deliberate driveline repositioning also promotes quality of life for the patient. Handling of controller, harness, and dressing can be optimized and personalized for each patient as per their daily habit. In case of a severe driveline exit site (DLES) infection, a well-established surgical path with a longer subfascial route may provide more options, for example, surgical revision [3].

This chapter provides existing information on the driveline positioning which is applicable to the currently available devices: HeartMate II, HeartMate III (both from/manufactured by St. Jude Medical, Inc.), HVAD (HeartWare, Inc.), HeartAssist5 (ReliantHeart, Inc.), and INCOR (Berlin Heart GmbH). When comparing the drivelines of these pumps, minor differences may be observed in driveline diameter or velour setting. While the HeartMate II, for example, shows two cable sections with the implantable part covered with velour and the external cable with a bar cable sheath, cables of HeartMate III and HVAD are divided into three sections: velour covers the cable's middle section, leaving a bar cable sheath near to pump in the implantable section and near the controller in the external section. This marginal distinction has nearly no effect on the surgical techniques for driveline positioning, described in this chapter. Only the pump geometry and driveline exit side on the pump may provide opportunities for driveline positioning.

28.2 Preparation/Planning of the Driveline Positioning and the Exit Site

The driveline course and the exit site position should be planned well before the surgery. The well-positioned driveline exit site is crucial for infection, cable wear and fracture prevention as well as patient's quality of life. The decision should accommodate patient's wish and behavior as well as anatomical considerations (see ◘ Table 28.1). The internal positioning and exit site of the driveline in

◘ **Table 28.1** Decisional aspects for driveline exit site (DLES) positioning and internal course

Aspects	Details
Patients anatomy and physical status	Obesity Size of abdominal region Avoid rib area Abdominal surgical history Diabetes mellitus type II
Patient preferences	Left or right hander Clothing habits Waistband positioning Sleeping side Preferred harness option Avoid sweaty areas for DLES DLES should be accessible for dressing/self-dressing
General aspects	Driveline course to the VAD system peripherals Prefer a long intrafascial course Avoid sharp bends at the intracorporeal course, e.g., at pump or rib Avoid sharp bends at the extracorporeal course when exiting the skin
Adverse events aspects	Surgical revision strategy: DLES position after revision

the coastal area as well as internal and external sharp bends should be avoided. In case of a history of abdominal surgery the opposite body side should be considered for tunneling and exit site. Patient preferences should be evaluated in a doctor/patient dialog involving a practical discussion with the patient standing and may include anatomic situation as well as patient's habits including sleeping side, right/left hander, waistband position, and clothing habits. Additionally, the external course of the cable should be taken into account and should affect the DL skin exit angle and direction: the thoughtful placing of the controller harness, immobilization dressing, and smooth cable bend toward the controller are important factors to avoid

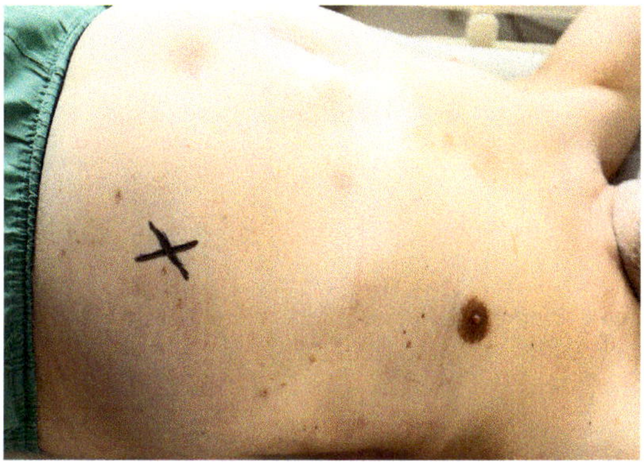

◻ **Fig. 28.1** Patient, whose driveline exit site was marked preoperatively

mechanical manipulation of the driveline exit site (DLES), which may promote wound fractures and contribute to DLES infection.

For documentation of the DLES and driveline course conclusion, the surgeon may consider marking the internal driveline course and exit site on the patient's body for the surgery process (◻ Fig. 28.1).

28.3 Surgical Procedure

There are different surgical procedures known in the field, all pursuing the goal to maximize the length of the velour-covered driveline being placed in the subcutaneous tissue, which promotes a reduced infection rate [4] as well as giving more options in case of surgical revision with DLES infection [3].

There are two main tunneling techniques for the driveline.

A. Single tunneling technique

This technique uses a single tunneling path for placing the driveline in the abdomen. ◻ Figure 28.2a, b gives a schematic view on the driveline course.

In one approach, the cable is placed in a U shape facing caudal from the pump toward the umbilicus, following the U bend again cranial toward the exit site at the midclavicular line below the right or left subcostal margin. This

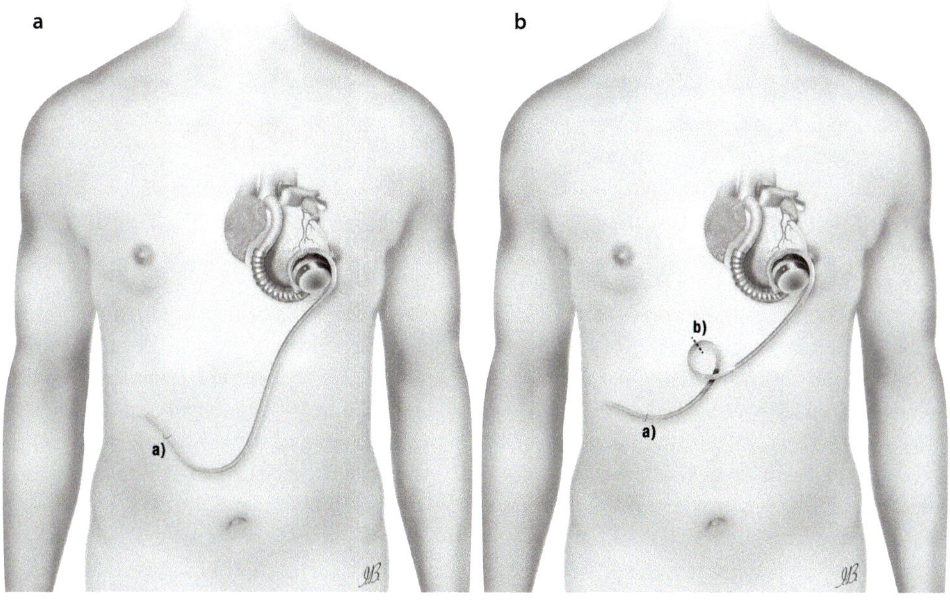

◻ **Fig. 28.2** **a**: (*a*) driveline exit site; **b**: (*a*) driveline exit site, (*b*) suture around driveline and peritoneum. (According to [7]) (*Pictures by Ilaria Bondi's Peppermint Advertising*)

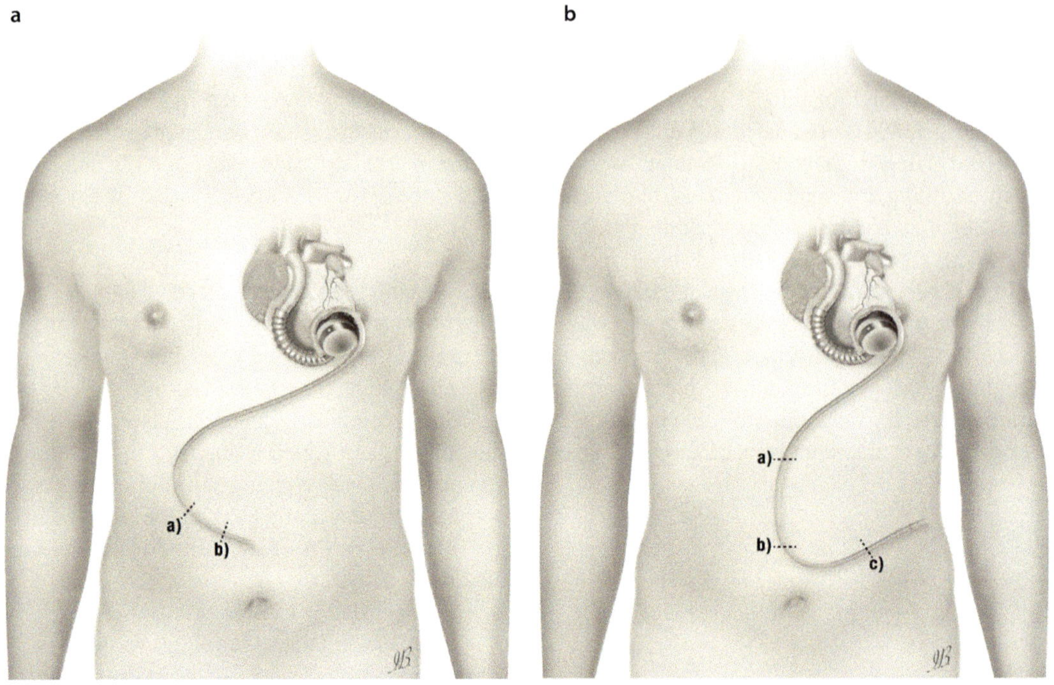

Fig. 28.3 **a**, **b** Driveline course and incision sites in double tunneling technique (According to [3, 4, 6]); **a**: (*a*) fascial transition, (*b*) driveline exit site; **b**: (*b*) fascial transition, (*c*) driveline exit site, which may be located on the left or right side. (*Pictures by Ilaria Bondi's Peppermint Advertising*)

surgical technique uses a U-shaped tunneling device. Some surgeons prefer a custom-made device bent into a U shape [7].

A second single tunneling approach uses a short tunneling track very lateral to the right or left exit site, which is again at the midclavicular line below the subcostal margin. The driveline is formed with a loop near the midline using the surgical pump implantation field to increase the intracorporeal part of the cable and act as a strain relief. The loop is fixed with a suture to the peritoneum. The driveline may exit in every abdominal quadrant, although the variables in DLES decisions mentioned in the previous section should be considered [7].

B. Doubled tunneling technique
This technique uses a tunneling path, which is set up in two to three steps. In Fig. 28.3a–c, respectively, the tunneling incisions and the driveline course can be seen; Fig. 28.4 gives an view of the intraoperative tunneling procedure.

In the two-step approach, the driveline is placed in a big C shape. The first tunneling step places the driveline with a long-curved course beneath the fascia of the abdominal muscles, transition the fascia through a small incision near the anterior axillary line, and 3 cm caudal of the subcostal line. The final DLES will be near the midline in the direction of the left lateral abdominal wall through a second small skin incision. Due to the design of the HeartMate II pump and its cable, this technique suits this pump type very well [3].

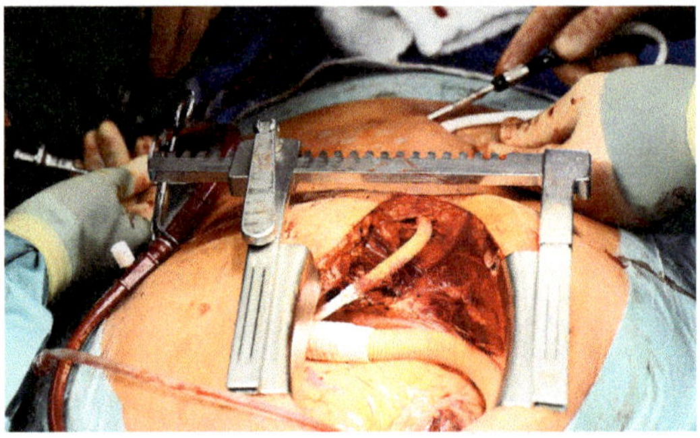

Fig. 28.4 Intraoperative image showing the last tunneling step in double tunnel technique to the designated driveline exit site

In the three-step approach, the driveline forms a long C-shape course with a more lateral exit site. Initially, the driveline is tunneled from the pump pocket through a small incision, approximately 5 cm medial of the anterolateral thoracotomy above the rectus abdominis muscle. Then the driveline is placed in the sheath of the musculus rectus abdominis and exits the muscle's fascia through a second small incision, which is placed caudal, median in umbilical direction. The third section of driveline course leads subcutaneously to the left or right upper abdominal quadrant [4, 6].

The standard tunneling device recommended by the pump manufacturer should ideally be used for this tunneling technique.

In case of the implantation of an HVAD (HeartWare Inc.), the cable may be placed around the pump before it finds its way through the fasciae. This is not necessary with the St. Jude Medical, Inc. devices HMII and HMIII, Berlin Heart's INCOR, or ReliantHeart's HeartAssist5.

There are some considerations which are applicable to all surgical tunneling techniques:

Sharp bends inside and outside the body (resulting from perpendicular skin exit direction) should be avoided. The skin incision for the tunneling exit site(s) should be prepared with the circular skin knife provided by the LVAD manufacturer or with a similar knife of comparable shape and size. The velour part of the driveline should end at skin level for any tunneling technique or LVAD type [4, 5, 7–9] or be completely covered inside the body. This might promote reduced DLES infection rates, which is described in literature in single center studies and a register study: Thoratec initiated a multicenter registry to investigate the outcome of HMII implantation with a longer part of the driveline so that the silicon part of the driveline exits the skin and the velour part is completely implanted [10]. Promising first results demonstrate a reduction of DLES infection with this DLES strategy, and prospective multicenter studies are ongoing to confirm this hypothesis with reliable statistical data.

In addition to these driveline-specific considerations for the surgical positioning, general guidelines for intraoperative infection prevention should be considered.

28.4 Dressing Procedure

Postoperative dressing of the driveline is an important part in driveline implantation procedure. Nevertheless, driveline fixation and dressing strategies vary from center to center.

After VAD implantation maximal immobilization of the driveline is mandatory to promote undisturbed wound healing and proper tissue ingrowth due to prevention of DLES trauma via mechanical manipulation [4, 10, 11]. For immobilization there are several systems available ranging from pump manufacturer provided (Thoratec/St. Jude Medical support binder) over anchoring devices from Hollister, Centurion, StatLock, or UniGrip and should be chosen to the patient's and clinic's best practice. Directly after surgery when the first wound dressing was applied, manipulation of the DLES should be avoided as long as possible for at least 10 days, and wound dressing changes should be minimized. This allows for an optimal initial anchoring of the driveline [4]. For detailed information on dressing change with regard to infection prevention, see the Infectious Complications chapter of this book. For optimal outcome, prevention of DLES infections, but also for improved quality of life, the patient and caregiver should be dedicated to LVAD "maintenance" including driveline dressing change. Extensive patient and caregiver education will prepare both for optimal home care and emphasize that patient behavior is an immense factor for infectious-free LVAD lifetime.

28.5 Explantation of the Driveline

An LVAD explantation may occur when the patient receives heart transplantation, the LVAD needs to be exchanged due to infections, pump thrombosis or other LVAD malfunction, or when the heart recovers from heart failure, and the LVAD is no longer needed for circulatory support. In these cases, the LVAD will be dissected in toto using full sternotomy or less invasive procedures [12]. The driveline is cut near the pump and completely, percutaneously removed.

28.6 What if a Driveline Damage or Infection Occurs?

Even with mindful surgical implantation, post-surgical handling, and dressing of the LVAD driveline, driveline infections and fractures may occur. In case of a cable injury with or without electrical functionality impairment, the surgeon in collaboration with the VAD manufacturer will find the optimal treatment solution for the specific patient case. This may result in a pump exchange as an ultima ratio treatment [13], although the driveline fracture may be successfully repaired, for example, with self-fusing tapes, latex tubing [14], or cable coupling [Hannover Medical School experience].

In case of a driveline infection, the physician has several surgical and nonsurgical options for treatment as extensively described in chapter Infectious Complications of this book. Nevertheless, a well-considered driveline positioning with a maximal long subfascial course will give the surgeon more options for surgical revision of the driveline.

References

1. Hanke JS, Rojas SV, Avsar M, Haverich A, Schmitto JD (2015) Minimally-invasive LVAD implantation: state of the art. Curr Cardiol Rev 11(3):246–251
2. Krabatsch T, Schweiger M, Stepanenko A, Kukucka M, Vierecke J, Lehmkuhl HB, Huebler M, Hennig E, Potapov E, Hetzer R (2011) Mechanical circulatory support—results, developments and trends. J Cardiovasc Transl Res 4(3):332–339
3. Schibilsky D, Benk C, Haller C, Berchtold-Herz M, Siepe M, Beyersdorf F, Schlensak C (2012) Double tunnel technique for the LVAD driveline: improved management regarding driveline infections. J Artif Organs 15(1):44–48
4. Fleissner F, Avsar M, Malehsa D, Strueber M, Haverich A, Schmitto JD (2013) Reduction of driveline infections through doubled driveline tunneling of left ventricular assist devices. Artif Organs 37(1):102–107
5. HeartWare, Inc. (2009) HeartWare® Ventricular Assist System Instruction for Use
6. Schmitto JD, Hanke JS, Rojas SV, Avsar M, Haverich A (2015) First implantation in man of a new magnetically levitated left ventricular assist device (HeartMate III). J Heart Lung Transplant 34(6):858–860
7. Slaughter MS, Pagani FD, Rogers JG, Miller LW, Sun B, Russell SD, Starling RC, Chen L, Boyle AJ, Chillcott S, Adamson RM, Blood MS, Camacho MT, Idrissi KA, Petty M, Sobieski M, Wright S, Myers TJ, Farrar DJ (2010) Clinical management of continuous-flow left ventricular assist devices in advanced heart failure. J Heart Lung Transplant 29(4):S1–S39
8. Schima H, Schloglhofer T, Dohna RZ, Drews T, Morshuis M, Roefe D, Schmitto JD, Struber M, Zimpfer D (2014) Usability of ventricular assist devices in daily experience: a multicenter study. Artif Organs 38(9):751–760
9. Thoratec Corporation (2012) Left ventricular assist system (LVAS) HeartMate II™. Instruction for Use
10. Dean D, Kallel F, Ewald GA, Tatooles A, Sheridan BC, Brewer RJ, Caldeira C, Farrar DJ, Akhter SA (2015) Reduction in driveline infection rates: results from the HeartMate II multicenter driveline silicone skin interface (SSI) registry. J Heart Lung Transplant 34(6):781–789
11. Pasque MK, Hanselman T, Shelton K, Kehoe-Huck B, Hedges R, Cassivi SD, Ewald GA, Rogers JG (2016) Surgical management of Novacor drive-line exit site infections. Ann Thorac Surg 74(4):1267–1268
12. Schmitto JD, Rojas SV, Hanke JS, Avsar M, Haverich A (2014) Minimally invasive left ventricular assist device explantation after cardiac recovery: surgical technical considerations. Artif Organs 38(6):507–510
13. Potapov EV, Kaufmann F, Stepanenko A, Hening E, Vierecke J, Löw A, Lehmkuhl E, Dranishnikov N, Hetzer R, Krabatsch T (2012) Pump exchange for cable damage in patients supported with HeartMate II left ventricular assist device. ASAIO J 58(6):578–582
14. Schima H, Stoiber M, Schlöglhofer T, Hartner Z, Haberl T, Zimpfer D (2014) Repair of left ventricular assist device driveline damage directly at the transcutaneous exit site. Artif Organs 38(5):422–425

Percutaneous Devices: Options

Melody Sherwood and Shelley A. Hall

© Springer International Publishing Switzerland 2017
A. Montalto et al. (eds.), *Mechanical Circulatory Support in End-Stage Heart Failure*,
DOI 10.1007/978-3-319-43383-7_29

29.1 Introduction

Percutaneous ventricular assist devices (pVADs) increasingly are being used in patients with cardiogenic shock (CS) as a bridge to recovery, decision, durable device, or cardiac transplantation [1]. By far the most common cause of CS is myocardial infarction. However, acute regurgitant valve failure, myocarditis, postcardiotomy shock, and acute or chronic heart failure also may present with end-organ dysfunction from hypoperfusion due to cardiac pump failure, the hallmark of this syndrome.

Though fibrinolytics and primary percutaneous coronary intervention (PCI) have improved mortality in patients who experience shock from acute myocardial infarction, little progress in the medical treatment of cardiogenic shock has been made over the last few decades; overall mortality remains greater than 40% [2]. The mainstay of medical treatment continues to be inotropes and vasopressors, but when used to temporize the patient hemodynamically in the short term, it actually contributes to end-organ dysfunction, arrhythmia, increased myocardial oxygen consumption, and increased mortality in the long term [3]. Frequently, they do not provide enough support to maintain adequate perfusion and hemodynamic stability. Unfortunately, once end-organ dysfunction occurs, it not only leads to increased mortality but can prevent the patient from being a candidate for advanced heart failure therapies such as durable ventricular assist devices or cardiac transplantation. In conditions where myocardial recovery is possible, medical therapy may not provide enough support to keep the patient alive and preserve end-organ function until recovery can occur.

While some pVADs have been studied for temporary support during "high-risk" PCI, there has been far less research on the role of these devices in the end-stage heart failure patient. This chapter strives to explain how these devices can be utilized in this patient population.

Currently, there are multiple percutaneous devices available for use in end-stage heart failure patients, and the choice of device or devices is dependent on multiple variables. Is RV failure, LV failure, or biventricular failure present? How much hemodynamic support is needed? Does the patient have respiratory failure, circulatory failure, or both? Does the patient have any absolute or relative contraindications for a particular device? What is the ease and rapidity of device deployment and what is the available operator's comfort deploying the device? What is the ancillary staff's level of comfort and experience caring for a patient with the device? What is the next step in management of the patient? The answer to each of these questions is important to determine the most appropriate device for the patient. There is no one-size-fits-all device, and there often is not a single solution to a patient conundrum.

Ultimately, all pVADs serve as a bridge to something, whether it is recovery, decision, durable device, or cardiac transplantation. If the patient has a condition at baseline that precludes them from bridging to advanced therapies or recovery, a pVAD should not be placed. A candid conversation about the possibility of failure to recover or about conditions that disqualify the patient from advanced therapies should take place with the patient and family beforehand whenever possible.

29.2 Intra-aortic Balloon Pump

The intra-aortic balloon pump (IABP) is the oldest and most widely used pVAD currently in use for left ventricular support. Invented in 1968, it works on the principle of counterpulsation to pressure unload the heart and, to a lesser extent, increase coronary perfusion [4–6]. The dual lumen catheter with a balloon at its distal end typically is inserted through the femoral artery and passed retrograde to the proximal descending aorta just distal to the ostium of the subclavian artery (■ Fig. 29.1). It is then connected to

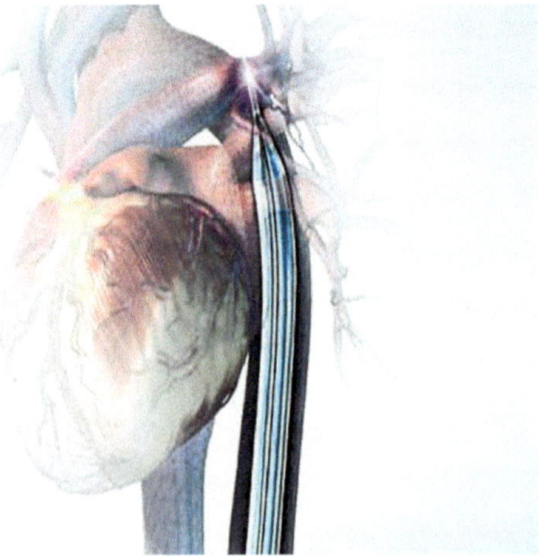

■ **Fig. 29.1** IABP

the controller which causes the balloon to inflate and deflate with the timing of the cardiac cycle. One lumen is the channel by which the balloon is inflated, and a second lumen facilitates a guide wire for placement and transduces an aortic pressure tracing when the catheter is in place. Helium is used to inflate and deflate the balloon due to its low viscosity, allowing rapid movement of the gas into and out of the balloon. Helium is able to be more rapidly absorbed by the body in the case of balloon rupture, decreasing the chance of occurrence of a fatal air embolism. Inflation of the balloon during diastole causes both retrograde and antegrade displacement of blood, augmenting diastolic blood flow and pressure. The retrograde flow into the coronary arteries increases coronary blood flow (CBF), and the antegrade displacement increases forward flow to the body, increasing the mean arterial pressure (MAP). Rapid deflation of the balloon at the onset of ventricular systole creates suction, dropping the pressure in the aorta and thus raising forward flow. This decrease in pressure and increase in flow results in a reduction in afterload, decreased LVEDP, rise in stroke volume, and therefore cardiac output. Myocardial ischemia is reduced through multiple mechanisms including decreasing oxygen consumption by lessening ventricular wall tension and coronary microvascular resistance and improving CBF both through a rise in diastolic pressure and a drop in LVEDP. IABP has been shown to increase cardiac output by 0.5 L/min in patients with cardiogenic shock [4].

Technically, the IABP is easy to place. It requires only one arterial access, most commonly 8F, though other sizes are available. A radiopaque tip allows placement under fluoroscopy, but bedside placement with "guestimate distance" is feasible with position later confirmed by the use of a chest X-ray. An experienced operator can insert a balloon in approximately10 min. Insertion via the femoral artery prohibits ambulation, though safety and efficacy have been demonstrated with insertion through the subclavian, axillary, or brachial arteries [7]. These approaches should be performed under fluoroscopic guidance.

The IABP has some limitations. Its performance is dependent on a relatively stable electrical rhythm, intrinsic heart function, vascular tone, correct placement of the balloon in the aorta, and timing of balloon inflation and deflation. It has limited, if any, support in right ventricular failure. It should not be used in patients with more than mild aortic insufficiency as increasing diastolic retrograde flow would raise LVEDP and thus worsen their hemodynamics. Severe atherosclerosis or tortuous vessels can also be a contraindication to IABP placement. Potential complications include bleeding, infection, thrombocytopenia, limb ischemia, embolization to distal vessels including stroke, and compromise of subclavian or renal artery perfusion by forward or backward migration of the balloon. Vascular injury can occur at the entry site or at any point along the aorta including the ostia of the visceral arteries.

Earlier studies on IABP use in patients with myocardial infarction showed improved mortality or a trend toward it. The SHOCK trial demonstrated lower in-hospital mortality of patients with myocardial infarction who received IABP in addition to thrombolytic therapy or early revascularization with PCI or coronary artery bypass graft surgery [8]. GUSTO-I showed a trend toward improved 30 day and 1 year mortality in early IABP and thrombolytic therapy, although this improved mortality comes with an increased risk in bleeding [9]. Subsequent analysis of registry data showed this mortality benefit only held in patients undergoing thrombolytic therapy and not in cases of primary PCI [10]. Meta-analyses of IABP use in infarct-related cardiogenic shock cases not only showed no improvement in mortality but also demonstrated an increased risk of complications including stroke [11]. In spite of the current data, IABP is still widely used and has some class II indications in the current guidelines [12].

The challenge arises with patient selection. With its limited CO augmentation of 0.5 lpm, IABP provides little support when end-organ perfusion is impaired. It is more effective in ischemic situations or acute instability, but it rarely provides adequate support for a prolonged period of time. Thus, while helpful in the post-MI patient, it is not a good durable bridge strategy for more than a day or two. Consequently, if the recovery of end-organ function is not significant, which would reflect adequate hemodynamic support, escalation to next stage therapy is often needed. Most evaluations for transplant or LVAD cannot occur in a day, and, more often than not, the next level of support is another pVAD.

29.3 TandemHeart®

The TandemHeart® (CardiacAssist, Inc., Pittsburgh, PA) is a continuous-flow pVAD that works in parallel with the heart to augment cardiac output and volume unload the heart. It is FDA approved for up to 6 h of support for procedures not requiring full bypass support, though there are reports of it being in excess of 3 weeks. The TandemHeart is a magnetically driven extracorporeal centrifugal pump that indirectly unloads the LV by transferring oxygenated blood from the left atrium to the iliac arteries and perfusing the aorta retrograde. Access to the left atrium is obtained by passing a catheter to the right atrium by femoral vein access and performing a transseptal puncture and dilation to place the 21F inflow cannula (Fig. 29.2). The outflow cannula is placed in the iliac artery via access of the femoral artery with either a 15F or 17F cannula. In patients with smaller femoral vessels or with peripheral vascular disease, two 12F cannulae can be placed bilaterally to decrease the potential for vascular compromise. The amount of flow can range from 2.5 to 4 L/min depending on the size of the cannulae and the speed of the pump.

The TandemHeart decreases LV preload, filling pressures, and wall stress and improves peripheral tissue perfusion. Due to its parallel circuit to the heart and its unloading distally, stroke volume is reduced, and the ventricular afterload is increased. Though myocardial oxygen demand is lowered due to lessened preload and wall stress, this increase in afterload leaves the absolute effect on myocardial oxygen consumption dependent on the hemodynamic severity of the cardiogenic shock [5, 6]. This device must be placed under fluoroscopy or with intracardiac or transesophageal echocardiographic guidance by an operator skilled in transseptal puncture, often limiting this technology to larger, tertiary centers. Aortography with runoff should be performed before placement to evaluate the iliac arteries. Placement of the device takes 30–45 min when done by an experienced operator. Systemic heparinization is required, and the device is FDA approved for the addition of an oxygenator to the circuit for gas exchange.

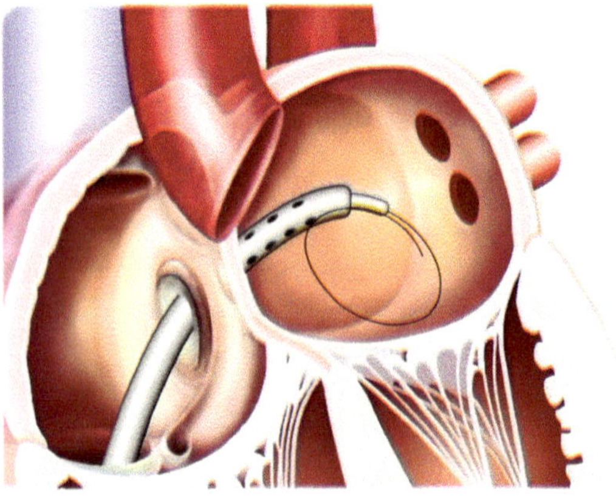

Fig. 29.2 Tandem inflow cannula across atrial septum

Contraindications to placement of the TandemHeart include right or left atrial thrombus, moderate or severe aortic insufficiency, ventricular septal defect, bleeding diathesis and coagulopathies, or significant peripheral vascular disease. Possible complications include bleeding at insertion sites, cardiac perforation and tamponade, infection, and embolic events – including stroke, limb ischemia, vascular injury, hemolysis, desaturation from migration of the left atrial cannula, or right to left shunting, paradoxical embolus, arrhythmia, or creation of an ASD from transseptal puncture.

Though studies of its use in cardiogenic shock after AMI show the TandemHeart provides more support and improves hemodynamics to a greater degree than IABP, no mortality benefit has been demonstrated [13]. In studies powered to detect mortality benefit, an increased risk of bleeding and vascular complications has been seen. Small case series demonstrated utility using the TandemHeart as a bridging device to advanced therapies such as durable device [14] and transplant and as bridge to recovery [15].

Moreover, TandemHeart has been used with limited success to provide RV support in certain clinical conditions such as isolated RV failure from RV infarct and pulmonary hypertension, in conjunction with other PVADs for biventricular failure and for temporary RV support after placement of a durable LVAD [16]. For RV support, both the inflow and outflow cannulae are placed by venous access, usually in the bilateral femoral veins. The inflow cannula is placed in the right atrium and the outflow located in the main pulmonary artery to support and offload the RV. When the distance from the femoral vein to the pulmonary artery is too long, the outflow cannula can be put in the pulmonary artery via the internal jugular. With its highly technical insertion needs, only high volume, tertiary centers are capable of maintaining the skill set necessary for proficiency. Its flexibility to potentially provide biventricular support is a plus. It does have a tendency to migrate over time, and, like all pVADs, risks of complications rise with prolonged support.

29.4 Impella®

The Impella Recover LP (Abiomed Inc., Danvers, MA) devices have become an increasingly popular pVAD option due to their ability to deliver a significant amount of support and their relative ease of deployment requiring only a single arterial access.

The Impella 2.5 and Impella CP are the most commonly used iterations of the Impella family of devices, and they are installed using the same platform [17, 18]. A miniature axial flow pump is mounted on a pigtail catheter, and using standard catheterization techniques, it is passed retrograde across the aortic valve and placed in the left ventricular cavity with TEE or fluoroscopic visualization (Fig. 29.3). Blood is pumped from the left ventricle through the inlet into the proximal ascending aorta by continuous flow. Up to 2.5 and 3.5 L/min of flow can be delivered by the Impella 2.5 and Impella CP, respectively. The amount of flow is dependent on the size of the pump, the speed of the impeller, and the pressure gradient between the ventricle (inflow) and aorta (outflow).

The Impella 2.5 is indicated for up to 6 h of use during high-risk PCI to prevent hemodynamic instability. The Impella CP is indicated for up to 6 h for partial circulatory support in procedures not requiring cardiopulmonary bypass. Studies comparing the Impella 2.5 and Impella CP with IABP in patients in cardiogenic shock associated with AMI showed superior hemodynamics in the Impella group, but to date there is no mortality benefit [17, 18].

The Impella 5.0 operates with the same type of pump as the Impella 2.5 and CP, but due to its large size it requires a surgical cut down for catheter placement. This procedure can be performed by the CV surgeon or a vascular surgeon in conjunction with a cardiologist. The Impella 5.0 generates a larger amount of flow, up to 5 L/min, than the Impella 2.5. Though the Impella 5.0 was

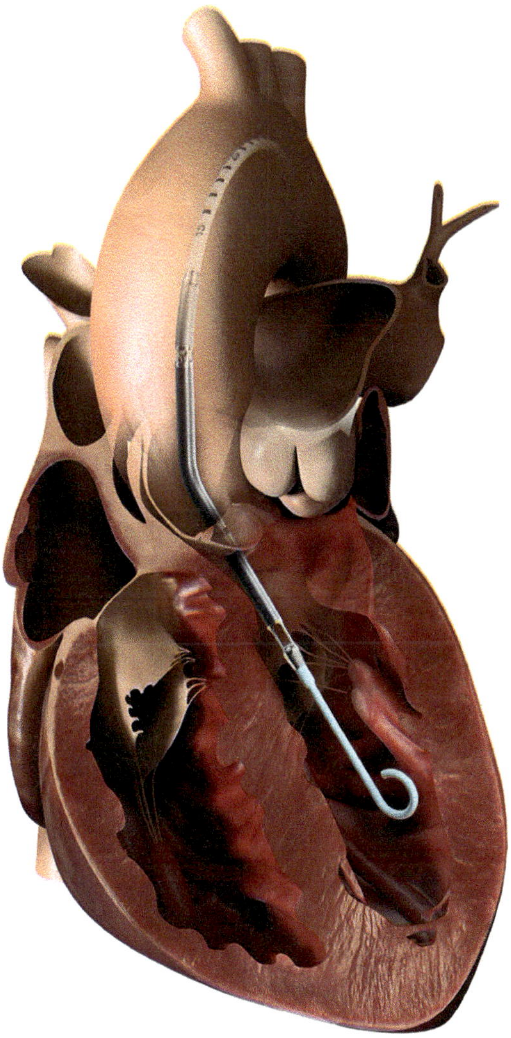

Fig. 29.3 All Impella left sided support placement across aortic valve

developed initially for femoral artery access, placement in the axillary or subclavian artery (Fig. 29.4) is safe and effective in providing support with the added benefit of allowing the patient to sit in a chair, ambulate, and rehabilitate while it is in place [17, 18].

Indications for the use of the Impella 5.0 are circulatory support with no cardiopulmonary bypass or circulatory support using an extracorporeal bypass control unit for up to 6 h, but it can provide adequate support for over 45 days [17, 18]. Case studies demonstrated successful utilization of the Impella 5.0 as bridge from ECMO to durable device [19], as support in acute rejection after orthotopic heart transplantation [20], for LV support in RV failure as a bridge to RV recovery

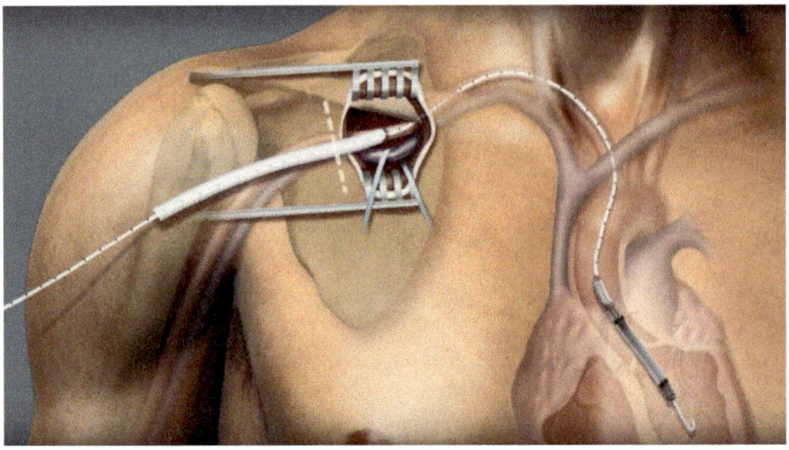

Fig. 29.4 Axillary access via placement of graft

and durable LVAD [21], as bridge to recovery in myocarditis [22], and as bridge to cardiac transplantation [23]. Results from some small case series suggest survival improved in patients with severe and profound shock after ST elevation myocardial infarction with immediate Impella 5.0 treatment compared to Impella 2.5 support alone [24].

Contraindication to placement of any of the Impella LP devices includes moderate or greater aortic insufficiency, the presence of a mechanical aortic valve, aortic stenosis with valve area less than 1.5 cm^2, a heart constrictive device, severe PVD that would impair the ability to place the device, or LV thrombus. The potential complications include bleeding, infection, vascular injury, hemolysis, stroke, cardiac perforation or tamponade, damage to the aortic valve, device malfunction, or arrhythmia. Hemolysis from mechanical shearing can also occur in 5–10% of patients but usually responds to device repositioning. If renal failure from persistent hemolysis occurs, the device should be removed.

Development of the Impella device greatly expanded the temporary support world for end-stage heart failure patients. With growing resistance to implanting durable VADs in the INTERMACS 1 patient, the Impella 5.0 allows adequate hemodynamic support for these patients, appropriate end-organ recovery of function, and a higher rate of success for the eventual cardiac replacement option. With the axillary implant option, these patients can also avoid the deconditioning that results from groin access mandatory bed rest restrictions. While the Impella 5.0 does require a mini-surgical approach, the single vessel access, no need to cross cardiac chambers and axillary implantation makes it poised to be the most currently balanced device for intermediate support in this patient population.

29.5 Extracorporeal Membrane Oxygenation (ECMO)

Extracorporeal membrane oxygenation (ECMO) offers pulmonary or cardiopulmonary support depending on its configuration. With its improved technology, it is having a "comeback" of sorts.

Venoarterial (V-A) ECMO provides both gas exchange and circulatory support through a continuous-flow pump. It is used in the setting of left ventricular or biventricular failure. In the V-A configuration, the inflow cannula is placed via a large central vein. Blood is circulated through the extracorporeal pump but is returned to the body after gas exchange through an arterial cannula. V-A ECMO can provide essentially physiologic flows up to 6 L/min without any intrinsic activity from the heart. It effectively decreases the preload of the right and left ventricles and increases MAP and end-organ perfusion, but it enhances the afterload on the left ventricle resulting in no real net change in myocardial oxygen consumption [5, 6]. The IABP or Impella devices are sometimes used concurrently with V-A ECMO for LV unloading when inotropes cannot produce enough LV contractility.

In pure pulmonary failure, veno-venous (V-V) ECMO circulates blood through an oxygenator outside of the body using a continuous-flow pump when gas exchange in the lung is impaired. The oxygenator not only oxygenates the blood but removes the waste carbon dioxide. In this configuration both the inflow cannula and the outflow cannula are placed through a venous access, sometimes even the same vein if a dual lumen catheter is used. Because blood is being removed from and returned to a vein, it offers no hemodynamic support and functions only for gas exchange in respiratory failure. The one exception to this rule is when the V-V ECMO outflow cannula is placed in the PA to provide ventricular unloading and RV support. In this case the PA cannula requires surgical placement.

V-V or V-A ECMO can be placed at the bedside without fluoroscopic guidance. The amount of flow generated is dependent on the size of the cannulae and the speed of the pump. ECMO also requires that the patient be heparinized. The degree of heparinization needed is determined by the type of oxygenator in the circuit. Management of the ECMO pump and circuit requires an experienced perfusionist, although high volume centers can appropriately train CVICU nurses to cover this responsibility. Contraindications to ECMO include severe PVD, significant aortic regurgitation, and bleeding diathesis. Potential complications include bleeding, vascular injury, limb ischemia, thromboembolic events, and pump failure. The risk of limb ischemia can be ameliorated by placement of a reperfusion cannula to provide additional blood flow to the limb distal to the cannulation site.

ECMO has resurged as a support technology for end-stage heart failure for recovery or bridge to more durable solutions. Yet the percutaneous approach is limited to groin access and all of the issues associated with prolonged bed rest. While upper vessel implantation can be done with limited surgical approaches, the durability is limited, and vascular complication rates are somewhat higher. However, unlike other technologies, it does have the ability to simultaneously support the RV and LV and provide oxygenation. Thus, when these conditions are present, it can be easier than multiple pVADs. ◘ Tables 29.1 and 29.2 summarize the comparative differences among the described devices in hemodynamics and technical issues.

◘ Table 29.1 Comparison of devices

Device	IABP	TandemHeart	Impella 2.5	Impella CP	Impella 5.0	ECMO
Cannula size	7.9 Fr	21 Fr inflow; 15–17 Fr outflow	13 Fr	14 Fr	22 F	Centrifugal
Pump mechanism	Pneumatic	Centrifugal	Axial flow	Axial flow	Axial flow	Centrifugal
Insertion technique	Descending aorta via the femoral artery	21 Fr inflow cannula into the left atrium via the left femoral vein and transseptal puncture and 15–17 Fr outflow cannula into the femoral artery	12 Fr catheter placed retrograde across the aortic valve via the femoral artery	14 Fr catheter placed retrograde across the aortic valve via the femoral artery	22 Fr catheter placed retrograde across the aortic valve via a surgical cut down of the femoral, axillary, or subclavian artery	Inflow cannula into the right atrium via the femoral vein, outflow cannula into the descending aorta via the femoral artery
Maximum hemodynamic support	0.5–1.0 L/ min	4 L/min	2.5 L/min	3.7 L/min	5.0 L/min	>4.5 L/min
Implantation time	+	+++	++	++	++++	++

(continued)

Table 29.1 (continued)

Device	IABP	TandemHeart	Impella 2.5	Impella CP	Impella 5.0	ECMO
Risk of limb ischemia	+	+++	++	++	++	+++
Anticoagulation	+	+++	+	+	+	+++
Hemolysis	+	++	++	++	++	++
Requires stable heart rhythm	Yes	No	No	No	No	No
Post-implantation management complexity	+	++++	++	++	++	+++
Optional cooling for hypothermia protocol	No	Yes	No	No	No	Yes
Optional extracorporeal oxygenation	No	Yes	No	No	No	Yes

Adapted from Ouweneel and Henriques [5]

Table 29.2 Percutaneous ventricular assist device effects on hemodynamics

Device	IABP	TandemHeart	Impella	ECMO
Afterload	Decreased	Increased	Neutral	Increased
LV Stroke volume	Slight increase	Decreased	Decreased	Decreased
Coronary perfusion	Slight increase	Not known	Not known	Not known
LV preload	Slight decrease	Decreased	Slight decrease	Decreased
PCW pressure	Slight decrease	Decreased	Slight decrease	Decreased
Peripheral tissue perfusion	No significant increase	Increased	Increased	Increased

Adapted from Werdan et al. [6]

29.6 Right Ventricular Support

Treatment of right ventricular failure in cardiogenic shock has been predominantly medical in nature. Volume administration to maintain adequate RV preload, vasodilators to reduce RV afterload, and inotropes to improve contractility are techniques that have been used for several decades. The consensus has been that if patients are able to survive their index hospitalization, their overall mortality is good. Though this remains true, the in-hospital mortality is high in patients with RV failure refractory to medical treatment. Previous options have been ECMO, surgical assist device, and atrial septostomy. Though IABP provided some support in RV infarction by increasing coronary blood flow, options for pVAD support had been extremely limited. With the development of the TandemHeart, percutaneous RVAD support has become a reality as discussed above.

More recently the Impella RP® (Right Percutaneous) was approved by the FDA under a Humanitarian Device Exemption for right ventricular failure refractory to medical therapy [25] . The device works using the same miniature axial flow pump mounted on a pigtail catheter as the Impella LP device with a few key differences. Access is obtained, again with standard catheter technique, via the right femoral vein using a series of upsizing dilators to final size of 24 FR tearaway sheath through which the pump is then inserted. It is passed through the right atrium, tricuspid valve, right ventricle, pulmonic valve, and into the pulmonary artery via a clockwise rotation of the entire device from the IVC. Once placed, the insertion sheath is torn off, and a graded smaller sheath is advanced and secured with a mattress suture. Blood travels in the opposite direction in the Impella RP; the inlet being more proximal and the outlet being more distal on the catheter. The inlet sits in the inferior vena cava where blood is aspirated and pumped into the proximal pulmonary artery (◘ Figs. 29.5 and 29.6). It provides up to 4 L/min of flow.

The RECOVER RIGHT trial was a prospective, multicenter single-arm study of patients with RV failure refractory to medical treatment after implantation of a durable LVAD, postcardiotomy or postmyocardial infarction who received RV support with Impella RP [25]. Hemodynamic benefit was observed using the Impella RP with an increase in cardiac index and a decrease in CVP both during support and after. Survival was 73% which suggested some benefit compared to prior studies, although there was no control arm to the study [25].

The Impella RP is indicated for support for up to 14 days in patients with BSA greater than or equal to 1.5 m^2 who develop acute right heart failure refractory to medical therapy following LVAD implantation, MI, heart transplant, or open-heart surgery. Contraindications include severe regurgitation, stenosis, or mechanical replacement of the tricuspid or pulmonic valves, anatomic conditions that preclude placement or correct positioning of the pump including disorders of the pulmonary artery, the presence of IVC filter unless there is clear access for a 21F catheter, or the presence of thrombus in IVC/RA.

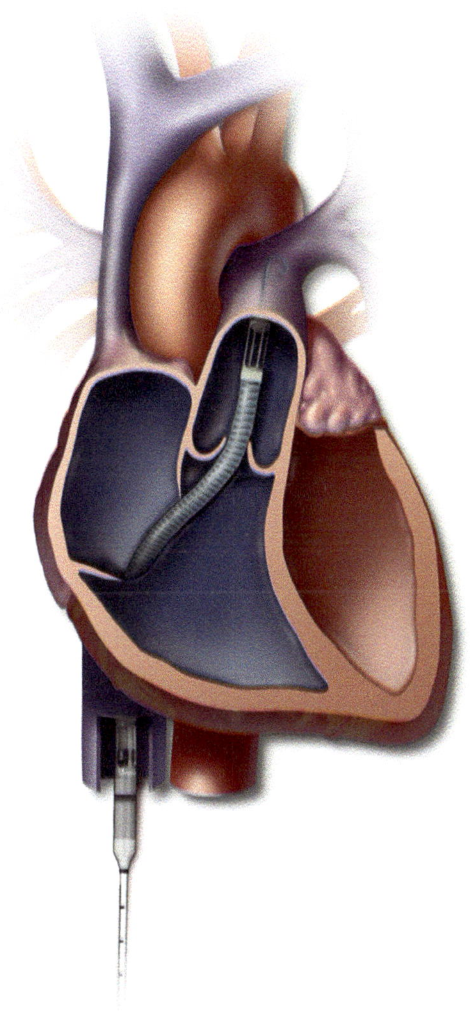

◘ **Fig. 29.5** Impella RP orientation across TV and PV

Potential complications with the use of the Impella RP include arrhythmia, bleeding, tamponade, vascular injury, hemolysis, thrombocytopenia, liver failure, device malfunction, or injury to the pulmonic or tricuspid valves. Insertion of this device requires a comfort level with percutaneous device implantation due to its rigid nature and somewhat technically challenging insertion. It can be limited by anatomy which often is not known until insertion is attempted.

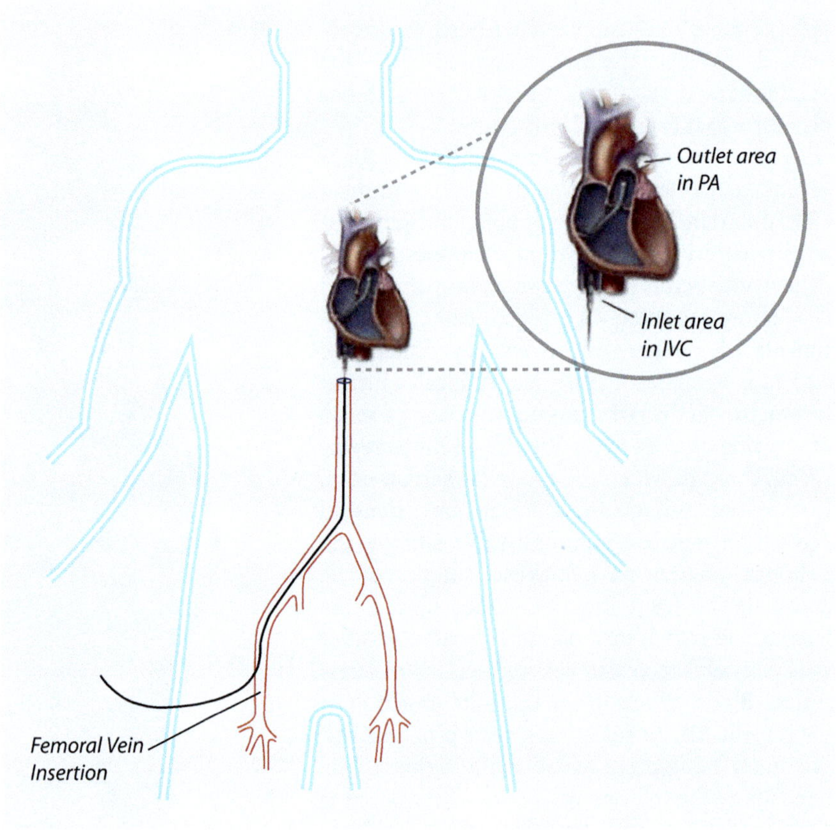

Fig. 29.6 Impella RP

29.7 Financial

Cost-effectiveness has increasingly become a focus in healthcare. As heart failure becomes more prevalent, the costs of taking care of heart failure patients is also steadily rising [26, 27]. Acute heart failure is one of the leading causes of hospital readmission in the USA making it a significant consumer of healthcare dollars [26]. A subset of these patients will present in cardiogenic shock and require a higher level of support than medical therapy provides. The availability of pVAD to bridge patients to recovery, durable device, transplant, or intervention gives the clinician another option at the expense of higher cost. Higher cost of an intervention over medical therapy is acceptable if it translates into survival benefit and improved quality of life at an acceptable cost-effectiveness ratio. The cost-effectiveness of pVADs is still being explored, but to date there are no randomized controlled trials in the primary PCI era demonstrating a mortality benefit of IABP over medical therapy or of pVAD (Impella 2.5 and TandemHeart) over IABP. There are no clinical trials comparing the benefit of pVADs with a higher level of support, like Impella 5.0, with IABP.

Retrospective analyses of cost comparisons of the use of IABP versus pVAD versus surgical VAD in patients have been made, the cost of IABP being the lowest and that of surgical VAD being the highest. Classification of these patients was based on coding, however, and not clinical assessment making it unknown if these were patients with similar clinical acuity [28, 29]. Large, randomized clinical trials assessing comparative outcomes in patients receiving pVADs for cardiogenic shock are needed before the cost-effectiveness of these therapies can be determined meaningfully. There is an element of common sense that can be applied. A preimplantation assessment of likelihood of recovery to next treatment should be made by the care provider. If the patient is not a candidate for advanced therapies, then implantation of these devices in an acute or chronic heart failure exacerbation may not be advisable unlike an acute event such as an MI.

29.8 Future

The technology of pVADs is still in its infancy. Research to develop new devices is ongoing as the industry works to make deployment easier, the size of access smaller, and the level of support greater. A potential example of this evolution is the HeartMate Percutaneous Heart Pump (St. Jude) now in clinical trials (NCT02156609). This pVAD is inserted through a single access via a 12F sheath placed in the femoral artery. The catheter is passed retrograde into the left ventricle where the distal end expands to 24F providing 4–5 L/min of flow. The impeller is caged, offering some protection to the surrounding structures. This device is now being trialed in comparison to Impella 2.5 in the high-risk PCI setting, but it has not been investigated as of yet in the more chronic heart failure situation. Additionally, a more durable pVAD that can provide support for a longer period of time allowing more time for recovery is needed.

29.9 Conclusion

Patients who present in cardiogenic shock continue to have high mortality. The utilization of pVADs for support in these critically ill patients continues to rise. Selection of an appropriate device should take into consideration the factors unique to each patient including the amount and type of support needed, the experience of the implanting center, and the presence of a potential end point including recovery, durable device, or transplant. Improvement in hemodynamic parameters has clearly been demonstrated though without mortality benefit in the limited studies to date. Early versus late implementation of support may prevent or ameliorate systemic inflammation and end-organ dysfunction in cardiogenic shock syndrome [30]. There is a clear need for randomized, prospective trials to evaluate the effect of these devices on mortality in patients with cardiogenic shock.

Acknowledgments We wish to thank Suneet Flora for her contributions in our literature search.

References

1. Khera R, Cram P, Lu X, Vyas A, Gerke A, Rosenthal GE et al (2015) Trends in the use of percutaneous ventricular assist devices: analysis of national inpatient sample data, 2007 through 2012. JAMA Intern Med 175(6):941–950
2. Goldberg RJ, Spencer FA, Gore JM, Lessard D, Yarzebski J (2009) Thirty-year trends (1975 to 2005) in the magnitude of, management of, and hospital death rates associated with cardiogenic shock in patients with acute myocardial infarction: a population-based perspective. Circulation 119(9): 1211–1219
3. Overgaard CB, Dzavik V (2008) Inotropes and vasopressors: review of physiology and clinical use in cardiovascular disease. Circulation 118(10):1047–1056
4. Scheidt S, Wilner G, Mueller H, Summers D, Lesch M, Wolff G et al (1973) Intra-aortic balloon counterpulsation in cardiogenic shock. Report of a co-operative clinical trial. N Engl J Med 288(19):979–984
5. Ouweneel DM, Henriques JP (2012) Percutaneous cardiac support devices for cardiogenic shock: current indications and recommendations. Heart 98(16):1246–1254
6. Werdan K, Gielen S, Ebelt H, Hochman JS (2014) Mechanical circulatory support in cardiogenic shock. Eur Heart J 35(3):156–167
7. Cochran RP, Starkey TD, Panos AL, Kunzelman KS (2002) Ambulatory intraaortic balloon pump use as bridge to heart transplant. Ann Thorac Surg 74(3):746–751 discussion 51-2
8. Sanborn TA, Sleeper LA, Bates ER, Jacobs AK, Boland J, French JK et al (2000) Impact of thrombolysis, intra-aortic balloon pump counterpulsation, and their combination in cardiogenic shock complicating acute myocardial infarction: a report from the SHOCK Trial Registry. SHould we emergently revascularize Occluded Coronaries for cardiogenic shocK? J Am Coll Cardiol 36(3 Suppl A):1123–1129
9. Anderson RD, Ohman EM, Holmes DR Jr, Col I, Stebbins AL, Bates ER et al (1997) Use of intraaortic balloon counterpulsation in patients presenting with cardiogenic shock: observations from the GUSTO-I Study. Global Utilization of Streptokinase and TPA for Occluded Coronary Arteries. J Am Coll Cardiol 30(3):708–715
10. Barron HV, Every NR, Parsons LS, Angeja B, Goldberg RJ, Gore JM et al (2001) The use of intra-aortic balloon counterpulsation in patients with cardiogenic shock complicating acute myocardial infarction: data from the National Registry of Myocardial Infarction 2. Am Heart J 141(6):933–939
11. Sjauw KD, Engstrom AE, Vis MM, van der Schaaf RJ, Baan J Jr, Koch KT et al (2009) A systematic review and

meta-analysis of intra-aortic balloon pump therapy in ST-elevation myocardial infarction: should we change the guidelines? Eur Heart J 30(4):459–468
12. Rihal CS, Naidu SS, Givertz MM, Szeto WY, Burke JA, Kapur NK et al (2015) 2015 SCAI/ACC/HFSA/STS clinical expert consensus statement on the use of percutaneous mechanical circulatory support devices in cardiovascular care: endorsed by the American Heart Assocation, the Cardiological Society of India, and Sociedad Latino Americana de Cardiologia Intervencion; Affirmation of Value by the Canadian Association of Interventional Cardiology-Association Canadienne de Cardiologie d'intervention. J Am Coll Cardiol 65(19):e7–e26
13. Burkhoff D, Cohen H, Brunckhorst C, O'Neill WW, TandemHeart IG (2006) A randomized multicenter clinical study to evaluate the safety and efficacy of the TandemHeart percutaneous ventricular assist device versus conventional therapy with intraaortic balloon pumping for treatment of cardiogenic shock. Am Heart J 152(3):469 e1-8
14. Bruckner BA, Jacob LP, Gregoric ID, Loyalka P, Kar B, Cohn WE et al (2008) Clinical experience with the TandemHeart percutaneous ventricular assist device as a bridge to cardiac transplantation. Tex Heart Inst J 35(4):447–450
15. Kar B, Adkins LE, Civitello AB, Loyalka P, Palanichamy N, Gemmato CJ et al (2006) Clinical experience with the TandemHeart percutaneous ventricular assist device. Tex Heart Inst J 33(2):111–115
16. Kapur NK, Paruchuri V, Korabathina R, Al-Mohammdi R, Mudd JO, Prutkin J et al (2011) Effects of a percutaneous mechanical circulatory support device for medically refractory right ventricular failure. J Heart Lung Transplant 30(12):1360–1367
17. Sassard T, Scalabre A, Bonnefoy E, Sanchez I, Farhat F, Jegaden O (2008) The right axillary artery approach for the Impella Recover LP 5.0 microaxial pump. Ann Thorac Surg 85(4):1468–1470
18. Bresson D, Sibellas F, Farhat F, Jegaden O, Kirkorian G, Bonnefoy E (2011) Preliminary experience with Impella Recover((R)) LP5.0 in nine patients with cardiogenic shock: a new circulatory support system in the intensive cardiac care unit. Arch Cardiovasc Dis 104(8–9):458–464
19. Hollander SA, Reinhartz O, Chin C, Yeh J, Maeda K, Mallidi H et al (2012) Use of the Impella 5.0 as a bridge from ECMO to implantation of the HeartMate II left ventricular assist device in a pediatric patient. Pediatr Transplant 16(2):205–206
20. Samoukovic G, Al-Atassi T, Rosu C, Giannetti N, Cecere R (2009) Successful treatment of heart failure due to acute transplant rejection with the Impella LP 5.0. Ann Thorac Surg 88(1):271–273
21. Samoukovic G, Rosu C, Giannetti N, Cecere R (2009) The Impella LP 5.0 as a bridge to long-term circulatory support. Interact Cardiovasc Thorac Surg 8(6): 682–683
22. Andrade JG, Al-Saloos H, Jeewa A, Sandor GG, Cheung A (2010) Facilitated cardiac recovery in fulminant myocarditis: pediatric use of the Impella LP 5.0 pump. J Heart Lung Transplant 29(1):96–97
23. LaRocca GM, Shimbo D, Rodriguez CJ, Stewart A, Naka Y, Weinberger J et al (2006) The Impella Recover LP 5.0 left ventricular assist device: a bridge to coronary artery bypass grafting and cardiac transplantation. J Am Soc Echocardiogr 19(4):468 e5-7
24. Engstrom AE, Cocchieri R, Driessen AH, Sjauw KD, Vis MM, Baan J et al (2011) The Impella 2.5 and 5.0 devices for ST-elevation myocardial infarction patients presenting with severe and profound cardiogenic shock: the Academic Medical Center intensive care unit experience. Crit Care Med 39(9): 2072–2079
25. Samuels L (2015) The RECOVER RIGHT™ trial: use of the Impella RP percutaneous right ventricular assist device: an Hde study. 5th international conference on clinical & experimental cardiology; April 27–29, 2015. Philadelphia, USA, J Clin Exp Cardiol 6:4
26. Heidenreich PA, Albert NM, Allen LA, Bluemke DA, Butler J, Fonarow GC et al (2013) Forecasting the impact of heart failure in the United States: a policy statement from the American Heart Association. Circ Heart Fail 6(3):606–619
27. Mozaffarian D, Benjamin EJ, Go AS, Arnett DK, Blaha MJ, Cushman M et al (2015) Heart disease and stroke statistics–2015 update: a report from the American Heart Association. Circulation 131(4):e29–322
28. Gregory D, Scotti DJ, de Lissovoy G, Palacios I, Dixon S, Maini B et al (2013) A value-based analysis of hemodynamic support strategies for high-risk heart failure patients undergoing a percutaneous coronary intervention. Am Health Drug Benefits 6(2): 88–99
29. Shah AP, Retzer EM, Nathan S, Paul JD, Friant J, Dill KE et al (2015) Clinical and economic effectiveness of percutaneous ventricular assist devices for high-risk patients undergoing percutaneous coronary intervention. J Invasive Cardiol 27(3):148–154
30. Chen JM, DeRose JJ, Slater JP, Spanier TB, Dewey TM, Catanese KA et al (1999) Improved survival rates support left ventricular assist device implantation early after myocardial infarction. J Am Coll Cardiol 33(7): 1903–1908

Paracorporeal Biventricular Assist Devices: The EXCOR® VAD System

Ares K. Menon and S. Ersel

© Springer International Publishing Switzerland 2017
A. Montalto et al. (eds.), *Mechanical Circulatory Support in End-Stage Heart Failure*,
DOI 10.1007/978-3-319-43383-7_30

30.1 Implantation Techniques

The EXCOR paracorporeal VAD can be utilized to provide biventricular or univentricular mechanical circulatory support from mid- to long term [1–3]. Its main application is bridging to heart transplantation, but also bridge to recovery or to candidacy is possible. The most common configurations for EXCOR BVAD cannulation are depicted in ◘ Figs. 30.1 and 30.2.

When planning an EXCOR implantation, concomitant procedures should be taken into consideration such as CABG or valve surgery. The exit sites for the EXCOR cannulas can be marked on the skin for better orientation during tunneling (see ◘ Fig. 30.6). A transesophageal echocardiography is mandatory for cardiac visualization and implantation guidance.

Under general anesthesia a median sternotomy is carried out, the pericardium is widely opened, and ECC is installed in standard fashion. In a BVAD patient or if other procedures are required (e.g., TVR), bicaval venous return using single-stage CPB cannulas is advantageous. Apart from a better access to the right atrium, the PA anastomosis can be performed without clamping when running on total CPB. The cannulation of the aortic CPB cannula should be done slightly more distally in the aortic arch. This leaves enough space for the EXCOR outflow aortic cannula. An alternative cannulation of the right subclavian artery for redo surgery is recommended. It allows for immediate CPB start to maintain hemodynamic stability while cardiac structures can be safely dissected and exposed. An LV vent can be inserted via the upper right pulmonary vein to unload the LV and prevent air entrapment. CO2 insufflation to the operatic field is optional. The EXCOR BVAD implantation has typically the following steps of cannulation: (1) LV apex, (2) right atrium, (3) main pulmonary artery, and (4) ascending aorta.

For the majority of EXCOR implantations, left ventricular apical cannulation is the standard access for sufficient LV decompression. However, left atrial cannulation is necessary in certain pathologies. For example, in a hypertrophic or restrictive cardiomyopathy, the LV cavity can be too small when compared to LA size. Thus, the blood flow needed to fill the EXCOR pump would be limited. Another reason could be a large myocardial infarction

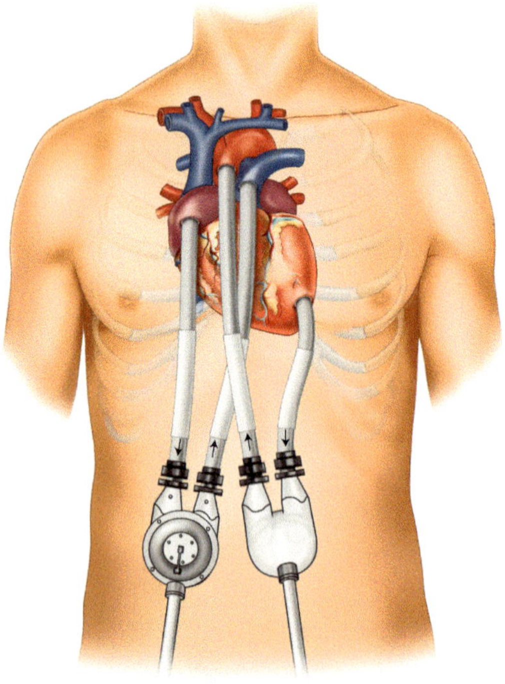

◘ **Fig. 30.1** BVAD (LVAD, inflow LV apical/outflow ascending Ao; RVAD, inflow RA/outflow PA)

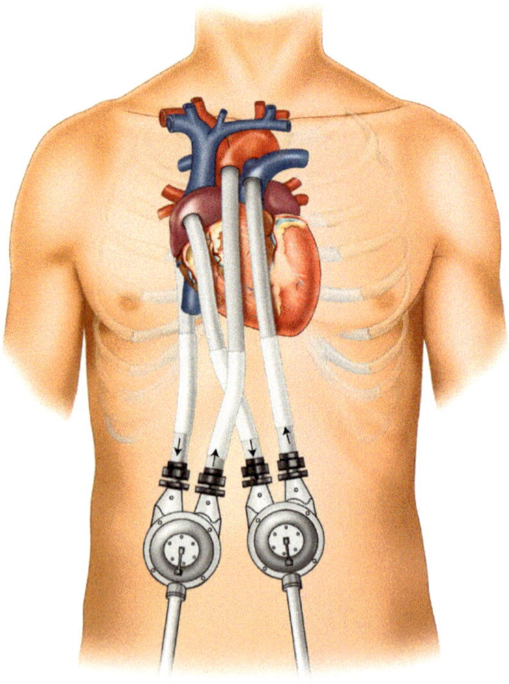

◘ **Fig. 30.2** BVAD (LVAD, inflow LA/outflow Ao; RVAD, inflow RA/outflow PA)

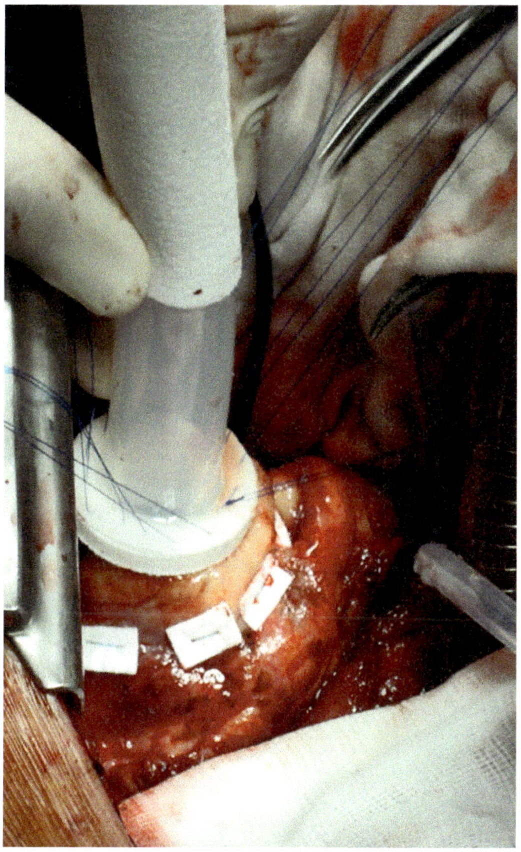

Fig. 30.3 Ventricular cannulation using PTFE-reinforced polypropylene 3–0 mattress sutures for fixation

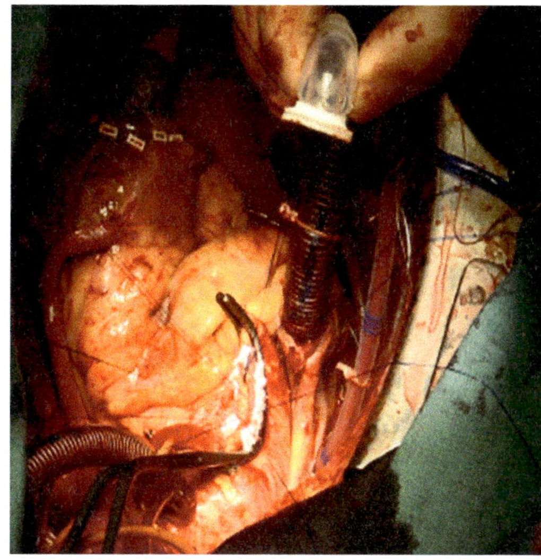

Fig. 30.4 End-to-side anastomosis of the 12 mm EXCOR outflow cannula (85° angle) to the aorta

prohibiting a safe anastomosis. In patients with severely diminished right ventricular function, RV apical cannulation instead of RA is a feasible modification, so-called biapical cannulation [4].

After the apex of the beating heart is luxated, the region for the ventriculotomy is located. The correct placement and alignment of the inflow cannula is a critical step in the procedure. Otherwise suction and insufficient pump flow will be encountered. The best area for the apical anastomosis is 2–4 cm apart from the LAD and 2–4 cm off-centered toward the anterior wall. Ideal position should be confirmed by TEE. After circular resection of myocardial tissue, 10–12 × pledgetted polypropylene 3–0 mattress sutures are placed around the apex whole (Fig. 30.3). Reinforcement of the sutures can also be achieved by using PTFE or bovine pericardial stripes instead. The apex whole is explored and residual trabeculae excised to avoid obstruction of the inflow cannula. During insertion the beveled tip is directed toward the orifice of the atrioventricular valve for optimal drainage. The apical inflow cannula should be in parallel to the interventricular septum.

Finally the sutures are passed through the sewing ring of the apex cannula and tied which should result in secure hemostasis. The apical anastomosis site can be covered by a GORE-TEX membrane to prevent adhesions.

In case of LA approach, the cannula insertion should be done at the back wall of the LA between RUPV and RLPV. A purse-string technique plus interrupted polypropylene 4–0 reinforced sutures can be used for proper fixation. The RA cannula is inserted at the free wall between IVC and SVC and fixed with the same technique as described for LA cannulation.

The anastomosis of the outflow cannulas to ascending aorta and PA is performed after site bite clamping (or alternatively for PA without clamping when on total bypass) in end-to-side fashion (Fig. 30.4). Adequate incision length is important to allow for tension-free suturing. Tear at the vascular wall can lead to bleeding complications especially at the aorta due to higher-pressure environment. Running or interrupted suture technique with polypropylene 4–0 or 5–0 can be used for cannula fixation.

Two different models of the arterial cannula with either a 85° or 60° angle of the tip are available. There is also a special graft adapter cannula which can be combined with any graft material for vascular anastomosis (Fig. 30.5).

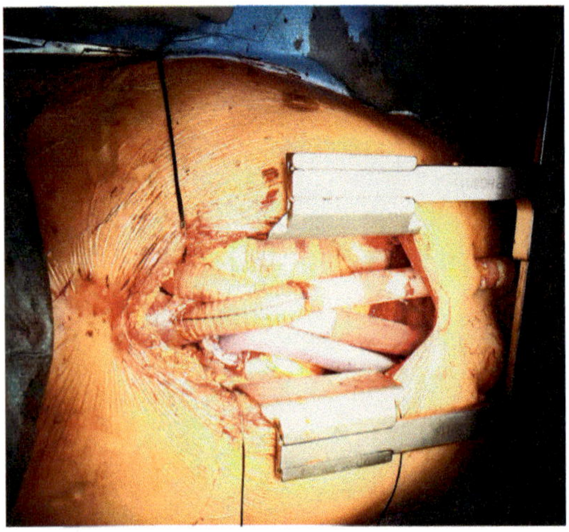

Fig. 30.5 12 mm EXCOR graft adapter cannulas in situ

In case of a small vessel anatomy, the use of the 9 mm EXCOR standard arterial or a graft adapter cannula should be considered.

The EXCOR cannulas are tunneled subcostally through the muscle fascia and the subcutaneous tissue. This is done before preparation of the anastomosis except for the apex cannula. Proper location of the exit site for each cannula is depicted in Fig. 30.6.

Preparation of the subcostal tunnel is done by blunt dissection. Some hospitals have used Hegar dilators to enlarge the tunnel for easier passing through the EXCOR cannulas. The size of the skin incision should approximately correspond to the length of the outer diameter of the cannula. A too small incision can cause tissue ischemia and subsequent necrosis. On the

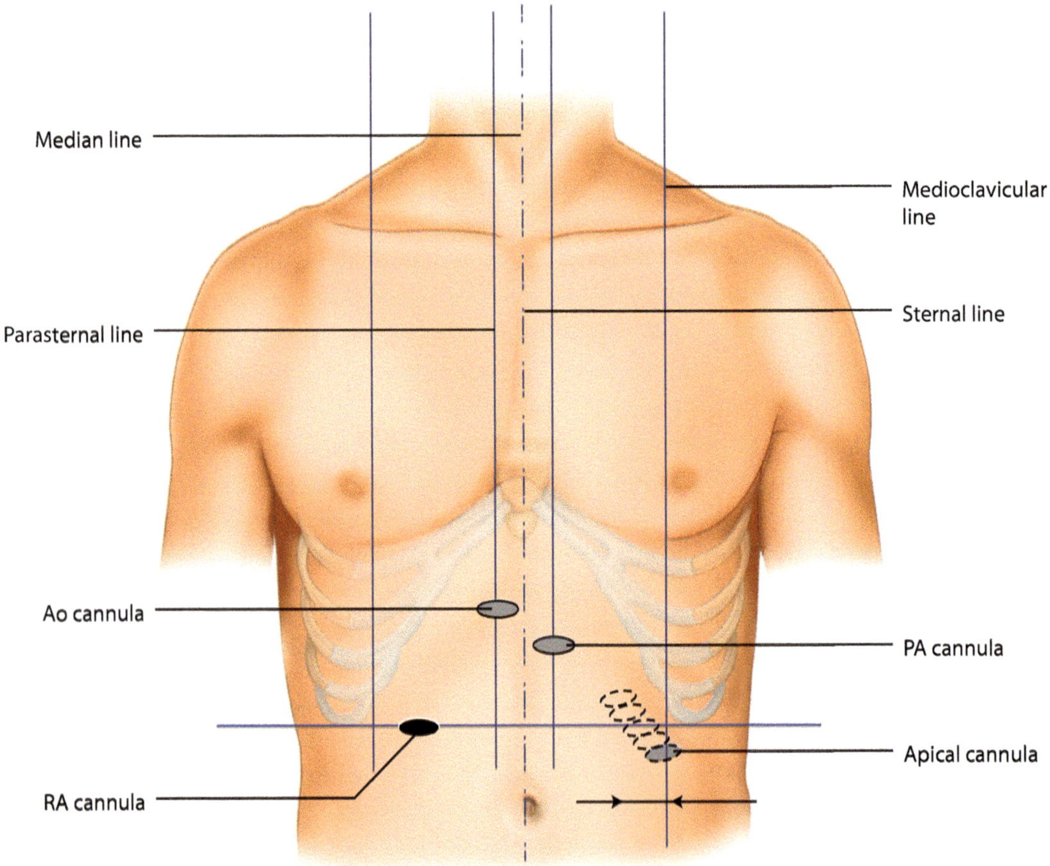

Fig. 30.6 Overview of the percutaneous exit sites for the EXCOR cannulas

other hand, a too large incision will leave a potential entry for pathogens causing infection. Finally the pump heads are connected to the EXCOR silicone cannulas and fixated by cable ties. Arrows on the pump mark the inflow and outflow direction. Two models of the 80 ml pump exist to expose the blood or air chamber on top. Visible air bubbles can be aspirated from the pump via the de-airing connector. The system can be started under low driving pressures, and gradual pump rate increase while coming off CPB.

In summary, the main strength of the EXCOR system is the high versatility based on a broad portfolio of different cannula types and sizes. It is worth to mention that even cases of successful creation of a total artificial heart with the EXCOR system have been reported [5, 6].

30.2 Outcome

Patients in INTERMACS level 1 or 2 with biventricular heart failure represent high-risk MCS candidates. According to the last INTERMACS report, 1-year survival for these patients is in the range of 50–60% (BVAD paracorporeal and LVAD plus centrifugal pump) [7]. Although it is desirable to implant an LVAD at first place, there is a significant amount of patients who require primary BVAD support. This accounts probably for 10–20% in the entire VAD population [8]. In addition, Takeda et al. found that patients receiving unplanned secondary RV support had much lower survival chances [9]. Another debated question is the success rate of temporary RVAD support. A recent study showed that only 19% of patients with temporary RVAD support could be successfully weaned [10]. In this regard primary BVAD support for patient with biventricular heart failure should be considered still as the adequate treatment option. Some centers have defined exclusive criteria which implicate BVAD support (see list).

Indications for EXCOR BVAD support:
- Acute cardiogenic shock with multiorgan dysfunction
- Intractable ventricular arrhythmia or persistent ventricular fibrillation
- Severe right heart failure on inotropic support
- Giant cell myocarditis [11]
- Acute biventricular myocardial infarction
- Acute postcardiotomy failure
- LVAD flow <2.0 l/min/m^2 and CVP $>$ 18 mmHg after LVAD implantation

With more experience better outcome for patients on EXCOR BVAD support has been accomplished during recent years. The group of the university hospital in Zurich retrospectively analyzed the outcome of 42 EXCOR BVAD patients [12]. Status of the patients at time of implantation was mainly INTERMACS level 1 or 2 with 31% being on previous MCS (ECMO) support. The overall survival rate seen in this cohort was 76%, whereof 69% were bridged to heart transplantation and 7% ongoing. Maximum support time reached 897 days. Comparable results were achieved at the Onassis Center in Greece. In their observational period from 2004 to 2013, a total of 53 EXCOR BVAD patients were evaluated [13]. They reported for this high-risk population a 1-year survival rate of 83%. Another study published by Bartfay et al. found a survival rate of more than 90% in selected younger patients supported by EXCOR BVAD [14].

Another concept is the installation of short-term centrifugal pumps in combination with EXCOR cannulas in postcardiotomy or cardiogenic shock patients. These patients are in the most critical status with a high mortality. Following this strategy optimal cardiac unloading can be achieved. It gives time to reevaluate the patient status including neurology after CPR, end-organ function, and myocardial contractility. If the patient is stable and suitable for heart transplantation, simple transition to EXCOR pumps for longer support can be done without repeated sternotomy. Despite the off-label approach, this strategy offers good success rates, lower invasiveness, and increased cost-efficiency [15].

References

1. Drews T, Krabatsch T, Huebler M, Hetzer R (2010) Paracorporeal biventricular mechanical circulatory support for more than 4 years. J Heart Lung Transplant 29(6):698–699
2. Ozbaran M, Yagdi T, Engin C, Erkul S, Balcioglu O, Baysal B, Nalbantgil S, Ertugay S (2013) Long-term paracorporeal ventricular support systems: a single-center experience. Transplant Proc 45(3):1013–1016
3. Schmid C, Tjan T, Etz C, Welp H, Rukosujew A, Klotz S, Drees G, Gogarten W, Scheld HH (2006) The excor

device - revival of an old system with excellent results. Thorac Cardiovasc Surg 54(6):393–399
4. Schmid C, Scheld HH, Tjan TDT (2005) Biapical cannulation for biventricular support with the pneumatically driven Excor system. ASAIO J 51(1):126–127
5. Tjan TDT, Klotz S, Schmid C, Scheld HH (2008) Creation of a self-made total artificial heart using combined components of available ventricular assist devices. Thorac Cardiovasc Surg 56(1):51–53
6. Valeske K, Yerebakan C, Mueller M, Akintuerk H (2014) Urgent implantation of the Berlin Heart Excor biventricular assist device as a total artificial heart in a patient with single ventricle circulation. J Thorac Cardiovasc Surg Volume 147(Issue 5):1712–1714
7. Kirklin JK et al (2015) Seventh INTERMACS annual report: 15,000 patients and counting. J Heart Lung Transplant 34(12):1495–1504
8. Boulate D, Marques MA, Ha R, Banerjee D, Haddad F (2014) Biventricular VAD versus LVAD for right heart failure. Ann Cardiothorac Surg 3(6):585–588.Z
9. Takeda K et al (2014) Outcome of unplanned right ventricular assist device support for severe right heart failure after implantable left ventricular assist device insertion. J Heart Lung Transplant 33(2):141–148
10. Oezpeker CCO et al (2013) Temporary RVAD support after LVAD – longterm outcome. J Heart Lung Transplant 32(4):S285
11. Bireta C, Tirilomis T, Grossmann M, Unsöld B, Wachter R, Perl T, Jebran AF, Schoendube FA, Popov AF (2015) Long term biventricular support with Berlin Heart Excor in a Septuagenarian with giant-cell myocarditis. J Cardiothorac Surg 10:14
12. Preliminary data presented by Prof. Wilhelm during the Journées de la Pitié 10/2015
13. Unpublished data, Berlin Heart Implant Registry
14. Bartfay SE, Liden H, Holmberg M, Karason K, Gabel J, Selimovic N, Dellgren G (2013) The BiVAD experience at the university hospital, results from the years 2010 to 2012 and comparison with contemporary LVAD patients. Eur Heart J 34(182):392–393
15. Loforte A, Potapov E, Krabatsch T, Musci M, Weng Y, Pasic M, Hetzer R (2009) Levitronix CentriMag to Berlin Heart Excor: a "Bridge to Bridge" solution in refractory cardiogenic shock. ASAIO J 55(5):465–468

Biventricular Circulatory Support with Two Implantable Continuous-Flow Pumps

Thomas Krabatsch

© Springer International Publishing Switzerland 2017
A. Montalto et al. (eds.), *Mechanical Circulatory Support in End-Stage Heart Failure*,
DOI 10.1007/978-3-319-43383-7_31

31.1 Background

Left ventricular assist devices (LVADs) have become a standard surgical therapy for end-stage heart failure during recent years [1, 2]. However, 10 to 30% of patients with end-stage heart failure suffer from biventricular failure requiring biventricular support [2]. For these patients only two approved long-term devices are available: the total artificial heart (TAH) CardioWest® (SynCardia, Tucson, AZ), requiring that the native heart be excised, and the biventricular pulsatile VAD, employing bulky extracorporeal or implantable displacement pumps. Both alternatives allow only limited quality of life for the patients, and the long-term results are dismal compared to those of patients with univentricular support [2]. The TAH is pneumatically driven and it requires a driver containing a noisy compressor. Furthermore, as the native heart of the patients is excised and cannot serve as a short-term backup, there are few chances of successful treatment in the case of device failure and of course no option for recovery of ventricular function.

The implantation of two pulsatile displacement pumps for biventricular long-term support requires either an extensive operation with the creation of large pockets in the abdominal wall to contain the pump chambers (Thoratec IVAD) or four blood cannulas penetrating the patient's skin and therefore carrying an excessive risk for cannula or even mediastinal infection (Berlin Heart Excor, Berlin Heart GmbH, Berlin, Germany; Thoratec BVAD, Thoratec Corp., Pleasanton, CA; Abiocor, Abiomed Inc., Danvers, MA).

31.2 History

Soon after the market launch of small miniaturized LVADs, attempts were published to use these devices for biventricular support. As early as 2004, Frazier et al. reported the successful use of two Jarvik 2000 FlowMaker pumps [3].

Since 2010 several VAD centers have been developing a method that allows the use of two implantable centrifugal LVADs of the type HeartWare HVAD® (HeartWare Inc., Framingham, MA) as a biventricular assist system. Two German VAD teams have been pioneers of this strategy, the groups in Berlin and Hannover [4, 5]. In making this attempt, three issues had to be solved:

1. As the HeartWare HVAD® is designed for use in the systemic circulation, in the pulmonary circulation without systemic afterload, even with the lowest recommended pump speed of 2200 rpm, the flow delivered by the HVAD® could be too high, theoretically resulting in severe pulmonary edema.
2. The inflow cannula of the HVAD® is 35 mm in length. Although the right ventricular dimensions are usually increased in right ventricular failure, this might be too long.
3. Because there was only little experience with connecting continuous-flow VADs to the right side of the heart, the optimal anatomical site for this connection had to be determined.

31.3 Patient Selection for Biventricular Long-Term Support

Patients who need biventricular long-term support either present with severe chronic biventricular failure or have developed persistent severe right ventricular failure in the support period after LVAD implantation, requiring additional long-term right-sided assistance. At our institution patients are considered for primary biventricular support mainly based on echocardiographic parameters. The degree of tricuspid regurgitation, right ventricular end-diastolic diameter, RV ejection fraction, right atrial diameter, and the sphericity index of the right ventricle together with the pulmonary resistance form the basis for the decision for biventricular support [6, 7] (Fig. 31.1). Clinical parameters of secondary renal or liver dysfunction are taken into consideration. However, there is a broad variety of factors published which could characterize patients in need for chronic biventricular support [8]. Here we recommend to follow each institution's guidelines.

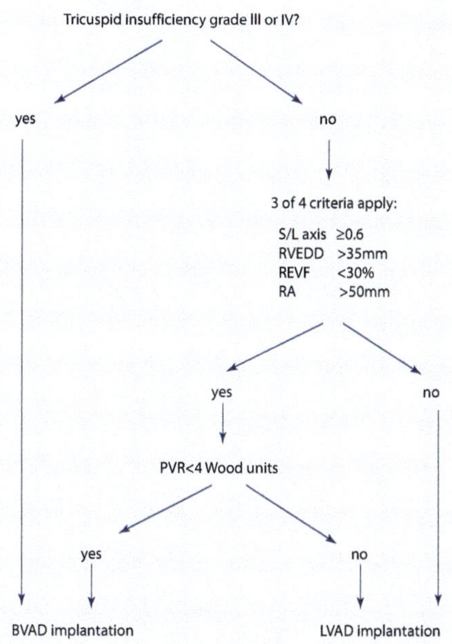

Fig. 31.1 Algorithm for decision between left ventricular and biventricular support in patients with terminal heart failure at our institution [8]. S/L axis indicates ratio of short-axis diameter to long-axis diameter. *RVEDD* right ventricular end-diastolic diameter, *RVEF* right ventricular ejection fraction, *RA* right atrium, *PVR* pulmonary vascular resistance, *BVAD* biventricular assist device, and *LVAD* left ventricular assist device

31.4 Operative Strategy

Only patients with extremely diminished RV function who are clear candidates for BVAD support receive implantation of a second HVAD as RVAD primarily. In all other patients, we recommend to implant first one HeartWare HVAD® device as an LVAD, and then to try to wean the patient from the heart-lung machine and to stabilize the hemodynamic situation. If this cannot be achieved without administering excessive catecholamine dosages, a second pump should be implanted into either the right ventricle or right atrium as an RVAD.

Alternatively, after implantation of one system as an LVAD and evaluation of whether the patient needs additional right ventricular support, a cost-effective temporary RVAD system (Levitronix CentriMag, Levitronix GmbH, Zurich, Switzerland) can be implanted. In the few patients who show no postoperative recovery of right ventricular function within a reasonable period of time, the temporary RVAD can later be replaced by a second HVAD system.

31.5 Implantation Procedure

Only in patients with a deep chest can connection of the pump to the free wall of the right ventricle be recommended (Figs. 31.2 and 31.3). In slim

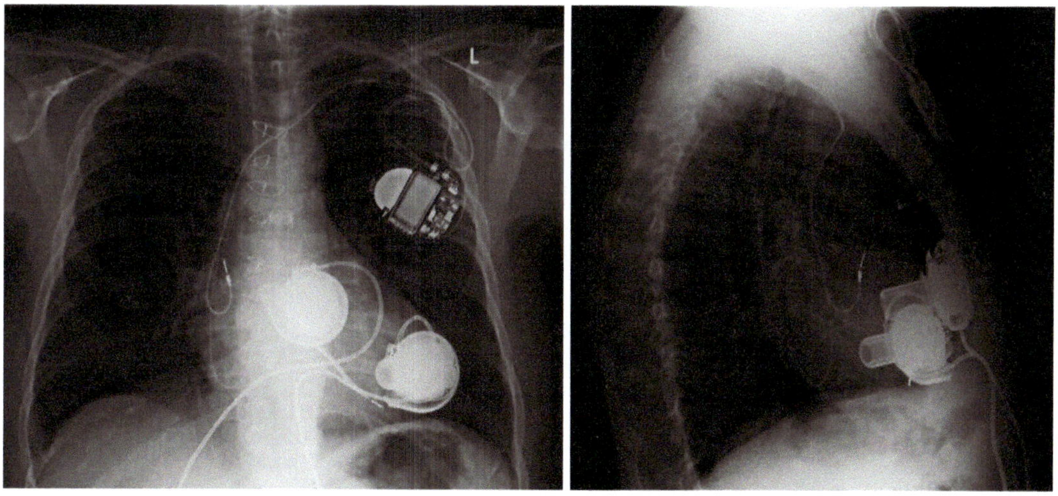

Fig. 31.2 Chest roentgenogram of a patient after implantation of two HeartWare HVAD® ventricular assist devices for biventricular support. The right pump is connected to the anterior free wall of the right ventricle

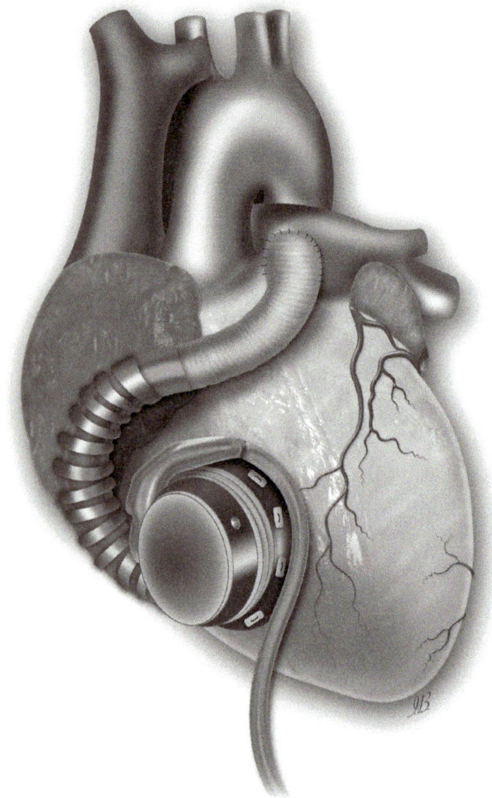

Fig. 31.3 The HVAD pump sewing ring is affixed with interrupted or running sutures to the anterior free wall of the right ventricle (RV) just below the outflow tract. The inflow cannula is then installed through the sewing ring into the RV. Outflow graft is attached to the main pulmonary artery (Picture by Ilaria Bondi's Peppermint Advertising)

patients with a small chest and in all small-framed patients, this would bear a significant risk for compression of the RV during and after chest closure. Therefore, in all small patients, we recommend connection of the pump to the right atrium (Figs. 31.4 and 31.5) or to the inferior (diaphragmatic) wall of the RV [9, 10].

To allow for a "physiological" flow range of 3 to 6 liters per minute within a pump speed setting of between 2200 and 3500 rpm, as usually set when the HVAD® is used as an LVAD and as recommended by the manufacturer, the afterload of the right pump should be artificially increased. We reduce the outflow graft diameter to such a degree that the afterload of the RVAD reaches the normal levels of the systemic circulation. This can be achieved by a reduction to an inner graft diameter of approximately 5 mm in patients with normal and to 6–7 mm in patients with elevated pulmonary vascular resistance. Diameter reduction can be performed by side clamping and narrowing the graft with a suture (6×0 Prolene) or by placement of titanium clips. To ensure definite and reproducible reduction of the diameter, Hegar bars are used for calibration. The length of the narrowed section should be about 35 mm as this length influences the added afterload according to the Hagen-Poiseuille equation.

To reduce the effective length of the inflow cannula, we add two 5 mm silicon suture rings covered with Dacron velour (in-house product

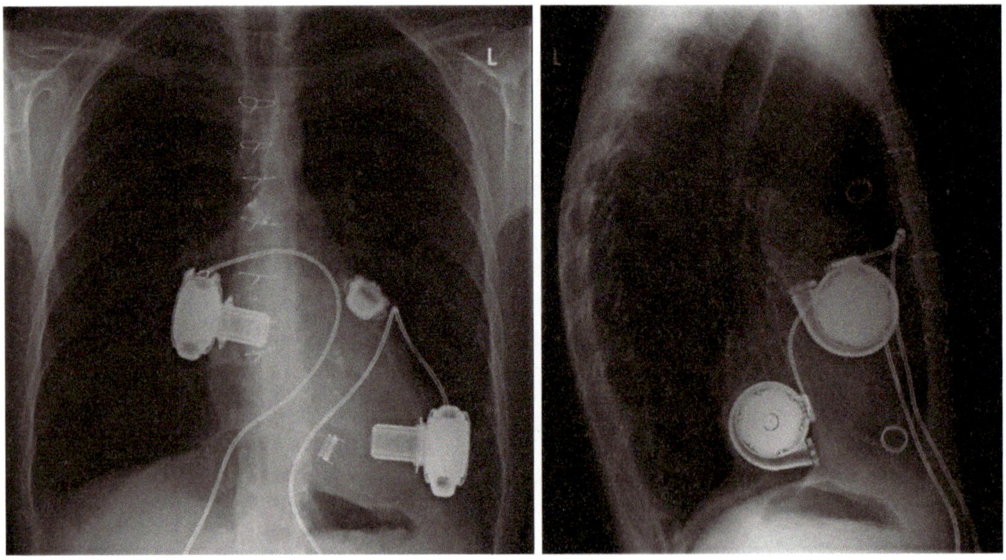

Fig. 31.4 Chest roentgenogram of a patient after switch of the right HeartWare HVAD® pump from the anterior free wall of the right ventricle to the right atrium

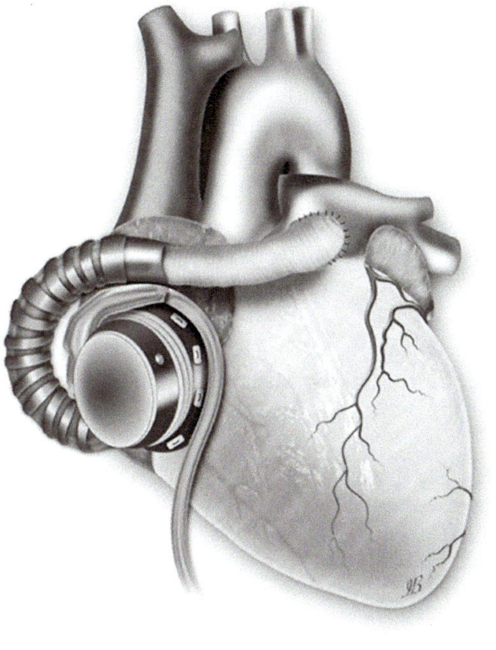

Fig. 31.5 Right ventricular support by cannulating the body of the right atrium (Picture by Ilaria Bondi's Peppermint Advertising)

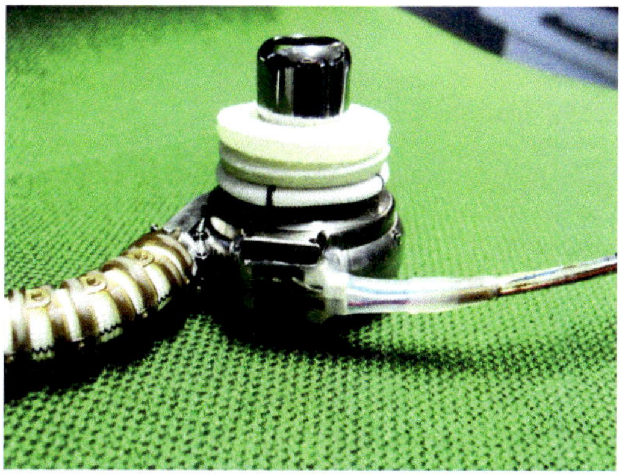

Fig. 31.6 Reduction of the effective length of the inflow cannula with two Dacron velour-covered 5 mm silicon suture rings

of the Deutsches Herzzentrum Berlin, made by Berlin Heart GmbH, Berlin, Germany) to the original HVAD® implantation ring. If this is not available, handmade rings of Dacron velour can be tailored (Fig. 31.6). The rings are fixed to the original "apical" fixation ring using BioGlue (CryoLife, Atlanta, GA). These additional rings prevent the cannula from deep penetration into the right ventricular cavity.

31.6 Postoperative Patient Management and Anticoagulation

All patients receive the standard postoperative care for VAD patients. Postoperative catecholamine support – if necessary – should consist of noradrenaline only.

Anticoagulation with IV heparin has to be started not earlier than 8 h postoperatively, after blood loss via drainage tubes has reached less than 50 ml per hour. Target aPTT level is increased from 50 to 55 s on postoperative day (POD) 1 to 55–65 s on POD 4. After removal of mediastinal drainage tubes and pacing wires, oral anticoagulation with Coumadin or warfarin is initiated. We set the target INR at 2.8–3.5. Additional platelet inhibition with 100 mg acetylsalicylic acid should be given.

Higher laboratory values for hemolysis have not been detected after cf-BVAD support [11] and would therefore be suspicious for pump thrombosis.

31.7 Further Considerations

Whether the outflow graft should be reduced in diameter or not is a matter of ongoing debate. In clinical practice the patient's pulmonary resistance is a dynamic value. During the weeks or months of left ventricular assistance, an initially increased pulmonary resistance can fall or can even drop to completely normal values. How far this process can go and which final level of pulmonary resistance will be reached is unpredictable. However, the reserve of the pump speed spectrum after a "banding" procedure should be sufficient to guarantee an appropriate flow within the recommended pump settings. Pump speeds below 2200 rpm should be avoided to ensure a stable rotor position.

Reduction of the effective length of the inflow cannula by simply increasing the thickness of the implantation ring using additional distance rings leads to increased height of the extraventricular part of the whole device. In this case the pump is not advanced as deeply into the right atrium or ventricle and therefore more of the device stays outside. This requires enough space. In our experience, especially in slim patients with a short distance between the sternum and the vertebral

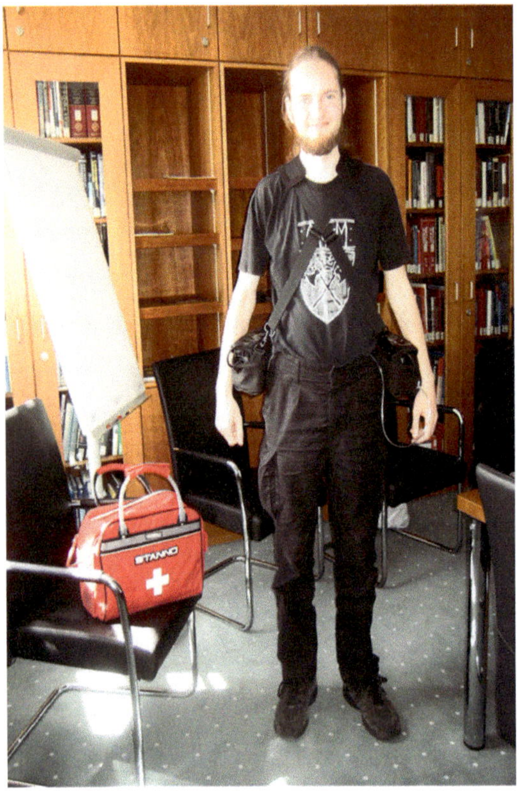

Fig. 31.7 Patient after implantation of two HeartWare HVAD® ventricular assist devices for biventricular support

body, this can be critical and in such cases atrial connection of the RVAD can be a solution.

Right ventricular dimensions vary during the postoperative course. As the left ventricle becomes smaller in most patients after LVAD implantation, this can also be expected for the right ventricle when supported by an RVAD. This can potentially lead to a situation where even the reduced effective length of the inflow cannula could be too long for the right ventricular diameter. However, we have seen in most of these cases an improved right ventricular function. These patients need less and less RV support. We have been able to stop RV support in a couple of patients after observing shrinkage of the RV with improvement of contractility. To avoid a further operation, we explanted the driveline only and left the (thrombosed) RVAD in place in these patients [12]. Compared to survival rates of LVAD patient populations, both 30-day and 6-month survival rates after continuous-flow BVAD implantations are lower. However, this is not significantly different from data on pulsatile BVAD patients in the literature.

Meanwhile, more than 200 cf-BVADs have been implanted worldwide, and this technique has proven to be feasible even in children [13, 14].

We consider the advantages of an implantable biventricular system to lie in the greater comfort and quality of life of the VAD patients (Fig. 31.7). The two systems run completely noiselessly, and, even if the patients have to carry two controllers and up to four batteries, they experience a higher degree of freedom and mobility.

Acknowledgment We gratefully thank Mrs. Anne Gale for editorial assistance.

References

1. Slaughter MS, Rogers JG, Milano CA, Russell SD, Conte JV, Feldman D, Sun B, Tatooles AJ, Delgado RM 3rd, Long JW, Wozniak TC, Ghumman W, Farrar DJ, Frazier OH (2009) HeartMate II Investigators. Advanced heart failure treated with continuous-flow left ventricular assist device. N Engl J Med 361:2241–2251
2. Kirklin JK, Naftel DC, Pagani FD et al (2015) Seventh INTERMACS annual report: 15,000 patients and counting. J Heart Lung Transplant 34:1495–1504
3. Frazier OH, Myers TJ, Gregoric I (2004) Biventricular assistance with the Jarvik Flowmaker: a case report. J Thorac Cardiovasc Surg 128(4):625–626
4. Krabatsch T, Potapov E, Stepanenko A, Schweiger M, Kukucka M, Huebler M, Hennig E, Hetzer R (2011) Biventricular circulatory support with two miniaturized implantable assist devices. Circulation 124(11 Suppl):S179–S186
5. Strueber M, Meyer AL, Malehsa D, Haverich A (2010) Successful use of the HeartWare HVAD rotary blood pump for biventricular support. J Thorac Cardiovasc Surg 140(4):936–937
6. Potapov EV, Stepanenko A, Dandel M, Kukucka M, Lehmkuhl HB, Weng Y, Hennig F, Krabatsch T, Hetzer R (2008) Tricuspid incompetence and geometry of the right ventricle as predictors of right ventricular function after implantation of a left ventricular assist device. J Heart Lung Transplant 27(12):1275–1281
7. Kukucka M, Stepanenko A, Potapov E, Krabatsch T, Redlin M, Mladenow A, Kuppe H, Hetzer R, Habazettl H (2010) Right-to-left ventricular end-diastolic diameter ratio and prediction of right ventricular failure with continuous-flow left ventricular assist devices. J Heart Lung Transplant 30(1):64–69
8. Fitzpatrick JR 3rd, Frederick JR, Hsu VM, Kozin ED, O'Hara ML, Howell E, Dougherty D, McCormick RC, Laporte CA, Cohen JE, Southerland KW, Howard JL, Jessup ML, Morris RJ, Acker MA, Woo YJ (2008) Risk score derived from pre-operative data analysis predicts the need for biventricular mechanical circulatory support. J Heart Lung Transplant 27:1286–1292
9. Krabatsch T, Stepanenko A, Schweiger M, Kukucka M, Ewert P, Hetzer R, Potapov E (2011) Alternative

technique for implantation of biventricular support with HeartWare implantable continuous flow pump. ASAIO J 57(4):333–335

10. McGee EC Jr, Ahmad U, Tamez D, Brown M, Voskoboynikov N, Malaisrie SC, Lee R, McCarthy PM (2011) Biventricular continuous flow VADs demonstrate diurnal flow variation and lead to end-organ recovery. Ann Thorac Surg 92(1):e1–e3
11. Stepanenko A, Krabatsch T, Hennig E, Kaufmann F, Jurmann B, Dranishnikov N, Lehmkuhl HB, Pasic M, Weng Y, Hetzer R, Potapov EV (2011) Retrospective hemolysis comparison between patients with centrifugal biventricular assist and left ventricular assist devices. ASAIO J 57(5):382–387
12. Potapov E, Schweiger M, Vierecke J, Dandel M, Stepanenko A, Kukucka M, Jurmann B, Hetzer R, Krabatsch T (2012) Discontinuation of HeartWare RVAD support without device removal in chronic BIVAD patients. ASAIO J 58(1):15–18
13. Stein ML, Yeh J, Reinhartz O, Rosenthal DN, Kaufman BD, Almond CS, Hollander SA, Maeda K (2016) HeartWare HVAD for biventricular support in children and adolescents: The Stanford Experience. ASAIO J 62(5):e46–e51
14. Schweiger M, Krüger B, Cavigelli-Brunner A, Dave H, Schmiady M, Hübler M (2015) Biventricular intracorporeal ventricular assist device in a 10-year-old child. Int J Artif Organs 38(4):233–235

The Total Artificial Heart

Jack Copeland, Francisco A. Arabia, Gero Tenderich, Antonella Marino, Oliver Voigt, Ciro Maiello, and Cristiano Amarelli

© Springer International Publishing Switzerland 2017

A. Montalto et al. (eds.), *Mechanical Circulatory Support in End-Stage Heart Failure*,
DOI 10.1007/978-3-319-43383-7_32

32.1 Rationale of the TAH

The TAH has been designed with the aim to give an effective circulatory support due to the possibility to both assure a high cardiac output (>9 L/min) and reduce venous congestion due to the low resistance of the inflows. The two 27 mm (25 mm in the 50 cc TAH) mechanical valves directly connected to the ventricular cuff (without the long cannulas of the paracorporeal BiVADs and without any uncontracting chamber at risk of thrombosis) permit to empty completely the venous circulation aiming to keep uncommonly low CVP, soon after implantation. These particular features well accomplish the clinical needs of patients in low cardiac output suffering of bad peripheral perfusion and of peripheral organ venous congestion reestablishing a high organ perfusion. The possibility to restore immediately after surgery a low venous pressure and an adequate perfusion pressure with a good mean arterial pressure warrants the possibility to restore a normal organ function.

32.1.1 Story and Development of TAH from First Experience Up to Now: Jack Copeland's Viewpoint

Kolff, Olsen, Kwan-Gett, Jarvik, and DeVries and colleagues laid the foundations for the clinical use of the current total artificial heart variously called: Jarvik-7-100, Jarvik-7-70, Symbion, CardioWest, and SynCardia (Table 32.1). The original intention for this heart was permanent cardiac replacement. It was designed and tested for a minimum of 4 years of durability.

As of 2015, more than 1584 implants and 520 patient years with the Jarvik-7, CardioWest, and SynCardia TAHs (all essentially the same device) account for >98% of the world experience with human total artificial heart implantation (reported in Table 32.1).

Table 32.1 Total artificial hearts implanted in humans from 1969 to 2015

TAH name	Timeline	No. of implants	Duration
Liotta	1969	1	64 h
Akutsu	1981	1	55 h
Jarvik-7100	1982–1992	44	6 years
Phoenix	1985	1	11 h
Penn State	1985–1989	4	1 year
Jarvik-7 70	1985–1992	159	11 years
Berlin	1986–1990	7	60 days
Unger	1986–1990	4	50 days
Vienna	1989	2	18 days
Brno	1988–1990	6	50 days
Poisk-IOM	1987–1990	16	100 days
CardioWest	1993–2002	218	31 years
Phoenix 7	1998	2	15 days
Abiocor	2001–2006	15	5 years
SynCardia	2002–2015	*1100*	464 years
Carmat	2013–2015	3	20 months
TOTAL	*1969–2015*	*1584*	*520 years*
"SynCardia type" Hearts	*1982–2015*	*1522 (96%)*	*512 years (98%)*

The first two TAH cases, the Liotta heart (1969) and the Akutsu heart (1981), were associated with device support for less than 3 days and patient survival after transplant of hours to 8 days with deaths from sepsis. Dr. William DeVries implanted the Jarvik-7 with 100 ml ventricular volumes in Dr. Barney Clark in 1982 followed by a celebrated 112 days of survival. Several other implants done by DeVries in Louisville were associated with adverse events causing public concern [1]. In 1984, the FDA limited the use of all mechanical circulatory support devices to bridge to transplantation.

By 1983 cardiac transplantation, survival results were improved, and length of hospital stay was shortened thus setting the stage for successful bridge to transplantation.

At the University of Arizona in March 1985, the lifesaving potential of total artificial heart technology appeared clear when we implanted emergently a "Phoenix TAH." Jack Copeland (JC) re-transplanted him after several hours of stable TAH support only to have the donor heart fail from sepsis. In the end JC and his staff were surprised with the excellent hemodynamic support provided by the Phoenix heart even in this septic patient.

On August 29, 1985, JC implanted a critically ill 25-year-old man with the Jarvik-7, 100 ml TAH. The device functioned very well and the patient survived to transplantation 9.5 days later and was discharged home. He lived 5.5 years with his transplanted heart enjoying excellent quality of life and return to work as a produce clerk in a grocery store. This case received worldwide public approval as the first successful bridge to transplantation with a total artificial heart [2]. JC's team and others began occasional implants in very sick patients realizing that there was much to be learned about this new technology because so little was known about issues of patient selection, fitting the device into the patient, anticoagulation, prevention of infections, biocompatibility, quality of life, explantation and subsequent transplantation, durability, and many other issues. Much has been learned in the past 30 years. From mid-1985 until late 2014, the size of the TAH has been 70 cc. The smaller 50 cc ventricle model for smaller patients has just been introduced in late 2014.

In the mid-1980s work with pulsatile left ventricular assist devices (LVADs) had been done in other centers and by 1988 LVADs, and biventricular support were implemented as options in the Arizona's center institutional surgical armamentarium, leading to formulation a selection protocol to select among the three types of devices [3].

The sicker patients that were considered for BiVAD or TAH implantation were not expected to live for more than hours to a few days. On maximal medical therapy, they had central venous pressures of 16–20 mmHg or greater, and some renal and hepatic dysfunction, but not enough that they would be eliminated as possible transplant candidates. They were on multiple inotropes and sometimes post-cardiac arrest, intubated, or on temporary device support such as cardiopulmonary bypass or ECMO.

Results with the TAH were good, also in a population of very sick patients. But when the FDA prohibited TAH use in the USA from 1991 through 1992, LVADs and BiVADs were used alternatively in the same patient population, and higher mortality rates were experienced, leading to the conclusion that patients experiencing rapid decompensation had better survival with TAH therapy than LVADs or BiVADs. In 1992, while a new IDE for study of the TAH was started (called CardioWest at the time) in five institutions, the implanted population received approximately 20% TAH, 20% BiVAD, and 60% LVAD.

In 2004 the FDA approved the SynCardia TAH-t as a bridge-to-transplant device for: "... temporary biventricular replacement for transplant eligible patients suffering from bi-ventricular failure and at imminent risk for death." Documentation of experience in the FDA study [4], in an institutional study of 101 consecutive patients headed by JC [5], in the area of anticoagulation [6], and in multivariate analysis of risk factors [7] has established evidence for the worldwide use of the TAH. Survival to transplantation in the FDA trial was 79% and in the 101 consecutive patient single institution trial of 69%. Strokes occurred in 8 of 99 consecutive patients. Four implant-related strokes were in the first 48 h following operation, and two were in the two chronic survivors that developed device endocarditis. There were two strokes in the remaining 93 patients (2%) for an event rate of 0.08 strokes/patient year in endocarditis-free patients after the first 48 h postimplantation. GI bleeding was found in two patients (2%) that is much lower than the risk with continuous-flow devices (15–40%). There were no valve failures, or pump thrombosis, and low rates of hemolysis (10 mg/dl plasma-free hemoglobin), only two device exchanges in >1500 patients (again in contrast to the exchange rates for the continuous-flow devices of about 5–15% per year), a small number of driveline perforations (estimate of <6), and eight diaphragm perforations in >1500 patients (>3000 ventricles or 0.003 events per ventricle [0.3%]). The mean time to perforation was 1.2 years (range 124–971d). Two of the eight patients were successfully transplanted and six died, with mortality from lack of durability of 0.4%.

In summary, the results of multiple studies have shown that the stroke rate is favorable when compared to LVAD stroke rates. The reasons for such a remarkably low stroke rate are most likely related to two independent factors. The first is that the flow rates of the TAH are high (7–9 l/ min) and do not allow stasis to occur. The second is that the shear stress created by this device, even with 4 mechanical valves, has been found to be low, >100 times less than with rotary pumps. This results in less platelet activation and in turn less activation of the final pathway of the coagulation cascade perhaps partially accounting for the absence of pump thrombosis. Likewise, pump exchange with the TAH is rare (2 in >1500 patients). GI bleeding is rare (2%). There are no arrhythmias. In patients with acute, not chronic, renal failure and/or hepatic failure, return to normal function commonly occurs within weeks.

Because of several historical restrictions, only a few centers were able to use the TAH while LVADs were much more widely available. In ▫ Fig. 32.1 the blue bar below the graph represents the time period when the only drivers for the TAH were too large for discharge and limited in number to 36 worldwide. This prevented widespread use. In 2009 the Freedom Driver trial started in the USA and has now led to >200 patient years of outpatient support. The SynCardia TAH-t has been approved by the FDA since 2004 and approved for funding by CMS (Centers for Medicare and Medicaid Services) in 2008.

Current use of the SynCardia TAH-t is at about 15 implants per month worldwide. As better selection criteria are used and smaller (6 pound/2.7 kg) quieter drivers improve quality of life, the true place of the TAH among MCS devices may become apparent (▫ Fig. 32.1). Right ventricular failure (RVF) with LVAD therapy and the management of INTERMACS I patients are among the challenges that have not been solved with LVAD therapy.

In 2015 a trial was started with a 50 cc ventricle pump that is 30% smaller and easier to fit into smaller patients perhaps down to 1.2 m^2 BSA. Over 20 have been implanted in the first few months primarily in females with good survival results. A destination therapy trial is also starting.

De facto long-term implants have resulted in >127 1-year, 63 1.5-year, and 27 2-year survivors. There are now two patients on TAH for over 4 years. Around 72% of 1-year survivors in a recent multi-institutional study were transplanted with 100% surviving to discharge and 73% of those on renal replacement therapy experiencing return of renal function.

The SynCardia TAH-t continues to demonstrate success in areas not covered by other options. The adverse event profile is favorable. Selection of appropriate patients in programs

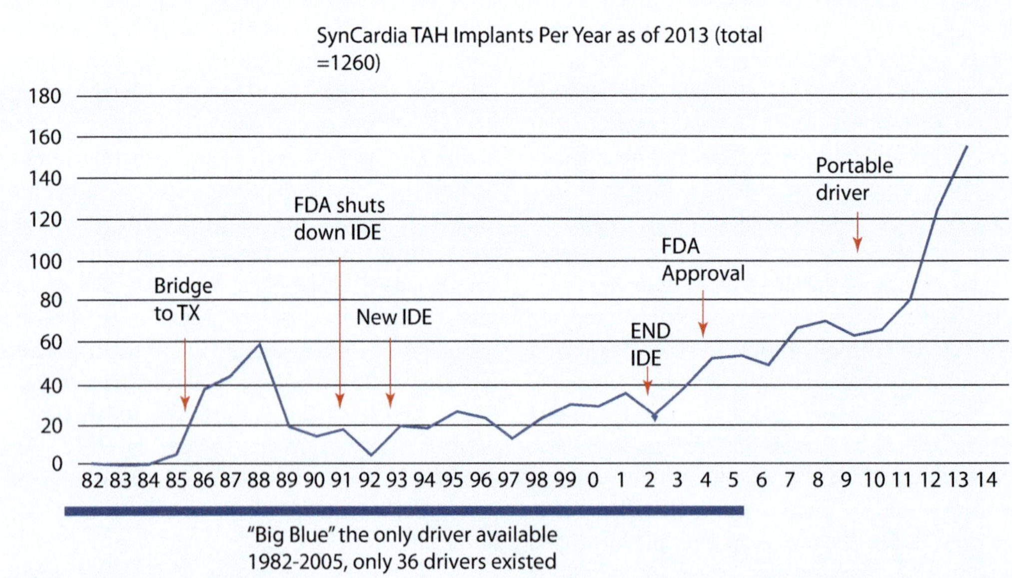

▫ **Fig. 32.1** Numbers of SynCardia TAH implants by year (Courtesy of SynCardia Systems, LLC)

that are new to the technology remains a problem that is slowly resolving. The overriding consideration in the mind of the author since he first used this device is that "it works." Major benefits include replacement of diseased native ventricles, high flow, low CVP, automatic left-right balancing, a Starling mechanism, pulsatility, and low shear pump characteristics. The 50 cc model may increase usage. The new DT trial may provide long-term support for sicker patients.

32.1.2 Engineering View of TAH and Technical Management of Drivers and System

Ventricular assist devices ("VADs") *assist* the native ventricle(s), while a total artificial heart ("TAH") *replaces* both native ventricles. In this respect a TAH eliminates global cardiac dysfunction (such as large myocardial infarction, rejection, stone heart, amyloid, cardiac tumor, Chagas, muscular dystrophy, etc.) and solves issues with arrhythmias, ventricular septal defects, ventricular thrombus, or others related to native ventricles. It can further be used as bailout for DT LVAD patients with failing right ventricle.

The SynCardia TAH is a pulsatile displacement pump system pneumatically driven and has three integral parts: the implanted two artificial ventricles, the external pneumatic driver, and the air tubes or drivelines (◘ Fig. 32.2).

The internal ventricle is made of segmented polyurethane solution (SPUS) and has two mechanical heart valves (SynHall™), identical to the original Medtronic Hall recently gone out of production. A flexible membrane of four layers separates air from blood (◘ Fig. 32.3). The ventricle has no sensors.

Drivelines for each ventricle are connected to the external driver. Currently two different external drive systems are in use: the "Companion 2" (C2) Driver System for initial implantation and in-hospital use which provides curves for the monitoring of the pumps (◘ Fig. 32.4). It weighs about 30 kg and fits on a hospital console with 360° rotatable screen or on a caddie resembling a carry-on suitcase. As of May 2015 the Companion 2 had been used in 367 patients for 72 years of support. The wearable Freedom Driver System for clinically stable patients at home weighs 6 kg and had supported 222 patients for 145 years. The noise of the driver still represents an issue that will be addressed in the near future by a new Freedom 2 Driver that is more portable weighing 3 kg and is very quiet.

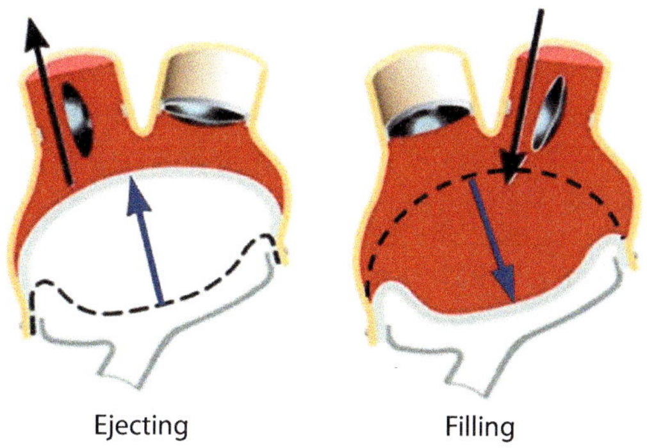

◘ **Fig. 32.3** SynCardia TAH ventricle (Courtesy of SynCardia Systems, LLC)

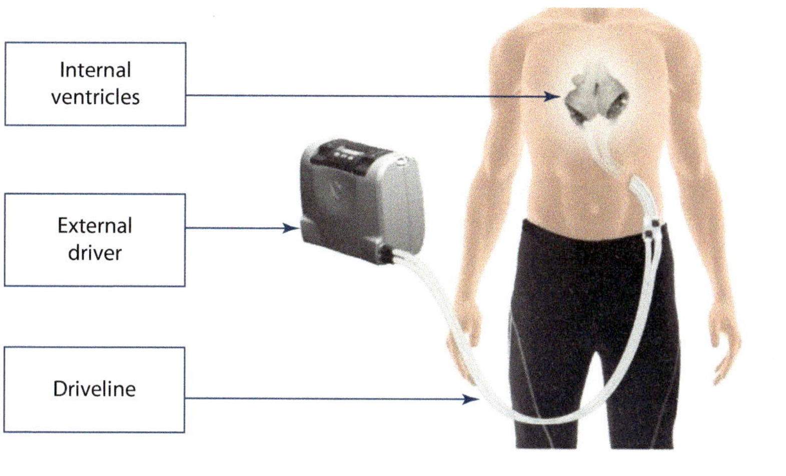

◘ **Fig. 32.2** SynCardia TAH components (Courtesy of SynCardia Systems, LLC)

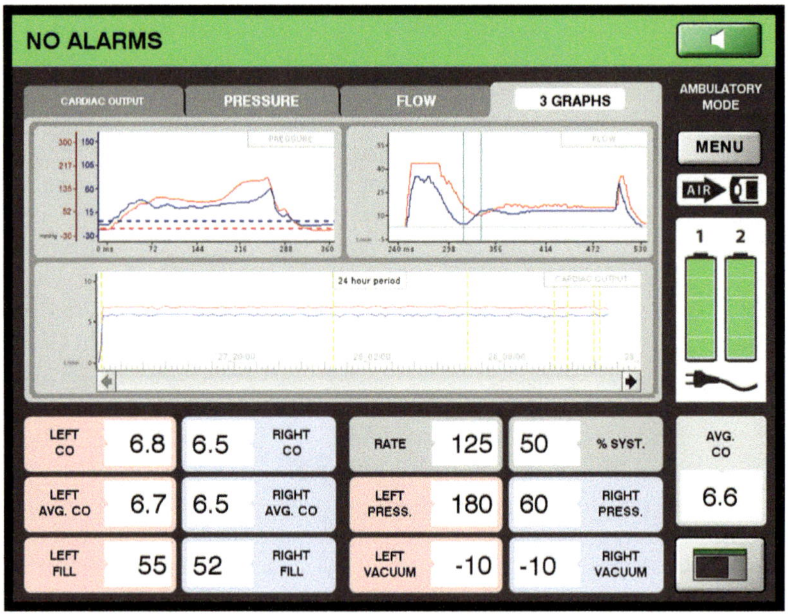

Fig. 32.4 Screenshot from "Companion 2" Driver – SynCardia TAH (Courtesy of SynCardia Systems, LLC)

The cardiac output in most adult patients runs at 7±1 l/min at a preload of 5–10 mmHg. Ejection pressures are preset to be about 30 mmHg > anticipated PA pressure and 60 mmHg above the anticipated systolic pressure. The C2 driver can be set to overcome any physiologic systemic vascular resistance (i.e., up to 200 mmHg). The Freedom Driver in the current iteration works best at systolic pressures under 150 mmHg, so careful systolic pressure control is desirable in outpatient recipients. Normal settings for the device include pump pressures of 80 mmHg, vacuum of −10 mmHg, percent systole of 50% on the right. On the left they are 180 mmHg pump pressure, −10 mmHg vacuum, and percent systole of 50%. The ventricles fill and empty simultaneously from 2 separate pumps and are generally run at a beat rate between 120 and 130/min.

As seen in Fig. 32.3, the ventricle is partially filled and fully ejected with each beat. Under this condition the pneumatic ventricles exhibit:

- Automatic balance between the left and right ventricles, preventing overflow to the lungs
- An increased pump output response to increase in preload (Starling response)

The limit of the device is about 140 beats/minute giving 9.8 l/min flow at a fill volume of 70 ml. Once this is exceeded by further increasing preload, increase in back pressure will occur. In this situation, volume reduction maneuvers such as dialysis, reverse Trendelenburg position, and therapeutic phlebotomy would be urgently indicated. To anticipate and thus avoid overload of the device, the operator may use the fill volume (stroke volume) reading from the driver (Fig. 32.5). In general, the fill volume serves as an index of the preload and is very helpful in dialysis patients to determine desired volume status. In all 70 cc ventricles, fill volumes of 50–60 cc are considered optimal and safe. Theoretically, this provides the possibility of increasing the stroke volume by 20 cc/beat for fill volume of 50 or 10 cc/beat for fill volume of 60. Thus the cardiac output reserve at a beat rate of 130 would be 2.6 l/min for the former and 1.3 l/min for the later. The fill volume is also directly related to the CVP. The fill volumes of the ventricles are adjusted by changing heart rate. If a lower fill volume is desired, the heart rate is increased and vice versa. In patients with intact renal function, changing any of the settings is rarely needed.

As one might expect with four mechanical valves, there is a low-grade hemolysis with a mean free hemoglobin of 10–12 mg/dl. Hematocrits are usually 25. Oxygen delivery is adequate at rest and with exercise. Also, there is some fragmentation of the von Willebrand protein, but platelet-collagen binding is not decreased [8].

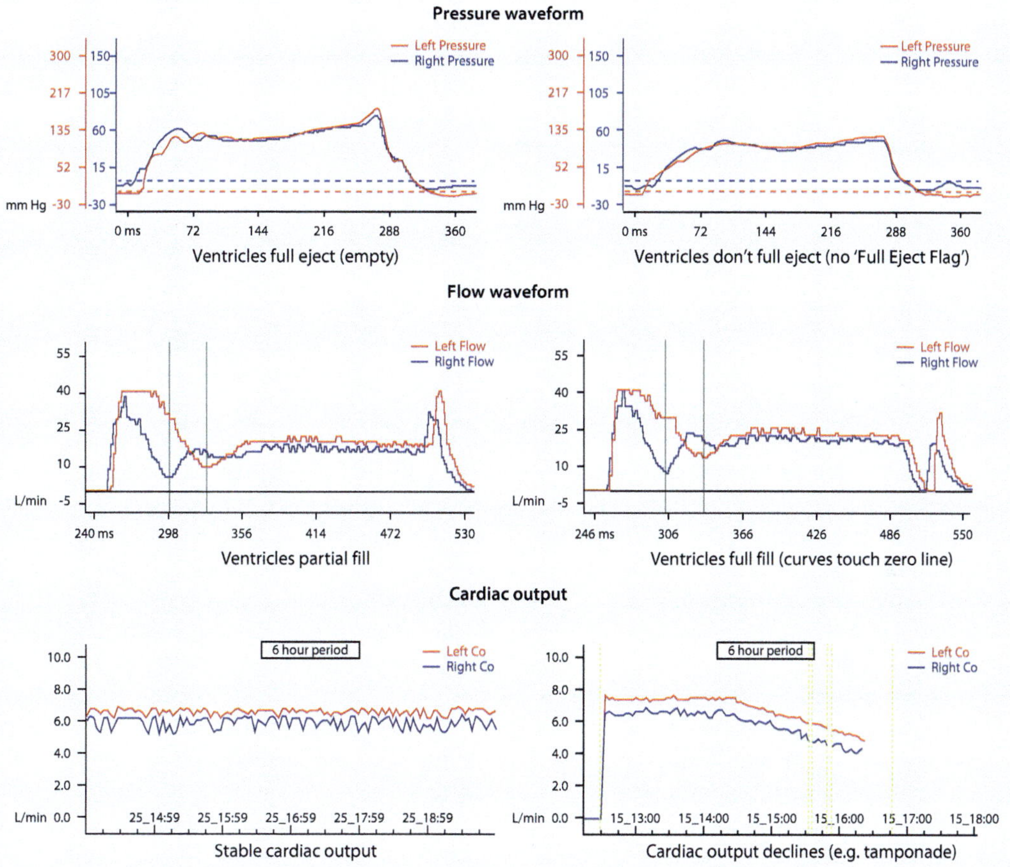

Fig. 32.5 Normal (*left*) and abnormal (*right*) wave forms for SynCardia TAH operation

32.1.3 Clinical and Surgical Issues

Indications

The TAH represents an alternative way to assist the patient suffering from an end-stage chronic or an acute biventricular heart failure, when LVAD support is predicted to be unsuccessful in providing adequate systemic flow to meet metabolic demands.

While a timely mechanical circulatory support aims at a desirable ventricular remodeling with a reversal of the severity of heart failure, the concept behind TAH is to completely replace the heart with a mechanical device. Of course, in patients who are potential cardiac graft recipients, the object is to remove the native heart. Thus for those hearts that appear to have no chance of reverse remodeling, cardiectomy with replacement is the therapy of choice when LVAD and medical therapies will not suffice.

This difference encompasses all the resistances and the fears of the clinicians related to eventual technical failures of such a machine. The principal concerns regarding the replacement with a TAH are related to the absence of a backup circulation in case of abrupt technical complications.

Long clinical experience with SynCardia TAH has shown excellent technical data with a remarkably low incidence of technical failures. However, the miniaturization of continuous-flow assist devices and the possible reversibility or even the healing of right ventricular dysfunction over the long term still represent an obstacle to the diffusion of the TAH technology to biventricular ES-CHF, and, as a consequence, during the last years, an increasing off-label use of devices designed to assist the left ventricle in a setting of a biventricular failure has been experienced.

On the other end, up to now the SynCardia TAH is the only device with a large experience over 1 year of support in biventricular failure whose data are validated both for bridge to transplant as for destination therapy. Unfortunately, there are no randomized clinical trials comparing TAH with other devices in the treatment of biventricular heart failure, and the principal obstacle to such a trial is the absence of a unique and safe "competitor" to the TAH.

However, in such a complex scenario, TAH has its principal benefits when the replacement of one or both ventricles is mandatory:

- Untreatable myocardial infarctions with or without complications
- Neoplasms of the heart without secondary lesions
- Irreversible post-transplant graft dysfunction
- Irreversible right ventricular failure after LVAD and PGF after transplants
- Untreatable severe arrhythmic cardiomyopathy
- Previous mechanical aortic valve in patients who are not candidates for LVAD
- Irreparable ventricular anatomical defects (e.g., ventricular rupture, significant ventricular septal defect following acute myocardial infarction, and so on)
- Ventricular failure with prior mechanical prosthetic valve replacement
- Severe biventricular failure
- Severe hypertrophic and restrictive disease
- Selected conventional operation misadventures

In these settings the risks of the replacement of the entire heart is justified in consideration of the actual lack of an alternative strategy. Biventricular failures that are not amenable to an intended implant of temporary RVAD+LVAD are a possible clinical indication for patients in INTERMACS class I/II. In this setting the implantation of a BiVAD with HVAD is preferred from many authors in light of an expected better quality of life and with the aim of a midterm reversal of right ventricular failure. Looking at the last INTERMACS report, it has to be noted how the risk of severe complications after BiVAD implantation remains significant, although reduced in the last era. However, clinical experience with the TAH as destination therapy has thus far been limited also if in this setting the implantation of a TAH appears at the moment the safest and easy solution. The principal advantages in favor of the TAH remain the extreme ease to manage TAH with respect to BiVAD and the low rate of technical failures during the long term.

Indication and Patient (and Model) Selection

Proper patient selection and timing of intervention are two of the most important factors in determining a successful outcome with the TAH. The main indication for the use of TAH is in patients who are heart transplant candidates with severe biventricular failure in imminent risk of death in whom a suitable donor heart is not available. LVADs have proven very effective in either bridging patient to heart transplantation or as destination therapy in those patients who are not candidates [9, 10] with near transplant survival outcomes but with a lower quality of life [11], higher incidence of adverse events, and with an incidence of RVF up to 40% [12]. However, the need for a right ventricular assist device (RVAD) identifies a patient population that has worse outcomes [13] and potentially manageable with a TAH.

The TAH continues to be used as a bridge-to-heart transplantation (BTT) in patients with severe biventricular failure, i.e., INTERMACS profile 1 and primarily profile 2 [14, 15]. However, the last few years has seen an increase in its use and better understanding of the indications for its implementation. Many potential indications for the use of a TAH have been conceptualized for many years; however, it has been in recent times that the TAH has been utilized for these very ill patients. For this reason, few of these cases have reached the medical literature and others are too early to report.

The need for re-transplantation is essential to provide long-term survival for a heart transplant recipient who is experiencing graft failure that is not responding to conventional therapy. If a donor has not become available and the patient is experiencing hemodynamic instability despite inotropic support, temporizing measures that will provide more time include the use of ECMO or biventricular support. The role of the TAH in this particular patient provides several advantages as long as the TAH is implanted prior to total cardiovascular collapse and end-organ damage. The TAH allows for immunosuppression to be discontinued and potentially lowers the increased risk of infection and kidney damage. Furthermore, it allows the patient to be ambulatory and potentially the benefit of being discharged home [16]. The use of the TAH for this indication is associated with a survival rate of 47%. However, the use of the TAH for hemodynamic collapse in the onset of acute rejection has not been described and is probably associated with a high rate of complications and poor outcomes. The role of the TAH in the chronic graft failure scenario will probably continue to increase as the transplant population has a mean survival of approximately 10 years and the donor shortage continues [17, 18].

The use of the TAH in the pediatric population with advanced heart failure as the result of an idiopathic, viral, or congenital structural abnormality provides significant advantages. In addition to correction of hemodynamic deterioration, it provides a surgical scenario that allows for the correction of some of the congenital abnormalities at the time of TAH implantation and prior to the time of transplantation. Although the 70 cc size of the SynCardia TAH dictates that the patient thoracic cavity has to be able to fit the device to allow sternal closure, the TAH has been until now utilized in children with BSA as small as 1.5 m^2. The requirement in this scenario is that there is significant cardiomegaly with an enlarged mediastinal space to allow for the device to fit in [19–22]. Although smaller LVAD's and biventricular assist devices have successfully been utilized in the small children, the 50 cc TAH is now available and may further expand the use of this technology in children and small adults with a BSA as low as 1.0–1.2 m^2 and the 50 cc appearing as a game changer in this field. Approximately 30 patients with congenital heart disease had been implanted with the SynCardia TAH by the end of 2013. The majority of these patients were implanted in the last few years and in multiple centers. Some of the congenital abnormalities in these patients include corrected transposition of the great vessels and single ventricle. Although reports are just starting to appear, some of these patients are experiencing from altered hemodynamics and physiology secondary to a failed Fontan procedure. It is the expectation that the next few years will provide more evidence-based medical literature regarding the management in this complex population with the TAH. The implantation of the SynCardia TAH or any newer TAH in patients with congenital heart disease will challenge the surgeons to develop surgical modifications to the conventional implantation of the device as the cardiac abnormalities dictate modification and design.

The outcome of the patient with a primary cardiac malignancy is usually dismal with poor survival. Although the majority of cardiac tumors are benign, however a malignant tumor carries a fatal prognosis if unresectable. Diagnosis of these malignant tumors usually includes a biopsy at the time of presentation or occurs at the time of an optimistic but failed surgical resection. Imaging studies (echocardiography, computerized tomography, and MRI) are usually helpful but in some if not most instances failed to accurately delineate the extent of the disease [23]. Chemotherapy and radiation therapy have been utilized in unresectable cases. Heart transplantation has been utilized to treat selected patients with cardiac malignancies; however series show poor outcomes. The use of ventricular assist devices has been reported, and more recently the use of the HeartMate II LVAD used in the TAH configuration was described in a patient. A very small number of patients with cardiac tumors have received the SynCardia TAH. Mostly literature is based on case reports, without enough scientific information to make any prediction on outcomes. The use of the TAH in this population will generate controversy in the medical field. However, long-term use of the TAH followed by transplantation may 1 day play a role.

Acquired or ischemic ventricular septal defect (VSD) as a complication of myocardial infarction remains a condition with significant morbidity. Surgical correction is the most common therapy that carries a significant morbidity and mortality [24]. The use of MCS has been reported in the management of ischemic VSDs [25]. The successful use of the SynCardia TAH has also been reported [26]. A very small number of patients have been done for this indication to have a series of patients. The procedure probably will continue to have a significant morbidity and mortality as these patient population is in significant hemodynamic and physiologic impairment.

The patient populations experiencing from infiltrative (i.e., amyloid) or hypertrophic cardiomyopathy are ideal candidates for the use of a TAH as this therapy eliminates the effect of the disease process in both affected ventricles. Although the use of left ventricular assist devices (LVADs) have been reported [27], the utilization of the TAH continues to increase in this population. Another population that benefit from the TAH technology are those patients who experience from ventricular tachycardia (VT) storm or malignant arrhythmias despite multiple ablations. Although LVADs have been used as a group, the TAH continues to find a role in this group. However, medical reporting in these two populations will increase in the next few years.

LVADs have been extremely successful in the management of congestive heart failure both in the BTT and destination therapy who are failing medical therapy. However, despite the best managements, a number of BTT patients who have received LVADs continue to or relapse with right ventricular failure (RVF). The TAH has been successful in re-bridging these patients and eliminating the effects of RVF despite an LVAD [28]. However, this has not been tested in the destination (DT) population.

32.1.4 50 cc TAH System

The SynCardia TAH-t 50 cc is an identical smaller version of the CE marked 70 cc TAH-t, originally designed for patients with smaller chest dimensions and or less need of consistent doses of cardiac output.

The TAH-t cannulas have colored bands on them to permit to the clinicians to distinguish the model 50 and 70 cc TAH-t also after implantation. The 50 cc TAH-t cannulas have two colored bands on each cannula, whereas the 70 cc TAH-t cannulas have one colored band on each cannula, as shown in the picture in ◘ Fig. 32.6.

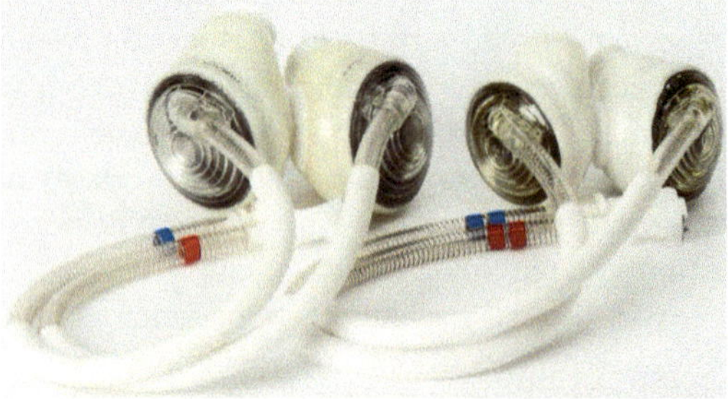

◘ **Fig. 32.6** SynCardia 70 and 50 cc systems (Courtesy of SynCardia Systems, LLC)

Until the introduction of the 50 cc model, TAH technology was restricted to patients with higher BSA, cardiothoracic ratio, and anteroposterior diameter at T10 level. A common problem, in oversizing, was the compression of the IVC by the RA quick connector and the compression of the left pulmonary veins by the LA quick connector. This problem may be often resolved by a delayed sternal closure waiting for the volume reduction of the lung after 24–48 h of effective perfusion and drying of the lung. Delayed sternal closure after the total artificial heart implantation might be beneficial for the outcomes preventing complications, as bleeding complications, tamponade, and sometimes several second-look operations. For that reason, delayed sternal closure after TAH-t implantation could be one option although it still has to be prospectively examined [29].

The new device has been designed as a pulsatile device similar to the 70 cc with the smaller dimensions, less stroke volume, and less cardiac output, as it shows in ◘ Table 32.2.

Ideal patients' characteristics for 70 cc TAH were BSA bigger than 1.7 square meter and a distance between the sternum and the tenth anterior vertebral body (T10) measured by CT scan, bigger than 10 cm. For 50 cc TAH the cutoff values have been reduced to approximately 1.2 m^2 and to 7.5 cm at T10 but further data need to be collected (◘ Fig. 32.7).

Concerning the surgical technique of 50 cc SynCardia TAH-t is the same compared to the 70 cc SynCardia TAH-t. Owing to the absence of deairing nipples, deairing procedure is more crucial and needs to be performed carefully. This is achieved as follows: the artificial ventricle is carefully filled with the patient blood by temporarily increasing venous return during extracorporeal circulation. Then, the lungs are inflated, and the artificial ventricle is allowed to perform three to four single beats in order to eliminate remaining air bubbles. After the deairing is completed, the outflow graft is connected to the ascending aorta. The same procedure is repeated for the right artificial ventricle. The 50 cc TAH-t system is then started at full support and the patient is weaned from extracorporeal circulation. Also the OR setting of the Companion Driver unit remain unchanged [30]. In relation to

Table 32.2 Comparison between 50 and 70 cc TAH-t

#	Characteristic	50 cc TAH-t	70 cc TAH-t	Comparison
1.	Type	Pulsatile	Pulsatile	Same
2.	Mechanism of action	Pneumatic	Pneumatic	Same
3.	Stroke volume (max)	50 ml	70 ml	20 ml reduction
4.	Cardiac output (max)	7.5 L/min	10.5 L/min	3.0 L/min
5.	Displacement volume (not including cannulas)	250 ± 25 ml	400 ± 20 ml	150 ml reduction
6.	Electrical power	External	External	Same
7.	Valves	25 M (mitral) and 23A (aortic) (titanium housing and pyrolytic carbon tilting disk)	27 M (mitral) and 25A (aortic) (titanium housing and pyrolytic carbon tilting disk)	Next available smaller valve sizes selected
8.	Diaphragms	Four diaphragms: one blood diaphragm and three redundant diaphragms (air and intermediate diaphragm assembly) Graphite between the diaphragms provides lubrification	Four diaphragms: one blood diaphragm and three redundant diaphragms (air and intermediate diaphragm assembly) Graphite between the diaphragms provides lubrification	Same number of diaphragm and same diaphragm thickness. Amount of graphite used for lubrification is scaled down
9.	Cannulas (connected to base of TAH-t)	Wire reinforced PVC tubing Internal diameter: 0,274″ +0/−0.010″ External diameter: 0.430″ +0.015/−0.010″ Wall thickness: 0.078″ Length: 18.0 ±.5 in.	Wire reinforced PVC tubing Internal diameter: 0,274″ +0/−0.010″ External diameter: 0.430″ +0.015/−0.010″ Wall thickness: 0.078″ Length: 18.0 ±.5 in.	Same
10.	Weight	Approximately 200 g	Approximately 240 g	Approximately 40 g lighter
11.	Approximate dimension (width × height)	Left ventricle: 66 × 77 mm Right ventricle: 80 × 75 mm	Left ventricle: 73 × 84 mm Right ventricle: 90 × 80 mm	Dimensions scaled down

the pediatric population, the device might not only offer a therapy in term of bridge to transplant but also an option regarding the failing Fontan population [31].

Early or late transplant failure can be treated by implanting the device, with the standard technique as long as the transplant procedure has been performed in Shumway technique [32], while JC has implanted it as usual leaving a small amount of the donor right atrium and cavae many times without complications.

In summary the 50 cc SynCardia TAH-t has the potential to expand the applicability of total artificial heart therapy for specific population and indication as well Kasirajan V, 2012, personal communication.

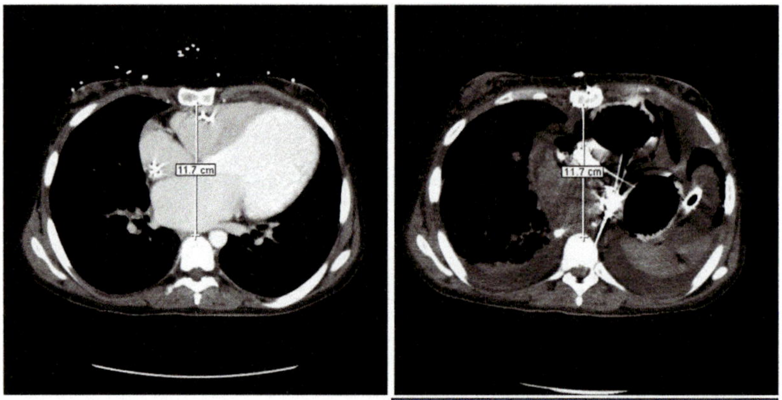

	70cc TAH-t	50cc TAH-t
BSA	≥ 1.70 m²	< 1.85 m²
Measurement at T10 CT scan: post. sternum to ant. spine	≥ 10 cm	TBD via study
LVEDD	≥ 70 mm	TBD via study
Cardio-thoracic ratio Chest X-ray	≥ .5	TBD via study

Fig. 32.7 Ideal patients' characteristics (Courtesy of SynCardia Systems, LLC)

In general, as implantation of total artificial heart is indicated in a very sick population of INTERMACS level 1 or 2, indication is mainly affecting the outcome. The amount of cardiac output needed to warrant end-organ recovery, specifically the renal and liver function, is a crucial point to guide the choice between a 50 cc TAH and a 70 cc TAH with delayed sternal closure. However, the availability of a TAH warranting higher flows means less risk of hemodynamic deterioration especially in the early period after implantation that might definitely influence the outcome. In patients with an earlier indication to support, flows over 7,5 L/min could be rarely needed, thus underlining the importance of the timing to tailor the approach on patient characteristics.

32.2 Virtual Fit Software Versus Intraoperative Surgical Decision

The CardioWest temporary total artificial heart (TAH-t; SynCardia Systems Inc., Tucson, AZ) is well suited for certain pediatric and young adult heart failure patients with previously limited MCS options. The standard fit criteria include a body surface area (BSA) of 1.7 m^2 and an anteroposterior distance greater than 10 cm from the sternum to the tenth thoracic vertebra (T10) [33]. On the basis of these criteria, most pediatric and small adult patients are excluded from TAH-t placement. Important limitations may be encountered in restrictive cardiomyopathies or in redo patients of congenital surgery where normal anatomic relationships may be lost during the multiple surgeries and during the long history of heart failure. Innovative imaging techniques have been proposed to improve eligibility for TAH-t placement in smaller patients, therefore, a novel technique using virtual TAH-t implantation in pediatric and small adult patients to compare with standard fit criteria has been recently described [34].

An accurately scaled three-dimensional (3D) surface rendering of the TAH-t was placed within a 3D reconstruction of the chest to assess for proper fit. Device compression of pertinent intrathoracic structures, including systemic veins, pulmonary veins, aorta, lungs, and diaphragm, was assessed.

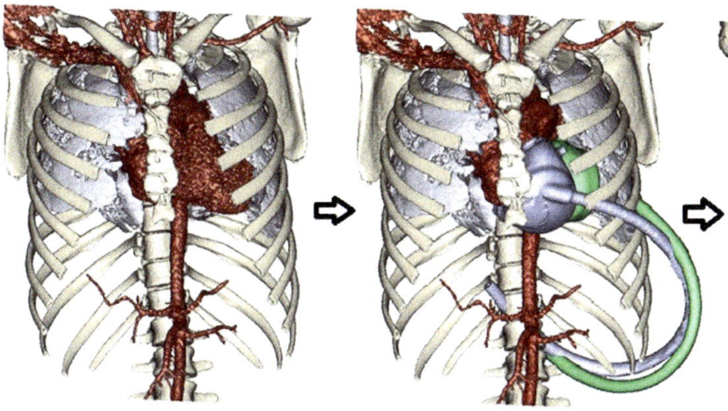

Fig. 32.8 Virtual and traditional evaluation of fitting and technical problems in case of suboptimal fitting of TAH (Reproduced with permission from Moore et al. [34])

A recent report discloses an excellent prediction of the fit in patients studied with such an approach: patients had successful virtual implantation also in patients with BSA <1.7 m^2, and the T10-sternum distance lower than 10 cm and post-device chest imaging showed no compression of pertinent intrathoracic structures, as predicted by the pre-device simulation.

This approach is still not used on a regular basis in the clinical field and requires time to receive an indication in a field in which time jokes a pivotal role and the availability of the 50-cc makes such an approach less needed. In the opinion of one of the authors (GT), the intraoperative measure of the anteroposterior diameter at the level of the diaphragm (Fig. 32.8) is alone capable to indicate the selection of the right machine for the patient.

32.2.1 Surgical Technique of TAH Implantation

The conventional median sternotomy incision is performed. A sternal retractor is placed with its base in the cephalad position. The pericardium is opened to expose the native heart. Purse-string sutures can be placed at this time in the ascending aorta, superior and inferior venae cavae. Umbilical tapes are also placed around the superior and inferior venae cavae for total control of venous return prior to removing the ventricles.

The tracks for each prosthetic ventricle drivelines are prepared. Two 1 cm stab wounds are made under the left costal margin. A surgical clamp is passed from the left upper abdominal quadrant, thru the stab wound and into the mediastinum with care not to enter the peritoneum. A 36 Fr. chest tube is then passed thru the track. The driveline from the prosthetic ventricle is then inserted into the chest. The chest tube is then pulled from the mediastinum and outward pulling with it the driveline. This is repeated a second time for the second prosthetic ventricle. Each driveline open tip is then covered to prevent fluid or any tissue from getting inside. The driveline from the prosthetic left ventricle is to the left of the midclavicular line, and the one for the prosthetic right ventricle is to the right.

The two atrial quick connects are brought to the surgical field. The excess ring is cut at this time leaving a ring width of about 4–5 mm. The arterial conduits are then preclotted using Coseal (Baxter Healthcare, Los Angeles, CA) or similar agent and allowed to dry.

Intravenous heparin is administered to bring the ACT to a therapeutic range to perform cardiopulmonary bypass. Aortic and bicaval cannulations are performed. Cardiopulmonary bypass is established, the heart is fibrillated, and the aorta is cross clamped. The patient is cooled to 32°F. A ventriculectomy is started about 1 cm distal to the AV grove at the right atrial level (Fig. 32.9). It is continued circumferentially, always staying 1 cm from the AV grove, around the right ventricle. This assures that some ventricular myocardium is left behind that will be utilized in the atrial suture lines. The tricuspid valve is excised leaving about 1–2 mm of valve tissue in the annulus of the valve. The ventricular septum is the excised. The ventriculectomy is then continued into the left ventricle.

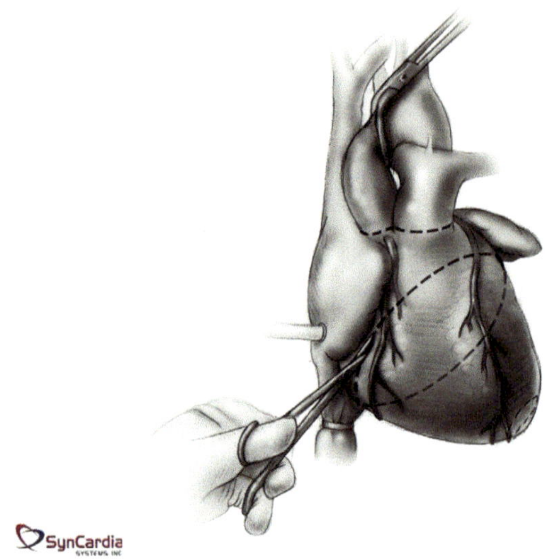

Fig. 32.9 A ventriculectomy is started about 1 cm. distal to the AV grove at the right atrial level

The mitral valve is then excised in a similar fashion as the tricuspid also leaving a rim of 1–2 mm of valve tissue attached to the annulus. The aorta and pulmonary arteries are then divided and excised above the semilunar valves. A C-clamp is passed from the aorta thru the aortic valve into the remaining left ventricular outflow tract (LVOT). An incision is then made thru the aorta, LVOT, and aortic valve with care not to enter the tricuspid or mitral valve annulus. The other leg of the V-shaped incision is now made, excising the right ventricular outflow tract with the pulmonic valve in toto with care not to enter the mitral or tricuspid valve annulus. This exposes the continuity of the anterior leaflet of the mitral valve with the left coronary cusp of the aortic valve. The coronary sinus is then closed with a running 3-0 or 4-0 polypropylene suture at this time. This will prevent back bleeding from all the veins that have been divided during the ventriculectomy.

The atrial quick connects are brought to the field. They are inverted to facilitate implantation. The left atrial quick connect is placed through the mitral valve annulus. A 3-0 polypropylene suture in an MH needle is used to suture the left atrial quick connect to the remnant ventricular muscle. The needle is passed from inside to outside, going through the “skirt” of the atrial quick connect, mitral valve annulus, and the muscle full thickness (Fig. 32.10). The suture is passed in a horizontal mattress fashion and tied. Another similar

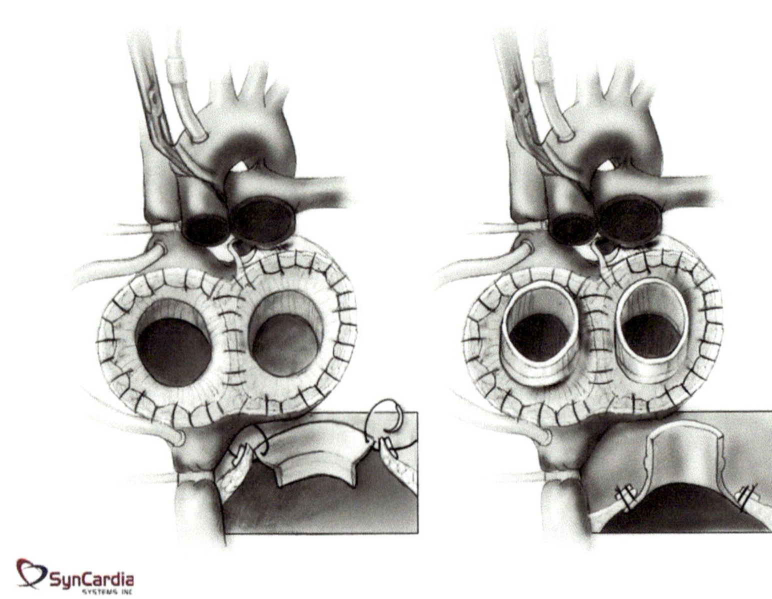

Fig. 32.10 The atrial quick connects are brought to the field. They are inverted to facilitate implantation. The atrial quick connects are placed through the valve annulus. A 3-0 polypropylene suture in an MH needle is used to suture the atrial quick connects to the remnant ventricular muscle. The needle is passed from inside to outside, going through the "skirt" of the atrial quick connect, valve annulus, and the muscle full thickness. The atrial quick connects are then reverted into their original configuration

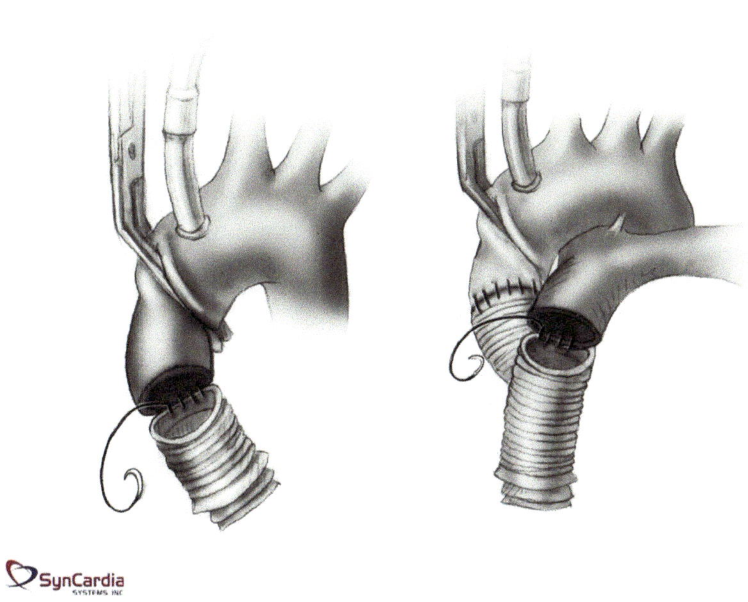

■ **Fig. 32.11** The arterial conduits are anastomosed to their respective artery with a running suture of 4-0 polypropylene

suture is passed in a similar fashion 180° from the first one and tied. This secures the quick connect in place and facilitates suturing. Each suture is then run to complete the circumference, advancing no more than 2 mm to avoid areas of separation in the suture line. The sutures are tied when they reach each other. When a separation between the skirt of the quick connects and the muscle occurs, a "scallop"-shaped deformity is created in the skirt. This is easily corrected by placing an interrupted 3-0 polypropylene suture in a horizontal mattress configuration. The suture line on the left side will go through the anterior leaflet of the mitral continuation with the left coronary leaflet of the aortic valves that was exposed earlier. The right atrial quick connect is placed thru the tricuspid valve annulus and sutured in a similar way. All "scallop" deformities are corrected. The atrial quick connects are then reverted into their original configuration.

The prosthetic left ventricle is placed in the mediastinum with its inflow resting over the left atrial quick connect. The ventricle is slightly rotated to the left, and its outflow aimed toward the aorta. This will provide the necessary length of the aortic conduit. The conduit can then be cut to this length. The prosthetic left ventricle is left in the mediastinum, and the right ventricle is brought in and allowed to rest on the right quick connect, aiming toward the pulmonary artery. This provides the length of the pulmonary artery conduit. In a patient with normal anatomy, the pulmonary artery conduit is usually 2–3 cm longer than the aortic conduit. The ventricles are then removed from the mediastinum and placed again over the surface of the left chest. The arterial conduits are anastomosed to their respective artery with a running suture of 4-0 polypropylene (■ Fig. 32.11). Rewarming is started at this time to bring the patient to normothermia.

Each suture line is checked for leaks. Two blunt-tipped needle drivers are placed side by side on the ring of the atrial quick connect or arterial conduit. A 27 mm tester could be used for the atrial quick connects and the 25 mm tester for the arterial conduits. The tester may be positioned at 180° from the needle drivers and gently pushed in. A 60 cc syringe with saline is connected to the tester and pressurized with one hand, placing the hand behind the left atrium and occluding the pulmonary veins. The left atrial quick anastomosis is the most difficult to test as not all the pulmonary veins can be occluded. A similar test may be performed in the right atrial, pulmonary artery, and aortic anastomosis. The pulmonary artery conduit requires placement of a cross clamp distal to the suture line to adequately test this suture line. Any leaks are corrected at this time with interrupted 3-0 or 4-0 polypropylene sutures. Coseal or BioGlue (CryoLife, Kennesaw,

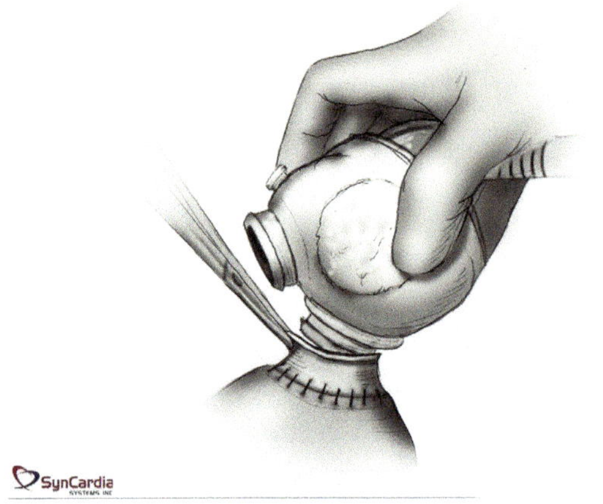

Fig. 32.12 The prosthetic left ventricle is brought back into the mediastinum again. The orientation of the ventricles has to be preset prior to the connection taking place. The ventricle is then connected to the aortic conduit in a similar fashion while installing saline to remove as much air as possible from the prosthetic ventricle. The prosthetic right ventricle is connected in a similar fashion; first to the right atrial quick connect. Blood volume is then passed from the CPB machine to the patient by removing one of the tourniquets in the cava until blood fills and deairs the right ventricle. The ventricle is then connected to the pulmonary artery conduit

GA) can be utilized to further secure the suture lines. A sheet of ePTFE membrane 20 × 15 × 0.1 mm is secured to the posterior pericardium, near the left pulmonary veins, with interrupted sutures. This will be used later to cover the left side of the device and will minimize adhesions at the time of the explantation.

The prosthetic left ventricle is brought back into the mediastinum again. The two blunt-tipped needle drivers are placed in the left atrial quick connect, and the inflow of the ventricle is connected to the quick connect. The orientation of the ventricles has to be preset prior to the connection taking place. The ventricle is then connected to the aortic conduit in a similar fashion while installing saline to remove as much air as possible from the prosthetic ventricle. The prosthetic right ventricle is connected in a similar fashion; first to the right atrial quick connect. Blood volume is then passed from the CPB machine to the patient by removing one of the tourniquets in the cava until blood fills and deairs the right ventricle. The ventricle is than connected to the pulmonary artery conduit (Fig. 32.12). A vent needle is placed in the ascending aorta, the patient is placed in the Trendelenburg position, and the aortic cross clamp is removed.

All tourniquets are removed from the cavae. Air is removed from the aorta TEE is used to visualize the aorta while air is removed. The Companion Driver is triggered on single shots to assist in removing air. Once no air is seen, the TAH is set at 40 beats/min as volume from the CPB machine is passed to the patient. If no air is seen, then the rate is increased by 20 beats/min up to 100–120 beats/min while the patient is weaned off the CPB machine. Once the patient is hemodynamically stable, protamine is administered to reverse the heparin. If an AICD is present, it can be removed along with the wires at this time.

Once bleeding has stopped, chest tubes are placed in the mediastinum and in the pleural cavities if necessary. The sternum and the chest are closed in the usual fashion. The two drivelines exiting the skin are secured to the skin at the surgeon's preference. If bleeding persists because of a coagulopathy, the mediastinum can be packed with laps and the sternum left open and covered with two layers of Ioban antimicrobial drape (3 M, St. Paul, MN). The patient might need daily mediastinal re-exploration until bleeding stops. Usually anticoagulation is started once bleeding has stopped and the chest is closed.

TEE is essential to verify that there is no compression of the cavae or pulmonary veins when the sternum is re-approximated. The most common evidence is compression of the IVC that usually improves with gentle rotation of the TAH toward the patient's left at the time of sternal re-approximation.

32.2.2 Technique for TAH Protection at the Time of Implantation

The technique to facilitate mediastinal re-entry utilizes three components: (1) blue polyisoprene bands (BBI; Bioseal, Placentia, CA), (2) GORE-TEX (PTFE) sheets (20 × 15 cm × 0.1 mm, W. L. Gore & Associates, Flagstaff, AZ), and (3) surgical-grade silicone membrane 0.060 in. thick (Bentec Medical, Woodland, CA) [35]. The blue polyisoprene bands (BB) have to be prepared in advance. They are placed into standard sterilization packaging and undergo gas sterilization

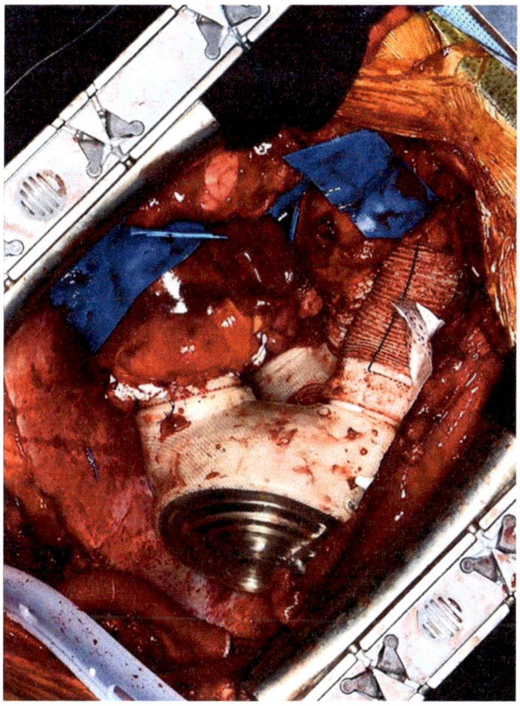

Fig. 32.13 The entire length of each vascular structure is covered in order to avoid adhesion formation, minimizing the necessity for dissecting the structure during the subsequent operation

(Sterrad 100S Sterilization System; Johnson and Johnson, Irvine, CA) for later use. After TAH implantation and at the time of chest closure, the surgical technique for future device explantation and transplantation starts. Blue bands are loosely placed circumferentially around the aorta and inferior vena cava (IVC). The entire length of each vascular structure is covered in order to avoid adhesion formation, minimizing the necessity for dissecting the structure during the subsequent operation (Fig. 32.13). The main advantage of this method is that no adhesions form around these latex-free bands. The BB for the SVC may be cut narrower to avoid possible SVC stenosis. Furthermore, the blue color facilitates identification of vascular structures and aids in timely preparation for cannulation. Care should be taken not to place the BB too tight around the vascular structures. Several centimeters of excess BB are left on top of the vascular structure and the free ends clipped together with Surgiclips (Autosuture Premium Surgiclip II M- 9.75; US Surgical, Norwalk, CT). The upper part of the most distal BB around the aorta is sutured down near the innominate vein to protect it from injury during re-entry. The upper part of the most proximal one placed around the aorta is folded down into the space between aorta and right atrium. Alternatively, a separate piece of BB can be the placed into that space. On occasion, a BB is placed around the pulmonary artery or placed between its posterior wall and a protruding (large) left atrial appendage.

Before the TAH is lowered into the mediastinal cavity, a 0.01 mm thick PTFE sheet is secured at the medial aspect of the mediastinum, by suturing the edges of the sheet with PROLENE sutures to areas lateral to the left pulmonary veins. During chest closure, one or two additional sheets of GORE-TEX, are utilized to cover the entire devices, as well as the right atrium and both venae cavae. The sheet over the right atrium can be tacked down with interrupted sutures to the pericardium near the venae cave to prevent migration. Chest and mediastinal drainage tubes are placed at this time in a routine fashion.

The edges of the various sheets are clipped together with Surgiclips. If appropriate, they are also clipped to the BBs already in place. For better drainage, several slit openings of about 0.5 in. in length are cut into the sheets with scissors to allow fluid or blood to reach the mediastinal drainage tubes.

A segment of surgical silicone membrane 1 cm wide and as long as the sternum is cut and placed above the sternal wires prior to sternal closure. When the sternum is re-approximated, care must be taken to make sure that the silicone membrane remains between the sternal wires and underside of the sternum and not be displaced between the blades of the sternum.

At transplant, a redo lateral oscillating blade saw is used to perform the sternotomy in a routine fashion at a level above the silicone membrane. The membrane serves as the first protective layer which can be easily removed, as no adhesions form around it. The BBs are identified around the encircled vessels. The clips on the BBs are removed and a small hole is cut into one end. An umbilical tape is threaded through that hole and subsequently placed around the vessel, as the BB is removed. As there are no adhesions around the encircled vessels (aorta, IVC, SVC), minimal dissection is required, and CPB can be initiated expeditiously, if required. The PTFE membranes are then removed from around the device the anterior surface of the heart or TAH. This facilitates exposure of the device as adhesions are minimized [35].

32.2.3 Perioperative Complications and Management of TAH

Postoperative

In the immediate postoperative period, the most important issue is bleeding and preventing tamponade of the TAH. Although the device is rigid, tamponade of the venae cavae and atria can occur resulting in a decrease in output with a rise in central venous pressure (CVP). This is the most common scenario for tamponade. Although initially most of the patients undergoing placement of a TAH had a sternotomy closure at the time, most recently the sternum is left open but with the wound sealed and drained with mediastinal tubes. This allows for further space to accumulate blood in the early period and decrease the deleterious effects of tamponade and hypoperfusion. Usually the chest is closed 24–48 h later, once bleeding has stopped, with no increase in infection rates [36].

32.3 Recovery of Renal Function After TAH

Although up to 52% of patients requiring TAH support have concomitant renal insufficiency, the renal function outcomes of such patients have not been well studied. In a recent series of 20 TAH [37], six of the 20 (30%) patients required preoperative dialysis [37]. Four recovered renal function (3 by day 30 and 1 by day 180), one remained on dialysis, and one died before 30 days of follow-up. Six of the 20 (30%) patients' renal insufficiency progressed after TAH implantation, resulting in a new dialysis requirement. Of these, 1 recovered renal function within 30 days; 2 were off of dialysis by 90 days. The remaining three patients died during the study period while on dialysis. Mortality in patients on new-onset dialysis was 50%. Overall, 75% (15 of 20) of the patients had renal insufficiency improved after TAH implantation, including 66% (4 of 6) of patients who were on dialysis at the time of surgery also if renal failure and replacement therapy are associated with an increased risk of multiorgan failure. In a study reported by Copeland et al. [20] where 19% of patients developed a new-onset dialysis requirement after TAH implantation, renal recovery was noted in 41% and 59% died. Thus, failure of renal recovery in patients with new-onset dialysis after TAH implantation is a marker of poor prognosis. Unfortunately, no data were available on the length of perioperative dialysis that could have probably a relevant role on the hazard of a recovery.

GT's experience seems to show that, as renal function, specifically in the chronic heart failure, is pretty much depending in B-type natriuretic peptide (BNP), early initiation of nesiritide might play a difference on recovery of renal and even liver function. The ideal timing to start the therapy [38], due to the possibility that liver and renal function could affect each other [39], could be immediately after ventriculectomy. Even after recovery of renal function, liver function may deteriorate specifically under high-volume output, as the liver was adapted to a low output status for a long time. With reference to the recovery of end-organ function, it might then be a difference between 50 cc TAH-t and 70 cc TAH-t. Also if the common view in the literature has always been that high flow combined with low CVP as it is seen with the TAH is the optimal way to improve dysfunctional kidneys and liver, there is not any evidence based on clinical data so far, GT has the impression that less cardiac output might be protective for the liver specifically in the early phase after implantation. It appears difficult to ascertain the differential impact of such strategies (and even devices) with respect to other factors driving the results such as the timing of the implantation.

32.4 Inpatient

The inpatient management usually focuses on anticoagulation (▶ see Sect. 32.8), nutrition, ambulation, driveline skin site management, blood pressure management, and end-organ function. Antibiotic prophylaxis is instituted based on each center protocols and infection control data. Specific infectious processes should be managed with antibiotic sensitivity data.

Most of the patients with advanced congestive heart failure experience some degree of nutrition impairment. Some patients may experience significant malnutrition, especially if the patient has been chronically ill and in an intensive care unit. Malnutrition is an independent predictor of mortality in this group of patients [40]. Different centers follow different nutritional parameters. Some of these include serum prealbumin, albumin, Mini Nutritional Assessment [41], and many more. There are multiple institutions working on the more consistent indicators including indirect calorimetry [42] and frailty scale. All patients need to have their nutritional status optimized before implantation if there is time and afterward to improve their chances of recovery with the TAH.

Early mobility, rehabilitation, and ambulation appear to be essential in the level of functionality and quality of life that patient experiences after placement of a mechanical circulatory device. The ventricular assist literature shows evidence that cardiac rehabilitation improves functional capacity [43] and quality of life [44]. Furthermore, patients with the SynCardia TAH have been shown to tolerate early rehabilitation and aerobic exercise training [45]. Further studies in the level of functionality and physiologic responses in patients who receive a TAH are much needed.

Blood pressure management is important in all patients with mechanical circulatory support (MCS). The total pump output in all MCSs is afterload dependent. If the afterload is high, then the pump output decreases. Furthermore, it places the patient at risk for a bleeding complication or stroke. Blood pressure control can usually be obtained with one or two agents in patients with continuous-flow LVADs [46]. In a similar fashion, the same appears to apply to patients with TAHs.

Normal end-organ function is essential for a successful patient outcome for any MCSs including TAH. Many of the patients who are evaluated for TAH are usually INTERMACS patient profiles 1 and 2. A significant subgroup is already experiencing some degree of end-organ dysfunction that may preclude the use of MCS. Initial evaluation of the patient needs to be critical with an emphasis on patient chances for recovery and rehabilitation. Two of the most important elements required for a successful outcome are patient selection and timing of surgical intervention. This translates in many ways to what is the overall function of the other organs. Hepatic and renal dysfunctions are common in patients who experienced cardiogenic shock prior to implantation. Liver dysfunction manifested by auto anticoagulation and/or elevated total bilirubin should be evaluated. A total bilirubin that continues to increase despite all attempts prior to implantation is a risk factor for poor outcome.

A significant number of patients who are considered for TAH are experiencing some degree of renal dysfunction as a result of the cardiac failure. Recently, it has been shown that TAH support improves renal function in 75% of patients with pre-existing renal insufficiency, including patients who required dialysis [36].

32.5 Preparation for Discharge Home

The management of patient with a TAH to the outpatient setting has occurred over the past few years. In the past, the EXCOR driver [47] was utilized in Europe, but more recently the Freedom Driver [48] has allowed a growing number of patients to be managed successfully at home. The patient who is a candidate to be trained for discharge meets the following criteria: no intravenous medications, ambulatory, no evidence of infections or ongoing adverse events, stable on oral medications including anticoagulation, and stable social support. Once identified, the patient as well as the designated social support, usually a family member, undergoes training. The training includes medication education, driveline skin care management, understanding of the Freedom Driver and alarms, close monitoring of anticoagulation, diet education, and required follow-up. Also the social support is trained on driver exchanged if necessary. A telephone number is provided to the patient and social support for emergency and routine access to the MCS staff.

32.6 Outpatient Management

The patient is usually followed in clinic once a week for the first month and then the visits progress to once a month. The patient keeps a record of medications, blood pressure, and any other important issues. At the time of the visit, vital signs are obtained; the Freedom Driver readings and history are examined. The patient undergoes a physical exam with attention to the driveline skin site. Anticoagulation parameters are reviewed and medications adjusted as indicated. The outpatient follow-up of a patient with a TAH is similar the outpatient follow-up of patients with other types of MCS. Listing for heart transplantation is considered like any other patient and follows the country's organ procurement organizations established rules.

32.7 Risk of Infection after TAH

There are several protocols used for the management of driveline skin site. The goals should be for a clean site and driveline immobilization. If the driveline site appears moist, the cleaning process and dressing change should be upgraded to a daily schedule. Erythema at the site requires further investigation and an active infection has to be ruled out. Antibiotics should be utilized when indicated. Immobilization of the SynCardia TAH drivelines can be a challenge as there are two of them; however, infections appear to be infrequent.

The large bore drivelines are subjected to infections as every device used in the clinical field of MCS. Local treatment is often necessary but a low incidence of infective complications appears to be due to the long pneumatic cannulas covered of Dacron velour offering an excellent sealing and healing thus preventing the possibility of ascending infections from the outside to inside. The worst clinical challenge remains left inflow valve infection that fails to respond to therapy. The setting of prosthetic endocarditis may cause multiple strokes and could require pump exchange. Luckily this complication appears very rare in the real-world clinical experience.

32.8 Anticoagulation

Device thrombosis, thromboembolism, and GI bleeding are not major issues with the SynCardia TAH-t. Stress accumulations in continuous-flow pumps are high [49] enough to cause platelet activation that currently available antiplatelet agents may not be able to inhibit. Further, when hemolysis occurs, the red cell ghosts contribute further to activation of the coagulation system [50]. Attempting to compensate for this problem with increased dosing of anticoagulants may lead to higher rates of hemorrhagic strokes.

In contrast, stress accumulations in the SynCardia TAH, in spite of having four mechanical valves, have been measured at hundreds of times less than those in continuous-flow pumps [51]. Stresses in the TAH are in the range that platelet activation can be controlled with currently available antiplatelet medications. In addition, flows with the TAH of 7–9 l/min average 2–3 l/min higher than those obtained with LVADs resulting in the "washing effect" of valves and foreign surfaces in any areas where stasis could occur. Still, withholding anticoagulation therapy will cause hypercoagulability and thromboembolism. What then is a reasonable protocol of anticoagulation?

The Arizona's center approach over a 15 year period [6] including our initial "learning curve" years was based upon a protocol involving: (1) adequate monitoring of platelet function and coagulation status and (2) therapy with medications tailored to platelet function and coagulation status targets.

32.9 Coagulation Monitoring and Anticoagulation Protocol (■ Table 32.3)

Careful daily assessment and therapy modulation based upon tests as well as clinical events is advised while the patient is hospitalized. In the Arizona's center protocol, transition from heparin to Coumadin is routine. Coumadin therapy is accompanied by aspirin, pentoxiphylline, and dipyridamole. Pentoxiphylline and dipyridamole are not commonly used in all TAH's programs around the world.

A review of 99 consecutive TAH recipients with this therapy disclosed that with these testing and treatment protocols, the chance of stroke is $\leq$ 0.08 per patient year without any case of pump thrombosis. High outputs and low shear accumulations with this device are forgiving enough that any combination of antiplatelet and anticoagulant therapy will yield good results if the patients are followed carefully.

Table 32.3 Anticoagulation management protocol Arizona center

Standard tests, daily
PT/INR (prothrombin time) useful in Coumadin-treated patients, target 2.5 ±0.5 s
PTT (partial thromboplastin time) useful in heparin-treated patients, target 45–50 s
Platelet count for all patients
Advanced tests, variable
TEG (thromboelastogram), daily for patients on heparin infusion, once or twice a week for patients off heparin and on Coumadin, target CI (coagulation index) in normocoagulable range, also useful for monitoring for hypercoagulability that can occur from inflammation, infection, trauma
Platelet aggregation studies, once or twice a week, target depressed response to ADP, epinephrine, arachidonic acid, but >50% response to collagen
Bleeding time, once or twice a week, target twice normal (e.g., normal of 10 min, target 20 min)
Therapy
Dipyridamole 100–250 mg every 6 h. Start per nasogastric tube immediately post-implant
Pentoxiphylline 400 mg every 8 h. Start per nasogastric tube immediately post-implant
Aspirin 81–325 mg every day. Start after platelet count exceeds 75,000 per cubic millimeter. Adjust dose according to platelet count (increase by 81–162 mg/d for each rise in platelet count of 100,000), platelet aggregation study, and bleeding time targets
Heparin 500 units per hour. Start after chest tube bleeding is <30 ml/h for 4 continuous hours. Adjust to keep TEG in normocoagulable range or PTT at 45–50 s
Coumadin 2.5–5 mg daily, adjust to INR of 2.5±0.5

32.10 Thromboembolic Risk of TAH

On 99 consecutive patients over a 15 year period treated with a consistent anticoagulation protocol, there were eight strokes (8%) [6]. The timing of the strokes is of interest: four were in the first 48 h after implantation and attributed to the patient's previous condition and the implant operation and two were associated with persistent positive blood cultures and the appearance of vegetations on the left-sided inflow valve as seen on transesophageal echo. Finally, for the remaining 93 patients over a period of 23 patient years, there were two strokes (0.08 strokes/pt. year), one middle cerebral artery embolus associated with hemiplegia, and one transient hemiplegia. Both of these patients were able to have cardiac transplants. From this experience the greatest hazard for thromboembolism is the implant operation. Extreme care has to be taken to eliminate left-sided particulate debris, with the aim to reduce these events. The worst clinical challenge has been left inflow valve infection in two cases that failed to respond to therapy. This prosthetic endocarditis caused multiple strokes. In one case the TAH was exchanged successfully, but both cases finally resulted in neurologic death. Finally, 2% rate of thromboembolism in 94% of the patients remains an outstanding result. Other studies have confirmed a low thromboembolic rate (NEJM multi-institutional study 2004: 81patients, strokes in 6%, Bad Oyenhausen 2005: 42 patients, strokes in 4.6%, La Pitie 2003: 127 patients, no strokes) [52]. The low rate of thromboembolism has been replicated in multiple institutions using multiple anticoagulation strategies suggesting that regardless of the anticoagulation protocol, there will be a low thromboembolic rate. In the study from Torregrossa [53], an incidence of 0.083 TE events per patient month was experienced, comparable with the previous international experience achieved within 1 year of support. Looking at the data, the risk of death following ischemic stroke was lower than the risk associated with hemorrhagic stroke, thus underlining the relative safety of TAH in term of thromboembolic risk.

Even the recent experience at La Pitie-Salpetriere Hospital in Paris illustrates that a simplification of the anticoagulation protocol of Szefner did not result in an increase in neurologic complications or thrombotic events [54]. Furthermore, the recent report from GRAM (Groupe de Relexion sur l'Assistance Mecanique) registry showed that SynCardia recipients experienced significantly fewer neurologic events compared with BiVAD recipients [55].

32.11 Long-Term Results of TAH

As of September 2015, numbers of long-term survivors have included 127, 26, 7, and 2 at 1–4 years. The longest survivors are over 4 years. In patients surviving at least 1 year, there have been 2 deaths from diaphragm rupture. The incidence of diaphragm perforation has been 0.5% per patient and 0.25% per ventricle over the history of the device. Two of the eight patients were successfully transplanted. Most deaths have been related to multiple organ failure. The yearly survival for each year has been 75%.

In the recent paper of Torregrossa et al. [53], resembling the experience of TAH with more than 1 year of survival, even after 1 year of support, the vast majority (72%) of patients underwent successful cardiac transplantation within a median support time of 563 days. Despite the long-term presence of the TAH, no intraoperative mortality is reported at the time of the cardiac transplantation when the device is removed from the chest. The outcome of heart transplantation could have benefited of selection bias because of the exclusion of all the patients supported for less than 1 year. The cohort might have included all patients with an excellent grade of rehabilitation transplanted in centers with better experience in the management of such patients.

Nevertheless, in the experience of Copeland et al., with 100 TAH implants (mean support time 87 ± 94.8 days), 70% of deaths occurred in the first 14 days, and 90% occurred within the first 40 days after implantation, underlining a substantial stabilization of patient death events over time. These data are confirmed also in the most recent experience in France where the actuarial estimates of survival under TAH support is constant between 120 and 360 days.

Nevertheless, in patients supported with TAH death generally arrive after a long-term period of ICU where the hemodynamic conditions are guaranteed by the mechanical device and infections superimposed a clinical scenario of multiorgan failure. These data highlight the need for maintaining an extremely high index of suspicion for infection in patients supported long term with a SynCardia TAH.

References

1. DeVries WC, Anderson JH, Joyce LD, Anderson FL, Hammond EH, Jarvik RK, Kolff WJ (1984) Clinical use of the total artificial heart. New Engl J Med 310: 273–278
2. Copeland JG, Levinson MM, Smith R, Icenogle TB, Vaughn C, Chang K, Ott R, Emery RW (1986) The total artificial heart as a bridge to transplantation. JAMA 256:2991–2995
3. Copeland JGIII, Smith RG, Arabia FA, Nolan P, Mehta VK, McCarthy MS, Chisholm KA (2001) Comparison of the CardioWest total artificial heart, the novacor ventricular assist system, and the thoratec ventricular assist system in bridge to transplantation. Ann Thorac Surg 71(3):S92–S97
4. Copeland JG, Smith RG, Arabia FA, Nolan PE, Sethi GK, Tsau PH, McClellan D, Slepian MJ (2004) Cardiac replacement with a total artificial heart as a bridge to transplantation. N Engl J Med 351:859–867
5. Copeland JG, Copeland H, Gustafson M, Mineburg N, Covington D, Smith RG, Friedman M (2012) Experience with more than 100 total artificial heart implants. J Thorac Cardiovasc Surg 143:727–734
6. Copeland J, Copeland H, Nolan P, Gustafson M, Slepian M, Smith R (2013) Results with an anticoagulation protocol in 99 SynCardia total artificial heart recipients. ASAIO J 59:216–220
7. Copeland JG, Smith RG, Bose RK, Tsau PH, Nolan PE, Slepian MJ (2008) Risk factor analysis for bridge to transplantation with the CardioWest total artificial heart. Ann Thorac Surg 85:1639–1644
8. Heilmann C, Geisen U, Beyersdorf F, Nakamura L, Benk C, Berchtold-Herz M, Trummer G, Schlensak C, Zieger B (2010) Acquired von Willebrand syndrome in patients with ventricular assist device or total artificial heart. Thromb Haemost 103(5):962–967
9. Park SJ, Kushwaha SS, McGregor CGA (2012) State-of-the-art implantable cardiac assist device therapy for heart failure: bridge to transplant and destination therapy. Clin Pharmacol Ther 91(1):94–100
10. Milano CA, Simeone AA (2013) Mechanical circulatory support: devices, outcomes and complications. Heart Fail Rev 18:35–53
11. Mulloy DP, Bhamidipati CM, Stone ML et al (2013) Orthotopic heart transplant versus left ventricular assist device: a national comparison of cost and survival. J Thorac Cardiovasc Surg 145:566–574
12. Hsu PL, Parker J, Egger C, Autschbach R, Schmitz-Rode T, Steinseifer U (2012) Mechanical circulatory support for right heart failure: current technology and future outlook. Artif Organs 36(4):332–347

13. Kormos RL, Teuteberg JJ, Pagani FD et al (2010) Right ventricular failure with the HeartMate II continuous-flow left ventricular assist device: Incidence, risk factors, and effect on outcomes. J Thorac Cardiovasc Surg 139:1316–1324
14. Kirklin JK, Naftel DC, Kormos RL et al (2013) Fifth INTERMACS annual report: Risk factor analysis from more than 6,000 mechanical circulatory support patients. J Heart Lung Transplant 32:141–156
15. Stevenson LW, Pagani FD, Young JB, Jessup M, Miller L, Kormos RL, Naftel DC et al (2009) J Heart Lung Transplant 28:535–541
16. Leibner ES, Cysyk J, Eleuteri K, El-Banayosy A, Boehmer JP, Pae WE (2013) Changes in the functional status measures of heart failure patients with MCS. ASAIO J 59(2):117–122
17. Kalya A, Jaroszewski D, Pajaro O, Scott R, Gopalan R, Kasper D, Arabia F (2013) Role of the total artificial heart in the management of heart transplant rejection and retransplantation: case report and review. Clin Transplant 27:E348–E350
18. Yoda M, El-banayosy A, Tendrich G, Koerfer R, Minami K (2009) The Cardio West artificial heart for chronic heart transplant rejection. Circ J 73:1167–1168
19. Morales LS, Khan MS, Gottlieb EA, Krishnamurthy R, Dreyer WJ, Adachi I (2012) Implantation of total artificial heart in congenital heart disease. Semin Thorac Cardiovasc Surg 24(2):142–143
20. Smith MC, Arabia FA, Tsau PH, Smith RG, Bose RK, Woolley DS, Rhenman BE, Sthi GK, Copeland JG (2005) CardioWest total artificial heart in a moribund adolescent with left ventricular thrombi. Ann Thorac Surg 80:1490–1492
21. Park SS, Sanders DB, Smith BP, Ryan J, Plasencia J, Osborn MB et al (2014) Total artificial heart in the pediatric patient with biventricular heart failure. Perfusion 29:82–88
22. Sharma MS, Forbess JM, Guleserian KJ (2012) Ventricular assist device support in children and adolescents with heart failure: the Children's Medical Center Dallas Experience. Artif Organs 36(7):635–648
23. Patel SW, Peterson A, Bartczak A et al (2014) Primary cardiac angiosarcoma – a review. Med Sci Monit 20:103–109
24. Yam N, Au TW, Cheng L (2013) Post-infarction ventricular septal defect: surgical outcomes in the last decade. Asian Cardiovasc Thorac Ann 21:539–545
25. Gregoric ID, Bieniarz MC, Arora H, Frazier OH, Kar B, Loyalka P (2008) Percutaneous ventricular assist device support in a patient with a postinfarction ventricular septal defect. Tex Heart Inst J 35(1):46–49
26. Ashfaq A, Jaroszewski DE, Pajaro OE, Arabia FA (2013) The role of the total artificial heart in the treatment of post-myocardial infarction ventricular septal defect. J Thorac Cardiovasc Surg 145:e25–e26
27. Swiecicki PL, Edwards BS, Kushwaha SS, Dispenzieri A, Park SJ, Gerts MA (2013) Left ventricular device implantation for advanced cardiac amyloidosis. J Heart Lung Transplant 32:563–568
28. Spiliopoulos S et al (2015) Delayed sternal closure after total artificial heart implantation. J Thorac Cardiovasc Surg 150:417–417
29. Spiliopoulos S et al (2015) Implantation technique of the 50 cc Syncardia Total Artificial Heart: does size make a difference? Multimed Man Cardiothorac Surg
30. Rossano JW et al (2014) Successful use of the total artificial heart in the failing Fontan circulation. Ann Thorac Surg 97:1438–1440
31. Lorver RR, Shumway NE (1960) Study on the orthotopic homotransplantations of the canine heart. Surg Forum 11:18
32. Spiliopoulos S et al (2015) Expanding applicability of Total Artificial Heart therapy: the 50 cc Syncardia TAH. Ann Thorac Surg 100:e55–e57
33. Copeland JG, Smith RG, Arabia FA et al (2004) Total artificial heart bridge to transplantation: a 9-year experience with 62 patients. J Heart Lung Transplant 23:823–831
34. Moore RA et al (2014) Virtual implantation evaluation of the total artificial heart and compatibility: beyond standard fit criteria. J Heart Lung Transplant 33(11):1180–1183
35. Ihnken K, Ramzy D, Esmailian F, Trento A, Arabia F (2016) Surgical technique to facilitate explantation of Mechanical Circulatory Devices (MCS): LVAD's, BiVAD's, and TAH's prior to heart transplantation. ASAIO J 62(2):211–213. doi:10.1097/MAT.0000000000000318
36. Quader M, LaPar DJ, Wolfe L, Ailawadi G, Rich J, Speir A, Fonner C, Kasirajan V (2016) Investigators for the virginia cardiac surgery quality initiative. Delayed sternal closure after continuous flow left ventricle assist device implantation: analysis of risk factors and impact on outcomes and costs. ASAIO J 62(4):432–437. doi:10.1097/MAT.0000000000000384
37. Quader M, Goodreau A, Shah KB, Katlaps G, Cooke R, Smallfield M, Tchoukina I, Wolfe L, Kasiraja V (2016) Renal function recovery with total artificial heart support. ASAIO J 62(1):87–91. doi:10.1097/MAT.0000000000000288
38. Wadei HM et al (2006) Hepatorenal Syndrome: pathophysiology and management. Clin J Am Soc Nephrol 1:1066–1079
39. Spiliopoulos S et al (2014) B-type natriuretic peptide therapy in total artificial heart implantation: renal effect with early initiation. J Heart Lung Transpl 33(6):662–663
40. Aggarwal A, Kumar A, Gregory MP, Blair C, Pauwaa S, Tatooles AJ, Pappas PS, Bhat G (2013) Nutrition assessment in advanced heart failure patients evaluated for ventricular assist devices or cardiac transplantation. Nutr Clin Pract 28:112–119
41. Yost G, Gregory M, Bhat G (2014) Short-form nutrition assessment in patients with advanced heart failure evaluated for ventricular assist device placement or cardiac transplantation. Nutr Clin Pract 29:686–691
42. Yost G, Gregory M, Bhat G (2015) Nutrition assessment with indirect calorimetry in patients for left ventricular assist device implantation. Nutr Clin Pract 30:690–697
43. Kerrigan DJ, Williams CT, Ehrman JK, Saval MA, Bronsteen K, Schairer JR, Swaffer M, Brawner CA, Lanfear DE, Selektor Y, Velez M, Tita C, Keteyian SJ (2014) Cardiac rehabilitation improves functional capacity and patient-reported health status with continuous-flow left ventricular assist devices. J Am Coll Cardiol Heart Fail 2:653–659

44. Rogers JG, Aaronson KD, Boyle AJ, Russell SD, Milano CA, Pagani FD, Edwards BS, Park S, John R, Conte JV, Farrar DJ, Slaughter MS et al (2010) Continuous flow left ventricular assist device improves functional capacity and quality of life of advanced heart failure patients. J Am Coll Cardiol 55:1826–1834
45. Kohli HS, Canada J, Arena R, Tang DG, Peberdy MA, Harton S, Flattery M, Doolin K, Katlaps GJ, Hess ML, Kasirajan V, Shah KB (2011) Exercise blood pressure response during assisted circulatory support: comparison of the total artificial heart with a left ventricular assist device during rehabilitation. J Heart Lung Transplant 30:1207–1213
46. Lampert BC, Eckert C, Weaver S, Scanlon A, Lockard K, Allen C, Kunz N, Bermudez C, Bhama JK, Shullo MA, Kormos RL, Dew MA, Teuteberg JJ (2014) Blood pressure control in continuous ventricular assist devices: efficacy and impact on adverse events. Ann Thorac Surg 97:139–146
47. El Banayosy A, Kizner L, Arusoglu L, Morshuis M, Brehm C, Koerfer R, Schuermann C, Smith RG, Copeland JG, Slepian MJ (2014) Home discharge and out-of hospital follow-up of total artificial heart patients supported by a portable driver system. ASAIO J 60:148–153
48. Shah N, Jaroszewski DE, Ashfaq A, Schroedl LA, Staley L, Pajaro O, Kasirajan V, Arabia F (2015) SynCardia portable freedom driver: a single-center experience with 11 patients. Innovations 10(3):188–194
49. Dimasi A, Rasponi M, Sheriff J, Chiu W-C, Bluestein D, Tran PL, Slepian MJ, Redaelli A (2015) Microfluidic emulation of mechanical circulatory support device shear-mediated platelet activation. Biomed Microdevices 17:117–128
50. Tran PL, Pietropaolo MG, Valerio L, Khalpey ZI, Redaelli A, Sheriff J, Bluestein D, Slepian M (2015) Perfusion 1:1–8
51. Marom G, Chiu W-C, Crosby JR, DeCook KJ, Prabhakar S, Horner M, Slepian M, Bluestein D (2014) Numerical model of full cardiac cycle hemodynamics in a total artificial heart and the effect of ots size on platelet activation. J Cardiovasc Transl Res 7:788–796
52. El-Banayosy A, Arusoglu L, Morshuis M et al (2005) CardioWest total artificial heart: Bad Oeynhausen experience. Ann Thorac Surg 80:548–552
53. Torregrosa G, Morshius M, Varghese R, Hosseinian L, Vida V, Tarzia V, Loforte A, Duveau D, Arabia F, Leprince P, Kasirajan V, Byersdorf F, Musumeci F, Hetzer R, Krabatsch T, Gummert J, Copeland J, Gerosa G (2014) Results with SynCardia total artificial heart beyond one year. ASAIO J 60:626–634
54. Szefner J (1995) Control and treatment of hemostasis in cardio- vascular surgery. The experience of La Pitie Hospital with patients on total artificial heart. Int J Artif Organs 18:633–648
55. Kirsch M et al (2012) Groupe de Réflexion sur l'Assistance Mécanique (GRAM). Survival after biventricular mechanical circulatory support: does the type of device matter? J Heart Lung Transplant 31(5):501–508 http://dx.doi.org/10.1016/j.healun.2011.11.024

Concomitant Cardiac Surgery During VAD Placement: When Is It Too Much?

Walter P. Dembistky, Karl K. Limmer, and Robert M. Adamson

© Springer International Publishing Switzerland 2017
A. Montalto et al. (eds.), *Mechanical Circulatory Support in End-Stage Heart Failure*,
DOI 10.1007/978-3-319-43383-7_33

33.1 Introduction

The aging of the global population has ushered in a new medical era where management of chronic degenerative diseases is becoming increasingly important. The growing global pandemic of heart failure is one component of that problem and remains, in the USA, as one of the most expensive to treat. To date, the treatments for terminal stages of heart failure are comfort care, cardiac transplantation, and support using ventricular assist devices. The overall impact of cardiac transplantation on the epidemiology of heart failure is "trivial" [1]. This shortcoming has placed greater emphasis on the use of mechanical devices to sustain patients. Initially, devices were used to support patients awaiting heart transplantation, but the ever-present shortage and the growing and aging population prompted their use as permanent devices or "destination therapy." In the 1980s, survival on a device for days was considered to be exemplary. In the 1990s, weeks of survival were an improvement, and in the 2000 era, a survival of months was considered to be uniquely poor.

At that time, studies were designed to test efficacy of devices as destination therapy using a 2-year metric. Now, with the evolution of device therapy and the continued growth of the heart failure population and contraction of the donor rates, a new time metric is being implemented, as indicated in ◘ Figs. 33.1 and 33.2.

Five- and 10-year survivals are becoming more common, with over 1000 patients surviving over 5 years using the HeartMate II in a recent analysis. Because of this new time metric, consideration has shifted from complications related solely to the implanted device and its durability and intrinsic thrombogenicity or local hematologic problems, to the relationship of the device to the retained native heart.

Our own philosophy has been to maintain the flow pathway by eliminating areas of recirculation and stasis and to ensure the maximum ability of the retained native heart to provide pulsations to be transmitted through the current generations of continuous-flow VADs [2, 3]. Our overriding philosophy has been to repair the native heart and then to add a left ventricular assist device.

To that end, we repair the mitral valve in approximately 40% of patients, we used aortic valve closure in approximately 17% of patients, and we have closed patent foramen ovale in approximately 15% of patients. We have used

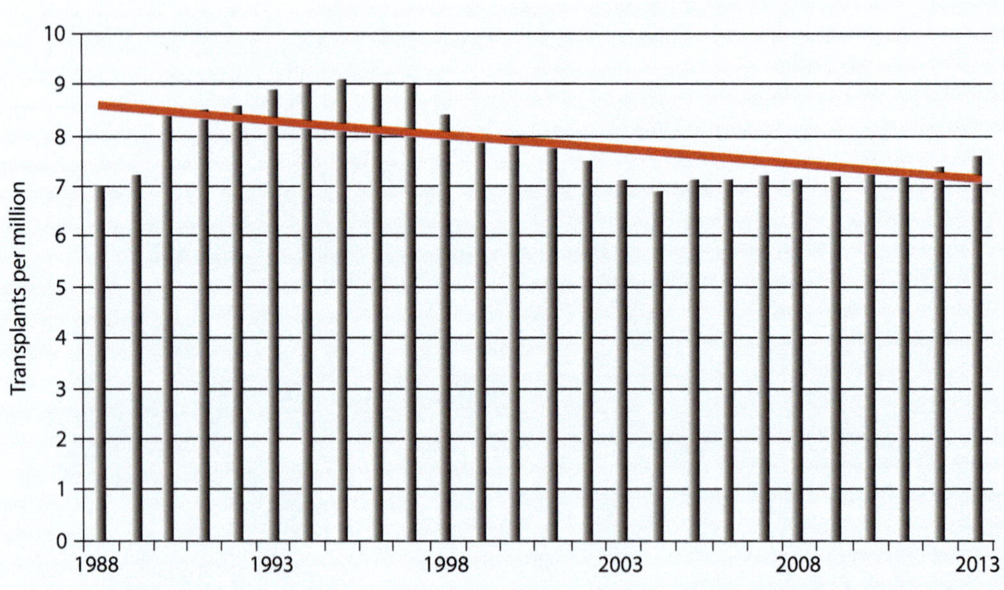

◘ **Fig. 33.1** Transplant/population ratio

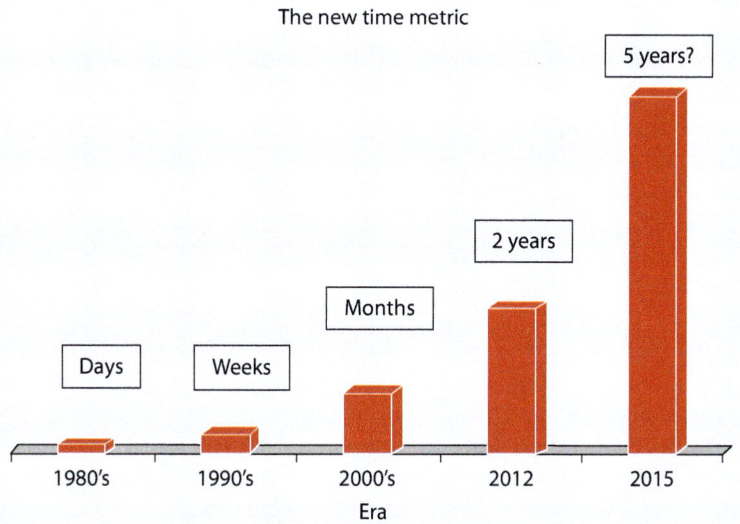

Fig. 33.2 The new time metric (Note: W. Dembitsky 2016)

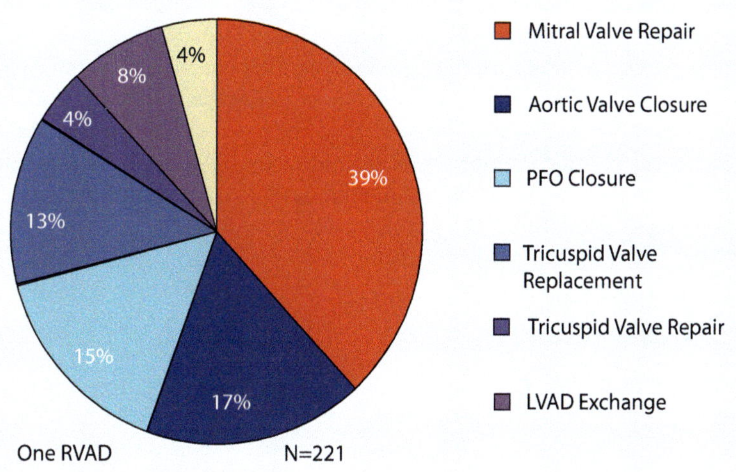

Fig. 33.3 Sharp Hospital-associated procedures (Note: Concurrent valvular procedures during HMII insertion are not associated with short- or long-term decreased survival. Adamson et al. [4])

tricuspid valve repair or replacement in approximately 17% of the patients. It is rare for us to only put in a HeartMate II (12% of patients), and usually one or more additional procedures are performed (Fig. 33.3) [4].

The discussion below will focus on patent foramen ovale management and valvular procedures, including the mitral valve, aortic valve, and tricuspid valve. Finally, there is a brief review of important miscellaneous procedures, including those on the aorta, left ventricle and atria, and coronary arteries.

33.2 Patent Foramen Ovale and LVAD Insertion

Patent foramen ovale can be difficult to diagnose with intraoperative transesophageal echo because left atrial pressures are usually greater than right atrial pressures. Even a bubble Doppler will fail to elucidate the potentially problematic patent foramen ovale. In the post-LVAD insertion patient, the left atrial pressures are lower than the right atrial pressures, which fosters a right-to-left shunt and produces a diagnostic triad of the missed patent foramen ovale: hypoxia, which is unresponsive to increased oxygen concentrations, a clear chest X-ray, and a bubble Doppler that shows a right-to-left shunt. Patent foramen ovale has certainly been closed during the postoperative period using both Amplatzer and BLANK devices, but is certainly much more complicated and potentially more of a thrombotic liability than simply opening the atrial septum to close the potentially problematic foramen.

We use a simple diagnostic test in the operating room prior to the insertion of LVAD. By compressing the pulmonary artery, the right atrial pressure increases and the left atrial pressure decreases and the atrial septum shifts to the left. Agitated saline, bubble Doppler, injected into the right atrium at that time will clearly demonstrate the presence of a potentially dangerous patent foramen. The incidence of patent foramen ovale in the general population is approximately 28%. If the atrium is inspected in every case, that is the approximate percentage that will be closed. Interestingly, in a reported analysis of multi-institutional results, only a 6% incidence of PFO closure is reported [5]. In our experience, using the pulmonary artery compression technique, we were able to reduce our patent foramen ovale closure significantly – down to approximately 20%, eliminating unnecessary pump time and incisions [4].

33.3 Mitral Valve

Mitral valve regurgitation is common in heart failure patients, but the need to correct mitral regurgitation in patients receiving LVADs remains controversial [6]. Insight comes from small, often single-centered, studies. Results of ongoing controlled studies are not yet available.

Most MR associated with cardiomyopathy is a consequence of LV dilation with resultant chordae tethering and mitral annular dilation. With LVAD decompression, LV dimensions decrease and may allow mitral leaflet coaptation and make MR insignificant during device support. Morgan [7] found that continuous-flow LVAD implantation significantly decreased the severity of MR (moderate-severe) from 76% preoperatively to 8% at 1 and 6 months postoperatively. However, there is still potential risk for residual MR when device support cannot be optimized to provide low, left-sided filling pressures, such as when there is suction of the interventricular septum over the inflow cannula at higher speeds or the need for intermittent AV opening [8]. Right ventricular failure is an important cause of early and late mortality and morbidity after LVAD implantation. Mitral regurgitation negatively affects RV function, LVAD filling, and possibly survival [9].

There are many proposed theoretical advantages of having a competent mitral valve in LVAD patients. In the early postoperative period when fluid balance is dynamic and often coupled with elevated pulmonary resistance, any contribution to the right ventricular afterload can result in increasing right heart failure. Early persistent mitral valve insufficiency is more likely to cause increases in afterload if the continuous-flow pumps are set to allow the ventricle to produce pulsatile pressure and guarantee adequate ventricular volumes for the LVAD to aspirate. The pressure can in turn be transmitted to the left atrium and reflected as an increase in the total pulmonary vascular resistance [10].

Experimentally, a competent valve can provide an increased pulsatility index [11]. LVAD filling and LVAD flow may affect pump thrombosis rates. In the presence of aortic insufficiency, a competent mitral valve will protect the pulmonary bed. If LVAD flows are kept low to permit aortic valve opening (in hopes of maintaining aortic valve integrity), pulsatility can again be transmitted retrograde to create a substrate for right ventricular failure. Finally, a competent mitral valve will facilitate weaning a patient with ventricular recovery.

Our bias has been to repair mitral valve regurgitation in any patient with greater than 2+ mitral regurgitation or in any patient with structural valvular problems (including ruptured chordae) or in functional regurgitation due to tethering of the leaflets and/or annular dilatation. Our technique for repairing the mitral valve is to perform the valve repair, almost always only requiring a posterior flexible annuloplasty in the beating heart, following the creation of an apical core for the LVAD. A vent placed through the apex and retractors on the annulus allows the heart to beat with no chance of embolization, excellent visibility, and only one case where aortic insufficiency necessitated the use of cardioplegia. A limited experience with transapical repair has been

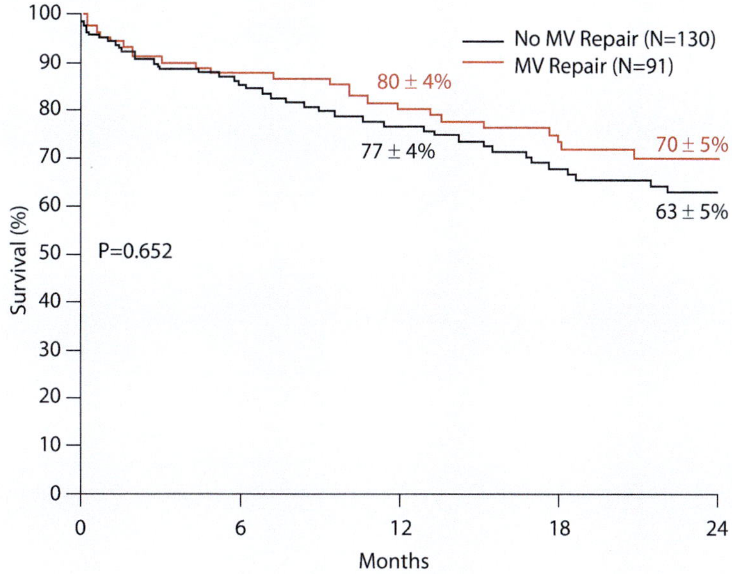

Fig. 33.4 Survival post-LVAD +/– mitral valve repair (Note: Mitral valve repair associated with HeartMate II insertion is not associated with increased operative mortality and may provide long-term survival advantage . Adamson et al. Jaski Presented ISHLT meeting San Diego 2014 JHLT abstract)

reported [12], and pre-existing mitral prostheses have been successfully left in place [13].

In our early experience from 1991 to 2008, we repaired approximately 17% of our mitral valves, and today our repair rate has risen to approximately 55%. As seen in the graph below (Fig. 33.4), a retrospective analysis of 221 HeartMate II patients, 41% of whom received mitral valve repair or replacement, the early survival was unchanged, and there is a tendency for late survival to separate with favoring the mitral valve group [14].

Some patients supported by LVADs will continue to have or develop mitral regurgitation after LVAD [15]. For us and others, mitral valve annuloplasty associated with an LVAD does not increase the operative mortality, reduces long-term mitral regurgitation, and may decrease immediate and long-term RV failure rates, possibly providing a long-term advantage [16].

33.4 Aortic Valvular Disease

Our first experience with aortic insufficiency at the time of LVAD insertion was in 1993 [17]. This was unexpected pre-op and was treated with a bioprosthesis replacement of the aortic valve. At the time of transplantation, the prosthesis was occluded, and there was red thrombus below the valve, demonstrating the risk of embolism. The 2013 ISHLT guidelines for mechanical support state that more than mild aortic insufficiency should prompt consideration for surgical intervention during device implantation. In the operating room, we assess the degree of aortic insufficiency preoperatively, then at intervals following institution of cardiopulmonary bypass, and finally during LVAD support. During each interval, aortic insufficiency can become increasingly more prominent. Initial echoes examining patients for aortic insufficiency may fail to demonstrate a significant regurgitant leak because of high end-diastolic pressures and low aortic diastolic pressures and the consequent low gradient jet. Cardiopulmonary bypass will reduce the left ventricular end-diastolic pressure significantly and increase the jet. With a functioning left ventricular assist device in place, aortic flows generally increase, and end-diastolic pressures decrease, making the gradient even more visible on an echo.

Any leak more than trace for us with the current technology prompts us to repair the valve. As seen in the table above, the incidence of aortic insufficiency at 12 months in LVAD patients ranges between 25 and 70% (Fig. 33.5). Although this is often not clinically significant, especially in the bridge to transplant population, these estimates are over a relatively short period

Fig. 33.5 Incidence of aortic insufficiency during LVAD support (Note: W. Dembitsky 2016)

author	Incidence %	population	Time interval	Risk factors
Soleimani	32	66 H MII Heart-Ware	12 mo	DT status Age >1 yr support
Toda	38	47	12 mo	Preop MR Less AoV opening
Pak	25	130 H M I II	12 mo	CF Pump Preop Ao root dil Less AoV opening
Hatano	70	37 CF & PF	2-18 mo	CF devices Lower EF Less AoV opening
Cowger	51	13 CF & PF	12-18 mo	AoV opening, Ao diameter, lower lv volumes

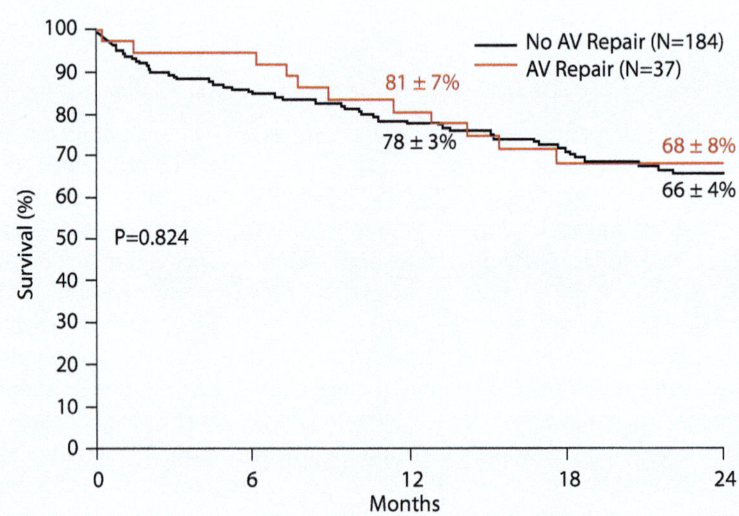

Fig. 33.6 Survival post-LVAD +/− aortic valve repair (Note: W. Dembitsky 2016)

of time. Aortic insufficiency tends to be progressive and is usually associated with older patients who have a natural tendency to develop valvular insufficiency over time.

Other risk factors are LVAD support for over 1 year, less aortic valve opening, preoperative aortic root dilatation, increased aortic diameters, and DT status [18]. Some have shown a potential advantage of pulsatility which occurs with left ventricular reverse remodeling which permits intermittent opening of the aortic valve [19]. Despite the fact that periodic aortic valve opening appears to reduce the incidence of insufficiency in LVAD patients, late de novo aortic insufficiency is known to have occurred (unsure incidence) in patients supported by the Jarvik 2000 FlowMaker device which allows opening of the native valve for 8 s every 64 s. The decision to repair or close an aortic valve should be made at the time of LVAD implantation, as severe AI may lead to heart failure and is not likely to be corrected without repeat surgery. Catheter interventions to correct late acquired aortic insufficiency have been used successfully, but not in a predictable way [20]. Amplatz catheters have embolized, as have Sapien valves [21] and Core valves. Although aortic insufficiency might be eliminated, it is unknown whether the architecture on the aortic side of the device will create the long-term liability of a thrombogenic profile and their durability is

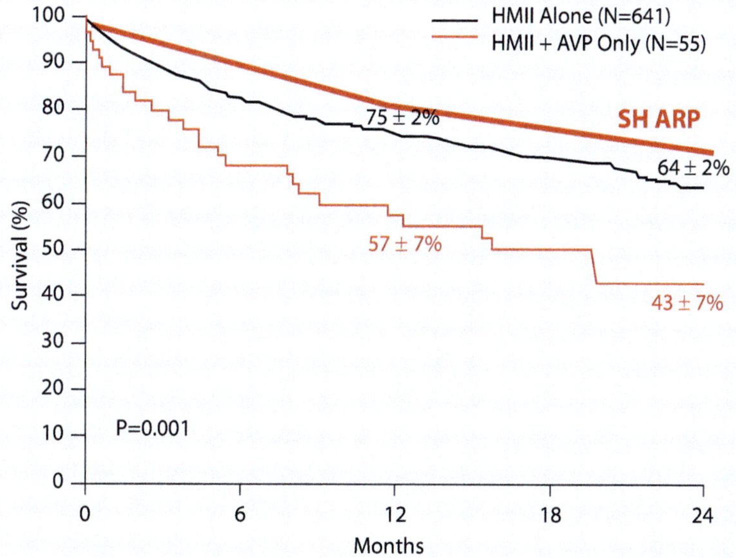

Fig. 33.7 Survival: LVAD alone versus LVAD + AVP only (Impact of concurrent surgical valve procedures in patients receiving continuous-flow devices. Ranjit et al. [5])

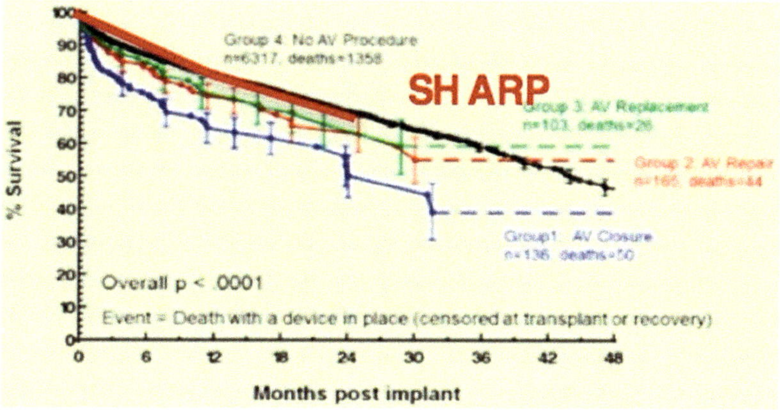

Fig. 33.8 Concomitant aortic valve procedures in patients undergoing implantation of continuous-flow LVADs. Sharp Hospital survival curve superimposed to INTERMACS database analysis (Note: W. Dembitsky 2016)

unknown in this situation. In our own examination of 221 patients with 17% aortic closure rate, there is no difference in early mortality between the groups and the survival of the two (closure and non-closure groups) (Figs. 33.6 and 33.7).

This is in contrast to the papers by John Robinson who used the INTERMACS database to illustrate a higher mortality in the AV closure group compared to repair and replacement. It is noteworthy that the observed mortality is in the early perioperative period, which brings management styles into question. Our own survival curve is superimposed over the no AV procedure with no early liability (Fig. 33.8).

A variety of aortic valve closure techniques have been used over time. Initial closure of the aortic valve leaflets at the nodule of Aranzio was used occasionally with some success, but was abandoned in the early days because of the periodic ejection of the heart, which would cause the valve to tear. The technique was modified by Soon Park who has had success using central closure with felt stitches with the intent of maintaining an outflow option for the ventricle in cases of LVAD failure. The procedure is especially recommended for patients expected to be supported for long periods of time, and based on Fukahara's [22] findings, consideration of CAVC as a prophylactic repair in DT, elderly, and female patients may be appropriate, even if they have mild-degree native AI with no increase in early mortality but with a possible late failure rate of 8% in a small series. Central stitches with felt can create a fibrous reaction which ultimately may seal the valve aperture, thereby eliminating the ventricular escape aperture.

This was further modified by Morgan [7] using multiple sutures. We have personally observed recurrent aortic insufficiency peripheral to the central closure following a "Park" stitch placed in a patient with a HeartMate I device. We subsequently successfully closed the valve surgically using our own evolved technique, described by Adamson [23], which incorporates three felt strips rather than individual pledges to expedite closure of the valve, as seen in the figure below (◘ Fig. 33.9).

Native aortic valve closure seen at 1 year shows a bio-friendly ventricular side of the closure and a well-healed, although pathologically irregular, aortic side (◘ Fig. 33.10). Previously placed aortic valve prostheses present a special condition. Unattended mechanical aortic prostheses in chronic LVAD patients have been reported. However, the often reduced flow across these devices is below the range they were intended to encounter. Critical washing, necessary to prevent thrombus formation on these valves, does not occur. Furthermore, the biomaterial interface is designed to be non-thrombogenic and therefore is no apt to be endothelialized, but more likely to be a source of constant thrombus generation [24]. For these reasons, we have used a modification of the technique originally described by Cohn [25] in patients with both bi-leaflet and mono-leaflet valves, using felt wafers above and below to assure their closure and subsequent sequestration by a firm, adherent biological cover. We no

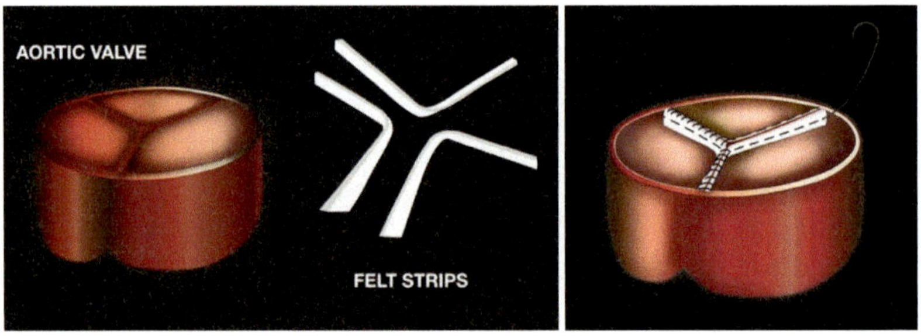

◘ **Fig. 33.9** Native aortic valve closure technique (Note: evolved technique, described by Adamson, which incorporates three felt strips rather than individual pledges to expedite closure of the valve, as seen in the figure below)

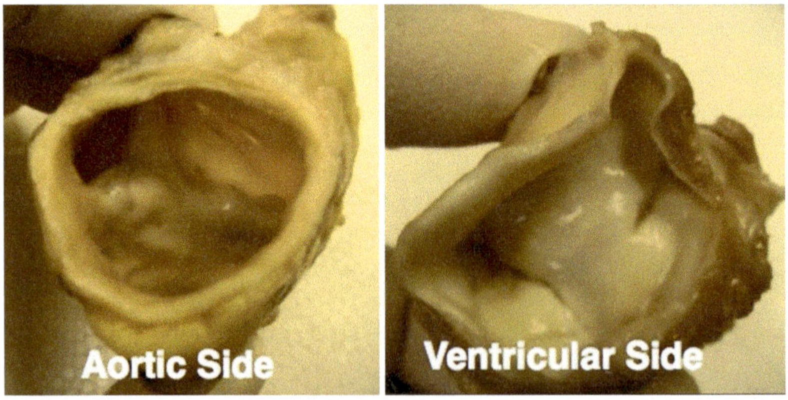

◘ **Fig. 33.10** Native aortic valve closure seen at 1 year (From Aortic valve closure associated with HeartMate left ventricular device support: technical consideration and long-term results. Adamson et al. [23])

longer use bioprosthetic valves to close the outflow trace, since they almost uniformly become occluded by tissue ingrowth from the ventricular side and they, like the native valve, can become insufficient.

33.5 Tricuspid Valve

Tricuspid regurgitation (TR) is common in patients with congestive heart failure and is usually due to annular enlargement caused by chronic pulmonary hypertension and the resultant right ventricular dilation. Continuous-flow LVADs can paradoxically exacerbate TR by restricting mobility of the septal leaflet and distorting the tricuspid annulus. However, chronically LVAD implantation usually results in left and right ventricular unloading and a consequent reduction in TV regurgitation [26].

The complex nature of the immediate postoperative clinical milieu creates a perfect storm for right heart failure with the continuously shifting fluid balances created by unstable cardiac outputs, transfusions, and varying reabsorption of chronically retained fluids. This is complicated by compromised perioperative myocardial function made worse, in the case of the right ventricle, by systemic arterial hypotension and venous hypertension, which are all added to the variably elevated right heart afterload.

In the early postoperative period, these factors often lead to RV overload, aggravation of TR, and subsequent RV failure. For these reasons, a competent tricuspid valve is most important in the early postoperative period. Subsequently, persistent or progressive TR is detrimental to the long-term outcome in other subsets of patients receiving other cardiac operations [27, 28]. It is reasonable to assume that tricuspid insufficiency is a likely culprit in the genesis of late right heart failure in 20% of LVAD recipients [2]. In the majority of patients, severe TR is functional and secondary to a left-sided pathology. Tricuspid leaflet anatomy is usually normal but leaflets are tethered, and the annulus is dilated by the enlarged right ventricle. These valves can usually be made competent using standard repair techniques [29].

Many patients undergoing LVAD implantation often have pacemaker or defibrillator leads traversing the tricuspid valve. Successful freeing of the lead from the septal lealet and fixation at the commissure to prevent re-entrapement with an annuloplasty has been successful. But these patients may have subvalvular chordal fusion, with leaflet perforations, which restricts motion and may require valve replacement rather than repair (◘ Fig. 33.11) [30].

Some published data indicates that, in case of LVAD implantation, the concomitant TV repair (TVR) has no additional benefit regarding clinical outcome. Robertson [31] retrospectively reviewed the STS database, between 2006 and 2012 containing 2196 patients with moderate-to-severe preoperative TR from 115 institutions, all of whom

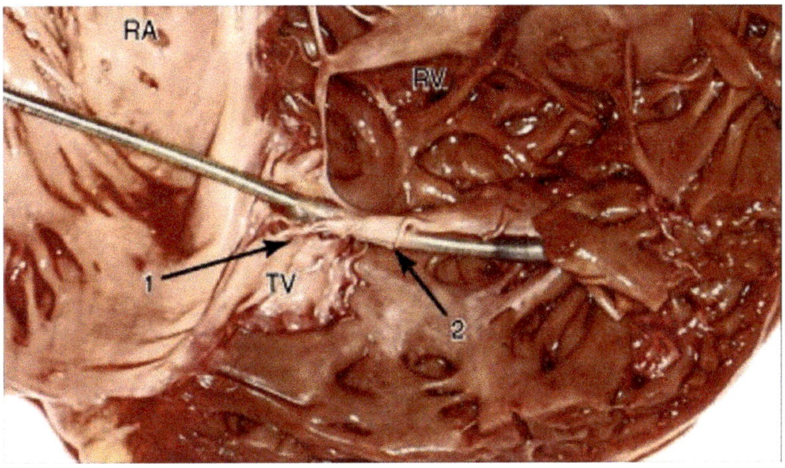

◘ **Fig. 33.11** Tricuspid leaflet entrapment (Note: W. Dembitsky 2016)

underwent implantation of a continuous-flow left ventricular assist device (LVAD) as reported by the Society of Thoracic Surgeons National Database. Of these, 588 (27%) underwent a concomitant TVP. Performing a concomitant TVP for continuous-flow LVAD patients with moderate-to-severe TR did not reduce early death or right VAD requirement and was in fact associated with worse early postoperative outcomes. The data cautions against routine concomitant TVP based solely on the degree of preoperative TR and suggests that additional selection criteria are needed to identify those patients in whom concomitant TVP may prevent postoperative right ventricular failure. Unfortunately, this analysis suffers from the liability of multi-institutional data with the widely known inter-institutional outcome variations [32].

However, other single-center reports consider TVR a reliable surgical option and suggest that TVR is able to reduce the incidence of postoperative right heart failure [33–37].

Their experience suggests that TVR reduces the volume overload of the right ventricle and results in better right heart function. Overall data on clinical outcomes concerning LVAD implants with or without concomitant TVR are inconclusive at present. In an attempt to clarify the issue, Oezpeker [38] reviewed their experience using right ventricular geometric propensity matching to predict outcomes. He analyzed 64 out of 345 LVAD recipients that had preoperative tricuspid regurgitation of over two plus or more and found that for them, end-stage heart failure LVAD patients with TV regurgitation grade greater than two did not benefit from concomitant TVR. They appropriately felt that their results are needed to be confirmed by prospective studies. Many centers feel that concomitant tricuspid valve surgery at the time of LVAD implant can be performed without any additional morbidity in the early postoperative period. The goal of concomitant tricuspid valve surgery should be to attain a competent tricuspid valve. This clearly leads to a significant fall in right-sided pressures with associated reduction in venous hypertension in the early postoperative period [32, 33]. Multiple techniques for eliminating tricuspid regurgitation at the time of LVAD implantation can be used. When leaflet integrity is unimpaired, a standard ring annuloplasty is preferred, although De Vega annuloplasty has been used with good short-term results in LVAD recipients [39]. However, in the general cardiac population, suture annuloplasty rather than a ring has been found to be a predictor of late recurrence of TR in patients with a functional TR [29]. In patients with destroyed leaflets, we and others have replaced the tricuspid valve using a tissue prosthesis inserted over the offending trans-valvular wires with good results [40]. Wires can also be transferred to the epicardium during the implantation procedure or later removed using laser techniques, in cases of infection. We have encountered one case of late tricuspid prosthetic stenosis which can be rectified using percutaneous valve technology.

33.6 Miscellaneous Procedures Performed During LVAD Insertion

The distorted intraventricular and intra-atrial flow architectures during continuous-flow LVAD can be prothrombotic [11], so minimizing the late stasis risk during the initial LVAD implantation is prudent. In patients with atrial fibrillation, the atrial appendage should be either occluded or amputated. We currently address the appendage in all LVAD recipient regardless of the presence of atrial fibrillation. We have also performed "cox-maze" procedures in some patients in hopes of maintaining long-term right ventricular functional integrity. Coronary artery bypass is performed to prevent postoperative angina, to minimize the genesis of ventricular arrhythmias, and to enhance right ventricular performance. In patients with monomorphic ventricular tachycardia, standard ablation techniques can be best easily applied thru the apical ventricular cannula access site. Ascending aortic pathologies require special attention to minimize systemic embolization. Patients requiring removal of atheroma or patients having complex aortic pathology such as aortic aneurysm, dissection, or previously placed grafts are treated using hypothermic circulatory arrest.

33.7 Concomitant Conclusions

The question of when is too much during LVAD implantation is dependent upon what the implanting surgical team and LVAD recipient expect. If the certain goal is short-term support and transplantation is an option, compromises in correcting native heart abnormalities (which can present long-term liabilities) are more attractive. Since cardiac transplantation or weaning from a device cannot be certain, it seems prudent to err on the side of correcting the maladies discussed above. Clinical decisions based on big data set analyses are subject to the errors infused by the wide variability of center-specific results. Big data conclusions are useful guides, but do not define excellence. Instead, they describe a median value, which in the current field of biomechanical support, must be considered to be mediocre.

References

1. Rose EA et al (2001) Long-term use of a left ventricular assist device for end-stage heart failure. N Engl J Med 345(20):1435–1443
2. Adamson RM, Mangi AA, Kormos RL, Farrar DJ, Dembitsky WP (2015) Principals of HeartMate II implantation to avoid pump malposition and migration. J Card Surg 30(3):296–299
3. Adamson RM, Bower BL, Sundareswaran KS, Farrar DJ, Dembitsky WP (2015) Radiologic assessment of HeartMate II position, minimal migration after long term support. J Heart Lung Transplant 34(12):1617–1623
4. Adamson RM, Limmer KK, Dembitsky WP, Mehta H, Jaski B, Hoagland P (2015) Single center, 23 year experience with PFO management during HeartMate LVAD implants. The Journal of Heart and Lung Transplantation. Presented at the ISHLT meeting in Nice, Apr 2015
5. Ranjit J, Naka Y, Park SJ, Sai-Sudhakar C, Salerno C, Sundareswaran KS, Farrar DJ, Milano CA (2014) Impact of concurrent surgical valve procedures in patients receiving continuous-flow devices. J Thorac Cardiovasc Surg 147(2):581–589
6. Patel JB, Borgeson DD, Barnes ME, Rihal CS, Daly RC, Redeld MM (2004) Mitral regurgitation in patients with advanced systolic heart failure. J Card Fail 10(4):285–291
7. Morgan JA, Brewer RJ, Nemeh HW, Murthy R, Williams CT, Lanfear DE, Tita C, Paone G (2012) Left ventricular reverse remodeling with a continuous flow left ventricular assist device measured by left ventricular end-diastolic dimensions and severity of mitral regurgitation. Am Soc Artif Int Organs 58(6):574–577
8. Wang TS, Hernandez AF, Felker GM, Milano CA, Rogers JG, Patel CB (2014) Valvular heart disease in patients supported with left ventricular assist devices. Circ Heart Fail 7(1):215–222
9. Stulak JM, Tchantchaleishvili V, Haglund NA, Davis ME, Schirger JA, Cowger JA, Shah P, Aaronson KD, Pagani FD, Maltais S (2015) Uncorrected pre-operative mitral valve regurgitation is not associated with adverse outcomes after continuous-flow left ventricular assist device implantation. J Heart Lung Transplant 34(5):718–723
10. Taghavi S, Hamad E, Wilson L, Clark R, Jayarajan SN, Uriel N, Goldstein DJ, Takayama H, Naka Y, Mangi AA (2013) Mitral valve repair at the time of continuous-flow left ventricular assist device implantation confers meaningful decrement in pulmonary vascular resistance. Am Soc Artif Int Organs 59(5):469–473
11. May-Newman K, Fisher B, Hara M, Dembitsky W, Adamson R (2016) The effect of mitral valve regurgitation on the hemodynamics of the LVAD-assisted heart. Manuscript submitted for publication
12. Russo MJ, Merlo A, Johnson EM, Akhter S, McCarney S, Steiman J, Anderson A, Jeevanandam V (2013) Transapical approach for mitral valve repair during insertion of a left ventricular assist device. Sci World J 2013(925310):4
13. Mohite PN, Zych B, Popov AF, Patil N, Luthra S, Hedger M, Simon AR, Amrani M (2013) Mitral commissurotomy through the left ventricle apical orifice with heart ware left ventricular assist device implantation. J Cardiothorac Surg 8(8):147
14. Schweiger M, Stepanenko A, Vierecke J, Drews T, Potapov E, Hetzer R, Krabatsch T (2012) Preexisting mitral valve prosthesis in patients undergoing left ventricular assist device implantation. Artif Organs 36(1):49–53
15. Yoon AJ, Sohn J, Grazette L, Fong MW, Bowdish ME (2015) Pan-cardiac cycle fixed mitral valve opening in an LVAD patient presenting with hemorrhagic shock (doi: 10.1111/echo.13150). Hoboken, NJ: Echocardiography. Retrieved from http://onlinelibrary.wiley.com/doi/10.1111/echo.13150/pdf
16. Krishan K, Pinney S, Anyanwu AC (2010) Successful use of continuous flow ventricular assist device in a patient with mechanical mitral and aortic valve prosthesis without replacement or exclusion of valves. Interact Cardiovasc Thorac Surg 10(2):325–327
17. Adamson RM, Dembitsky WP, Jaski BJ, Daily PO, Moreno-Cabral RJ, Kim JC, Sono J, Akasaka T, Hoagland PM, Gordon JB (1997) Left ventricular assist device support of medically unresponsive pulmonary hypertension and aortic insufficiency. ASAIO J 43(4): 365–369
18. Deo SV, Sharma V, Cho YH, Shah IK, Park SJ (2014) De novo aortic insufficiency during long-term support on a left ventricular assist device: a systematic review and meta-analysis. Am Soc Artif Int Organs 60(2):183–188
19. Imamura T, Kinugawa K, Nitta D, Hatano M, Kinoshita O, Nawata K, Ono M (2015) Advantage of pulsatility in left ventricular reverse remodeling and aortic insufficiency prevention during left ventricular assist device treatment. Circ J 79(9):1994–1994
20. Grohmann J, Blanke P, Benk C, Schlensak C (2011) Trans-catheter closure of the native aortic valve with an amplatzer occluder to treat progressive aortic regurgitation after implantation of a left-ventricular assist device. Eur J Cardiothorac Surg 39(6):181–183
21. Kornberger A, Beiras-Fernandez A, Fichtlscherer S, Assmus B, Moritz A, Stock UA (2015) Percutaneous SAPIEN S3 transcatheter valve implantation for post-left ventricular assist device aortic regurgitation. Ann Thorac Surg 100(4):67–69

22. Fukuhara S, Takeda K, Chiuzan C, Han J, Polanco AR, Yuzefpolskaya M, Mancini DM, Colombo PC, Topkara VK, Kurlansky PA, Takayama H, Naka Y (2016) Concomitant aortic valve repair with continuous-flow left ventricular assist devices: results and implications. J Thorac Cardiovasc Surg 151(1):201–210
23. Adamson RM, Dembitsky WP, Baradarian S, Chammas J, May-Newman K, Chillcott S, Stahovich M, McCalmont V, Ortiz K, Hoagland P, Jaski B (2011) Aortic valve closure associated with HeartMate left ventricular device support: technical considerations and long-term results. J Heart Lung Transplant 30(5):576–582
24. Tanawuttiwat T, Zelinger AB, Trivedi DA, Tatooles AJ (2011) Massive aortic thrombus in patient with mechanical prosthetic valve supported with left ventricular assist device. J Cardiovasc Comput Tomogr 5(1):66–67
25. Cohn WE, Demirozu ZT, Frazier OH (2011) Surgical closure of left ventricular outflow tract after left ventricular assist device implantation in patients with aortic valve pathology. J Heart Lung Transplant 30(1):59–63
26. MacGowan GA, Schueler S (2012) Right heart failure after left ventricular assist device implantation: early and late. Curr Opin Card 27(3):296–300
27. Nath J, Foster E, Heidenreich PA (2004) Impact of tricuspid regurgitation on long-term survival. J Am Coll Card 43(3):405–409
28. Anyanwu AC, Chikwe J, Adams DH (2008) Tricuspid valve repair for treatment and prevention of secondary tricuspid regurgitation in patients undergoing mitral valve surgery. Curr Card Rep 10(2):110–117
29. Pinney SP (2012) The role of tricuspid valve repair and re- placement in right heart failure. Curr Opin Cardiol 27(3):288–295
30. Al-Mohaissen MA, Chan KL (2012) Prevalence and mechanism of tricuspid regurgitation following implantation of endocardial leads for pacemaker or cardioverter-defibrillator. J Am Soc Echocardiography 25(3):245–252
31. Robertson JO, Grau-Sepulveda MV, Okada S, O'Brien SM, Matthew Brennan J, Shah AS, Itoh A, Damiano RJ, Prasad S, Silvestry SC (2014) Concomitant tricuspid valve surgery during implantation of continuous-flow left ventricular assist devices: a Society of Thoracic Surgeons database analysis. J Heart Lung Transplant 33(6):609–617
32. Saeed D, Kidambi T, Shalli S, Lapin B, Malaisrie SC, Lee R, Cotts WG, McGee EC Jr (2011) Tricuspid valve repair with left ventricular assist device implantation: is it warranted? J Heart Lung Transplant 30(5):530–535
33. Deo SV, Hasin T, Altarabsheh SE, McKellar SH, Shah IK, Durham L 3rd, Stulak JM, Daly RC, Park SJ, Joyce LD (2012) Concomitant tricuspid valve repair or replacement during left ventricular assist device implant demonstrates comparable outcomes in the long term. J Card Surg 27(6):760–766
34. Piacentino V 3rd, Troupes CD, Ganapathi AM, Blue LJ, Mackensen GB, Swaminathan M, Felker GM, Stafford-Smith M, Lodge AJ, Rogers JG, Milano CA (2011) Clinical impact of concomitant tricuspid valve procedures during left ventricular assist device implantation. Ann Thorac Surg 92(4):1414–1418
35. Krishan K, Nair A, Pinney S, Adams DH, Anyanwu AC (2012) Liberal use of tricuspid-valve annuloplasty during left-ventricular assist device implantation. Eur J Cardiothorac Surg 41(1):213–217
36. Piacentino V 3rd, Williams ML, Depp T, Garcia-Huerta K, Blue L, Lodge AJ, Mackensen GB, Swaminathan M, Rogers JG, Milano CA (2011) Impact of tricuspid valve regurgitation in patients treated with implantable left ventricular assist devices. Ann Thorac Surg 91(5):1342–1346
37. Fujita T, Kobayashi J, Hata H, Seguchi O, Murata Y, Yanase M, Nakatani T (2014) Right heart failure and benefits of adjuvant tricuspid valve repair in patients undergoing left ventricular assist device implantation. Eur J Cardiothorac Surg 46(5):802–807
38. Oezpeker C, Zittermann A, Paluszkiewicz L, Piran M, Puehler T, Sayin AO, Ensminger S, Milting H, Morshuis M, Gummert JF (2015) Tricuspid valve repair in patients with left-ventricular assist device implants and tricuspid valve regurgitation: propensity score-adjusted analysis of clinical outcome. Interact Cardiovasc Thorac Surg 21(6):741–747
39. Akhter SA, Salabat MR, Philip JL, Valeroso TB, Russo MJ, Rich JD, Jeevanandam V (2014) Durability of De Vega tricuspid valve annuloplasty for severe tricuspid regurgitation during left ventricular assist device implantation. Ann Thorac Surg 98(1):81–83
40. Adamson RM, Dembitsky WP, Chammas J, Baradarian S, Hoagland B, Jaski B, Stahovich M, Chillcott S, Ortiz K, McCalmont V (2009) Tricuspid valve replacement coincident with HeartMate LVAD insertion. J Heart Lung Transplant, Presented at the ISHLT meeting in Paris, FR. February 2009

Pump Removal After Myocardial Recovery During Left Ventricular Assist Device Support

E. Potapov, M. Kukucka, and T. Krabatsch

© Springer International Publishing Switzerland 2017
A. Montalto et al. (eds.), *Mechanical Circulatory Support in End-Stage Heart Failure*,
DOI 10.1007/978-3-319-43383-7_34

Myocardial recovery occurs in up to 5–10% of patients supported with continuous-flow left ventricular assist devices (LVAD). Most experience has been gained in patients with dilative cardiomyopathy and acute myocarditis. Predictors of recovery are younger age and short duration of the disease [1].

Myocardial recovery is not likely to occur in patients with ischemic cardiomyopathy; therefore, close attention should be paid to patients with dilative cardiomyopathy of different etiology – myocarditis or postpartum. Unfortunately, only few cases of myocardial recovery in patients suffering from toxic cardiomyopathy (mostly after chemotherapy) have been reported. Our limited experience shows recurrence of heart failure and dilatation of the left ventricle months after LVAD removal in patients with toxic cardiomyopathy. Therefore, we do not reccomed scheduled LVAD removal in such patients. However, in the case of LVAD-associated complications LVAD removal may be justified. Myocardial recovery should be monitored during outpatient visits. First, echocardiography on pump should be performed. If echocardiography shows normal size of the left ventricle with satisfactory contractility, echocardiography at reduced pump speed and then an off-pump study should be scheduled during outpatient visits. We do not recommend special "training" of the left ventricle by reducing the speed. However, in the case of suction events due to LV ejection, the speed should be reduced. After myocardial recovery has been demonstrated in off-pump studies, the patient should be admitted to the hospital for pump-stop studies with outflow graft occlusion, to eliminate the backflow through the pump. After the oral anticoagulation has been switched to intravenous, the patient is transferred into the catheter laboratory. The occlusion balloon (10 mm for HeartWare HVAD [HeartWare International Inc., Framingham, MA], 16 mm for HeartMate 2 [Thoratec Corp., Pleasanton, CA], and 14 mm for HeartMate 3) should be placed retrogradely into the outflow graft. Additionally, a Swan-Ganz catheter is placed and echocardiography is also set up. After an anticoagulation bolus, the balloon is inflated for 3–4 min and the pump stopped. During this period, serial measurements of cardiac output, arterial and pulmonary artery blood pressures, wedge pressure, and blood mixed venous saturation should be taken. The balloon should be deflated after 3–4 min and the pump started for 10–20 s, and then the procedure may be repeated 3–5 times, to obtain stable results of all measurements.

The criteria for sustained myocardial recovery in patients with dilative cardiomyopathy have been meticulously described by Dandel [1]. Briefly these criteria are sinus rhythm, absence of significant valve pathology, and normal function and geometry of both the left and right side of the heart together with stable systemic and pulmonary hemodynamics and mixed venous saturation during pump stop with balloon occlusion of the outflow graft [2].

After the VAD team determines that existing myocardial recovery is likely to be sustained for a longer time, in the next step, the strategy for withdrawal of ventricular support should be discussed. There are several options:

1. Complete removal of the LVAD, including the pump, fixation ring, outflow graft, and driveline through a redo median sternotomy or left lateral thoracotomy, depending on the primary approach during LVAD implantation. This option requires oversewing of the apex of the left ventricle and of the prosthetic anastomosis to the ascending or descending aorta. In the case of anastomosis to the ascending aorta median sternotomy and in the case of anastomosis to the descending aorta left lateral thoracotomy is necessary as a redo procedure. Because of the oversewing of the apex, the cardiopulmonary bypass (CPB) must be employed. For safety reasons, the CPB should, if possible, be installed through peripheral vessels, mostly in the groin.
2. Partial removal of the LVAD, with the pump and complete driveline being retrieved. Because of the oversewing of the apex, this approach also requires the cardiopulmonary bypass (CPB), installed, if possible, through peripheral vessels, mostly in the groin. In this case a minimally invasive approach is used, through a small incision above the pump in the sixth intercostal space for the HeartMate III, HeartWare HVAD or MVAD and through a subcostal incision with partial dissection of the margo cartilage of the rib cage for the HeartMate II or HeartAssist5 (ReliantHeart Inc., Houston, TX).
3. In the case of HeartMate II, the pump body and the driveline can be removed, with the inflow and outflow grafts ligated and the inflow cannula left in situ. This approach allows a smaller subcostal incision, with partial

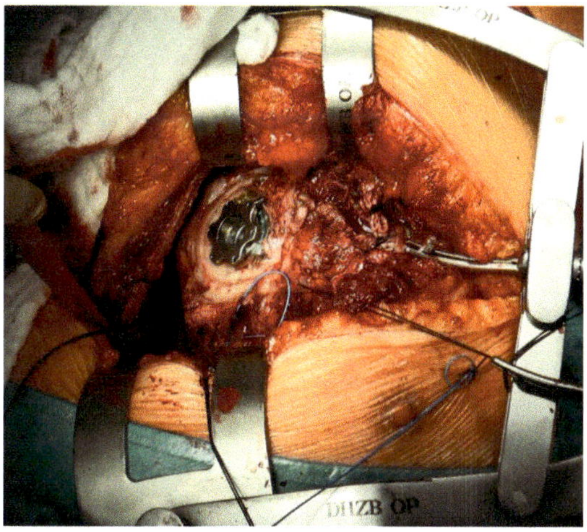

Fig. 34.1 Intraoperative view of individually designed titanium plug inserted after HeartWare HVAD explantation through left lateral thoracotomy

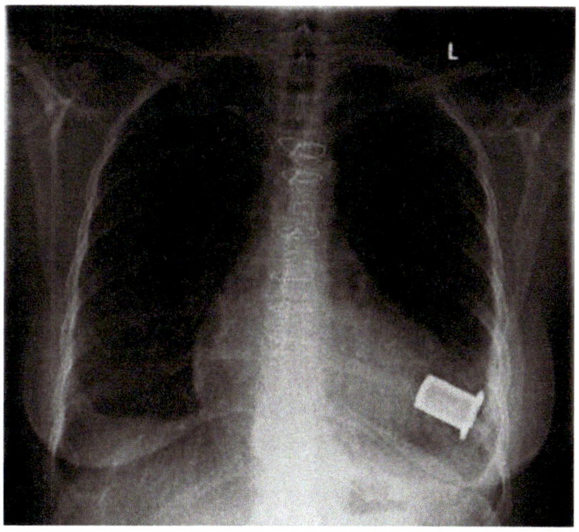

Fig. 34.2 Thoracic X-ray after removal of HeartMate II showing the titanium plug inserted into the original fixation ring "chimney"

dissection of the margo cartilage and reduced volume of dissection in areas of severe adhesion, and avoids the use of CPB [3].

4. In the case of the HeartMate II, HeartMate III and HeartWare HVAD, a specially designed titanium plug allows complete removal of the inflow cannula from the left ventricle, while the myocardium in the apical area is preserved and CPB use is avoided [4] (see Figs. 34.1 and 34.2).
5. Ligation of the outflow graft is also possible through a small subcostal incision to stop backflow, with transection of the driveline below the skin, while the outflow graft, pump, and driveline remain in situ [3].
6. Percutaneous interventional closure of the outflow graft and trannsection of the driveline below the skin.
7. Withdrawal of anticoagulation, letting the pump thrombose, and transsection of the driveline below the skin.

Table 34.1 shows the advantages and disadvantages of these approaches.

In some patients general anesthesia may lead to depression of myocardial function, which precludes removal of the pump. It is unclear whether reevaluation of the myocardial recovery some months later would be helpful. Interventional closure of the outflow graft or ligation of the outflow graft and shortening of the driveline under local anesthesia would avoid this phenomenon, but it is still unclear whether the recovery in such patients would be long lasting.

In patients supported with Heart Mate II, HeartMate III and HeartWare HVAD, we recommend partial removal employing the individually designed plug. This approach is less invasive and eliminates from the body the potentially contaminated driveline and the inflow cannula as a potential source of thrombi from the LV cavity [3]. Removal of the inflow cannula also avoids the need for life-long anticoagulation. The inserted individually designed titanium plug (Fittkau GmbH, Berlin, Germany) is sintered with titanium spheres and becomes overgrown with tissue [6], therefore requiring anticoagulation with a vitamin K antagonist for 6 months only. If heart failure recurs and an LVAD is needed for the second time, the fixation ring may be reused after removal of the plug [7]. The now commercially available HeartMate III has unfortunately been released on the market without the company supplying its own plug. Therefore Fittkau GmbH is designing a plug suitable for HeartMate III. The HeartWare MVAD is currently still under investigation but will be brought on to the market with a titanium plug included in the kit on request.

In all cases except ligation or interventional closure of the outflow graft, we recommend complete removal of the driveline because of the potential risk of infection [3].

In a small series of 27 HeartMate II deactivations, all methods were feasible and were found to produce similar early and late survival and clinical outcomes [3].

Table 34.1 Advantages and disadvantages of approaches to LVAD removal

Approach	Advantage	Disadvantage	Indication
1. Complete removal	No foreign material remains in the body	Redo surgery, use of CPB, risk of damage or bleeding	Infected LVAD
2. Partial removal without plug	Less invasive approach, reduced risk of damage and bleeding	Use of CPB, outflow graft remains in the body	Non-infected LVAD, type Incor, HeartAssist5, Jarvik 2000
3. Partial removal of HeartMate II pump	Less invasive approach, no need for CPB, low risk of damage and bleeding	Outflow graft remains in the body. Inflow cannula remains in the cavum of the LV. Life-long anticoagulation	For HeartMate II only
4. Partial removal employing specially designed plug	Less invasive approach, no need for CPB, minimal risk of damage and bleeding. Possible reuse of the apical ring if 2nd pump becomes necessary	Outflow graft remains in the body	Non-infected LVAD, type HeartWare HVAD and HeartMate II
5. Ligation of the outflow graft	Minimally invasive approach, no need for CPB, minimal risk of damage and bleeding	Driveline remains in the body. Inflow cannula remains in the cavum of the LV. Life-long anticoagulation	Patients with high risk for major surgery
6. Percutaneous interventional closure of the outflow graft [5]	No risk of damage or bleeding	Driveline remains in the body. Inflow cannula remains in the cavum of the LV. Life-long anticoagulation	Patients with high risk for major surgery

Manufacturers: Berlin Heart INCOR (Berlin Heart GmbH, Berlin, Germany); Jarvik 2000 (Jarvik Heart Inc., New York, NY)

References

1. Dandel M, Weng Y, Siniawski H, Stepanenko A, Krabatsch T, Potapov E et al (2011) Heart failure reversal by ventricular unloading in patients with chronic cardiomyopathy: criteria for weaning from ventricular assist devices. Eur Heart J 32(9):1148–1160
2. Potapov EV, Schweiger M, Krabatsch T (2011) Percutaneous balloon occlusion of a left ventricular assist device outflow cannula to facilitate evaluation of myocardial recovery. J Heart Lung Transplant 30(11):1300–1301
3. Baldwin AC, Sandoval E, Letsou GV, Mallidi HR, Cohn WE, Frazier OH (2016) Surgical approach to continuous-flow left ventricular assist device explantation: a comparison of outcomes. J Thorac Cardiovasc Surg 151(1):192–198
4. Potapov EV, Stepanenko A, Hennig E, Hetzer R, Krabatsch T (2010) A titanium plug simplifies left ventricular assist device removal after myocardial recovery. J Heart Lung Transplant 29(11):1316–1317
5. Pettit SJ, Shapiro LM, Lewis C, Parameshwar JK, Tsui SS (2015) Percutaneous withdrawal of HeartWare HVAD left ventricular assist device support. J Heart Lung Transplant 34(7):990–992
6. Potapov EV, Huebler M, Morawietz L, Hetzer R (2011) Connective tissue overgrowth on a titanium plug inserted to facilitate left ventricular assist device explantation. J Heart Lung Transplant 30(2):235–236
7. Saito T, Potapov E, Dandel M, Hetzer R, Krabatsch T (2014) Reimplantation of left ventricular assist device late after weaning of device using a titanium plug. J Heart Lung Transplant 33(9):972–974

MCS in Pediatric Population

Contents

Mechanical Circulatory Support in Pediatric Population: Clinical Considerations, Indications, Strategies, and Postoperative Management

O. Miera, F. Berger, and K.R. Schmitt

© Springer International Publishing Switzerland 2017
A. Montalto et al. (eds.), *Mechanical Circulatory Support in End-Stage Heart Failure*,
DOI 10.1007/978-3-319-43383-7_35

The main etiologies leading to end-stage heart failure requiring mechanical support in children are dilated cardiomyopathy, myocarditis, and congenital heart disease. Since end-stage heart failure is rather uncommon in the pediatric population, very few randomized controlled trials have been conducted due to the small number of patients available. Therapeutic guidelines are mainly derived from large adult terminal heart failure studies [1]. Regardless of the underlying etiology, terminal heart failure may present acutely as cardiac arrest or cardiogenic shock or more prolonged in a child with signs of low cardiac output in spite of maximal medical therapy. With failure of the medical therapy, the question arises if mechanical support can/should be applied to save the patient's life. The clinician has to assess whether short support can be expected to be sufficient or if long-term support is likely needed, if an oxygenator is required, and if only left ventricular support is adequate, or if mechanical support for both ventricles is necessary.

Extracorporeal life support (ECLS, venoarterial extracorporeal membrane oxygenation) is generally accepted as the preferred mode of circulatory support for the first few days to weeks in children presenting with hyperacute heart failure, especially after cardiac surgery, and in children with unknown etiology of the heart failure. However, during the child's treatment, the clinician may be confronted with the question if the child is a candidate for ventricular assist device (VAD) support either primarily or after ECLS.

35.1 Indication and Timing

Exact timing of intervention is a clinical challenge: early VAD implantation improves outcome, but at the same time poses a risk for adverse events. Waiting too long before VAD implantation means undue stress on secondary organs and on the right ventricle. As a consequence, the probability of biventricular support or even ECLS may increase [2]. Generally accepted indications are critical cardiogenic shock and progressive decline despite inotropic support. The most challenging clinical presentation is a child who is hemodynamically stable but inotrope dependent. The patient's condition must frequently be reevaluated for signs of secondary organ failure. Signs indicating the need for VAD support can be application of mechanical ventilation, escalation of inotropic support, inability to tolerate enteral feeds, rise of liver function tests, increase in creatinine levels, altered mental status, low central venous saturation (<60%), or elevated lactate [3].

35.2 Preoperative Considerations

A meticulous evaluation before implantation of a VAD is a prerequisite for improving outcome and reducing morbidity, as dictated by the following steps:

1. Definition of the underlying pathology and exclusion of any residual defect or coronary injury in children with congenital heart disease. In patients with cardiomyopathy or suspected myocarditis, an endomyocardial biopsy should be obtained, at the latest before implantation of the VAD, to better evaluate a potential for recovery.
2. Assess organ function with a focus on the kidneys, liver, coagulation system, central nervous system, and lungs.
3. Rule out any contraindications to VAD therapy such as lung failure, severe neurological injury, severe liver failure, bleeding tendency, or inborn error of metabolism. Since heart transplantation may become necessary, contraindications for transplantation must be considered.
4. Informed consent of parents or legal guardians and if suitable of the patient. Obtaining consent is time consuming but extremely important in establishing a trustful patient-physician relationship. Issues to be addressed should not only include the immediate postoperative course but also long-term prognosis, everyday life on VAD that can persists for many months to more than a year and, finally, the possibility and consequences of heart transplantation.
5. An echocardiographic evaluation should be performed before implantation to define whether the intra-atrial septum is intact or the aortic and pulmonary valves are competent. An intracardial thrombus must be ruled out. Additionally, the right ventricular function is of special concern in patients scheduled for LVAD implantation, and evaluation of the size of cardiac chambers is important for selection of cannulas.

6. The extent of pulmonary vascular disease has to be determined. Pulmonary hypertension secondary to left ventricular diseases is not necessarily a contraindication to LVAD alone, as the pulmonary pressure can drop substantially with unloading of the left ventricle. However, the need for right ventricular support becomes more likely with pronounced elevation of pulmonary vascular resistance. VADs in patients with idiopathic or hereditary pulmonary hypertension cannot be recommended [4].
7. Define a strategy. Short-term support may be suitable for diseases with a high probability of recovery, such as coronary anomalies after surgical correction, myocarditis, or graft rejection. If the need for long-term support is likely implantation of a long-term VAD, it should be the primary preference, as VAD support has been proven to be superior to ECLS in bridging children to transplantation [5]. Although the vast majority of patients needing a long-term device are candidates for heart transplantation (bridge to transplantation), recovery of myocardial function is possible (bridge to recovery). In patients with elevated pulmonary vascular resistance, left ventricular support combined with specific therapy may lower pulmonary pressures, allowing for heart transplantation alone (bridge to candidacy). Implantation of a VAD as destination therapy, i.e., without listing for heart transplantation or chance for recovery, is a rare exception in the pediatric population.
8. Selection of a suitable device. For short-term VAD support, extracorporeal centrifugal pumps are preferred. The use of EXCOR cannulas combined with a temporary centrifugal pump switched to a pulsatile device (EXCOR) in small children requiring permanent support has been previously described [6]. Long-term VAD support in small children is achieved with the Berlin Heart EXCOR pediatric device (see ◘ Fig. 35.1). For LVAD support cannulation of the ventricular apex is recommended to completely unload the ventricle, to minimize the risk of thromboembolic events, and to achieve the best possible unloading of the heart with a potential focus on myocardial recovery. Atrial cannulation may become necessary if the cardiac chamber is small, e.g., in restrictive cardiomyopathy. Children with a body surface area larger than 1–1.2 m^2 can be supported successfully with continuous-flow VADs [7]. To date these devices are not approved for right or biventricular support, which is necessary in about one third of children [8]. VADs suitable for long-term support in children are summarized in ◘ Table 35.1.

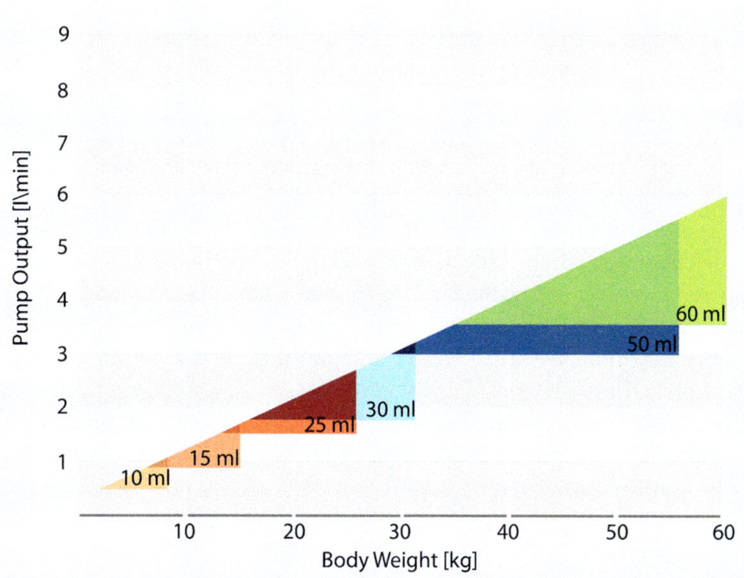

◘ **Fig. 35.1** Pump output of Berlin Heart EXCOR pediatric at common clinical use. Depending on body size and patient's needs, pump chambers of different sizes can be chosen

Table 35.1 Ventricular assist devices for long-term support in children and adolescents

Device	Manufacturer	Principle	Patient size
EXCOR pediatric	Berlin Heart	Paracorporeal pulsatile	>2.5 kg – adult
HeartMate II	Thoratec	CF, axial	>1.2 m^2 BSA
HeartMate III[a]	Thoratec	CF, centrifugal	>1.2 m^2 BSA
HVAD[a]	HeartWare	CF, centrifugal	>1 m^2 BSA
MVAD[b]	HeartWare	CF	Under investigation

CF continuous flow. The EXCOR pediatric device is the only being approved for use in children
[a]Not approved in patients <18 years
[b]MVAD: device not approved, ongoing clinical trial

9. Considerations in children with congenital heart disease. For children with congenital heart diseases, an individualized approach is mandatory. Support for children with a univentricular heart is possible at every stage of palliation (aortopulmonary shunt, superior caval vein anastomosis, and Fontan circulation) [9]. However, the prognosis is worse in patients with a univentricular physiology as compared to patients with normal heart anatomy.

35.3 Postoperative Management

Postoperative management starts in the operating room. To support the right ventricle during weaning from cardiopulmonary bypass, inhaled nitric oxide, milrinone, and epinephrine are recommended. Mechanical ventilation with normoventilation (pCO_2 35–40 mmHg) and long expiratory times are helpful to lower right ventricular afterload. Transesophageal echocardiography is used to rule out inflow obstruction of the cannula, to confirm adequate unloading of the left ventricle without septal shift, and to analyze right ventricular geometry and function. If right ventricular function is severely impaired despite maximal medical therapy and optimal left ventricular pump settings, the implantation of an RVAD is mandatory. Directly after bypass the heparin effect should be completely antagonized. Initial accurate hemostasis is necessary to minimize the need for blood products and avoid volume overload of the right ventricle. Closure of the chest allows for early extubation, and medical support of right ventricular function in the intensive care unit is crucial to avoid secondary heart failure.

A standard protocol for antithrombotic therapy has been proposed [10]. Anticoagulation is withheld during the first 24 h until bleeding has completely stopped. Antithrombotic therapy is initiated with unfractionated heparin and switched to low molecular heparin in infants or warfarin in children older than 1 year of age. Dual antiplatelet therapy is introduced during the first or second week of VAD support. Due to the substantial rate of early thromboembolic events, modifications of this protocol are used in many centers. Examples of strategies to lower the adverse event rate include earlier initiation of unfractionated heparin, higher target ranges for low molecular heparin and warfarin, higher dosages of antiplatelet drugs, and introduction of a third agent. Additionally, various efforts such as timely extubation, early removal of the central lines, early enteral feeding, and early mobilization should be made to reduce the risk for adverse events such as infections or thromboembolic events.

After the acute postoperative course, the child should be checked regularly for recovery of cardiac function. Thereby, the unloading of the left ventricle is mandatory and must be verified not only directly after cardiopulmonary bypass but also during follow-up examinations. Any evidence of incomplete unloading such as mitral valve insufficiency or increased left ventricular dimensions must prompt a careful reassessment to rule out incorrect position of the cannula, suboptimal pump settings, aortic regurgitation, or obstruction of the inflow cannula. A pump stop procedure with echocardiographic and/or invasive examinations can then be initiated after signs of ventricular recovery to identify children in whom the device can be explanted [11].

A child on support has many different needs which can only be met by an interdisciplinary team dedicated to the many different aspects of VAD therapy, including surgical, cardiologic, and technical aspects of VADs; knowledge in antithrombotic therapy; growth on assist with adequate nutrition, mobilization, and physiotherapy; special dressings to avoid infections; social issues; outpatient management; as well as pretransplantation issues.

References

1. Kirk R, Dipchand AI, Rosenthal DN (2014) The international society of heart and lung transplantation guidelines for the management of pediatric heart failure: executive summary. J Heart Lung Transplant 33:888–909
2. Karimova A, Pockett CR, Lasuen N, Dedieu N, Rutledge J, Fenton M, Vanderpluym C, Rebeyka IM, Dominguez TE, Buchholz H (2014) Right ventricular dysfunction in children supported with pulsatile ventricular assist devices. J Thorac Cardiovasc Surg 147:1691–1697 e1
3. Jaquiss RDB, Bronicki RA (2013) An overview of mechanical circulatory support in children. Pediatr Crit Care Med 14:S3–S6
4. Keogh AM, Mayer E, Benza RL, Corris P, Dartevelle PG, Frost AE, Kim NH, Lang IM, Pepke-Zaba J, Sandoval J (2009) Interventional and surgical modalities of treatment in pulmonary hypertension. J Am Coll Cardiol 54:S67–S77
5. Fraser CD Jr, Jaquiss RDB, Rosenthal DN, Humpl T, Canter CE, Blackstone EH, Naftel DC, Ichord RN, Bomgaars L, Tweddell JS, Massicotte MP, Turrentine MW, Cohen GA, Devaney EJ, Pearce FB, Carberry KE, Kroslowitz R, Almond CS (2012) Prospective trial of a pediatric ventricular assist device. N Engl J Med 367:532–541
6. Maat APWM, van Thiel RJ, Dalinghaus M, Bogers AJJC (2008) Connecting the centrimag levitronix pump to Berlin heart excor cannulae; a new approach to bridge to bridge. J Heart Lung Transplant 27:112–115
7. Miera O, Potapov EV, Redlin M, Stepanenko A, Berger F, Hetzer R, Hübler M (2011) First experiences with the HeartWare ventricular assist system in children. ATS 91:1256–1260
8. Almond CS, Morales DL, Blackstone EH, Turrentine MW, Imamura M, Massicotte MP, Jordan LC, Devaney EJ, Ravishankar C, Kanter KR, Holman W, Kroslowitz R, Tjossem C, Thuita L, Cohen GA, Buchholz H, St Louis JD, Nguyen K, Niebler RA, Walters HL, Reemtsen B, Wearden PD, Reinhartz O, Guleserian KJ, Mitchell MB, Bleiweis MS, Canter CE, Humpl T (2013) Berlin heart EXCOR pediatric ventricular assist device for bridge to heart transplantation in US children. Circulation 127:1702–1711
9. VanderPluym CJ, Rebeyka IM, Ross DB, Buchholz H (2011) The use of ventricular assist devices in pediatric patients with univentricular hearts. J Thorac Cardiovasc Surg 141:588–590
10. Fraser CD Jr, Jaquiss RDB, Rosenthal DN, Humpl T, Canter CE, Blackstone EH, Naftel DC, Ichord RN, Bomgaars L, Tweddell JS, Massicotte MP, Turrentine MW, Cohen GA, Devaney EJ, Pearce FB, Carberry KE, Kroslowitz R, Almond CS (2012) Prospective trial of a pediatric ventricular assist device supplement. N Engl J Med 367:532–541
11. Stiller B, Dähnert I, Weng YG, Hennig E, Hetzer R, Lange PE (1999) Children may survive severe myocarditis with prolonged use of biventricular assist devices. Heart 82:237–240

Continuous-Flow Pumps in Pediatric Population

Martin Schweiger, Daniel Zimpfer, Gaetano Gargiulo, and Michael Hübler

© Springer International Publishing Switzerland 2017
A. Montalto et al. (eds.), *Mechanical Circulatory Support in End-Stage Heart Failure*,
DOI 10.1007/978-3-319-43383-7_36

36.1 Introduction

To overcome death on the heart transplantation waiting list, specially designed VADs for children have been introduced and successfully implanted in adolescents [1] and babies [2]. These systems work with a pulse and the pump chambers are extracorporeal. While extracorporeal VADs are vastly superior to ECMO in terms of surviving transplantation, the devices are far from perfect due to the high risk of thromboembolic events, and the design limits mobilization and precludes discharge from hospital [3, 4]. Also, a shift has occurred from not only to save a child's life but to quality of life (QoL) on VAD support as well. Implantation of cf-VADs may be a promising option to reduce morbidity, to overcome the need for hospitalization, and to improve QoL in young patients. These devices work with a "nonphysiological" continuous flow; are small, fast, and easy to implant; and have a better reliability compared to pulsatile-flow devices. With miniaturization of pump design and increasing applications of cf-VADs in adults, implantation in smaller patients became feasible [3, 5, 6]. Experience in older children with these cf-VADs has been promising [7–12], and the quest goes to children even below BSA 1m^2. This chapter summarizes the experiences gained so far with the most commonly used cf-VADs.

36.2 Intracorporeal LVADs

36.2.1 HeartWare HVAD (Table 36.1)

The HeartWare HVAD (HeartWare Inc., Framingham, MA, USA), which was developed in the mid-1990s, is a third-generation rotary blood pump generating a continuous flow, with magnetically levitated rotor and hydrodynamic bearings with the hope to improve pump durability. This small compact design allows direct implantation into the left ventricle, and the pump remains housed within the pericardial space. It was initially designed for diaphragmatic implantation [13], but when first implanted in Europe as LVAD, the apical placement became the standard technique [14, 15]. Due to its size, it is applicable to children in supporting congenital or acquired systemic circulation [16]. Although the ventricle has to be large enough to provide sufficient space for the inflow cannula (see Figs. 36.1 and 36.2), implantation in patients as young as a 2-year-old child has been done (by D. Zimpfer, Vienna, see Fig. 36.3). The first reports form Miera et al. listed seven children with an 86% success rate of bridging to HTx. Two years later, Padalino et al. reported three adolescent patients had all successfully bridged to transplant. The first use within the USA was on a 13-year-old girl for 11 days [17]. Similar to adult patients, these

Table 36.1 Selection of the most relevant pediatric experience with HVAD HeartWare as implantable left ventricular assist devices

Author	Year	No. of patients	Age (year)	Weight (kg)	BSA (m^2)	Support time (days) (range)	BTT (%)	BTR (%)	Died on support (%)
Miera et al. [8]	2011	7	6–16	17–79	0.7–2.0	1–136	86	0	0
Schweiger et al. [9]	2015	12	8–15	18–81	0.76–1.96	42–790	83	8	0
Sparks et al. [31]	2015	6	10–16	36–82	1.2–1.8	61.3–195	83	0	0
Padalino et al. [32]	2013	3	11–15	26–65	1.05–1.68	17–49	100	0	0

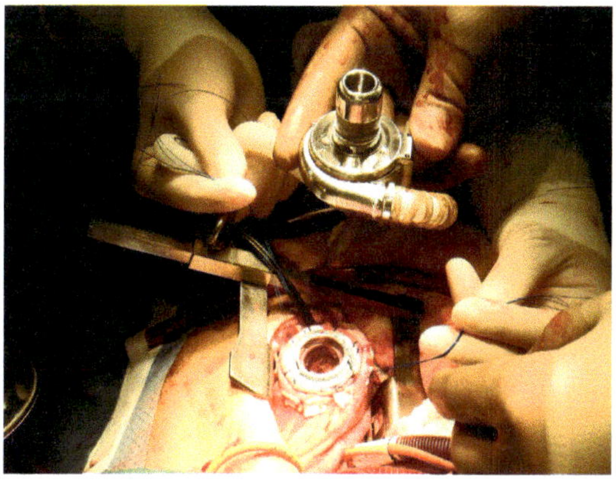

■ **Fig. 36.1** Intraoperative view of apical ring positioning

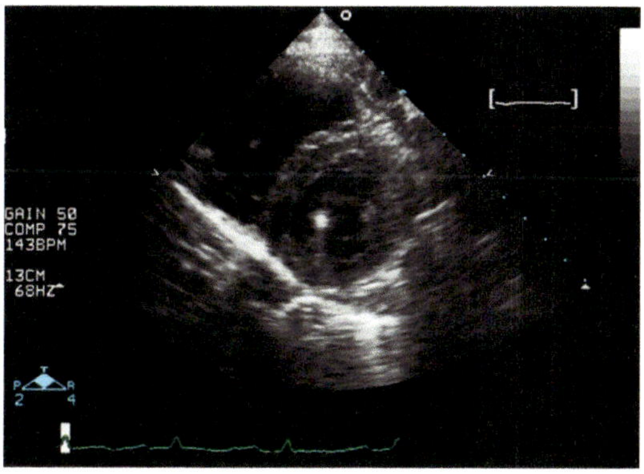

■ **Fig. 36.2** Transversal Echocardiographic image of ventricles in young patient

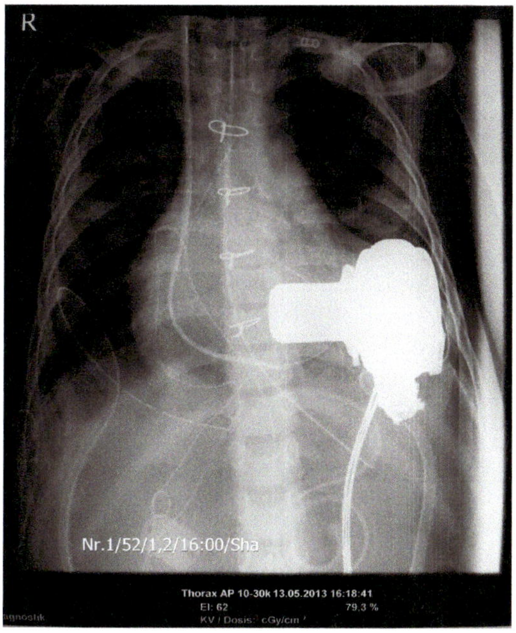

■ **Fig. 36.3** Chest Radiography showing HVAD implantation in a 2 years old child

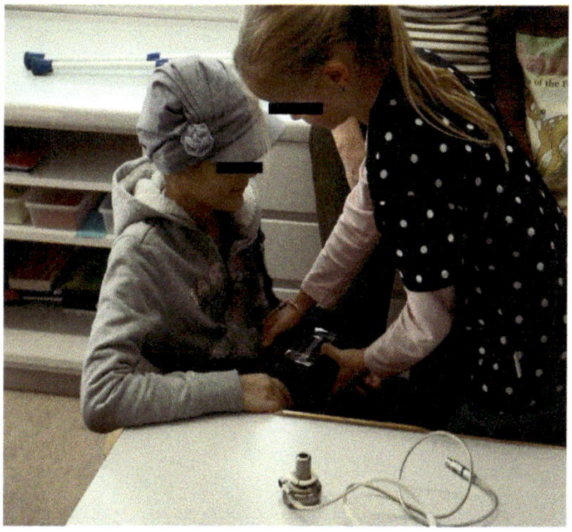

■ **Fig. 36.4** Children can be discharged home, resume schooling and resume regular activities of daily living

children can be discharged home, resume schooling, and resume regular activities of daily living (see ■ Fig. 36.4). In a multicenter experience from nine participating sites, Schweiger et al. reported that 12 pediatric patients were successfully discharged from hospital and managed as outpatients (60% of all pediatric HVAD patients from these nine centers were discharged). No severe adverse events occurred during outpatient management, and the readmission rate was low with 0.02 per patient month (2.1 per patient). The largest series in the USA included six children above 10 years of age.

36.2.2 DeBakey VAD Child (■ Table 36.2)

The DeBakey VAD Child (MicroMEd Cardiovascular, Inc., Houston, Texas) is an axial flow pump which is based on the technology of the adult DeBakey VAD with minor modifications. The inflow and outflow cannula are shortened and a reduced size of the flow probe on the outflow tract is used. The first clinically implanted axial flow pump in the world was the MicroMed DeBakey VAD [18] and gained FDA approval as DeBakey VAD Child (MicroMed Technology Inc., Houston, TX) for children older than 5 years or having a body surface area between 0.7 and 1.5 m^2. The first successful BTT after 56 days in support with the Debakey VAD Child was done on a 14-year-old boy [19]. A very aggressive anticoagulation was necessary to prevent pump

Table 36.2 Selection of the most relevant pediatric experience with DeBakey VAD Child as implantable left ventricular assist devices

Author	Year	No. of patients	Age (year)	Weight (kg)	BSA (m^2)	Support time (days) (range)	BTT (%)	BTR (%)	Died on support (%)	Notes
Fraser et al. [20]	2006	6	6–15	–	0.81–1.7	8–84	50	0	50	
Padalino et al. [33]	2006	1	10	–	1.2		100	0	0	
Morales et al. [34]	2005	1	6	–	0.7	16	0	0	100	Own experience
Morales et al. [34]	2005	9	10–17	42–110	1.3–2.2	–	56	0	44	Overview of experiences worldwide
Imamura et al. [19]	2005	1	14	–	–	56	100	0	0	

thrombosis in the DeBakey VAD Child [20]. Today, the DeBakey VAD Child is known as the HeartAssist5 Pediatric VAD.

36.2.3 Thoratec HeartMate II

The HeartMate II is an FDA-approved (does not specify the age) cf-LVAD which has also been adopted for use in children like other devices. It is implantable in patients with a BSA > 1.2 m2. Especially, the favorable adverse event rate profile concerning anticoagulation makes this an attractive LVAD in adolescents. The largest series was published by Cabrera et al. in 2013. The authors reported their experience of 28 pediatric patients (11–18 years, 50–132.8 kg, 1.47–2.65 BSA). Mean support time was 10.8 months. Thirty-six percent of the patients underwent transplantation, four patients died on support, and the others were still ongoing at the end of follow-up [7]. Owens et al. reported four patients with favorable outcome (either transplanted or 50% recovery). The smallest patient was 53 kg and had a 1.5 m2 BSA [5].

36.2.4 Infant Jarvik

The infant Jarvik 2000 is a small, hermetically sealed, axial-flow device which has shown promising results in animal testing [21]. The pump is part PumpKin (pumps for kids, infants, and neonates) Trail which was funded with $20 million by NHLBI in 2010. The pump is entering its clinical phase for IDE approval. The study protocol aimed at 44 patients with a weight from above 4 to 15 kg or a BSA ≤0.8 m2. So far, the pump has been implanted in Italy in a 16-month-old child, keeping the baby alive for 13 days before a switch back to the Berlin Heart was necessary due to technical problems [22].

36.2.5 VentrAssist

Ruygrok and coworkers published their experience with the VentrAssist in three patients (10–16 years, 36–80 kg, 1.1–1.5 BSA) with a support time of 375 to 954 days. One patient was successfully transplanted, one died on support, and one showed signs of recovery, and the pump was explanted [23]. The device is no longer available on the market.

36.3 Congenital Anomalies and cf-Implantable VAD Support

Congenital heart anomalies/defects (CHD) pose unique challenges for pediatric MCS, especially in the setting of single ventricles and Fontan

Table 36.3 Selection of the experience using cf-VAD in CHD patients

Author	Year	No. of patients	Age (year)	Diagnoses	Support time (days) (range)	BTT (%)	DT (%)	Died on support (%)	Devices
Shah et al. [35]	2013	6	23–54	ccTGA (n:3) dTGA (n:3)[a]	27–988	33.3	33.3	33.3	HeartMate II, HM XVE, Jarvik 2000, HVAD
Joyce et al. [36]	2010	3	25, 33, 35		Up to 2 years	100	0%	0	HeartMate II, DeBakey LVAD
Huebler et al. [16]	2011	2	24, 59	ccTGA (n:1) dTGA (n:1)[a]+	140–180	100	0	0	HAVD
Schweiger et al. [9]	2015	1	47	dTGA[a]		100	0	0	HVAD
Rajagopalan et al. [37]	2013	1	38	ccTGA	61	100	0	0	HeartMate II

ccTGA congenitally corrected transposition of the great arteries, *dTGA* dextro-transposition of the great arteries
aAll patients suffering from dTGA underwent Mustard or Senning (+) procedure in childhood

circulation. CHD patients with VAD support have a significantly higher postoperative mortality and inferior outcome [12, 24, 25] compared to patients suffering from cardiomyopathy. Furthermore it has to be recognized that an "adult-designed VAD" (like the cf-VAD) is not the optimal solution for single ventricle physiologies and failing Fontan circulations. On the other hand, there are patients, who after biventricular CHD repair in childhood may benefit greatly from intracorporeal VAD support. Patients who had Mustard or Senning operations may suffer from heart failure of the systemic ventricle decades later. In such patients, the anatomical right ventricle serves as the systemic heart chamber, and it is likely to fail before the pulmonary, anatomically left ventricle deteriorates [16, 26] (Table 36.3).

Nevertheless, the increase in anatomical complexity, limited and difficult selection of the proper device, correct surgical placement, and clinical management still constitute major challenges, resulting in the low utilization of VAD among adults with CHD listed for HTx [27].

36.4 Intracorporeal BVADs

Whereas the number of BVAD implantations is declining in adult patients, the incidence of biventricular failure among children remains high, ranging from 29–43%. In children, despite the paracorporeal Berlin Heart EXCOR® and the complete excision of the native heart and replacement by a total artificial heart (TAH), the implantations of two miniaturized cf-VADs is a feasible option for biventricular support. Successful implantations have been reported in young adults with the HeartWare HVAD [28] and the Jarvik 2000 FlowMaker® pumps [29, 30]. Recently, we bridged a 10-year-old child (BSA $1 m^2$) with two implanted HeartWare HVAD pumps to cardiac transplantation (see Fig. 36.5).

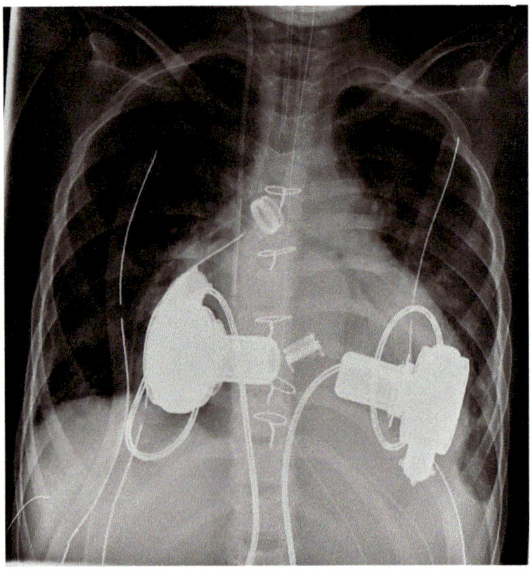

Fig. 36.5 Chest Radiography showing a 10-year-old child implanted with two Heartware HVAD pumps

36.5 Decision Algorithm

(See Fig. 36.6)

Patient selection and timing remain crucial factors for improving outcomes in VAD recipients. There are accepted indications when to consider MCS, and there are only a few contraindications for MCS like ongoing malignant neoplastic diseases with a very limited life expectancy, advanced multiorgan failure, complex congenital heart lesions involving intracardiac shunts or irreversible pulmonary failure, or severe extracardiac malformations such as chromosomal and genetic syndromes with poor quality of life prognosis. Although there is no broad consent what kind of MCS or what kind of VAD to use, there are advantages and disadvantages for each device, and the decision may be tailored to the patient's need and the experience of the physician team. If long-term

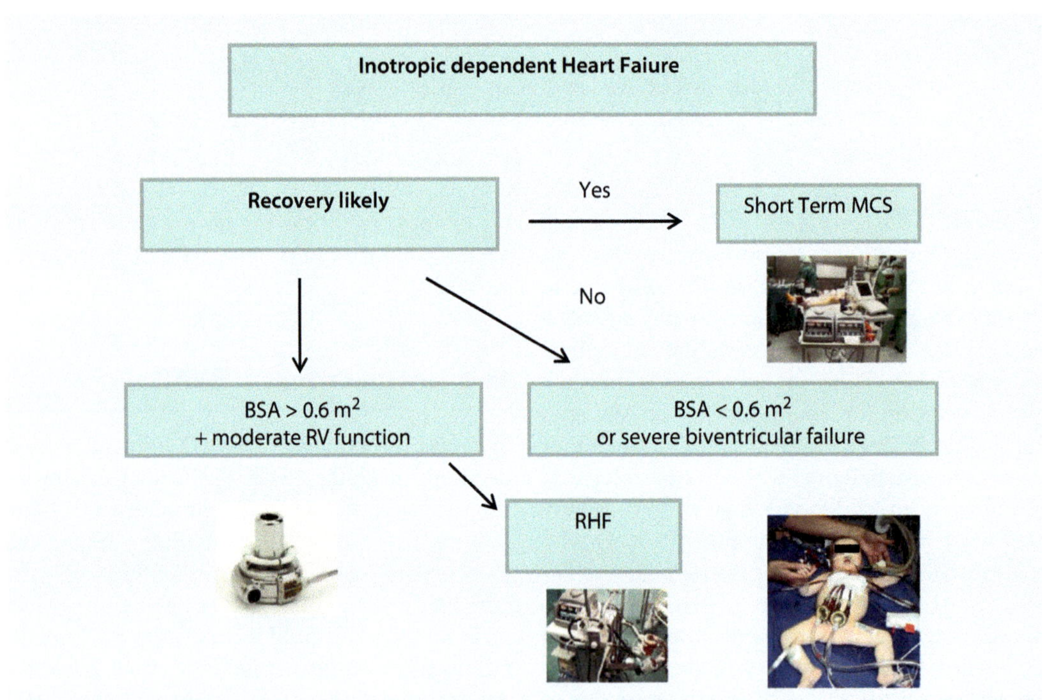

Fig. 36.6 Decision algorithm for ventricular assist device implantation in children used at the Children's Hospital Zurich. *BSA* body surface area, *RHI* right heart failure

VAD support is aimed for, it has to be kept in mind that the child should to be suitable for HTx. If a contraindication for HTx like pulmonary hypertension or successful treated malignancy but with a too short observational period for HTx is diagnosed, a concept known as bridge to candidacy should be considered.

At the our Department for Congenital Cardiovascular Surgery at the Children's Hospital Zurich, we use the following published approach: we try to differentiate between acute and chronic heart failure; in children under inotropic support without the possibility to wean them off or in case of deterioration of clinical status, MCS will be evaluated. If there are no absolute contraindications, MCS will be initiated; once again if a fast recovery may be expected (i.e., acute myocarditis or postcardiotomy failure), ECMO will be implanted. In chronic heart failure VAD implantation will be done; regarding the BSA and the right ventricular (RV) function of the child, either an intracorporeal VAD (BSA > 0.6 m^2 and acceptable RV function) or an extracorporeal VAD will be chosen (BSA < 0.6 m^2 or severe biventricular failure).

36.6 Anticoagulation

It is clear that patients on VAD support should receive anticoagulation (class I recommendation) [31]. While there is no debate for the need of anticoagulation, there are no standardized protocols. Anticoagulation is tailored to different types of VAD and individualized by different centers. Most of the protocols used propose a two- or three-drug regimen involving oral anticoagulation with additional antiplatelet therapy (i.e., aspirin, clopidogrel, Persantine).

In contrast to extracorporeal VAD where thrombus formation can be visualized and if necessary the pump chamber easily exchanged, pump thrombus formation in a cf-LVAD remains a devastating complication, associated with high morbidity and mortality. To achieve a balance between minimizing thromboembolic events and bleeding complications, an anticoagulation strategy involving the international normalized ratio (INR), the thrombocyte aggregation test (TAT), and the thromboelastography (TEG) has been proposed. Despite the development of new anticoagulant agents, unfractionated heparin (UFH) continues to be the anticoagulant of choice, especially in the early postoperative phase in which close titration is required [32]. UFH is given guided by aPTT (target, 1.5 times the baseline) or anti-factor Xa (target, 0.3–0.7 IU/ml). While still no uniform evidence-based guidelines exist on the optimal method for monitoring UFH therapy, especially in young children and in pediatrics, data suggest that anti-Xa monitoring achieves therapeutic anticoagulation more rapidly, maintains the values within the goal range for a longer time, and requires fewer adjustments in dosage and repeated tests [33, 34]. Recently it was shown that anti-Xa assay was better correlated with heparin dosing than the aPTT or ACT in pediatric ECMO [35]. Further, the aPTT is impacted more frequently by preanalytic compared to anti-Xa [33]. After removal of invasive lines and drainages, oral anticoagulation (i.e., warfarin) with a targeted INR from 2.0 to 3.5 depending on device type can be started. Additional antiplatelet therapy including aspirin and Persantine is monitored with TAT and TEG, respectively.

36.7 Myocardial Recovery: Device Explantation

In some patients after LVAD placement, myocardial recovery can be expected. To evaluate cardiac recovery under continuous axial flow pumps, a "three-step" approach (regularly echocardiography, cardiopulmonary exercise testing, and right heart catheterization) has been established by Dandel et al. [36, 37]. In contrast to the adult population, these criteria are so far not established for congenital heart diseases, and no guidelines for echocardiographic and hemodynamic criteria have been established. Nevertheless, there have been case reports of successful device explantation published [38]. One of these approaches proposes if echocardiographic parameters normalize (normal EF, normal dimensions of ventricular chambers, no valve regurgitation) and remain stable under full pump assistance; further evaluation with reduced pump flow (CAVE: optimal anticoagulation) can be done. Finally, a complete pump stop (CAVE: anticoagulation) and temporary catheter blocking of the outflow graft of the device to impede retrograde backflow to the LV in the catheter labor to test invasive hemodynamics and echocardiographic evaluation might be considered.

References

1. Warnecke H et al (1991) Mechanical left ventricular support as a bridge to cardiac transplantation in childhood. Eur J Cardiothorac Surg 5(6):330–333
2. Hetzer R et al (2006) Mechanical cardiac support in the young with the Berlin Heart EXCOR pulsatile ventricular assist device: 15 years' experience. Semin Thorac Cardiovasc Surg Pediatr Card Surg Annu 99–108
3. Fraser CD Jr et al (2012) Prospective trial of a pediatric ventricular assist device. N Engl J Med 367(6):532–541
4. Jeewa A et al (2010) Outcomes with ventricular assist device versus extracorporeal membrane oxygenation as a bridge to pediatric heart transplantation. Artif Organs 34(12):1087–1091
5. Owens WR et al (2010) Initial clinical experience with the HeartMate II ventricular assist system in a pediatric institution. Artif Organs 34(7):600–603
6. Almond CS et al (2011) Berlin Heart EXCOR pediatric ventricular assist device investigational device exemption study: study design and rationale. Am Heart J 162(3):425–435. e6
7. Cabrera AG et al (2013) Outcomes of pediatric patients supported by the HeartMate II left ventricular assist device in the United States. J Heart Lung Transplant 32(11):1107–1113
8. Miera O et al (2011) First experiences with the HeartWare ventricular assist system in children. Ann Thorac Surg 91(4):1256–1260
9. Schweiger M et al (2015) Outpatient management of intra-corporeal left ventricular assist device system in children: a multi-center experience. Am J Transplant 15(2):453–460
10. Fan Y et al (2011) Outcomes of ventricular assist device support in young patients with small body surface area. Eur J Cardiothorac Surg 39(5):699–704
11. Reinhartz O et al (2005) Thoratec ventricular assist devices in pediatric patients: update on clinical results. ASAIO J 51(5):501–503
12. Reinhartz O et al (2001) Multicenter experience with the thoratec ventricular assist device in children and adolescents. J Heart Lung Transplant 20(4):439–448
13. Gregoric ID, Cohn WE, Frazier OH (2011) Diaphragmatic implantation of the HeartWare ventricular assist device. J Heart Lung Transplant 30(4):467–470
14. Wieselthaler GM et al (2010) Initial clinical experience with a novel left ventricular assist device with a magnetically levitated rotor in a multi-institutional trial. J Heart Lung Transplant 29(11):1218–1225
15. Strueber M et al (2011) Multicenter evaluation of an intrapericardial left ventricular assist system. J Am Coll Cardiol 57(12):1375–1382
16. Huebler M et al (2012) Mechanical circulatory support of systemic ventricle in adults with transposition of great arteries. ASAIO J 58(1):12–14
17. D'Alessandro D et al (2012) First reported use of the heartware HVAD in the US as bridge to transplant in an adolescent. Pediatr Transplant 16:E356–E359
18. Potapov EV et al (2000) Pulsatile flow in patients with a novel nonpulsatile implantable ventricular assist device. Circulation 102(19 Suppl 3):III183–III187
19. Imamura M et al (2005) The first successful DeBakey VAD child implantation as a bridge to transplant. ASAIO J 51(5):670–672
20. Fraser CD Jr et al (2006) Preliminary experience with the MicroMed DeBakey pediatric ventricular assist device. Semin Thorac Cardiovasc Surg Pediatr Card Surg Annu 109–114
21. Wei X et al (2013) Pre-clinical evaluation of the infant Jarvik 2000 heart in a neonate piglet model. J Heart Lung Transplant 32(1):112–119
22. Schweiger M et al (2013) Paediatric ventricular assist devices: current achievements. Swiss Med Wkly 143: w13804
23. Ruygrok PN et al (2008) Pediatric experience with the VentrAssist LVAD. Ann Thorac Surg 86(2):622–626
24. Conway J et al (2015) Delineating survival outcomes in children <10 kg bridged to transplant or recovery with the Berlin Heart EXCOR Ventricular Assist Device. JACC Heart Fail 3(1):70–77
25. Blume ED et al (2006) Outcomes of children bridged to heart transplantation with ventricular assist devices: a multi-institutional study. Circulation 113(19):2313–2319
26. Schweiger M et al (2015) Biventricular failure in dextro-transposition of the great arteries corrected with the Mustard procedure: VAD support of the systemic ventricle is enough. Int J Artif Organs 38:233–235
27. Gelow JM et al (2013) Organ allocation in adults with congenital heart disease listed for heart transplant: impact of ventricular assist devices. J Heart Lung Transplant 32(11):1059–1064
28. Krabatsch T et al (2011) Biventricular circulatory support with two miniaturized implantable assist devices. Circulation 124(11 Suppl):S179–S186
29. Frazier OH, Myers TJ, Gregoric I (2004) Biventricular assistance with the Jarvik FlowMaker: a case report. J Thorac Cardiovasc Surg 128(4):625–626
30. Yoshioka D et al (2014) Over 1200-day support with dual Jarvik 2000 biventricular assist device. Interact Cardiovasc Thorac Surg 19(6):1083–1084
31. Sparks J et al (2015) Continuous flow device support in children using the HeartWare HVAD: 1,000 days of lessons learned from a single center experience. ASAIO J 61(5):569–573

32. Padalino MA et al (2014) HeartWare Ventricular Assist Device as Bridge to Transplant in Children and Adolescents. Artif Organs 38:418–422
33. Padalino MA et al (2006) Bridge to transplant using the MicroMed DeBakey ventricular assist device in a child with idiopathic dilated cardiomyopathy. Ann Thorac Surg 81(3):1118–1121
34. Morales DL et al (2005) Lessons learned from the first application of the DeBakey VAD Child: an intracorporeal ventricular assist device for children. J Heart Lung Transplant 24(3):331–337
35. Shah NR et al (2013) Clinical outcomes after ventricular assist device implantation in adults with complex congenital heart disease. J Heart Lung Transplant 32(6):615–620
36. Joyce DL et al (2010) Mechanical circulatory support in patients with heart failure secondary to transposition of the great arteries. J Heart Lung Transplant 29(11):1302–1305
37. Rajagopalan N et al (2013) Successful ventricular assist device placement in transposition of the great arteries with pulmonary hypertension. Ann Thorac Surg 95(2):E47–E47
38. Cavigelli-Brunner A et al (2014) VAD as Bridge to Recovery in Anthracycline-Induced Cardiomyopathy and HHV6 Myocarditis. Pediatrics 134:e894–e899

The Berlin Heart EXCOR Experience in the USA

Chet R. Villa and David L.S. Morales

© Springer International Publishing Switzerland 2017
A. Montalto et al. (eds.), *Mechanical Circulatory Support in End-Stage Heart Failure*,
DOI 10.1007/978-3-319-43383-7_37

Heart transplantation is the final therapeutic option in children with end-stage heart failure due to cardiomyopathy or congenital heart disease. Approximately 11,000–14,000 children are admitted to the hospital with heart failure [1] each year in the USA. A proportion of these patients will require heart transplantation due to end-stage heart failure. Prior to FDA approval of the Berlin Heart EXCOR, there was no reliable mechanical circulatory support option for children. Historically, children with end-stage heart failure were bridged to transplant with extracorporeal membrane oxygenation (ECMO). The outcomes of this approach were suboptimal as only ~47% of patients bridged to transplant survived to hospital discharge [2]. Early experience with the off-label use of adult ventricular assist devices (VADs) in children was promising as 76% survived to transplant; however, the outcomes in children <10 years of age and with congenital heart disease were less encouraging [3]. The Food and Drug Administration (FDA) granted a humanitarian device exemption (HDE) for the continuous-flow DeBakey VAD Child in 2004; however, use of the device in children was limited by concerns about device fit within the chest wall of small children and thrombotic complications [4].

37.1 The Pre-IDE Experience

The first implants with the EXCOR device occurred in Europe in 1992. The development of a pediatric-sized VAD raised the possibility that both infants and children could be supported with the device [5]. The first use of the device in the United States (US) occurred in 2000; however, only three devices were placed between 2000 and 2004. However, in 2004, multiple things occurred which marked the dawn of VAD support for children in the USA. The US government for the first time awarded monies to develop a pediatric-specific VAD, and the Berlin EXCOR began to have widespread acceptance as a potential bridge to transplant with over 40 VADs placed that year in the USA [6]. EXCOR use continued to increase despite being used under a compassionate use exemption that required significant paperwork and for the device/supporting hardware to be shipped to the center for each use from Germany. In spite of these logistical issues, the device was implanted 100 times between June 2000 and May 2007 (97% of the implants occurred from 2004 to 2007). The initial, multicenter North American experience showed that 77% of children implanted with the EXCOR were successfully bridged to transplant or recovery [7]. This, even though this was often the first VAD placed by most pediatric centers, and that patients were commonly placed on ECMO until the device arrived at each center. This clinical momentum along with multiple discussions with the FDA [8] gave rise to a prospective, multicenter, single-group clinical cohort investigational device exemption (IDE) study [9]. The clinical data from the IDE study as well as data from the patients who were implanted via compassionate use access in the pre-IDE era formed the North American experience with the EXCOR device. This review will summarize these data and will briefly discuss future directions with the EXCOR in the USA.

37.2 The IDE Trial

The IDE study began enrolling children in May 2007 and continued enrolling through December 2010 [9]. Eligible patients were ≤16 years of age, weighed between 3 and 60 kg, had two-ventricle circulation, and were on a weight list for transplantation at one of the 17 study sites. The final study included 48 patients 0–16 years of age, stratified into two cohorts by body surface area (BSA), and enrolled at one of the 17 IDE study centers in the USA and Canada. Cohort 1 included patients with a BSA <0.7 m^2, while cohort 2 included patients with a BSA 0.7–1.5 m^2. Patient outcomes were compared to historical matched ECMO patients from the Extracorporeal Life Support Organization (ELSO) registry. Consideration was given to a randomized trial comparing the EXCOR and ECMO; however, this was deemed infeasible given the lack of clinical equipoise in many of the centers [8]. Given the early positive outcomes with the EXCOR, clinical equipoise was lacking as many centers did not feel randomizing patients to ECMO as a bridge to transplant was appropriate as the benefits of the EXCOR were clinically obvious. The study included devices with a stroke

Table 37.1 EXCOR IDE study patient characteristics

Variable	Cohort 1 (BSA < 0.7 m²)	Cohort 2 (BSA 0.7–1.5 m²)
Age in months – median (range)	11.7 (2.6–45.6)	111.2 (50.8–191.8)
Weight in kilograms – median (range)	9.2 (3.6–13.6)	30.7 (16–58.1)
Congenital heart disease – number (%)	3 (12)	6 (25)
Dilated cardiomyopathy/myocarditis – number (%)	19 (79)	17 (71)
INTERMACS profile – number (%)		
1	11 (46)	13 (54)
2	13 (54)	11 (46)
Preoperative ECMO – number (%)	6 (25)	8 (33)
VAD configuration – number (%)		
LVAD	17 (71)	14 (58)
Biventricular VAD	7 (29)	10 (42)

BSA body surface area, *ECMO* extracorporeal membrane oxygenation, *IDE* investigational device exemption, *INTERMACS* Interagency Registry for Mechanically Assisted Circulatory Support, *VAD* ventricular assist device

volume of 10, 25, 30, 50, or 60 ml (the 15 ml pump which is currently available was not developed at this time).

The most common diagnosis in each size cohort was dilated cardiomyopathy (Table 37.1). The implant characteristics of the EXCOR patients reflect the state of the pediatric VAD community at that time. The patients quite ill as 50% were INTERMACS profile 1 and 29% had preoperative ECMO. Biventricular VAD use was also significantly more common than in the current era. It should also be noted that over 70% of the study cohort was implanted at two institutions.

Survival was significantly higher for each of the EXCOR cohorts than for the historical ECMO control groups (log rank $p < 0.001$ for cohort 1 and 2 compared to ECMO) (Fig. 37.1). Furthermore, 90% of patients supported with the EXCOR survived to transplant or were weaned from the device compared to 67–75% of ECMO matched controls. The most common serious adverse events were major bleeding (46%), infection (56%), and stroke (29%). Adverse events rates were 0.07 events/patient day for cohort 1 and 0.08 events/patient day for cohort 2. The cumulative survival benefit and adverse event profile of the EXCOR met the burden of proof for HDE approval by the FDA of probable benefit and safety, and thus the EXCOR was given HDE approval in December 2011. HDE approval requires less than 4000 implantations a year and that the implanting institutions keep an active IRB protocol. The official approval stated, "EXCOR is intended to provide mechanical circulatory support as a bridge to cardiac transplantation for pediatric patients…..who are candidates for cardiac transplant…." One should note that the FDA chose not to limit the use of the EXCOR to the parameters of the study cohort and allowed wide application of the EXCOR (i.e., patients with complex congenital heart disease). It also did limit the use of the device to transplantation centers.

Subsequent analyses of the IDE cohort and patients who did not meet the study inclusion criteria and who received the device under compassionate use protocols further explored risk factors for poor outcome including the complex congenital heart disease and the impact of device use on post-transplant survival.

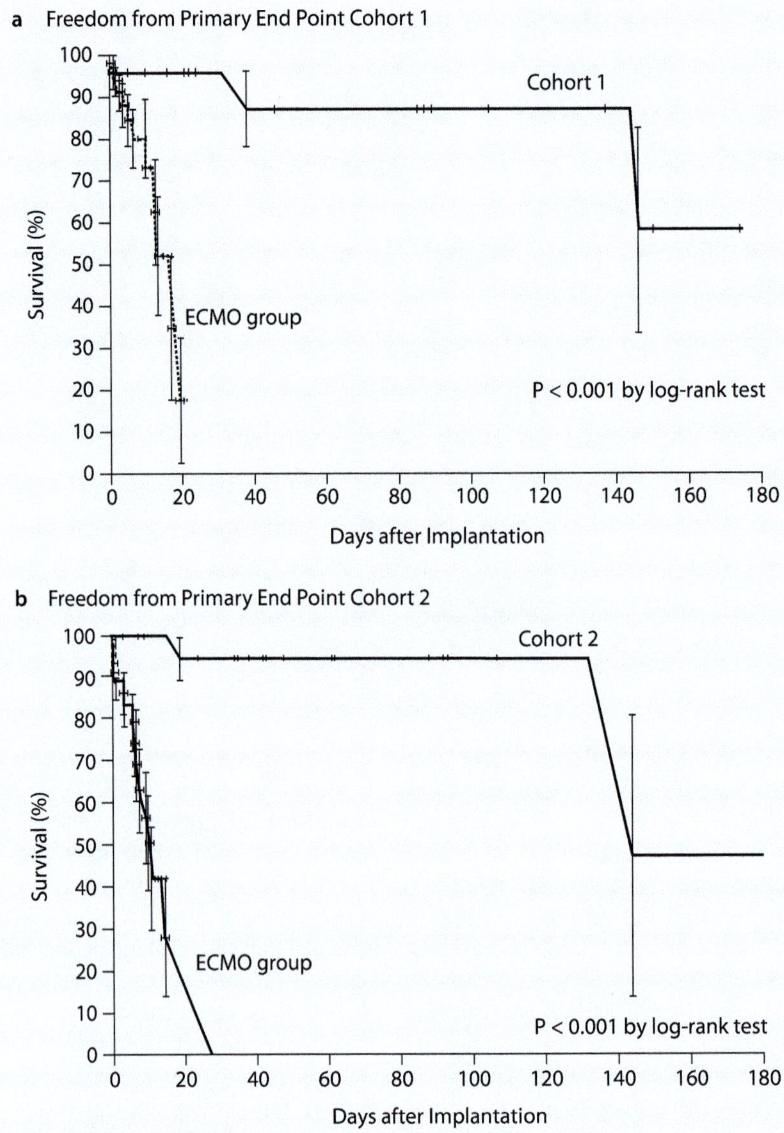

Fig. 37.1 Kaplan-Meier estimates of freedom from primary end point (death for ECMO cohort, death or weaning from device with unacceptable neurologic outcome for EXCOR cohorts). Cohort 1 includes patients with a body surface area < 0.7 m^2, and cohort 2 includes patients with a body surface area 0.7–1.5 m^2 (From Fraser et al. [9])

37.3 Combined IDE and Compassionate Use Data

The data from the IDE study was quite definitive to demonstrate the superiority of the EXCOR over ECMO in bridging patients to transplantation. However, it did not provide a complete picture of the US EXCOR experience, "the real-world experience," as it only reported on a third of all the patients implanted with the EXCOR during the study period. Also, it did not include important patient cohorts such as those with complex congenital heart disease or with significant end-organ dysfunction. Nor did it represent a wide sample of all institutions placing the device. The broader perspective was provided by a comprehensive analysis of the combined IDE and compassionate use data [6].

This study included all children who received an EXCOR in the USA or Canada between May 2007 and Dec 2010. The pump sizes available and adverse event definitions were the same as for the IDE study.

Two hundred and four children were enrolled (only one in Canada) during the study period, of which 95 (47%) patients received the EXCOR at a non-IDE center. Compassionate-use patients comprised 67% of the entire cohort and were younger, smaller, more likely to have congenital heart disease, more likely to be supported on ECMO and had worse end-organ function (◘ Table 37.2).

Of the 204 children supported with the EXCOR during the study, 75% survived to transplant or recovery. Children in the compassionate use cohort were less likely to reach transplantation (53% versus 85%) and were more likely to die (34% versus 7%; $p < 0.01$). Predictors of early mortality while supported on the EXCOR included lower weight, higher bilirubin, and BiVAD support, while bilirubin extremes and decreased glomerular filtration rate (GFR) predicted late mortality. Decreased GFR was the strongest overall predictor of death. Of note, death also occurred more commonly in children with congenital heart disease, children on ECMO at the time of implantation, at non-IDE centers, and at centers with lower volume; however, these differences were not statistically significant after adjusting for the other risk factors for mortality.

◘ Table 37.2 Patient characteristics for IDE criteria and compassionate use EXCOR cohorts

Variable	IDE criteria cohort ($n = 68$)	Compassionate use cohort ($n = 136$)
Age in years – median (IQR)	2.1 (0.6–7.1)	1.4 (0.4–4.4)
Weight in kilograms – median (IQR)	10 (6.5–16.6)	9.4 (5.7–14.8)
Congenital heart disease – number (%)	10 (15)	49 (36)
Single Ventricle – number (%)	0 (0)	19 (14)
Preoperative ECMO – number (%)	18 (27)	65 (48)
GFR categories – number (%)		
<30% predicted	0 (0)	11 (8)
30–99% predicted	11 (16)	32 (24)
>99% predicted	57 (84)	93 (68)

ECMO extracorporeal membrane oxygenation, *IDE* investigational device exemption, *GFR* glomerular filtration rate estimated from Schwartz formula [10]

The most common cause of death ($n = 51$) in the study was neurologic insult ($n = 17$, 33%), with thromboembolic strokes significantly outnumbering hemorrhagic stroke. Stroke severity data was only available for the IDE cohort; thus, further information regarding stroke severity could not be gleaned from this data. Neurologic insult was followed by respiratory failure ($n = 6$, 12%), bleeding ($n = 3$, 6%), multisystem organ failure ($n = 3$, 6%), right ventricular failure ($n = 3$, 6%), and other less common events. Of note, death due to device malfunction occurred in only one patient.

Most interesting is that even though mortality differed significantly between the IDE and non-IDE patients, the incidence of all morbidities was not different, in fact almost identical. Centers with increased experience (VAD implants >5 for an institution) was associated with significantly improved survival compared to institutions with less experience. Therefore, it was not the avoidance of complications but the recognition of complications and the ability to mitigate them in experienced centers that was associated with improved outcomes. This experience, we hypothesize, was a result of the formation of a multidiscipline team with protocol-driven care.

This study [6] was not only notable for providing the largest, most comprehensive analysis of EXCOR support to date, but it also identified the importance of neurologic insults on clinical outcomes in addition to identifying risk factors for mortality while supported on the EXCOR. Subsequent analyses would provide more in-depth analysis of neurologic events [10], patient size [11], and BiVAD use [12] on outcomes.

37.4 Neurologic Events

Neurologic insult was the most common cause of mortality among patients supported with an EXCOR in both the IDE study [9] and combined IDE/compassionate use study [6]. Neurologic dysfunction was also a frequent cause of morbidity (29% of patients suffered a neurologic insult) among patients who survived to transplant in these cohorts. Given the importance of this topic, Jordan et al. [10] specifically analyzed the stroke data available from the combined IDE and compassionate use cohorts.

Of the 204 children included in the study, 59 (29%) experienced at least one neurologic event (total of 73 events) for a total event rate of 0.51 events/100 patient days. The majority of events were ischemic strokes (n = 47, 89%) with few hemorrhagic strokes (n = 5, 9%). The risk for a neurologic event was not evenly dispersed as the majority of events (45 [62%]) occurred during the first month of support. Hazard function analysis showed the risk per patient day was highest during the perioperative period and slowly decreased to "baseline" by day 50 of support.

Assessing the severity of neurologic impairment following the events was limited to some degree by the lack of chronologic neurologic testing, only 25 of the patients who experienced a neurologic event had at least one Pediatric Stroke Outcome Measure (PSOM) completed, and only 15 had PSOM data following the event. That said, gross estimates of the severity could be gleaned from what data did exist. Of the patients with long-term PSOM data following the event, 11 of 22 (50%) had no or mild PSOM abnormalities. Furthermore, 56% of patients who experienced an event subsequently underwent heart transplantation.

Attempts to identify risk factors for stroke using pre-implant demographic and clinical variables yielded limited results. Female gender and a history of pump change due to thrombus were the sole risk factors for neurologic insult identified in the final multivariable model. The pump exchange data was further limited by the lack of data regarding the timing of pump change and the neurologic insult. Single centers have demonstrated improvement in stroke-related outcomes with increased institutional experience [13]. Centers have also explored alternate management strategies including anti-inflammatory therapy [14] and more frequent device pump exchanges [15] to try to decrease the risk of stroke; however, the success of these interventions have not yet been demonstrated. Finally, recent data from the Berlin database demonstrates there is considerable variation (tenfold) in the incidence of stroke [16] and the risk was not explained by center volume. This suggests it may be possible to improve outcomes through shared learning and establishing best practices from centers with the lowest risk of stroke.

37.5 BiVAD Versus LVAD Support

Seventy-six (37%) of the 204 patients that comprised the combined IDE and compassionate use cohorts were placed on BiVAD support [6]. This was an incremental improvement from the 43% of patients who received a BiVAD during the pre-IDE North American experience [7]. The relatively high BiVAD rates were notable given patients who received BiVADs had significantly higher mortality in each of these studies, as in numerous adult and single-center pediatric studies. While there are clearly some patients who benefit from BiVAD support, identifying these patients remains a challenge. This prompted a focused analysis regarding BiVAD support in the 204 patient combined IDE/compassionate use cohorts.

Patients who received BiVADs had generally similar preimplantation and implantation characteristics. BiVAD patients were more commonly Caucasian (76% versus 55%; p = 0.003) and INTERMACS profile 1 (63% versus 46%; p = 0.018). They also more commonly had an elevated bilirubin level (56% versus 37%; p = 0.015). As expected, survival was significantly lower in BiVAD versus LVAD patients (100-day survival 60% versus 80%; log rank p = 0.03). There was no difference in serious adverse events or total days on support. Patients who were implanted at a site with <5 implantations, had an abnormal GFR, and who had a pump size of 10 mL were more likely to experience mortality on BiVAD. Furthermore, there was no patient subgroup (based on pre-implant characteristics) that showed improved survival on BiVAD support. This last point is significant and should be underscored. While there may be a subgroup of patients who require BiVAD support, the widespread use of BiVADs in this era did not confer a survival advantage and may have worsened outcomes. This is consistent with single-center studies which show decreased BiVAD use with similar or improved outcomes as a program matures [17].

37.6 The EXCOR in Univentricular Hearts

The analysis of combined IDE and compassionate use cohorts identified a number of risk factors for death while supported with the EXCOR [6]. The presence of congenital heart disease was not identified as a risk factor in the final multivariable model; however, a specific analysis examining the outcomes of patients with a univentricular heart was not performed, but was rather the focus of a subsequent study by Weinstein et al. [18].

The study by Weinstein et al. was largely the same cohort as in the Almond [6] and Jordan [10] studies, though the study endpoint was extended to December 2011. Twenty-six of the 281 identified via the Berlin EXCOR database were single ventricles (15 of 26 had hypoplastic left heart syndrome) (■ Table 37.3). Only 42% of single-ventricle patients were bridged to transplant compared to 73% of biventricular patients. There was a significant difference in survival according to stage of palliation. Only one of nine stage I patients and none of the neonatal Norwood patients survived. The one stage I patient that survived had a Norwood-like procedure at 17 months of age and was supported via BiVAD placement. Survival was better for stage II (7 of 12) and stage III patients (three of five).

Unlike the stage I patients, less of these patients were salvage VADs (VADs placed after failed palliation and usually proceeded with post-cardiotomy ECMO) probably explaining their increased survival. A handful of case reports describing the use of the EXCOR in single ventricles have also been described [19–22]. Given the outcomes to date, EXCOR support following Glenn and Fontan procedures should be approached cautiously, while support of a failed neonatal Norwood procedure does not appear prudent [11] looking at the worldwide experience.

■ **Table 37.3** Diagnosis, palliative stage, and VAD configuration among single ventricles supported with the EXCOR

Variable	Number (%)
Primary diagnosis	
Hypoplastic left heart syndrome	15 (58)
Unbalanced atrioventricular canal	2 (8)
Double inlet left ventricle	2 (8)
Ebstein's double outlet right ventricle	2 (8)
Transposition, hypoplastic left ventricle	2 (8)
Tricuspid atresia	1 (4)
Pulmonary atresia with intact septum	1 (4)
Palliative stage	
1	9 (35)
2	12 (46)
3	5 (19)
VAD configuration	
Systemic VAD	24(92)
BiVAD	2 (8)

VAD ventricular assist device

37.7 Post-transplant Outcomes

While survival to transplantation on the EXCOR is important, survival following bridge to transplantation is no less relevant. This is reflected in outcome data for patients bridged to transplant with ECMO where a significant component of cumulative mortality occurs following transplantation [2, 23]. Patients bridged to transplant between 2007 and December 2011 were identified via the Berlin EXCOR database. Outcomes were compared to patients within the Organ Procurement and Transplant Network (OPTN) database between May 2007 and December 2011 who were listed 1a and those bridged to transplant on ECMO. Patients bridged with EXCOR had similar early post-transplant survival to the status 1a patients, and both had higher survival than patients bridged with ECMO.

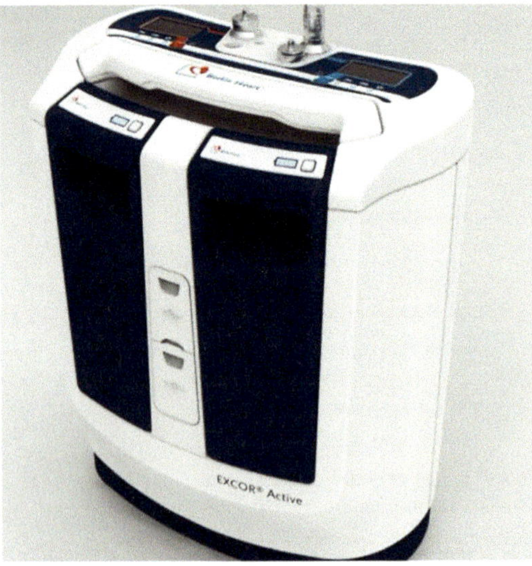

Fig. 37.2 Prototype EXCOR active mobile drive

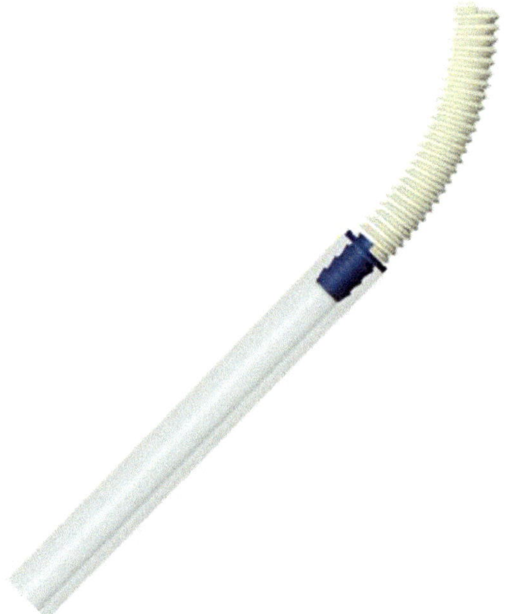

Fig. 37.3 Prototype EXCOR Graft Cannula

Congenital heart disease was the only univariate predictor of death after transplant among patients bridged with the EXCOR. Furthermore, none of the INTERMACS defined serious adverse events predicted post-transplant mortality in EXCOR patients. These data were also confirmed using a matched cohort of EXCOR patients and non-MCS patients [24]. Importantly, these data also showed that there was no difference in midterm post-transplant outcomes.

37.8 Future Directions

The IKUS driving unit is designed for in-house mobility as the driver is heavy, difficult to direct, and cannot be maintained safely without healthcare providers. The EXCOR active mobile driving system is a much more user-friendly driver that will allow for out of hospital support, which will change the use of the device tremendously if outpatient therapy is possible. The drive may be available in the USA as early as 2017 and is suitable for all EXCOR pumps (Fig. 37.2).

The use of any ventricular assist device requires positional flexibility given the myriad anatomic variations present in congenital heart disease. With this in mind, EXCOR is developing the graft cannula (likely in 6, 8, and 12 mm variations) which will allow greater flexibility in cannulation to accommodate innovative, individualized implantation strategies (Fig. 37.3). The cannula may be available in the USA as early as late 2017.

The EXCOR has greatly improved outcomes for children with end-stage heart failure; however, opportunities for improvement exist. In particular, the rate of neurologic dysfunction and mixed outcomes associated with device use in patients with congenital heart disease provide opportunities for improvement. Recent data from the USA and internationally have demonstrated the benefits of VAD support on waitlist mortality and post-transplant outcome [2, 23, 25–28]. The EXCOR remains the standard of care-to-bridge children less than 25–30 kg to cardiac transplantation and clearly revolutionized the treatment of children with end-stage heart failure.

References

1. Rossano JW, Kim JJ, Decker JA, Price JF, Zafar F, Graves DE, Morales DL, Heinle JS, Bozkurt B, Towbin JA, Denfield SW, Dreyer WJ, Jefferies JL (2012) Prevalence, morbidity, and mortality of heart failure-related hospitalizations in children in the United States: a population-based study. J Card Fail 18:459–470
2. Almond CS, Singh TP, Gauvreau K, Piercey GE, Fynn-Thompson F, Rycus PT, Bartlett RH, Thiagarajan RR (2011) Extracorporeal membrane oxygenation for bridge to heart transplantation among children in the united states: analysis of data from the organ

procurement and transplant network and extracorporeal life support organization registry. Circulation 123:2975–2984
3. Blume ED, Naftel DC, Bastardi HJ, Duncan BW, Kirklin JK, Webber SA (2006) Outcomes of children bridged to heart transplantation with ventricular assist devices: a multi-institutional study. Circulation 113:2313–2319
4. Morales DL, Dibardino DJ, McKenzie ED, Heinle JS, Chang AC, Loebe M, Noon GP, Debakey ME, Fraser CD Jr (2005) Lessons learned from the first application of the DeBakey VAD Child: an intracorporeal ventricular assist device for children. J Heart Lung Transplant 24:331–337
5. Hetzer R, Loebe M, Potapov EV, Weng Y, Stiller B, Hennig E, Alexi-Meskishvili V, Lange PE (1998) Circulatory support with pneumatic paracorporeal ventricular assist device in infants and children. Ann Thorac Surg 66:1498–1506
6. Almond CS, Morales DL, Blackstone EH, Turrentine MW, Imamura M, Massicotte MP, Jordan LC, Devaney EJ, Ravishankar C, Kanter KR, Holman W, Kroslowitz R, Tjossem C, Thuita L, Cohen GA, Buchholz H, St. Louis JD, Nguyen K, Niebler RA, Walters HL, Reemtsen B, Wearden PD, Reinhartz O, Guleserian KJ, Mitchell MB, Bleiweis MS, Canter CE, Humpl T (2013) Berlin heart EXCOR pediatric ventricular assist device for bridge to heart transplantation in US children. Circulation 127:1702–1711
7. Morales DL, Almond CS, Jaquiss RD, Rosenthal DN, Naftel DC, Massicotte MP, Humpl T, Turrentine MW, Tweddell JS, Cohen GA, Kroslowitz R, Devaney EJ, Canter CE, Fynn-Thompson F, Reinhartz O, Imamura M, Ghanayem NS, Buchholz H, Furness S, Mazor R, Gandhi SK, Fraser CD Jr (2011) Bridging children of all sizes to cardiac transplantation: the initial multicenter North American experience with the Berlin Heart EXCOR ventricular assist device. J Heart Lung Transplant 30:1–8
8. Almond CS, Buchholz H, Massicotte P, Ichord R, Rosenthal DN, Uzark K, Jaquiss RD, Kroslowitz R, Kepler MB, Lobbestael A (2011) Berlin heart EXCOR pediatric ventricular assist device investigational device exemption study: study design and rationale. Am Heart J 162:425–435 e6
9. Fraser CD, Jaquiss RDB, Rosenthal DN, Humpl T, Canter CE, Blackstone EH, Naftel DC, Ichord RN, Bomgaars L, Tweddell JS, Massicotte MP, Turrentine MW, Cohen GA, Devaney EJ, Pearce FB, Carberry KE, Kroslowitz R, Almond CS (2012) Prospective trial of a pediatric ventricular assist device. N Engl J Med 367:532–541
10. Jordan LC, Ichord RN, Reinhartz O, Humpl T, Pruthi S, Tjossem C, Rosenthal DN (2015) Neurological complications and outcomes in the Berlin heart EXCOR® pediatric investigational device exemption trial. J Am Heart Assoc 4:e001429–e001429
11. Conway J, St Louis J, Morales DL, Law S, Tjossem C, Humpl T (2015) Delineating survival outcomes in children <10 kg bridged to transplant or recovery with the Berlin heart EXCOR ventricular assist device. JACC Heart Fail 3:70–77
12. Zafar F, Jefferies JL, Tjossem CJ, Bryant R 3rd, Jaquiss RD, Wearden PD, Rosenthal DN, Cabrera AG, Rossano JW, Humpl T, Morales DL (2015) Biventricular Berlin heart EXCOR pediatric use across the united states. Ann Thorac Surg 99:1328–1334
13. Byrnes JW, Prodhan P, Williams BA, Schmitz ML, Moss MM, Dyamenahalli U, McKamie W, Morrow WR, Imamura M, Bhutta AT (2013) Incremental reduction in the incidence of stroke in children supported with the Berlin EXCOR ventricular assist device. Ann Thorac Surg 96:1727–1733
14. Byrnes JW, Bhutta AT, Rettiganti MR, Gomez A, Garcia X, Dyamenahalli U, Johnson C, Jaquiss RD, Imamura M, Prodhan P (2015) Steroid therapy attenuates acute phase reactant response among children on ventricular assist device support. Ann Thorac Surg 99:1392–1398
15. Maeda K, Almond C, Hollander SA, Rosenthal DN, Kaufman B, Yeh J, Gowen MM, Shuttleworth P, Reinhartz O (2015) Refining of the pump exchange procedure in children supported with the Berlin heart EXCOR ventricular assist: device: 10 years experience at a single institution. J Heart Lung Transplant 34:S88–S89
16. Almond CS, Lorts A, Rossano JW, Jordan LC, VanderPluym C, Price JF, Daly KP, Maeda K, Shin AY, Rosenthal DN (2015) Abstract 19540: US center variability in the incidence of stroke for the Berlin heart EXCOR pediatric ventricular assist device. Circulation 132:A19540
17. Hetzer R, Potapov EV, Stiller B, Weng Y, Hübler M, Lemmer J, Alexi-Meskishvili V, Redlin M, Merkle F, Kaufmann F, Hennig E (2006) Improvement in survival after mechanical circulatory support with pneumatic pulsatile ventricular assist devices in pediatric patients. Ann Thorac Surg 82:917–924 ;discussion 924-5
18. Weinstein S, Bello R, Pizarro C, Fynn-Thompson F, Kirklin J, Guleserian K, Woods R, Tjossem C, Kroslowitz R, Friedmann P, Jaquiss R (2014) The use of the Berlin heart EXCOR in patients with functional single ventricle. J Thorac Cardiovasc Surg 147:697–705
19. Halaweish I, Ohye RG, Si MS (2015) Berlin heart ventricular assist device as a long-term bridge to transplantation in a Fontan patient with failing single ventricle. Pediatr Transplant 19:E193–E195
20. Niebler RA, Shah TK, Mitchell ME, Woods RK, Zangwill SD, Tweddell JS, Berger S, Ghanayem NS (2016) Ventricular assist device in single-ventricle heart disease and a superior cavopulmonary anastomosis. Artif Organs 40:180–184
21. Hoganson DM, Boston US, Gazit AZ, Canter CE, Eghtesady P (2015) Successful bridge through transplantation with berlin heart ventricular assist device in a child with failing fontan. Ann Thorac Surg 99:707–709
22. Mackling T, Shah T, Dimas V, Guleserian K, Sharma M, Forbess J, Ardura M, Gross-Toalson J, Lee Y, Journeycake J, Barnes A (2012) Management of single-ventricle patients with Berlin heart EXCOR ventricular assist device: single-center experience. Artif Organs 36:555–559
23. Dipchand AI, Mahle WT, Tresler M, Naftel DC, Almond C, Kirklin JK, Pruitt E, Webber SA (2015) Extracorporeal membrane oxygenation as a bridge to pediatric heart transplantation: effect on post-listing and post-transplantation outcomes. Circ Heart Fail 8:960–969

24. Bryant R, Zafar F, Castleberry C, Wilmot I, Jefferies JL, Chin C, Lorts A, Morales DL (2013) Post transplant survival using the berlin heart pediatric ventricular assist device as a bridge to cardiac transplantation. Circulation 128:A15991
25. Cassidy J, Dominguez T, Haynes S, Burch M, Kirk R, Hoskote A, Smith J, Fenton M, Griselli M, Hsia TY, Ferguson L, Van Doorn C, Hasan A, Karimova A (2013) A longer waiting game: bridging children to heart transplant with the Berlin Heart EXCOR device--the United Kingdom experience. J Heart Lung Transplant 32:1101–1106
26. van der Meulen MH, Dalinghaus M, Maat AP, van de Woestijne PC, van Osch M, de Hoog M, Kraemer US, Bogers AJ (2015) Mechanical circulatory support in the dutch national paediatric heart transplantation programme. Eur J Cardiothorac Surg 48:910–916 ; discussion 916
27. Zafar F, Castleberry C, Khan MS, Mehta V, Bryant R, Lorts A, Wilmot I, Jefferies JL, Chin C, Morales DLS (2015) Pediatric heart transplant waiting list mortality in the era of ventricular assist devices. J Heart Lung Transplant 34:82–88
28. Jeewa A, Manlhiot C, McCrindle BW, Van Arsdell G, Humpl T, Dipchand AI (2010) Outcomes with ventricular assist device versus extracorporeal membrane oxygenation as a bridge to pediatric heart transplantation. Artif Organs 34:1087–1091

Ventricular Assist Device Support for Hypoplastic Left Heart Syndrome, Fontan Failure, and End-Stage Systemic Right Ventricular Dysfunction

Fabrizio De Rita, Antonio Amodeo, and Asif Hasan

© Springer International Publishing Switzerland 2017
A. Montalto et al. (eds.), *Mechanical Circulatory Support in End-Stage Heart Failure*,
DOI 10.1007/978-3-319-43383-7_38

38.1 Introduction

The successful treatment of wide-ranging congenital abnormalities by sustained and progressive development in intensive care, cardiology, and congenital cardiac surgery has resulted in burgeoning number of patients who are left with either uncorrectable lesions or heart failure. We now face the hurdle of providing durable, safe, and effective mechanical circulatory support (MCS) to this group. There are several challenges to overcome. Salient among them include anatomical difficulties and avoidance of morbidities associated with previous multiple operations. In addition the presence of high sensitization and worldwide shortage of donor organs would imply that these patients would require prolonged support. These factors contribute toward making these patients a high-risk group not only during but also before transplantation.

It would not be an exaggeration to stipulate that patients with failing single ventricle with its variety of manifestation is the first group which deserves our attention to find a suitable MCS strategy. Secondly, the growing aging population of patients where the morphological failing right ventricle (RV) provides the systemic circulation, after atrial switch operations for transposition of great arteries (TGA) and in palliated variants (physiological repair) of congenitally corrected transposition of the great arteries (ccTGA), is another group where MCS is increasingly being sought.

To follow here is a discussion on technical approach of MCS in failing HLHS circulation, Fontan failure, and end-stage systemic right ventricle dysfunction.

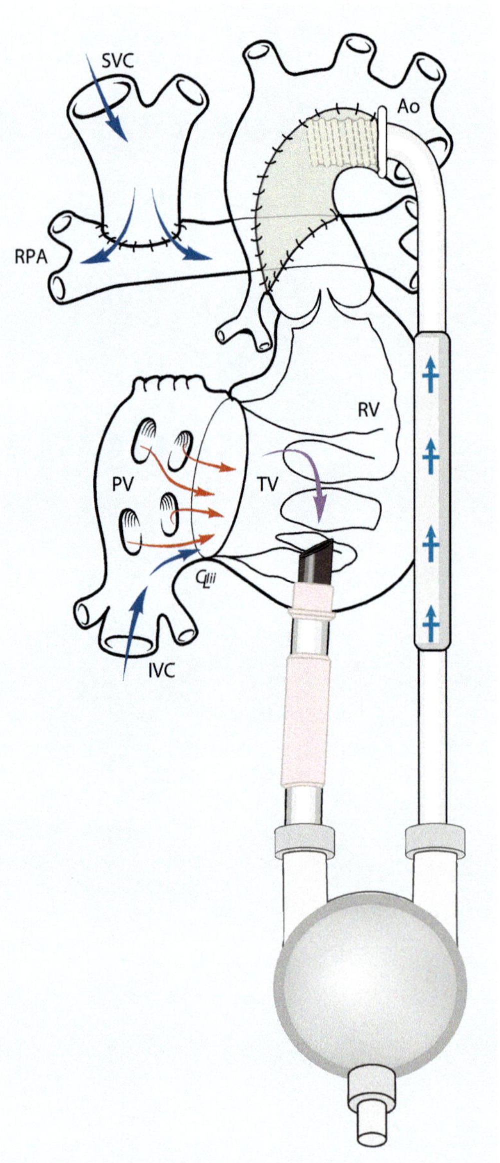

Fig. 38.1 Schematic view of UVAD placement in single ventricle anatomy after first-stage palliation (Norwood with modified BT shunt) of HLHS. The inflow cannula is inserted in the apex of the single right ventricle and the outflow cannula at the level of the Damus-Kaye-Stansel anastomosis, leaving the shunt open to allow the pulmonary circulation. *UVAD* univentricular assist device, *HLHS* hypoplastic left heart syndrome

38.2 VAD for Failing HLHS

The surgical strategy to implant a VAD is adapted to anatomical and hemodynamic variables with two different approaches [1, 2]. A univentricular VAD (UVAD) implantation with Berlin Heart (BH) EXCOR (Berlin Heart, Berlin, Germany) device in surgically palliated HLHS anatomy is displayed in Figs. 38.1 and 38.2. The correct landmark of apical cannulation must be carefully identified, as previous surgical adhesions and coronary abnormalities can distort the anatomy. Right orientation of the inflow cannula to the septum and accurate resection of right single ventricle inner trabeculation are also mandatory for an optimal drainage of the heart. The single systemic atrium can also be used as site for inflow cannulation in case of inadequate drainage with the apical cannula. The outflow cannula placement results are likewise challenging due to the previous surgically reconstructed aorta via Norwood patch and Damus-Kaye-Stansel anastomosis, so that an extension with prosthetic graft can be used to obtain a better alignment and orientation avoiding compression by the sternum. The

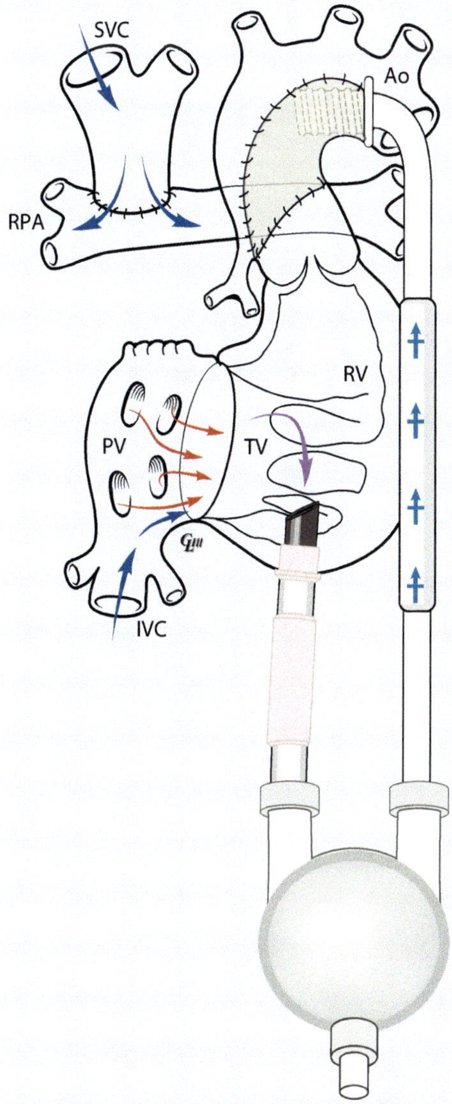

Fig. 38.2 Schematic view of UVAD placement in single ventricle anatomy after second-stage palliation (Glenn circulation) of HLHS. The inflow cannula is inserted in the apex of the single right ventricle and the outflow cannula at the level of the Damus-Kaye-Stansel anastomosis. *UVAD* univentricular assist device, *HLHS* hypoplastic left heart syndrome

pulmonary perfusion is provided either by a systemic to pulmonary shunt, that can be narrowed down to regulate the pulmonary blood flow (Fig. 38.1), or by the bidirectional cavopulmonary Glenn connection already in place (Fig. 38.2).

A biventricular VAD (BiVAD) configuration can also be used using BH EXCOR for HLHS as shown in Fig. 38.3. The fundamental requirement is to create a systemic venous reservoir by joining the superior vena cava to the right atrium and thereafter separating the systemic venous from the pulmonary venous drainage. The left-sided VAD is implanted as described above, and the right-sided VAD is inserted with inflow cannula in the new artificial systemic venous atrium and the outflow cannula in the right pulmonary artery. The systemic to pulmonary shunt is finally ligated or disconnected.

Additional pulmonary artery obstruction, intracardiac shunts, and both atrioventricular and semilunar valve incompetence must be addressed and repaired at time of VAD implantation.

Patients with failing single ventricle are likely to have multiorgan dysfunction before VAD implantation with minimal response to medical treatment and hemodynamic instability with signs of end-organ dysfunction [1–6]. Invasive ventilation and ECMO support are required in nearly 50% of the cases prior to VAD insertion, respiratory failure being the commonest cause of death on MCS. Veno-venous and aortopulmonary collaterals that cause high pulmonary vascular resistance (PVR) must be closed in the first instance to avoid both chronic lung disease and systemic venous hypertension. Pre-existing renal and liver dysfunction is also associated with poor prognosis. Complications related to excessive bleeding are likely to be encountered in these patients and are due to a combination of multiple previous operations and coagulation abnormalities related to multisystem failure.

A palliated HLHS fails due to ventricular dysfunction, elevated pulmonary resistance, or a combination thereof [1, 3]. Horne and colleagues from Edmonton, Canada, rationalized an approach to VAD decision in univentricular circulation based on mechanisms of failure and patient weight (Fig. 38.4). In the setting of primary ventricular dysfunction and normal PVR, standard UVAD may be adequate. A higher flow is required to cope with the increased load of the systemic single ventricle so that, equal to patient's body surface area, a larger BH size pump is often required in shunt and Glenn physiology compared to the predicted left VAD size pump in biventricular circulation [2]. Instead, the presence of high PVR, high-end diastolic pressure, or mixed pathophysiological mechanisms may require the addition of a right-sided VAD ("pushing" pump) to adequately push blood in the pulmonary circulation.

When the single ventricle physiology fails at the early stages of the palliation, the small size of the patients (most likely less than 15 kg) limits the

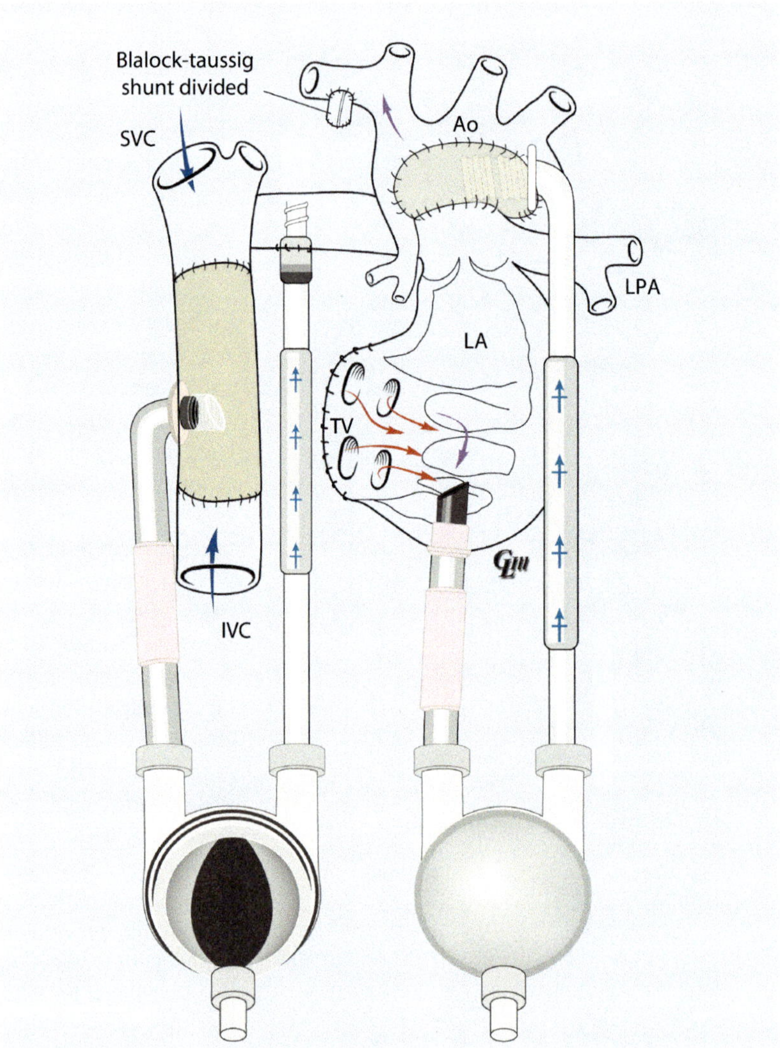

Fig. 38.3 Schematic view of BiVAD placement in single ventricle anatomy after first-stage palliation (Norwood with modified BT shunt) of HLHS. The physiology is converted to a biventricular circulation dividing the systemic venous return from the pulmonary venous return. *BiVAD* biventricular assist device, *HLHS* hypoplastic left heart syndrome

	Systolic dysfunction	Diastolic dysfunction	Increased PVR/fontan failure	Mixed type
	Elevated EDP, low CO	**Elevated EDP, normal CO**	**Elevated CVP, hepatic congestion**	**Elevated CVP + EDP, pulmonary congestion, low CO**
< 15 kg	Para-corporeal pulsatile VAD (systemic ventricle-aortic cannulation)	Extra-corporeal continues flow VAD Para-corporeal pulsatile VAD (atrio-aortic cannulation)	Glenn ± extra-corporeal continuous-flow VAD transitioned to a Para-corporeal pulsatile VAD	Glenn ± extra-corporeal continuous-flow VAD transitioned to a Para-corporeal pulsatile VAD
15-50 kg	Long-term intra-corporeal centrifugal VAD	Long-term intra-corporeal centrifugal VAD	Glenn ± long-term intra-corporeal centrifugal VAD TAH	Glenn ± long-term intra-corporeal centrifugal VAD TAH
> 50 kg	Long-term intra-corporeal axial flow VAD	Long-term intra-corporeal axial flow VAD TAH	Bi-ventricular para-corporeal VAD	Bi-ventricular para-corporeal VAD

Fig. 38.4 Approach to device decision in the univentricular heart based on patient weight and mechanism of failure. *CO* cardiac output, *EDP* end-diastolic pressure, *PVR* pulmonary vascular resistance, *CVP* central venous pressure, *EXCOR* Berlin heart EXCOR, *VAD* ventricular assist device, *TAH* total artificial heart

VAD option to paracorporeal devices, with BH EXCOR and Levitronix (Thoratec Corporation, Pleasanton, CA) pumps providing pulsatile and continuous flow, respectively (Fig. 38.4). The initial connection of CentriMag pump to the BH EXCOR cannulas is strongly recommended in case of transition from ECMO support, allowing the option of adding an oxygenator in the VAD circuit in case of persistent poor lung function [1–4]. In the acute phase, continuous flow is preferable as it can also allow a better unloading of the systemic ventricle, can occur throughout the entire cardiac cycle, and can consequently provide higher flow than pulsatile pumps at the same filling pressure [1, 3–5]. Furthermore, it can reduce pulmonary venous congestion avoiding pulmonary vein blood flow reversal that occurs with a pulsatile device in the absence of a compliant pulmonary venous atrium [1]. Finally, the anticoagulation management results easier in the setting of continuous VAD flow reducing the thromboembolic risk associated with BH EXCOR.

Two large series worldwide, a single institution experience from Newcastle upon Tyne, UK [2], and a multicenter study from the USA [4], demonstrated the feasibility of bridge to transplantation MCS in single ventricle physiology, using the combination of BH EXCOR, Levitronix, and ECMO. However, the success is limited compared to the congenital biventricular pediatric MCS population, with decreased overall survival to transplantation or VAD explantation. The complex anatomical and physiological nature of single ventricle in infants still remains a challenging proposition. In fact it could be argued that patients undergoing successful transplantation in these cohorts were lucky to have received a donor organ in a relatively short period of time, with none of the survivors mechanically assisted for longer than 21 days. Cerebrovascular events, bleeding, infective and multiorgan failure complications [2, 4, 6], and requirement of ECMO-type circulation post-VAD implantation due to persisent respiratory dysfunction are harbingers of adverse prognostic factors for death during MCS [2].

38.3 VAD for Fontan Failure

The interplay of various cardiovascular factors leading to failure of Fontan circulation is highlighted in Fig. 38.5 [7]. The Fontan failure is either due to

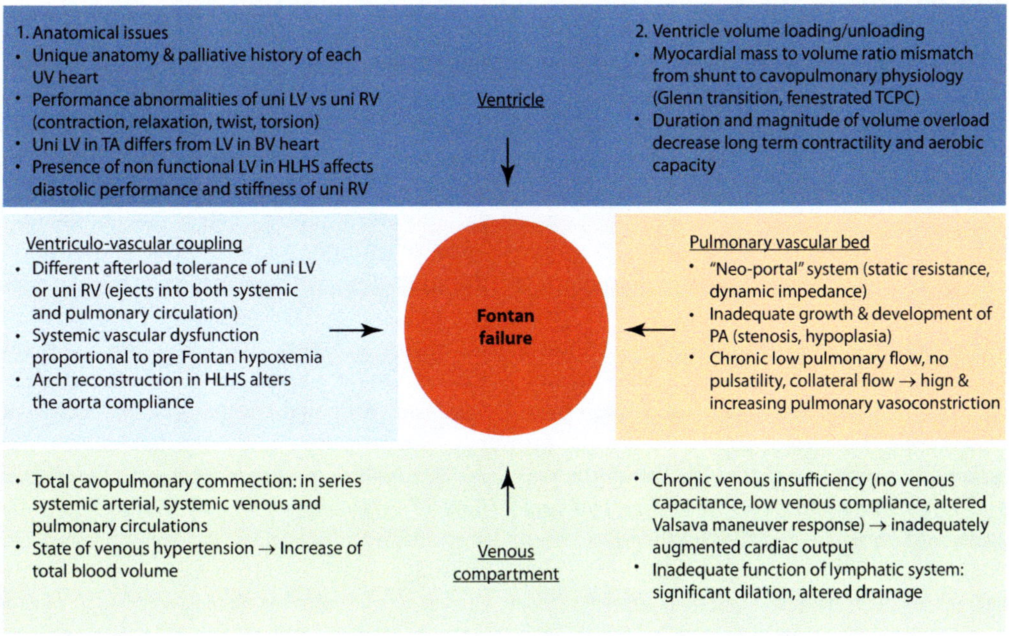

Fig. 38.5 Cardiovascular system components and alterations in failing Fontan circulation. *UV* univentricular, *BV* biventricular, *LV* left ventricle, *RV* right ventricle, *TCPC* total cavopulmonary connection, *HLHS* hypoplastic left heart syndrome, *PA* pulmonary artery (Reprinted with permission of De Rita et al. [7])

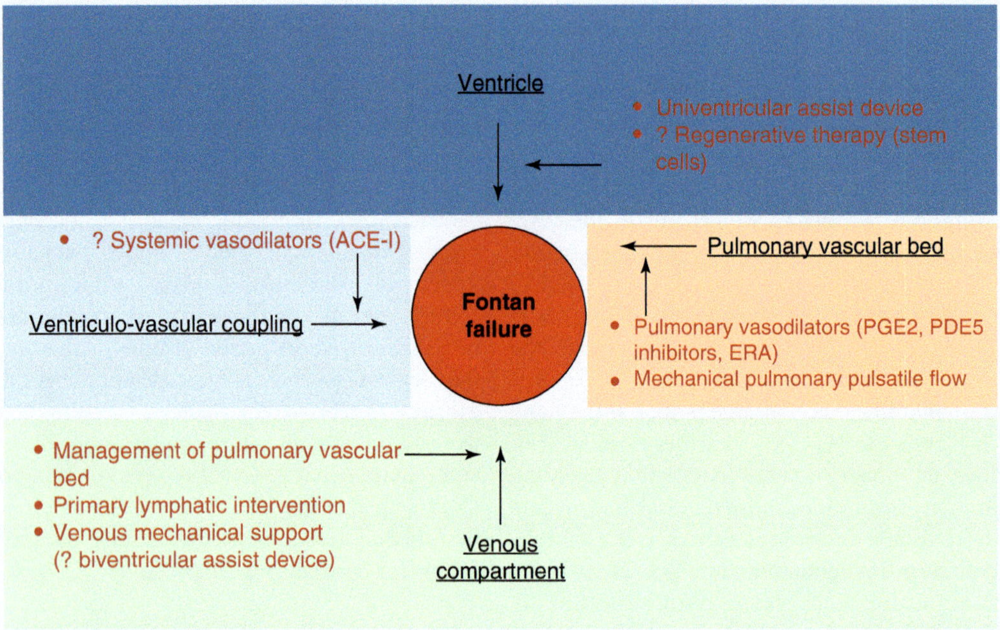

Fig. 38.6 Represents the wide spectrum of tools at our disposal to achieve this (Reprinted with permission of De Rita et al. [7])

ventricular dysfunction or as a consequence of failure of the Fontan circulation with preserved ventricular function. The principle of management of Fontan failure is to prolong the state of Fontan circulation and make these patients better candidates for heart transplantation. A wide variety of medical, catheter-based, or surgical intervention including MCS (Fig. 38.6) represents the wide spectrum of tools at our disposal to achieve this.

As general presumption, the identification of predominant etiology of failure may direct the most suitable approach to mechanically support the circulation (Fig. 38.4). A standard "pulling" left-sided UVAD with ventricle to aorta connection may be adequate to unload the systemic single ventricle and decrease Fontan pressure in case of isolated or combined systolic and diastolic dysfunction [1, 3, 8, 9]. When the elevated systemic venous pressure is mainly a consequence of unusually isolated high PVR without evident pump failure, a single "pushing" right-sided system can be established to support only the pulmonary circulation, with surgical construction of a new venous reservoir joining the venae cavae to allow VAD filling and restitution of blood to the pulmonary arteries via the disconnected Fontan conduit (Fig. 38.7) [10]. The BiVAD configuration is instead reasonable in case of the mixed mechanism of failure where the use of a single "pushing" UVAD might cause pulmonary congestion if a "pulling" system is not used in combination [11].

The feasibility and outcome of MCS support in Fontan failure remain largely anecdotal [8–11], with just single reports described. Fontan-failing patients are commonly bigger size children, adolescents, and young adults, allowing the option to use adult-designed implantable devices in pediatric population (Fig. 38.4). Third-generation HeartMate II (Thoratec Corporation, Pleasanton, CA) axial-flow pump and the HeartWare (Heart ware Inc., Framingham, MA) centrifugal devices have been successfully reported as UVAD in Fontan failure pediatric patients. Continuous-flow UVADs compared to pulsatile flow pumps seem to promote a more favorable unloading of the single ventricle and a more significant decrease of systemic venous pressure avoiding the pulmonary congestion [1]. When both systemic and pulmonary circulation requires mechanical support, a pulsatile paracorporeal BiVAD with separate BH EXCOR pumps can be established as

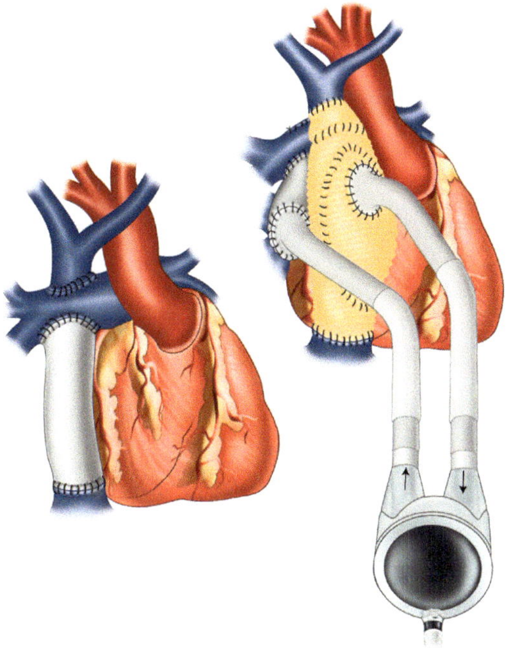

Fig. 38.7 Schematic view of the implantation of the Berlin Heart on the right circulation. *Left* sketch shows the cavopulmonary anastomosis and the extracardiac conduit. *Right* sketch shows the implantation of the arterial cannula in the proximal stump of the extracardiac conduit, the capacity chamber created with an enlarging patch, and the connection of the superior vena cava in the capacity chamber with enlargement patch. The venous cannula is inserted in the capacity chamber. Both cannulas are brought percutaneously and connected to a paracorporeal ventricle

previously described. To date, total artificial heart implantation (SynCardia, Tucson, AZ) for failing Fontan adults or children has not been reported, but the recent introduction in the market of the 50 ml device may allow implant of intracorporeal biventricular system in a pediatric population, provided first the construction of an adequate systemic venous chamber to accommodate the SynCardia inflow sewing cuff.

38.4 VAD for End-Stage Systemic RV Dysfunction

Systemic RV failure usually appears late after previous physiological repair (Mustard or Senning operation) of TGA and in individuals with ccTGA, in whom their size allows the use of intracorporeal devices. Third-generation continuous-flow pumps have been increasingly implanted in the last decade to support the failing systemic RV either as bridge to transplantation (in patients too sick to wait for a suitable donor) or as bridge to decision (where immediate listing was not possible) [12–14]. Indication to VAD implant takes place when medical treatments and surgical and interventional procedure do not improve heart failure symptoms, not infrequently with patient on inotropic support and mechanically ventilated experiencing biventricular dysfunction. Therefore, the concomitant pre-, peri- and post-procedural optimization of the sub-pulmonic ventricular function is crucial to achieve MCS just of the systemic ventricle.

VAD implantation requires mild hypothermic cardiopulmonary bypass preferentially via bicaval cannulation (mandatory in the presence of intracardiac shunt and previous atrial baffle) and venting of the left heart [12]. Device implantation can be performed on a beating heart or inducing ventricular fibrillation, with cardioplegic arrest established when a concomitant systemic atrioventricular or semilunar (aortic) valve operation and intracardiac shunt repair are required.

The implantation of ventricular assist device is facilitated by the loss of tripartite configuration of systemic right ventricle. However, there could be difficulties related to the presence of trabeculae in the body of morphological right ventricle. The choice of the optimal device implantation site must be carefully evaluated, by using intraoperative transesophageal echocardiography and most appropriately with the heart still full before going on cardiopulmonary bypass, if possible [12].

The device is then inserted to the inferior diaphragmatic surface of the morphologic RV free wall. Resection of an adequate amount of coarse muscle trabeculation, muscle bands, and obstructive chordae is mandatory to prevent obstruction to the inflow cannula. Figure 38.8 illustrates the anatomical constraints of the inflow placement in TGA and ccTGA anatomies [13]. Figure 38.9 instead shows HeartWare position at chest radiogram in TGA (rightward systemic morphologic RV) and ccTGA (leftward systemic morphologic RV) variants [12].

The outflow graft is normally sutured in end-to-side fashion to the ascending aorta. Multiple previous operations might have produced dense adhesions to first of all compel peripheral cannulation for cardiopulmonary bypass and to also

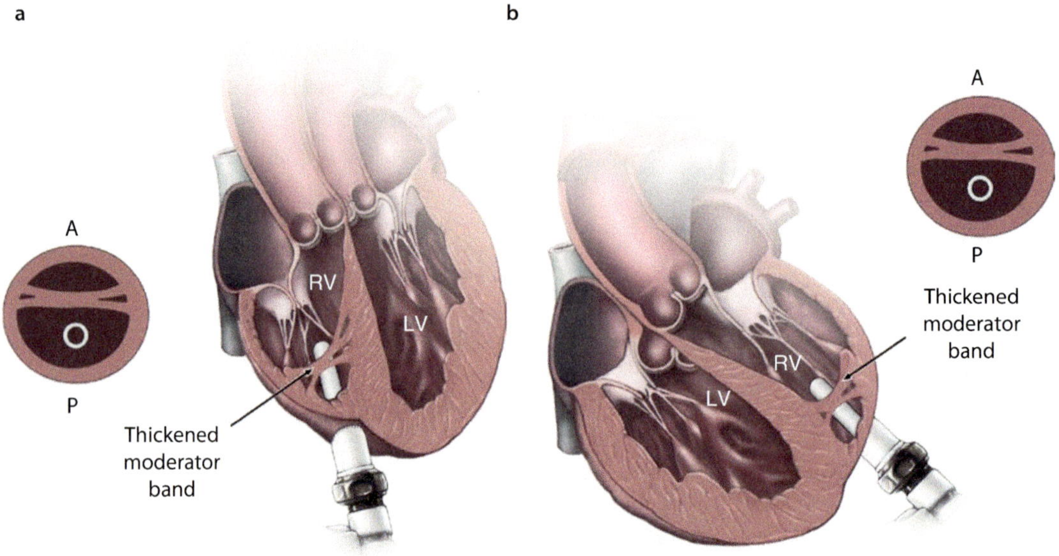

Fig. 38.8 Anatomic challenges associated with ventricular assist device implantation in a morphologic RV. *RV* right ventricle, *LV* left ventricle. (**a**) Transposition of the great arteries. (**b**) Congenitally corrected transposition of the great arteries (Reprinted with permission of Joyce et al. [13])

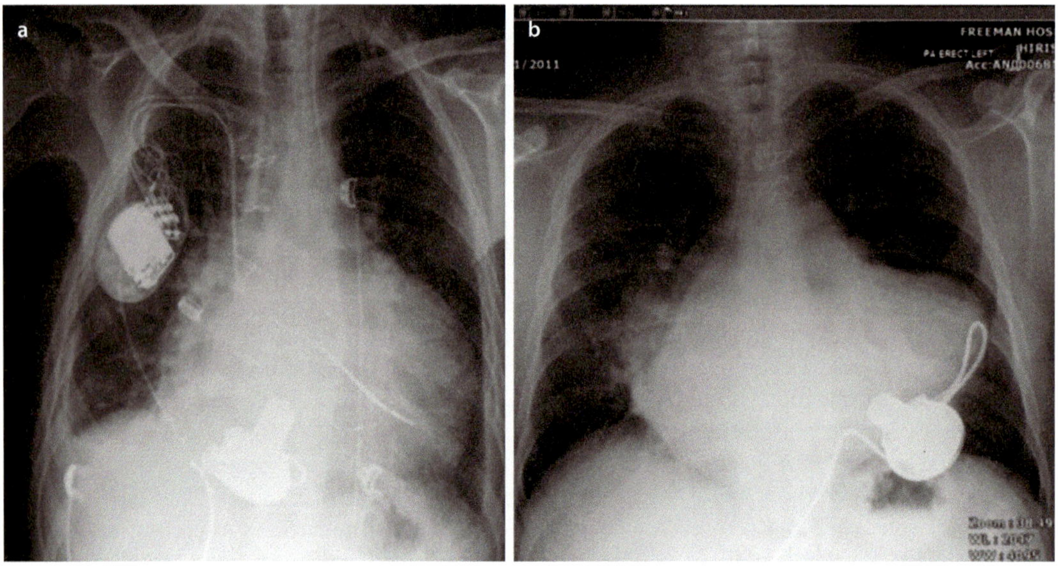

Fig. 38.9 (**a**) A chest radiogram after HeartWare implantation for a patient with Mustard operation for TGA with an intact septum. The device was inserted to the inferior surface of the rightward, systemic, morphologic RV. (**b**) A chest radiogram after HeartWare implantation in a patient with ccTGA. The device was inserted to the inferior surface of the leftward, systemic, morphologic RV. *TGA* transposition of the great arteries, *RV* right ventricle, *ccTGA* congenitally corrected transposition of the great arteries (Reprinted with permission of Peng et al. [12])

preclude easy access for graft placement to the ascending aorta. The outflow graft can be then sutured onto the innominate artery that can be safely reached via extended suprasternal notch incision, even before sternotomy completion [12].

In addition to several anecdotal reports from the USA [13, 14], our group in Newcastle upon Tyne, UK, recently published the largest series of VAD support for failing systemic morphologic RV, showing the durability and effectiveness and safety of third-generation device implantation as both bridge to transplantation and bridge to decision [12]. However, the challenge to provide MCS in this growing sick population is not free from risks, with bleeding, thrombosis, and sepsis as the most represented, even if the overall outcome does not appear to differ from our experience with HeartWare support in non-congenital population.

None of our patients required BiVAD implantation and this is borne out by experience of others. One can argue that a left morphologic sub-pulmonic ventricle is stronger and more durable without the need of mechanical support. Most importantly, the accurate strategy adopted to optimize the sub-pulmonic ventricular function resulted essential in our experience [12]. All patients received aggressive dehydration with diuretics (and elective hemofiltration if required) with or without combination inotropic therapy (most commonly milrinone) prior to VAD implantation, aiming a target central venous pressure of less than 10 mm Hg. Measures to protect the sub-pulmonic ventricle before and after cardiopulmonary bypass weaning were considered, including nitric oxide inhalation and continuous measurement of pulmonary artery pressure. Finally, the use of newer generation continuous-flow devices used as a left-sided VAD seems to perform better than the pulsatile pumps in assisting the pulmonary circulation; they have the ability to unload the systemic ventricle during the entire cardiac cycle, thus reducing end-diastolic pressure and avoiding pulmonary congestion. In case of early left ventricular dysfunction, a temporary addition of less invasive sub-pulmonic Levitronix VAD to allow right-sided ventricle recovery always remains a fallback option. This is usually achieved with percutaneous cannulation of the right jugular vein for the right heart drainage and return of blood in the pulmonary circulation using a graft sutured to pulmonary artery and tunneled through the chest wall anteriorly (◘ Figs. 38.10 and 38.11). This approach allows weaning and decanulation of the sub-pulmonic VAD with minimal anesthesia and without chest reopening.

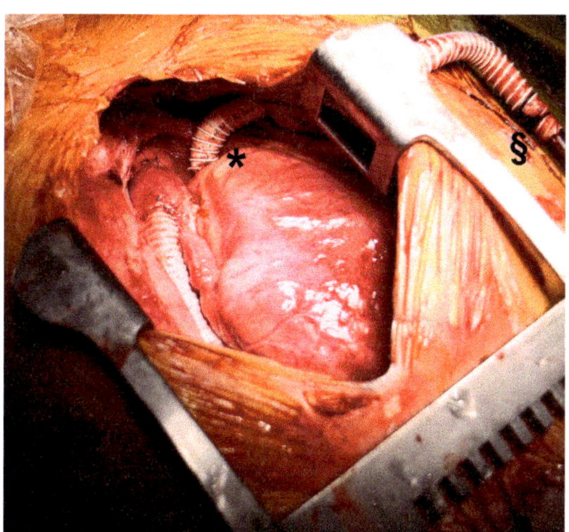

◘ **Fig. 38.10** Surgical view of an intraoperative right-sided VAD pulmonary arterial cannulation in the setting of a HeartWare implantation. (§) The outflow cannula stays outside the chest and is inserted in a graft previously anastomosed to the pulmonary artery (*) and tunneled throughout the skin. *VAD* ventricular assist device

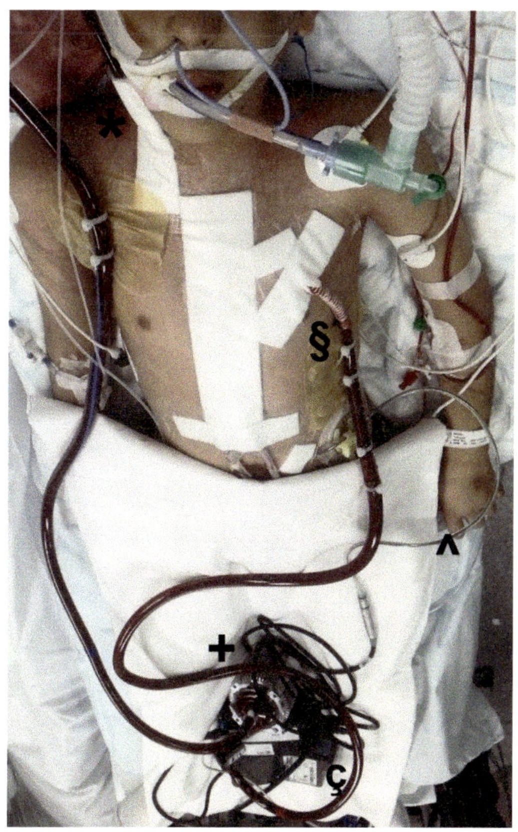

◘ **Fig. 38.11** Postoperative view after implantation of a HeartWare device and a temporary Levitronix right-sided VAD. (*) Percutaneously inserted Levitronix inflow cannula in the right jugular vein, (§) Levitronix outflow cannula inserted in the graft outside the chest, (+) Levitronix pump, (ç) HeartWare transport console and batteries, and (^) HeartWare driveline. VAD, ventricular assist device

As already mentioned, the competence of the systemic atrioventricular and aortic valves and absence of intracardiac shunts are mandatory before HeartWare implantation. The status of aortic valve following implantation of continuous-flow pumps has been a cause for concern. We noticed de novo aortic regurgitation in two out of the seven patients receiving MCS. In one patient aortic valve replacement was eventually undertaken.

References

1. Horne D, Conway J, Rebeyka IM et al (2015) Mechanical circulatory support in univentricular heart: current management. Semin Thorac Cardiovasc Surg Pediatr Card Surg Annu 18(1):17–24
2. De Rita F, Hasan A, Haynes S et al (2014) Mechanical cardiac support in children with congenital heart disease with intention to bridge to heart transplantation. Eur J Cardiothorac Surg 46(4):656–662
3. Kirklin JK, Bennett Pearce F, Dabal RJ et al (2014) Mechanical circulatory support: strategies and outcomes in pediatric congenital heart disease. Semin Thorac Cardiovasc Surg Pediatr Card Surg Annu 17(1):62–68
4. Weinstein S, Bello R, Pizarro C et al (2014) The use of the Berlin Heart EXCOR in patients with functional single ventricle. J Thorac Cardiovasc Surg 147:697–705
5. VanderPluym CJ, Rebeyka IM, Ross DB et al (2011) The use of ventricular assist devices in pediatric patients with univentricular hearts. J Thorac Cardiovasc Surg 141:588–590
6. Brancaccio G, Gandolfo F, Carotti A et al (2013) Ventricular assist device in univentricular heart physiology. Interact Cardiovasc Thorac Surg 16(4):568–569
7. De Rita F, Crossland D, Griselli M et al (2015) Management of the failing Fontan. Semin Thorac Cardiovasc Surg Pediatr Card Surg Annu 18(1):2–6
8. Niebler RA, Ghanayem NS, Shah TK et al (2014) Use of a HeartWare ventricular assist device in a patient with failed Fontan circulation. Ann Thorac Surg 97(4):e115–e116
9. Morales DL, Adachi I, Heinle JS et al (2011) A new era: use of an intracorporeal systemic ventricular assist device to support a patient with a failing Fontan circulation. J Thorac Cardiovasc Surg 142:e138–e140
10. Prêtre R, Häussler A, Bettex D et al (2008) Right-sided univentricular cardiac assistance in a failing Fontan circulation. Ann Thorac Surg 86:1018–1020
11. VanderPluym CJ, Khoo NS, Rebeyka IM (2013) Unique case of total artificial cardiac support in failed Fontan circulation after cardiectomy: is continuous flow better than pulsatile flow? J Thorac Cardiovasc Surg 145:e62–e63
12. Peng E, O'Sullivan JJ, Griselli M et al (2014) Durable ventricular assist device support for failing systemic morphologic right ventricle: early results. Ann Thorac Surg 98(6):2122–2129
13. Joyce DL, Crow SS, John R et al (2010) Mechanical circulatory support in patients with heart failure secondary to transposition of the great arteries. J Heart Lung Transplant 29:1302–1305
14. Shah NR, Lam WW, Rodriguez FH 3rd et al (2013) Clinical outcomes after ventricular assist device implantation in adults with complex congenital heart disease. J Heart Lung Transplant 32(6):615–620

Continuous-Flow Pumps in Infants, Jarvik Infant System, and Destination Therapy in Pediatrics

Antonio Amodeo, Sergio Filippelli, Arianna Di Molfetta, Gianluigi Perri, and R. Jarvik

© Springer International Publishing Switzerland 2017
A. Montalto et al. (eds.), *Mechanical Circulatory Support in End-Stage Heart Failure*,
DOI 10.1007/978-3-319-43383-7_39

39.1 Introduction

The need for long-term mechanical support in the pediatric population has been recognized for many years. Annually, about 300–500 pediatric heart transplants are performed worldwide, but many more could be done if donors were available. The US National Institutes of Health (NIH) estimates that in the USA there are ~1800 infant deaths from congenital heart defects annually and several hundred additional pediatric patients under 5 years old who develop heart failure. Left ventricular assist devices (LVADs) in pediatrics are frequently implanted as a bridge to transplantation (BTT) and rarely for recovery or as destination therapy (DT). The number of pediatric patients suffering from end-stage heart failure is continuously increasing, and assisting smallest ones in a long-term strategy remains an unsolved problem. This is mainly because today only one-labeled VAD is available for neonates and infants, namely, the Berlin Heart EXCOR (BHE) that is a paracorporeal pulsatile pneumatic-driven system. This has substantially limited the system's portability which has been a barrier to hospital discharge. BHE is a second-generation device, and neurological complications vary between 25 and 30% with a survival rate approaching 80% [1–4].

On the other side, there are teenagers with Duchenne muscular dystrophy (DMD) with end-stage cardiomyopathy who are not eligible for orthotropic heart transplant (OHTx) but can be addressed for VAD as destination therapy [5–8].

In these two settings, the development of new assisting devices is strongly required, and here we present an overview of the state of the art of the infant Jarvik continuous-flow pump and the use of VAD as DT in pediatrics.

39.2 Continuous-Flow Pump

Blood pump miniaturization has made an amazing progress, reducing pump diameter to one-tenth the size of previous positive displacement pumps. In particular, axial-flow pump technology allows tiny pumps running at high speed to deliver from 2 to 10 L/min.

The Jarvik 2000® (Jarvik Heart Inc.®, NY, USA) Ventricular Assist System development began in 1987 and has been refined over the last 25 years [9, 10]. It is a continuous-flow pump allocated inside the left ventricle close to the apex. The blood flows into the device and then forced by a magnetically driven axial rotor into a tubular graft anastomosed to the ascending aorta. The pump has only one moving component: the rotor containing a permanent magnet of a brushless direct current motor and an axial flow impeller. The rotor is supported by ceramic bearings and floats into the bloodstream.

The impeller is powered by electromagnetic fields across the motor "air gap," through which the blood flows. The flow provided by the pump depends on the pump speed set by the operator and on the pressure drop across the pump.

39.3 Infant Jarvik

In 2004 NIH initiated the PumpKIN program (Pumps for Kids, Infants, and Neonates) to develop mechanical support systems for pediatric patients. Jarvik Heart proposed miniaturization of the adult Jarvik 2000, which had achieved patient support over 3 years at the time, with excellent quality of life.

Under the NIH contract that Jarvik Heart was awarded, child- and infant-size blood pumps were designed as closely as possible to the successful adult Jarvik 2000 system. The new pumps appeared to be direct scale-down versions of the adult model, but actually required redesign of almost every component part. The physiological requirements for children included lower flow, but not lower outflow pressure. If we were to scale down the pump size without changing blade geometry, and were to operate the pumps close to the presently used speed in rpm, the pumps would produce insufficient pressure. If we were to increase the speed to maintain the necessary pressure, with the same blade shapes, the matching of motor peak efficiency and torque with pump requirements would not be optimized, the system efficiency would be poor, and hemolysis would be high. In the smaller pumps, the flow channels become very small, and the fluid interactions based on surface roughness and boundary layer effects are more pronounced (Fig. 39.1).

There were also a number of practical manufacturing considerations including the high precision required to maintain very close tip clearances in the axial pump designs. Some parts must have

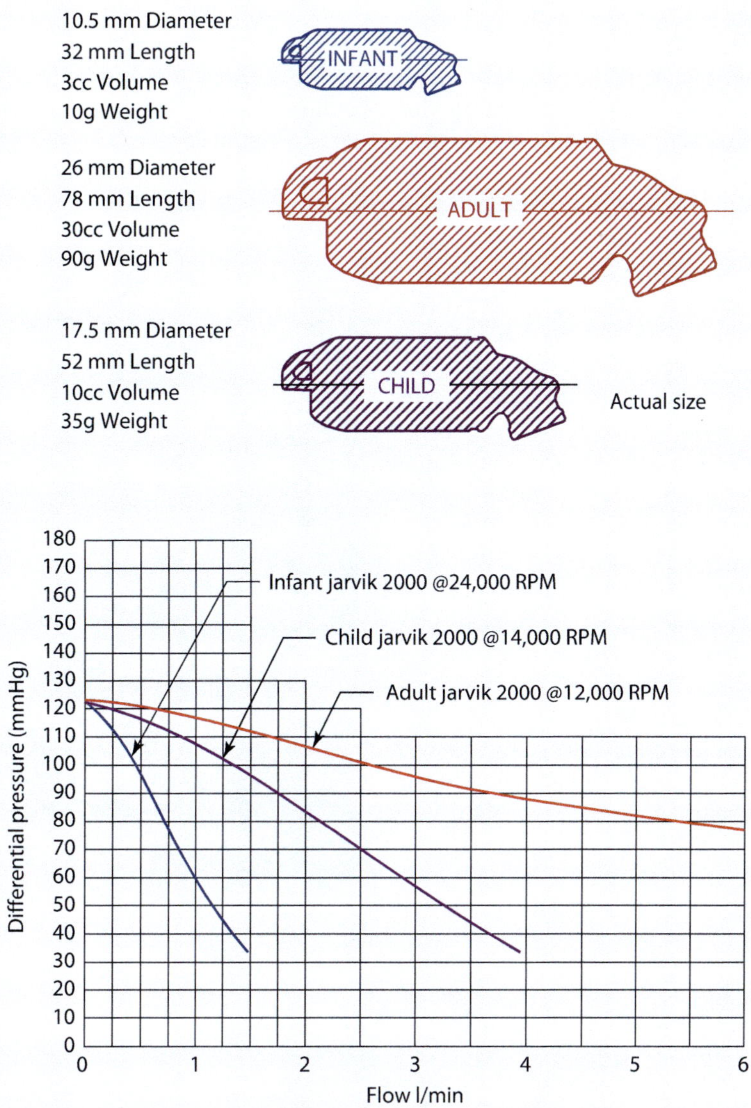

Fig. 39.1 Projected characteristics of infant and child size pumps based on the adult Jarvik 2000

very thin wall sections. Machining methods and quality assurance were critical to success.

The approach we used was to calculate motor power requirements based on reasonable assumptions about pump and motor size and efficiency, design the motor for peak efficiency at the nominal pump operating point, and seek to maximize motor efficiency within the physical size constraints of the planned device layout and available battery voltage. Only last after most of the physical dimensions of the device had been determined, did we optimize the blade shapes. Our approach to optimization of the blade shapes for the proposed pediatric pumps utilized CFD methods much more than we had done previously with the adult model. The initial blade designs were based on two-dimensional theory, but also used three-dimensional CAD modeling of the blade and flow channel shapes and CFD modeling to identify high shear regions, areas of potential stasis and thrombus formation, and to predict pump hemolysis.

Using data available from the adult model Jarvik 2000, and the many small pumps we have tested, we made initial calculations to establish the sizes of the child and infant models. Major hydrodynamic parameters that determine pump flow and pressure including the rotor hub and tip velocity and the cross-sectional area of the flow path through the blade system were selected. The child and infant models keep the hub and tip velocity almost the same as with the adult model and reduced the cross-sectional flow area in proportion to the lower flow requirements. This established the physical dimensions of the motor, by establishing the motor ID and OD and the motor air gap dimension through which the blood flows. The speed and torque requirements of the motor are determined by the required impeller tip velocity and the required output power of the motor. With these values known, the motors were designed using computer modeling techniques.

The infant pump that we developed was 11 mm diameter, small enough to fit a newborn, but this proved to be too small to achieve enough flow for infants over 10 kg, unless speed was increased to 32,000 rpm (◘ Fig. 39.2).

We submitted our animal data together with extensive other design and validation data for the infant Jarvik 2000 system to the FDA. The agency informed us that the hemolysis that occurred was unacceptably high, and the condition of the in vivo animals was not good enough for approval. At that speed the pump produced excessive hemolysis, so after extensive efforts to lower hemolysis using redesigned pump blades, we abandoned the 11 mm design.

We decided to optimize the design with CFD studies done by Dr. Jingchun Wu of Advanced Design Optimization, LLC. Jarvik Heart provided a 3D CAD model of the 11 mm pump and Dr. Wu analyzed it (◘ Fig. 39.3).

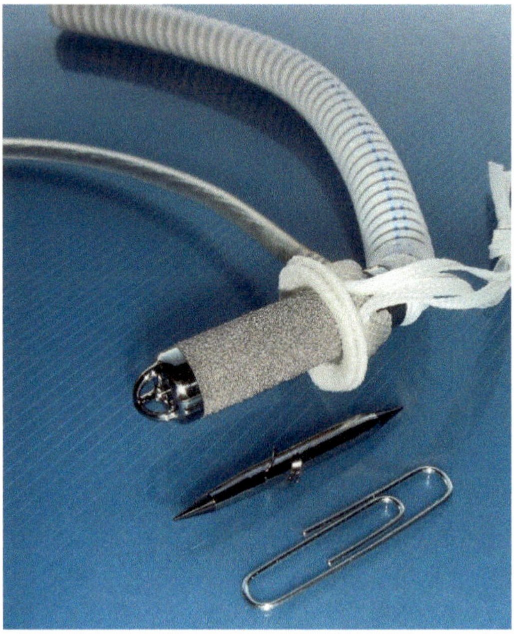

◘ **Fig. 39.2** Infant Jarvik 11 mm

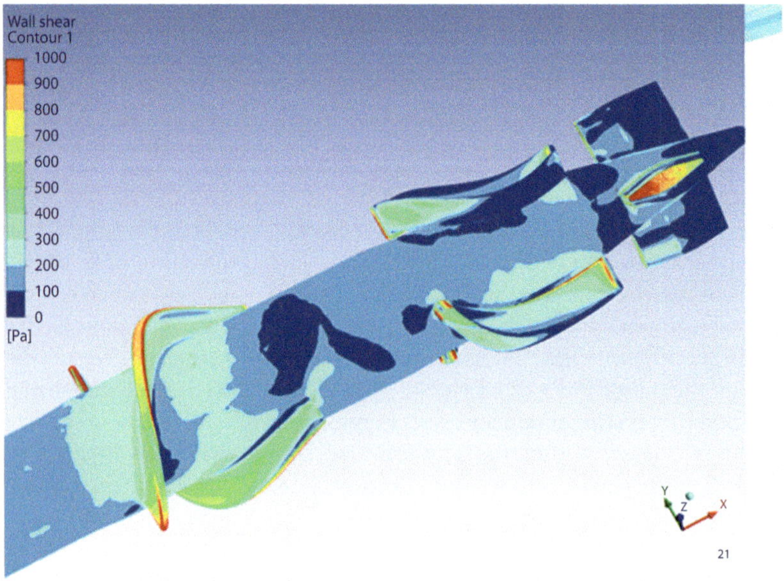

◘ **Fig. 39.3** The model predicted that the highest shear would occur at the blade tips and gaps between stationary and rotating components

We postulated that much of the hemolysis might be originating from the bearings at the high speeds, which were needed to obtain sufficient flow and pressure from the 11 mm design. We fabricated pumps that had no impeller blades and no stator blades. Thus the only sites of high shear that remained were the gaps between the rotating conical ceramic bearing shaft and the tips of the supporting posts. Hemolysis caused by the bearings increased substantially at speeds above 18,000 rpm and at 30,000 rpm would be too high as confirmed by normalized index of hemolysis (NIH) and in vivo experiments.

To keep the speed as low as possible, we decided to increase the diameter of the pump from 11 to 15 mm, named infant Jarvik 2015 (◘ Fig. 39.4a, b). This proved to be a major improvement.

Increasing the diameter of the pump increases the cross-sectional area of the flow path, reduces resistance, and increases flow. Increasing the diameter also increases the tip speed at a given rotational speed, which allows the pump to operate at a lower speed for a given pressure. Lower speed permits the pump to avoid blood damage caused by high shear at the bearings. The new pump gave an excellent flow from .5 to 3 L/min at a maximum speed of 18,000 rpm with an NIH (normalized index of hemolysis) <.05 g/100 L and good pressure/flow curves (◘ Fig. 39.5) and proper power consumption (◘ Fig. 39.6).

In vivo tests are now under way with the infant Jarvik 2015. To date we have conducted three non-GLP implants in 20–30 kg sheep, sacrificed at 30 days. The animals showed low hemolysis.

Additionally we have begun a series of GLP animals for 60-day survival. Since these animal experiments are still under way at the time of writing this chapter, details are unavailable, but in general the hemolysis is low, and the animal's condition has been excellent except in

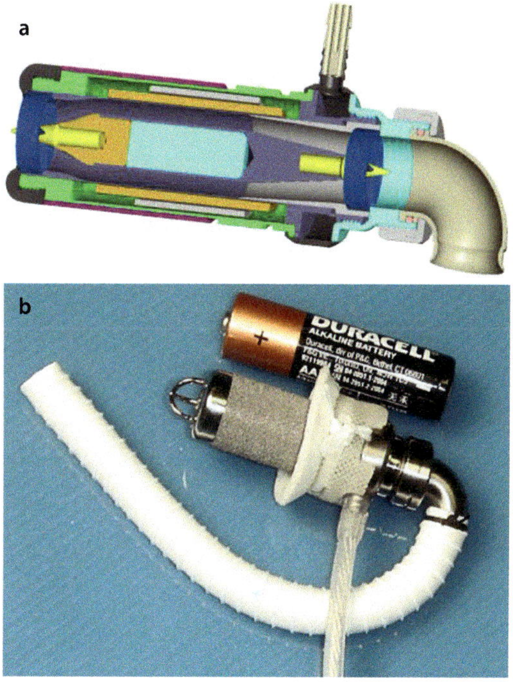

◘ **Fig. 39.4** **a** Sectioned view of the infant Jarvik 2015 blood pump with adjustable outflow elbow. **b** The final design infant Jarvik 2015

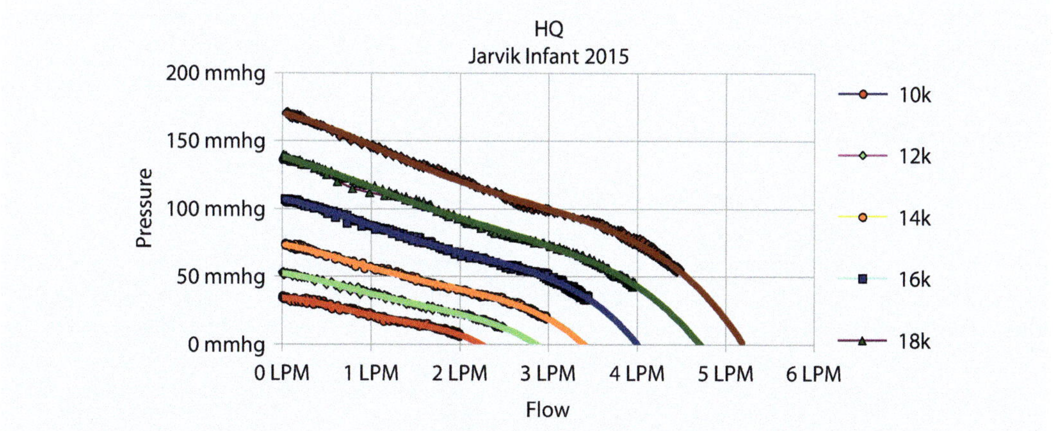

◘ **Fig. 39.5** Flow/pressure curves show that the device can pump up to 3 L/min at 18,000 rpm

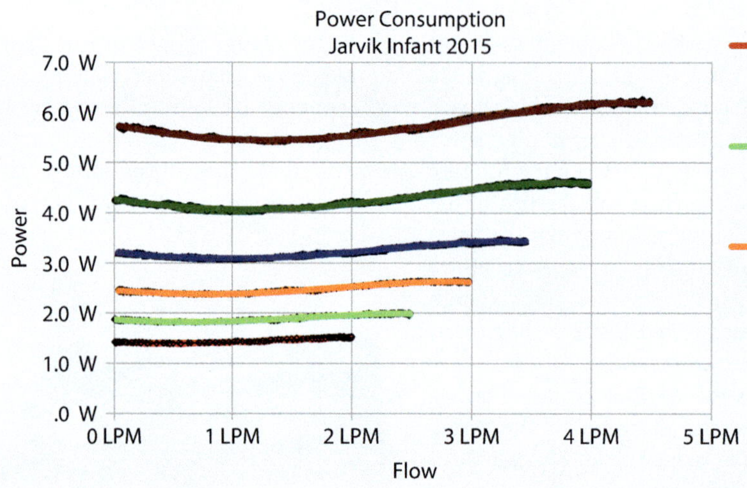

Fig. 39.6 Power consumption remains below 5 watts for speeds up to 18,000 rpm

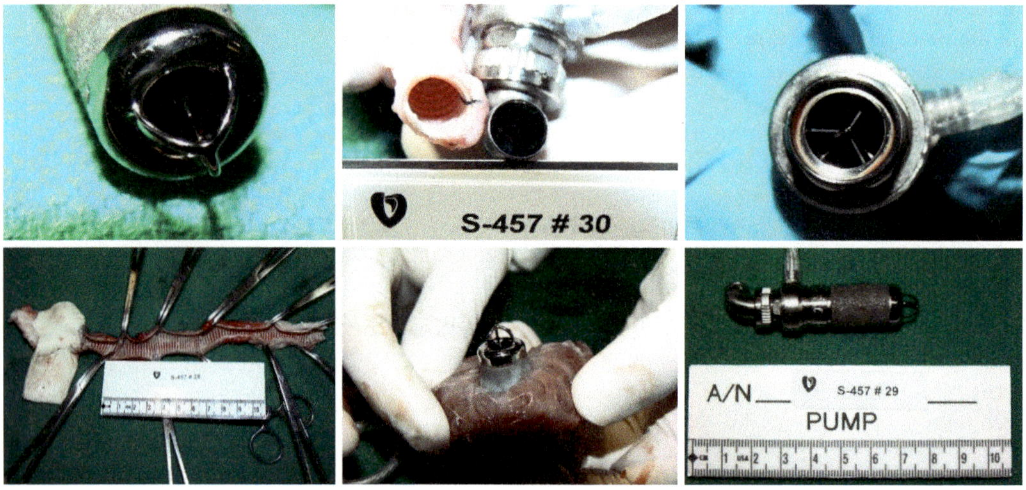

Fig. 39.7 Clockwise from *upper left*: clean inflow cage and bearing, clean outflow elbow, clean outflow bearing, clean outflow graft, microsphere housing well healed to the endocardial tissue, pump removed from the heart. This pump is typical of all of the infant Jarvik 2015 pumps implanted up to 60 days

two cases of surgical problems unrelated to the pump.

Plasma Hb values were mostly below 5–10 mg/dl. There was no thrombus in the pumps or grafts. The kidneys and other organs were free of infarcts (Fig. 39.7). Most animals were healthy, appeared normal, and were free of any serious pump-related problems. Lab values were also essentially normal and unremarkable.

FDA approval is still ongoing and the procedure will be over at the end of August 2016. Once the FDA approval will be gained, the clinical trial will be started within 2016.

Clinical Experience

The infant Jarvik pump (11 mm) was used at Bambino Gesù Hospital in Rome for a compassionate use in a 1-year-old male affected by an idiopathic dilated cardiomyopathy in 2012. Patient was preliminary treated implanting a 10 ml Berlin Heart EXCOR LVAD when the patient was 11 months old with a weight of 5 kg.

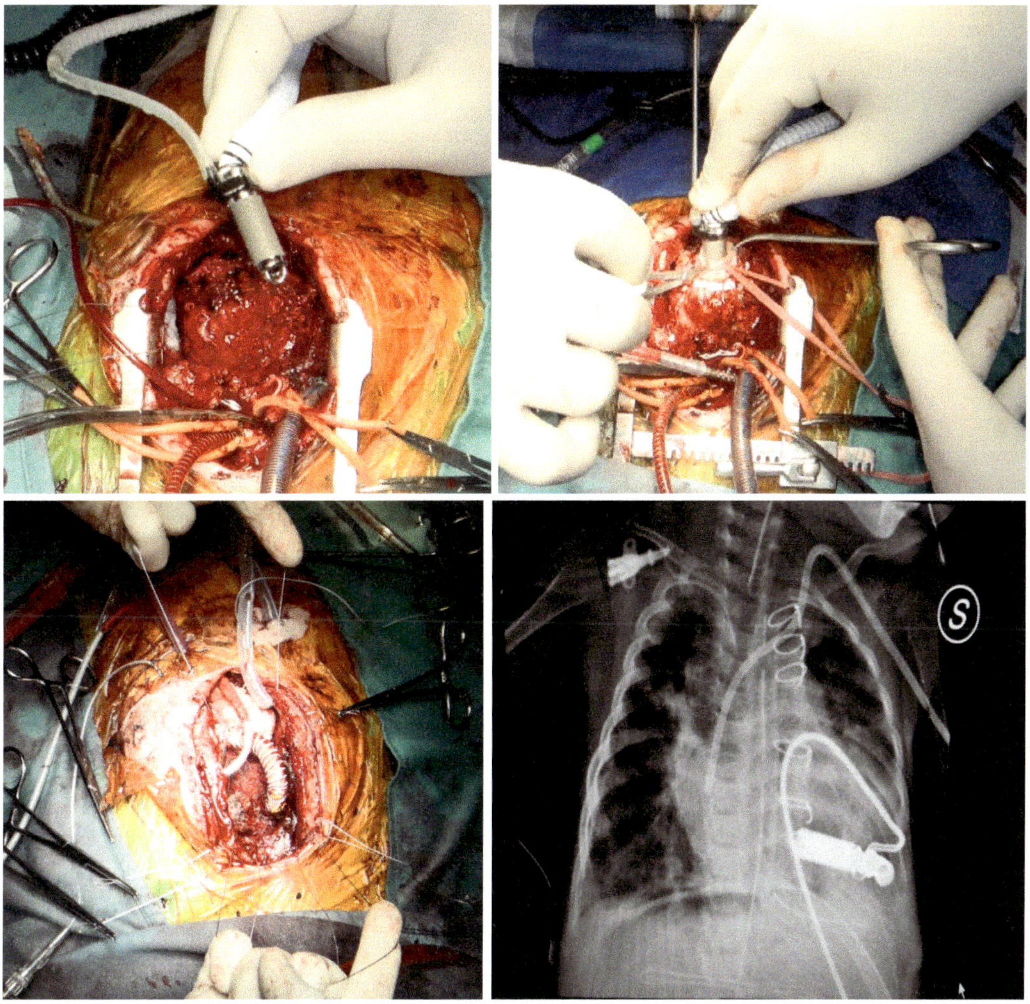

Fig. 39.8 Implantation of an infant Jarvik in a 1-year-old patient

Patient was supported for 123 days. Finally, he experienced severe Berlin Heart EXCOR cannula infection leading to mediastinitis and requiring the device explantation. He was on LVAD (Levitronix) from the left atrium to the ascending aorta for 25 days with sternum open and mediastinal irrigation. Therefore, for compassionate use, the patient was treated implanting an infant Jarvik pump (Fig. 39.8). After 13 days during battery exchange, the pump stopped, for a pump electric blackout, and it was back on ECMO. In the meantime the patient recovered from the infection, and 7 days later it was possible to implant another 10 ml Berlin Heart EXCOR LVAD. After 20 days, the patient underwent successfully Heart Transplantation, and he is currently alive 4 years after heart transplant.

39.4 VAD as Destination Therapy in Pediatrics

A merging matter of debate is the treatment of teenagers suffered from end-stage cardiac failure not eligible for cardiac transplant due to the shorten expectancy of life related to the primary disease such as Duchenne's patients and other form of muscular dystrophies. End-stage dilated cardiomyopathy (DCM) is currently one of the most challenging elements in the management of patients affected by Duchenne muscular dystrophy. DCM is a complication of DMD and leads to advanced heart failure and premature death. Until the last decade, cardiomyopathy in Duchenne muscular dystrophy accounted for only 20% of deaths because respiratory failure occurred earlier than cardiac failure [11]. Due to recent technological advances, respiratory care has greatly improved, and life expectancy has increased to 30–40 years. The efficacy of standard heart failure treatment for improving the clinical outcome of these patients has been proven, but more than 40% will die of heart failure. Duchenne syndrome has generally been considered a contraindication for cardiac transplantation due to the associated progressive skeletal myopathy leading to limited functional capacity [6]. This concern has resulted in a reluctance to offer cardiac transplantation to these patients in an era of donor shortage. The recent advances in left ventricular assist devices, used as destination therapy, have made feasible the use of such devices for the treatment of DCM in Duchenne patients [7, 8, 12].

Cardiac Evaluation in DMD The early detection of DMD cardiomyopathy is relevant, since the institution of cardioprotective medical therapies may slow adverse cardiac remodeling and attenuate HF symptoms. Baseline assessments of the cardiac involvement should be performed first at the age of 6 years and once every 2 years until the age of 10. Annual complete cardiac assessments should begin at the age of 10 years or at the onset of cardiac signs and symptoms if they occur earlier [11]. After the age of 10, many boys will begin to develop a cardiomyopathic process, initially in the form of asymptomatic regional wall motion abnormalities with the posterobasal and lateral walls of the left ventricle most commonly involved. Although the quality of echocardiographic scans in DMD patients can be affected by the presence of the scoliosis, the current standard of care guidelines still recommend echocardiography as the preferable imaging tool to evaluate the left ventricle (LV) function. Cardiovascular magnetic resonance (CMR) with gadolinium is emerging as the gold standard for cardiac monitoring, although sedation is required in children, limiting the widespread use of this methodology.

VAD in DMD At Bambino Gesù Hospital in Rome was first implanted in 2011 a Jarvik 2000 as DT in a DMD teenager with end-stage heart failure. In 5-year time, we implanted seven VAD as DT (six in DMD) and one being affected by β2 sarcoglycan deficit. Median age and weight at surgery were 16.5 years and 44 kg, respectively. [12]. In DMD patients suitable for LVAD as DT, a specific multidisciplinary approach is necessary including: orthopedic, gastroenterology, radiologic, respiratory, psychological, anesthesiological, ethical, and cardiac assessments. The central goal of a patient-centric care requires that the patient and the family are sufficiently educated about the alternatives available so that their expectations can be met as fully as possible. A CT scan of head is routinely performed to assess the area of the skull where the pedestal should be inserted (bone thickness should be at least 5 mm). We believe that the use of pedestal in patient on wheelchair is preferable and more comfortable, thus reducing the cable infection [13]. Two reasons for the low infection rate are that the scalp tissue is immobile relative to the skull and the connector post-exit site is therefore protected from trauma if the cable is accidentally pulled. Moreover, the scalp skin is more resistant to infection than the skin of the abdomen.

In our series of patients, LVAD surgery was performed on beating heart cardiopulmonary bypass except in one case carried out by minimally invasive approach through left mini-thoracotomy and mini-sternotomy. All patients preoperatively and after extubation required noninvasive positive pressure (NIV) ventilation and cough machine cycles. Early extubation and the use of NIV during the preoperative and postoperative period in DMD are essential. Postoperative patient management in DMD patients undergoing LVAD is challenging and should be multidisciplinary and patient tailored [8, 12]. At median follow-up time of 22 months (range 6–44.8), we have three late deaths, only one pump related. Since the first report, other centers started to implant LVAD as DT in dystrophinopathies [14, 15].

39.5 Clinical Perspective

Future practical clinical use of infant version of Jarvik 2000 will open a new frontier in assisting smallest child in order to discharge them home while waiting for heart transplantation, with an improvement in patient and caregiver quality of life.

The prolonged life expectancy in DMD patients up to third/fourth decade of life poses the DCM the main cause of death. Our experience showed the possibility to use VAD as DT in dystrophinopathy patients with end-stage DCM. Intensity of care is very high even when discharged home because of all comorbidities (non-deambulating adolescent, scoliosis, etc.). Our results suggest that the use of VAD as DT may be a palliative time-limited therapy for the treatment of these patients with otherwise no therapeutic options.

References

1. Alvarez JA, Orav EJ, Wilkinson JD et al (2011) Pediatric Cardiomyopathy Registry Investigators. Competing risks for death and cardiac transplantation in children with dilated Cardiomyopathy: results from the pediatric cardiomyopathy registry. Circulation 124(7): 814–823
2. Almond CS, Morales DL, Blackstone EH, Turrentine MW, Imamura M, Massicotte MP, Jordan LC, Devaney EJ, Ravishankar C, Kanter KR, Holman W, Kroslowitz R, Tjossem C, Thuita L, Cohen GA, Buchholz H, St Louis JD, Nguyen K, Niebler RA, Walters HL 3rd, Reemtsen B, Wearden PD, Reinhartz O, Guleserian KJ, Mitchell MB, Bleiweis MS, Canter CE, Humpl T (2013) Berlin Heart EXCOR pediatric ventricular assist device for bridge to heart transplantation in US children. Circulation 127(16):1702–1711
3. Sandica E, Blanz U, Mime LB, Schultz-Kaizler U, Kececioglu D, Haas N, Kirchner G, zu Knyphausen E, Lauenroth V, Morshuis M (2016) Long-term mechanical circulatory support in pediatric patients. Artif Organs 40(3):225–232
4. Feldman D et al (2013) The 2013 International Society for Heart and Lung Transplantation Guidelines for mechanical circulatory support: Executive summary. J Heart Lung Transplant 32:157–187
5. Brancaccio G, Filippelli S, Michielon G, Iacobelli R, Alfieri S, Gandolfo F, Pongiglione G, Albanese S, Perri G, Parisi F, Carotti A, Amodeo A (2012) Ventricular assist devices as a bridge to heart transplantation or as destination therapy in pediatric patients. Transplant Proc 44:2007–2012
6. Wu RS, Gupta S, Brown RN et al (2010) Clinical outcomes after cardiac transplantation in muscular dystrophy patients. J Heart Lung Transplant 29:432–438
7. Amodeo A, Adorisio R (2012) Left ventricular assist device in Duchenne cardiomyopathy: can we change the natural history of cardiac disease? Int J Cardiol 161(3):e43
8. Iodice F, Testa G, Averardi M, Brancaccio G, Amodeo A, Cogo P (2015) Implantation of a left ventricular assist device as a destination therapy in Duchenne muscular dystrophy patients with end stage cardiac failure: management and lessons learned. Neuromuscul Disord 25(1):19–23
9. Westaby S, Banning AP, Jarvik R et al (2000) First permanent implant of the Jarvik 2000 Heart. Lancet 356(9233):900–903
10. Frazier OH, Myers TJ, Gregoric ID et al (2002) Initial clinical experience with the Jarvik 2000 implantable axial-flow left ventricular assist system. Circulation 105(24):2855–2856
11. Bushby K, Finkel R, Birnkrant DJ, Case LE, Clemens PR, Cripe L, Kaul A, Kinnett K, McDonald C, Pandya S, Poysky J, Shapiro F, Tomezsko J, Constantin C, DMD Care Considerations Working Group (2010) Diagnosis and management of Duchenne muscular dystrophy, part 1: diagnosis, and pharmacological and psychosocial management. Lancet Neurol 9(1):77–93
12. Perri G, Filippelli S, Adorisio R, Iacobelli R, Iodice F, Testa G, Paglietti MG, D'Amario D, Massetti M, Amodeo A (2017) Left ventricular assist device as destination therapy in cardiac end stage dystrophinopathies: midterm results. J Thorac Cardiovasc Surg 153(3):669–674
13. Siegenthaler MP, Martin J, Pernice K, Doenst T, Sorg S, Trummer G, Friesewinkel O, Beyersdorf F (2003) The Jarvik 2000 is associated with less infections than the HeartMate left ventricular assist device. Eur J Cardiothorac Surg 23(5):748–754 discussion 754-5
14. Ryan TD, Jefferies JL, Sawnani H, Wong BL, Gardner A, Del Corral M, Lorts A, Morales DL (2014) Implantation of the HeartMate II and HeartWare left ventricular assist devices in patients with duchenne muscular dystrophy: lessons learned from the first applications. ASAIO J 60(2):246–248
15. Seguchi O, Kuroda K, Fujita T, Fukushima N, Nakatani T (2016) Advanced heart failure secondary to muscular dystrophy: Clinical outcomes after left ventricular assist device implantation. J Heart Lung Transplant 35(6): 831–834

Postoperative Recommendations

Contents

Physiotherapy and Rehabilitation Management in Adult LVAD Patients

L. Compostella, M. Polastri, M. Lamotte, Fabio Bellotto, and M. Antoine

© Springer International Publishing Switzerland 2017
A. Montalto et al. (eds.), *Mechanical Circulatory Support in End-Stage Heart Failure*,
DOI 10.1007/978-3-319-43383-7_40

40.1 Introduction

Increasing numbers of patients require implantation of permanent ventricular assist devices (VADs) for treatment of refractory end-stage heart failure [1, 2], as confirmed by surveys conducted in several European hospitals [3, 4]. VADs have been initially employed either as a bridge to recovery or bridge to transplantation [5]. It has been reported that 78% of VAD implants (between 2002 and 2004) have been used as bridge to transplantation, 11.9% as destination therapy, and 5.3% as bridge to recovery [6]: rehabilitation management, if we consider these data, would be centered on maintaining motor abilities in order to prepare patient for a future transplantation when VADs are used as bridge treatment. Such a trend is nowadays differing since, due to the donor crisis, VADs are increasingly used as destination therapy. Although this practice is widely experienced in end-stage heart failure populations, mortality remains high: appropriateness of enrollment criteria is determinant in order to avoid inappropriate patient selection. In this regard, it has been found that patient's frailty reduce the left ventricular assist devices (LVADs) outcomes; mortality at 1 year after implantation is higher in frail patients when compared with not frails [7]. Earlier reviews examined indications for LVAD use, LVAD suitability, cost-effectiveness, and the utility of the devices when used to treat refractory end-stage heart disease [8–16]. VAD implantation is indicated in order to augment or replace left ventricle (LVAD), right ventricle (RVAD), or both ventricle (BiVAD) function [6]. Postoperative complications of physiotherapic interest are mainly represented by infections, bleeding, thromboembolic events, device malfunction, and depression [17]. Indeed, postoperative rehabilitation in VAD recipients does not substantially differ from common cardiac surgery patients, as the main goals are related to the treatment/prevention of postoperative pulmonary complications, in the early phase. One of the major differences between common surgery patients and LVAD recipients consists in the complexity of the preoperative general conditions, being LVAD patients more prone to physical deconditioning often determined by forced bed rest and physical inactivity. Another substantial difference concerns the safety issues related to the device management, either by patients or by those providing care, including caregivers.

Herein, we aim to discuss emerging aspects of the physiotherapeutic intervention in LVAD patients, dividing the rehabilitation pathway in several steps from the acute phase to discharge home.

40.2 Before Implantation

Some of the patients sent for an LVAD implantation are chronic patients suffering from heart failure and who are slowly deteriorating. A program of revalidation is frequently proposed: it is now evident that there are clinical benefits in this type of population. Recommendations for physical exercises are established: they propose mixed training to obtain central and peripheral effects – dynamic training, resistive training, and work on the respiratory muscles [18, 19]. Another aspect of this rehabilitation is that all these cardiac patients (heart failure, LVAD, heart transplantation) are following their training in the same sports hall: they are progressively familiarized with the post-LVAD implantation or even the post-transplantation program.

40.3 Intensive Care Unit Stay and Related Patient Goals: Early Postoperative Physiotherapy in a High Intensity Level of Care (The First Ten Days)

Physiotherapeutic intervention takes place at every phase during the postoperative recovery, starting in the intensive care unit (ICU), as early as the subject is awake. Physiotherapists are actively involved in the pathway of care, and they are recognized as a key figure within the multidisciplinary team in order to achieve patient recovery and manage postoperative complications in those subjected to cardiac surgical procedures [20]. Rehabilitation pathway in LVAD patients can be divided into some phases according to the patient's clinical status, and intensity of care characteristics (◘ Fig. 40.1). The early recovery phase, after implantation, consists of the treatment and/or prevention of pulmonary complications and

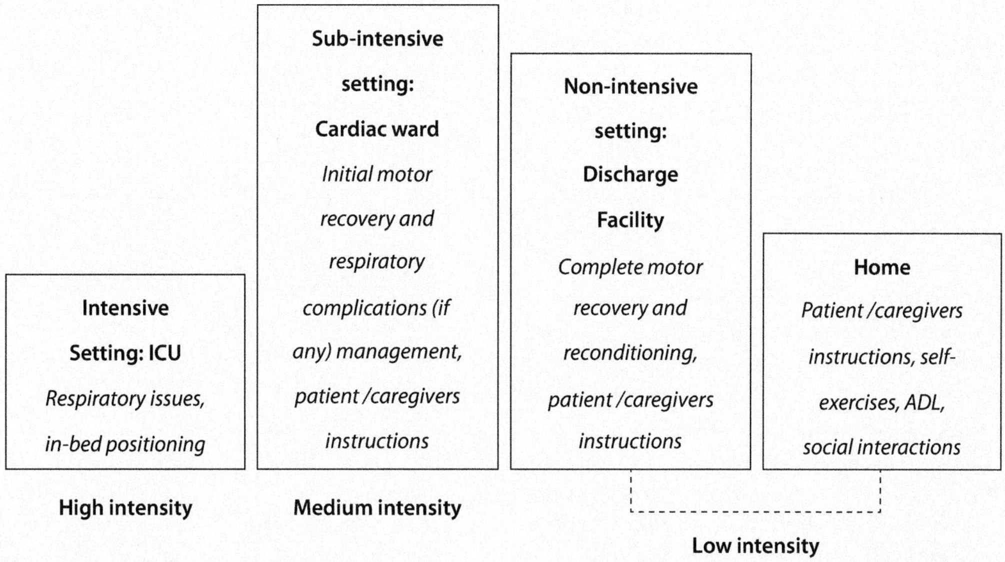

Fig. 40.1 Rehabilitation phases and intensity of care. *ICU* intensive care unit, *ADL* activities of daily living

improvement of respiratory function if compromised by surgery (i.e., pulmonary atelectasis, oxygenation impairment, pleural effusion). To this end, in the first 24/48 h or after extubation, and/or when sedation is reduced and then stopped, an early physiotherapeutic evaluation process should start. The bedside evaluation will consist in observing the respiratory pattern: Is chest dynamic altered? Is the patient breathing spontaneously? How much oxygen support is needed and, if yes, which kind of support is provided? Is pain preventing appropriate breathing? Are pulmonary secretions present, and, if yes, is patient able to eliminate them by means of effective cough?

All of these issues should be checked in order to obtain a global view of the pulmonary condition and function, postoperatively. Indeed, ICU is the safer place in a hospital since intensive monitoring and staff allocation usually guarantee the highest degree of assistance to the patient. The physiotherapeutic approach must be oriented to share clinical information with the multidisciplinary team: multidisciplinarity in ICU is not an option rather a true need. Physiotherapy intervention must take place both according to the patient's clinical status and team shared decisions: a certain degree of personal attitude and the willingness to cooperate must identify a physiotherapist in such a setting. Physiotherapeutic evaluation must be oriented to identify red flags and appropriateness of care, considering the patient mental status, the patient's cooperation, and stability of the vital signs. It should not be forgotten that physiotherapeutic duties can be different around the world: in example, respiratory treatment is usually carried out by respiratory therapist, and physical rehabilitation is instead provided by physical therapist in the USA. Within the Eurozone countries, physiotherapists are normally entitled to provide both respiratory and physical rehabilitation. Returning back to the matter, ICU timeframe is an exciting phase since the planning of an appropriate treatment can pave the way for further improvements along the whole postoperative recovery.

LVAD recipients, while in ICU, are initially confined to bedrest: in the first postoperative days, the patient configuration will be characterized by the presence of the Swan-Ganz catheter, infusion lines, heavy monitoring, urinary catheter, oxygen support systems (goggles or facial mask), and the VAD equipment – batteries and controller. Early mobilization and wound care play a key role in the initial management of VAD patients already in the ICU. Early physiotherapy is initiated to prevent complications of bedrest and minimize loss of mobility [21] by means of range of motion (ROM) exercises, and in-bed positioning: once hemodynamically stable, patient is assisted out of the bed to a chair [22]. In such a configuration – in uncomplicated patients – ROM exercises can be done in order to evaluate if any deficit is present and to stimulate further active movements. Indeed, enhancing patient in-bed positioning can play an important role with the aim to stimulate the first patient's movements. Mobilization in ICU of patients on mechanical circulatory support is considered a standard of care and it can begin with simple activities such as turning in bed [23]. The ICU phase is generally protective against pulmonary complications; they are more frequently seen in the sub-intensive setting as they become more evident at 48–72 h, because a certain amount of time is necessary to develop and, consequently, observe imaging alterations and related clinical findings. As previously observed, an important ICU physiotherapeutic goal is to prevent the onset of pulmonary complications and enhance the respiratory pattern, if altered. On the other hand, pleural effusion and dysventilation phenomena, requiring physiotherapeutic intervention, are common after cardiac surgical procedures [24, 25]. To this end, respiratory therapy should be proposed including deep breathing exercises and secretions clearance techniques. Deep breathing exercises and resistive breathing are commonly carried out in ICU patients, postoperatively [26]. The major objective to be pursued by means of respiratory exercises is to encourage patients to perform deep breathings in order to treat atelectasis, improve hypoxemia, and prevent worsening of the pulmonary function more in general [24]. To this end, in uncomplicated patients, the blow-bottle device can be used as soon as the subject is awake and sedation stopped. Blow bottle is a respiratory device used to allow lung expansion in postsurgical setting. It consists of a set that can be built up using material commonly available in hospital wards, such as a saline bottle and a chest drain tubing (length 20–30 cm, >30 cm) [25, 26] (◘ Fig. 40.2). The patient is asked to make an inspiration and then blow into the tube: during the expiration, the water contained in the bottle provides an expiratory resistance. The blow-bottle respiratory exercises, a simple and feasible technique, can be used in the first postoperative days, when needed. This exercise can be repeated – several daily sessions by a defined set of repetitions according to the patient's status – and it can be performed either in a sitting or in a supine position. Patient must be awake and cooperative. Effective coughing can also play an important role in the secretions clearance: the subject is instructed to effective coughing in order to facilitate the secretions clearance. A pillow embraced with the arms while coughing is usually well accepted in order to reduce chest pain during cough.

40.4 Sub-intensive Setting Stay and Related Patient Goals: Postoperative Physiotherapy in a Medium Intensity Level of Care (From Tenth to Thirtieth/Fortieth Day)

At the ICU discharge, VAD recipients are usually transferred to a sub-intensive setting where the principal objectives of the physiotherapeutic intervention are improving safe movements and postural passages and improving autonomy of daily activities. Monitoring of the pulmonary function still remains an important aspect. To this end, continuing evaluation of the chest imaging, together with the clinical observation, should be adopted to avoid worsening of the respiratory function if it has been already jeopardized during the ICU stay. Pleural effusion, atelectasis, and lung dysventilation must be also prevented/treated by means of a respiratory program focused on respiratory exercises (◘ Fig. 40.3). Particularly in those showing pulmonary alterations, and that do not require a more intense treatment, respiratory therapy can be continued by means of incentive spirometry exercises, in order to encourage deep breathings and enhance diaphragmatic excursion and chest wall expansion. This practice, during the initial postoperative timeframe, also contributes to obtain the active patient involvement. Respiratory exercises can be scheduled during the day in more than one session; once the patient is trained on the use of the incentive spirometry device, the exercise can be performed autonomously. Furthermore, since the degree of patient's mobility normally increases during this phase, there is also the need to plan a specific device training activity in order to preserve and guarantee the patient's safety. Thus, the main goals of the initial rehabilitation treatment are centered on patient's autonomy and device management: exercise sessions are a

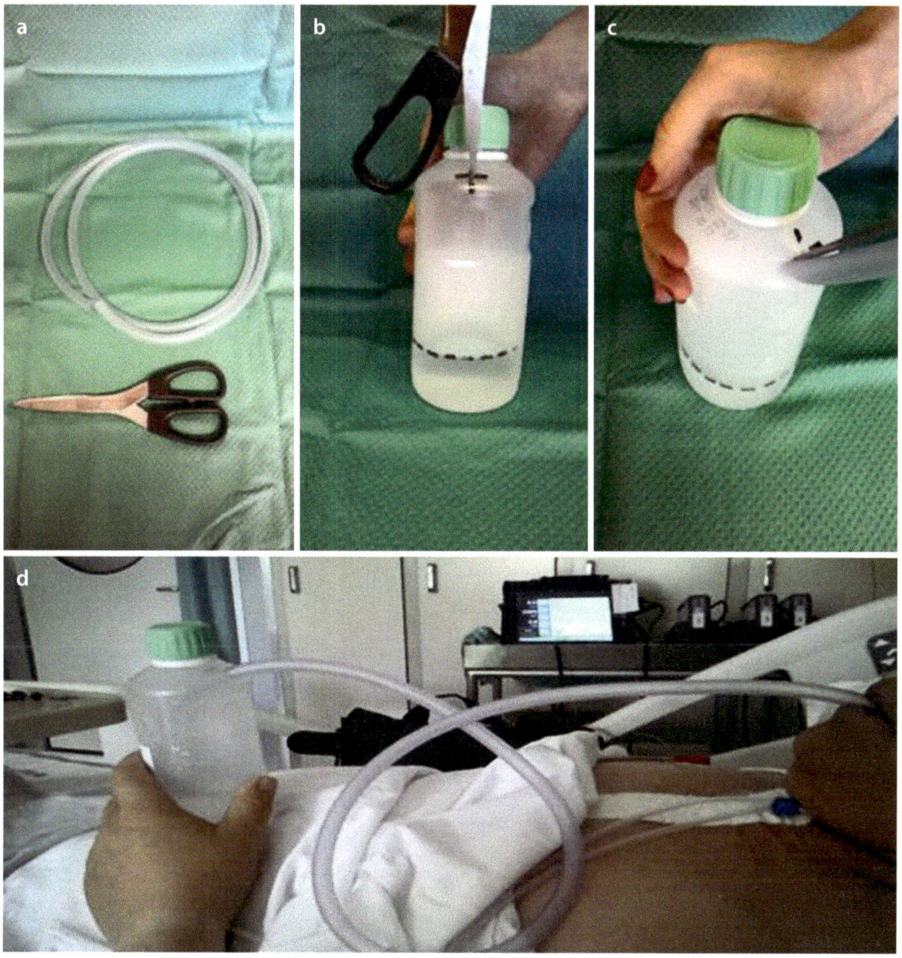

Fig. 40.2 Exercises with blow-bottle device. **a–c** The blow-bottle device can be made using common material available in hospital wards. A saline bottle (500 ml) is opened and drained to the desired level of water **b**, and then the bottle is closed and a tube is inserted into the water through a slot **b**, **c** formed on the container. **d** A patient is performing the respiratory exercise while in a supine position. The device shown in this figure can be closed preventing exit of water even while patient is resting. The set should be replaced frequently in order to guarantee adequate sanitation

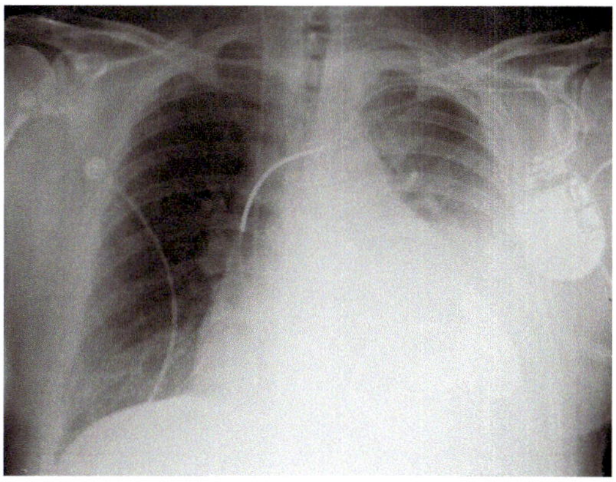

Fig. 40.3 Pulmonary complications after surgery. A left pleural effusion in a patient after LVAD implantation

good way also to teach the patient how to handle an alarm and a change of batteries. At this stage, active ROM exercises, ambulation, and stair climbing are implemented [27], and flexibility exercises are also encouraged and tailored on patient characteristics. Upper body exercises are delayed until 6–8 weeks to ensure sternal healing. Exercise is stopped in case of subjective intolerance or drop in systolic pressure. Physiotherapist must be trained in emergency procedures in case of device malfunctioning and must be also aware of patient hemodynamic instability and device dislodgement during mobilization [22].

Initial postural passages should be performed and the subject instructed how to change the position safely. These activities, for those patients who have not yet started, should be encouraged beginning with the maintenance of a sitting position at the edge of the bed, progressing toward the sitting position in a chair. Then, the patient can start a more intensive muscular program oriented to develop the ability to gain autonomously an upright position. When postural passages, upright position, and in-bed movements are carried out autonomously, patient is ready to walk with or without a walking frame. Walking, lifting on toes, bending knees, cycling, climbing stairs, and other exercises should be supervised (■ Figs. 40.4 and 40.5). At this stage, the patient

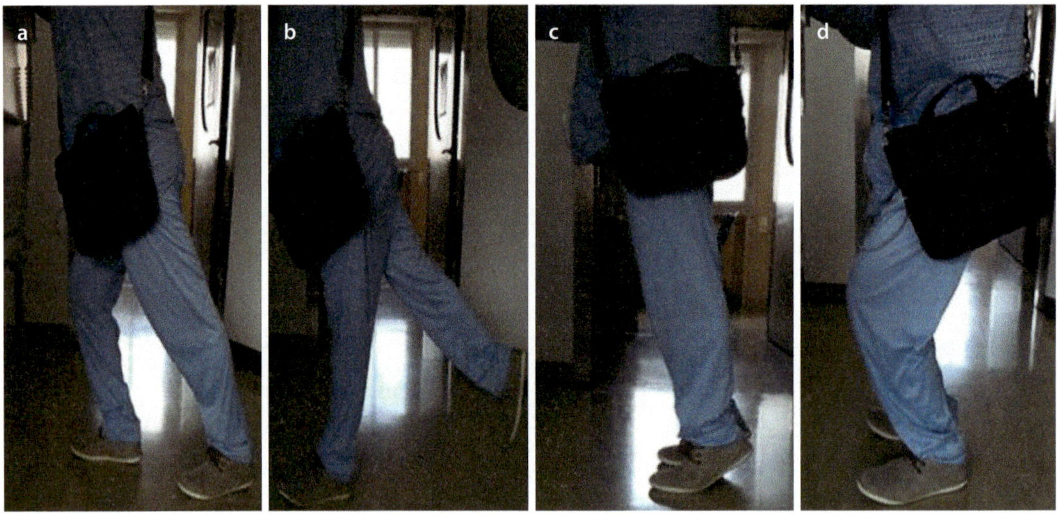

■ **Fig. 40.4** Supervised lower limb exercises. **a** Stretching of the left leg posterior muscles. **b** Strengthening of the gluteus. **c** Strengthening of calves. **d** Bending on the knees and quadriceps strengthening

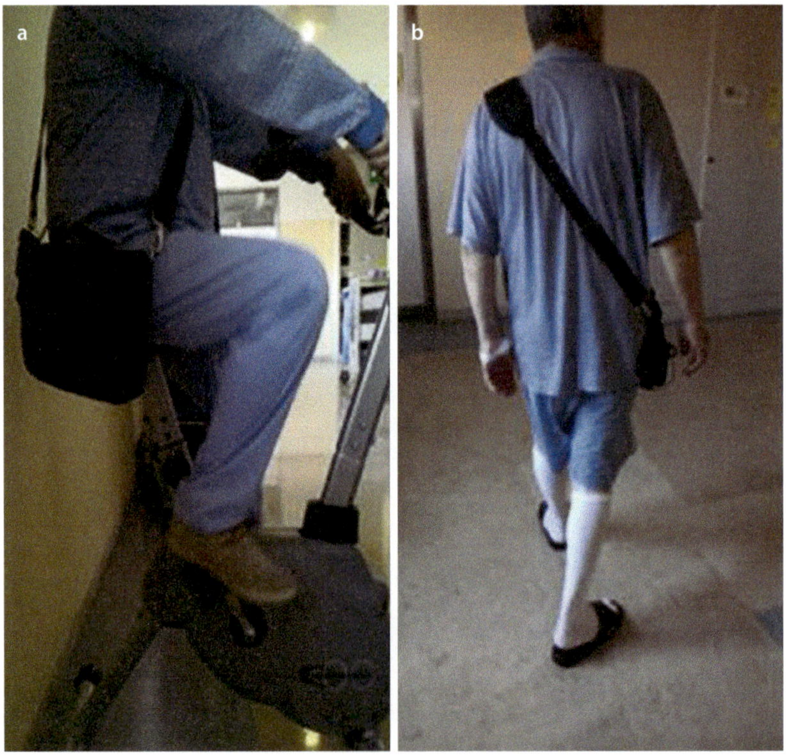

■ **Fig. 40.5** Supervised cycling and walking. **a** A patient is cycling. **b** Walking onward

must be confident with the device and must be able to dress it, safely. Pre-LVAD conditions can play a major role during the postoperative rehabilitation. Patients who were already confident with the exercise may be facilitated; hemodynamic stability is needed in order to proceed with the exercise's intensity [28]. Physical activity can be made also in small groups and the duration can range between 5 and 30 min. Group activities are important as patients need to gain confidence in the equipment and become comfortable with the reactions of those who look at the device. Indeed, facilitation of LVAD acceptance is an important component of rehabilitation. At discharge, it is advisable to set up a follow-up period which comprises sessions of supervised exercise [29]. At the end of the hospitalization, the patient must be able to walk alone and to climb the stairs.

40.5 Outcome Measures, Evaluation Tools, and Treatment Progression in LVAD Recipients

No official guidelines or even recommendations exist to determine the training modality for the patients with a LVAD. It seemed appropriate to build the program on the established recommendations for heart failure since many problems are common to both populations. Therefore, we decided to take care of two aspects of the rehabilitation:

1. The aerobic metabolism: we know that there is an interaction between the pulmonary, cardiovascular, and skeletal systems during exercise. There is an improvement of the aerobic metabolism, of the autonomic regulation, and on the peripheral perfusion. This will lead to an improvement of the respiratory control and an improvement in the quality of life. A very demonstrative benefit is the decreasing of hospital readmissions.
2. The reinforcement of the resistance training: due to the usual previous physical inactivity, this part of the rehabilitation is mandatory in order to increase muscle strength and muscle endurance. Due to increased blood flow, there are an increased mitochondrial ATP production rate, a better oxidative capacity, and a relative increase of flow distribution in the area of type I fibers. Again with those physiological benefits, we will obtain an increased quality of life and probably an increased VO_2 peak but certainly no adverse events and no deterioration of the ventricular function. Based on the physiological understanding of the Fick equation, O_2 consumption per minute = pulmonary blood flow × (pulmonary artery O_2 blood concentration – pulmonary vein O_2 blood concentration) [$VO_2 = Q\ (CaO_2 - CvO_2)$], we know that we have to work on the flow (LVAD) and the muscular extraction of O_2.

Following the Fick principle, the VO_2 depends from the flow and the peripheral extraction. After LVAD implantation the improvement of VO_2 values is not concomitant with an improvement of the hemodynamic parameters given by the device: this confirms the need of a training oriented to the peripheral muscles [30, 31]. There is a common conclusion in literature to agree on the benefit of revalidation after implantation. With a well-oriented training program and combined exercises, the patients will have a better quality of life; those patients who may still develop an aortic flow during exercise could most probably be able to generate greater efforts.

Physiotherapeutic intervention is planned considering a certain degree of progression along the recovery pathway. Activities should progress from passive ROM to ambulation and resistive ROM exercises [32]. Safety during mobilization is implemented by means of the physiotherapeutic intervention as patient can be instructed how to realize postural passages and how to achieve a safe mobility program considering the safety issues related to the driveline and device management [33]. In the ICU, implanted patient is not able to manage autonomously the device, and safety is completely delegated to the staff.

The LVAD used today has a continuous flow, which does look to be an improvement [34]. The absence of pulse and the measurement of a mean arterial pressure (not always easy) have created the necessity to design the training on the maximal charge obtained during cardiopulmonary exercise testing (CPET). The rehabilitation program must propose a combined training.

The *dynamic training* is based on a CPET practiced on bicycle, treadmill, or other similar ergometers. The feasibility of a maximal test is well demonstrated in the literature, proved by the respiratory quotients (RQ) reached [35–41]. It is mandatory to obtain this maximal test in order to optimize the structure of the training and also to obtain a unique scale to compare results (intra- and inter-studies).

When this CPET is maximal with a RQ >1.15 and without anomaly, the workload will be fixed to 70–80% of the Watts max. The dynamic training must be completed by muscular reinforcement: the principal muscular groups (arms, legs, back, abdominal) must be trained with specific tools [40, 42–44]. Those specific exercises address qualitative and quantitative muscular changes which are met in the heart failure patients and increased by a prolonged bedrest [45, 46]. Based on the one repetition maximum (RM, charge that the patient can lift one time), exercises are planned at 75% of RM, and performed as two sets of ten repetitions.

Some authors define the limited zone of exercise around 60–70% of the VO2max [47] or 50% of the VO2reserve [45], but they do not explain how the training is adapted afterward.

The *interval training* has not shown this benefit, in any study, for these types of patients. Anyway, the improvements obtained in patients suffering from cardiac failure, via the peripheral pathway, and the higher workload developed with this type of training, give us the impression that this interval training should be proposed as a complementary modality. For the same reason, a training with work period above the respiratory level 1 seems to be pertinent and feasible [42–48]: cycling, walking, rowing, etc., session of 45–60 min, frequency 3–5 per week, duration 8–10 weeks.

We did not find in the literature any publication and of course no recommendation for the use of neuromuscular electrical stimulation for these patients; this technology is very limited and is more about addressing noncompliant patients. It is the same for stretching and relaxation.

A single study proposes a training of the respiratory muscles [39].

On the contrary, in multiple studies, as for heart failure patients, there is a major interest of a multidisciplinary team in close collaboration with the VAD team [34, 42, 43, 48, 49].

Patient's progress and rehabilitation outcomes of LVAD recipients admitted to a sub-intensive care setting after ICU discharge should be evaluated. To this end, the Functional Independence Measure (FIM) scale has been described as a suitable tool during in-patient rehabilitation [50–53]. The FIM scale consists of the evaluation of 18 functional and cognitive items: eating, grooming, bathing, upper body dressing, lower body dressing, toileting, bladder, bowel, toilet transfer, bed/chair/wheelchair transfer, tub/shower transfer, walking or wheelchair mobility, stair climbing, comprehension, expression, social interaction, problem solving, and memory. FIM, more than other evaluation tools (i.e., Barthel Index), better intercept the treatment progress thanks to the presence of a number of items that explore various functional areas: the cognitive items also contribute to the evaluation of the social and personal interactions. During in-patient rehabilitation, treatment intensity should be also established in order to guarantee appropriateness and safety of care (◘ Fig. 40.6). In LVAD patients, the use of the Borg scale has been proven effective to check patient's status while exercising [29, 32, 40]. An exertion of somewhat hard intensity on the Borg scale should be used as a limit to interrupt the exercise [39, 40, 43].

A further evaluation tool consists in the measurement of the daily walking distance which should improve over the rehabilitation treatment: this is a simple, immediate measure which can be obtained in order to verify patient's progressions [54]. Ambulation distance can be fixed on meters or time and must take into account adverse symptoms [55].

6-min walk test has been shown, at 3.6 months postoperatively, to be a predictor of LVAD

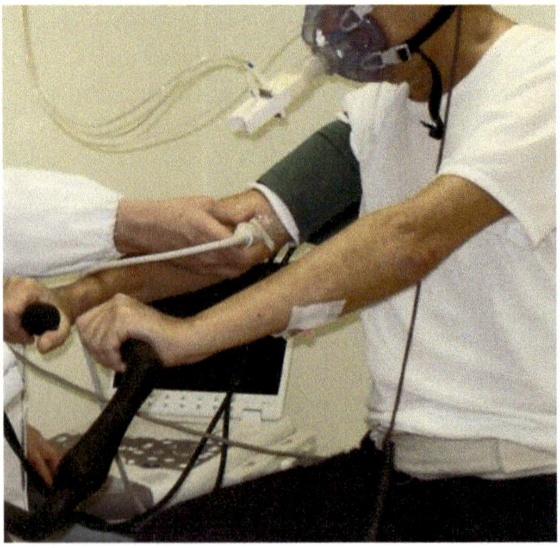

◘ **Fig. 40.6** The work intensity is being evaluated in an LVAD patient (Jarvick). Ergometric stress test and pressure measurement (by means of Doppler technique)

mortality, since poor performance (<300 m) on the test is associated with increased mortality [56].

To our best knowledge, there is not yet any specific study in LVAD-supported patients that investigated how to best afford gait and balance problems during cardiac rehabilitation (CR). Some useful suggestions could be derived by a study on aged individuals submitted to CR after coronary bypass heart surgery [57]. In that study, besides other physical and functional evaluations, patients were assessed by a Timed-Up-and-Go (TUG) test, aimed at documenting the time taken to rise from a 43 cm high chair, walk as fast as possible to a mark on the floor 3 m away from the chair, and turn, walk back, and sit down again; [58] a TUG test taking longer than 16 s is considered a predictor of falls in older individuals. In order to improve patients' balance, in the cited study, the usual aerobic and callisthenic exercises and resistance training aimed at reinforcing legs strength have been complemented by exercises on unstable devices, such as balls and loose platforms, under progressively increasing difficulties. The intervention group showed a highly significant improvement in the TUG test, without any complication linked to the exercises. Similar positive results have been reported also by a study on rehabilitation of chronic pulmonary disease patients, [59] in which balance assessment was performed by the cited TUG test and integrated with four more evaluations: the Berg balance scale (a 14-item scale evaluating activities such as transfers, reaching, turning around, and single-leg stance, graded on a scale ranging from 0 = unable/unsafe to 4 = independent/efficient/safe) [60], the unipedal stance test (patient's ability to stand on one leg for 45 s) [61], the Tinetti test (a 16-item test divided into two sections: balance (9 items) and gait (7 items), for a total score of 28, where scores <26 indicate high risk of falling) [62], and the activities-specific balance confidence scale (it describes patient's confidence in performing 16 activities without losing their balance or becoming unsteady, on an 11-point scale) [63]. Although no study evaluating such tests and specific interventions has yet been conducted in LVAD-supported patients, the cited tests and the balance training interventions seem to be possibly useful in the particularly new group of chronic patients represented by LVAD patients. Device education and self-care management must be achieved prior to discharge and are basic conditions for admission to an outpatient rehabilitation program. A multidisciplinary approach including cardiac rehabilitation and prevention staff, contributing staff, and consultant staff is strongly recommended in order to guarantee effectiveness and appropriateness of care in VAD patients [64].

40.6 Discharge Facility: Advanced Rehabilitation in a Low Intensity Level of Care Setting (Over the Thirtieth Day)

After device implantation, a progressive reduction of left ventricular pressure and volume and a decrease of mean pulmonary artery and wedge pressures are usually observed [37]. Such modifications result in reduction and disappearance of dyspnea. The increased output obtained with the support of the LVAD leads to better perfusion of muscle masses, gradual anatomical and functional muscle fibers reverse modifications, and smoothening of neurohormonal mechanisms, which result in progressive reduction of fatigue. Thus, the majority of patients gradually improve their clinical status, from preimplantation NYHA class IV to class I or II; this improvement is most often noticed after 1 month from implantation, as reported by the HeartMate II Investigators [34]. As soon as the LVAD-supported patient is hemodynamically stable, comprehensive (mainly exercise-based) rehabilitation may begin, aimed at restoring an adequate level of mobility independence [21, 22, 65, 66]. The optimal time to start exercise training is yet to be defined. Some recent studies report beginning of exercise training after 27 ± 15 days [52], after 38 ± 18 days [67], and after 48 ± 38 days [40] when patients are considered clinically stable; this kind of rehabilitation is usually conducted as in-patient rehabilitation. Exercise-based rehabilitation is also advocated in the following period, as long-term ambulatory rehabilitation, with the aim of adequately addressing the challenges that influence patients' independence and quality of life [68]. What is known nowadays is that exercise training, as part of a multimodal intervention, is safe and effective in LVAD-supported patients, both in those ones waiting for heart transplantation (in which exercise training favorably impacts clinical course and improves post-transplant recovery) and in patients implanted with an LVAD as destination therapy [39, 42, 43, 49, 50, 69, 70]. In LVAD-supported patients, it is well known that regular physical exercise has the potential to progressively reverse – at least partially – the pre-existing negative physical and functional modifications [71]. At the beginning of more intensive rehabilitative activities, some care must be given to the fact that the device could create an obstacle to physical, mainly exercise-based, rehabilitation in a still debilitated patient. Patients supported by LVAD come usually from a long and troublesome history of low cardiac output; one of the main features they often present for weeks or months after beginning of LVAD support is sarcopenia. The reduced muscle masses cause a direct limitation on individual's capacity to stand and walk with correct balance; the effects are worsened by concomitant presence of autonomic dysfunction that may contribute to orthostatic hypotension and to reduced efficiency of receptor-integrator-effector system with consequent reduced balance/stability control.

During the most common rehabilitative activities practiced in the initial phases of CR, such as walking, treadmill, cyclette, and stepping, there is the risk of accidental falls of the patient or the device. Little is reported in literature about complications linked to such falls. It must be remembered that, in the majority of continuous-flow LVAD (cf-LVAD) models in use, the driveline (from skin to controller) is rather short, and a fall of the device (or a fall of the patient with the driveline caught in the handlebars of the ergometer or treadmill) could lead to disconnection of the LVAD's external power supply, with awful consequences [72]. In some models of cf-LVADs, spring wire extensions are used between the body cable and the external controller, which could be rather long (up to 2 m or more); patients should be instructed to avoid cable swing while cycling, a situation that could lead to trapping or stretching of the cable by the cycle treadle. In a similar way, patients should be instructed to avoid carrying by hand the bag containing batteries and controller, as the long extension cables could swing near their feet and be accidentally stump. In patients with heart failure, all training intensities have been shown to be effective in improving exercise capacity, while moderate to high intensity aerobic training seems to be more effective to induce reverse left ventricular remodeling [73]. In LVAD-supported patients, we would suggest that exercise training could be conducted at individual anaerobic threshold. A cardiopulmonary exercise test should thus be performed as soon as the patient is able to cycle and repeated by time to time; the effort could be limited to the amount necessary to identify the anaerobic threshold (or slightly more), with greatest attention paid to patient's symptoms (dyspnea, fatigue, sense of fainting) or clinical signs possibly indicating low peripheral perfusion (paleness, cold sweating, reduction – even small – of mean blood pressure). Performing exercise training at individual's anaerobic threshold has demonstrated to be safe and effective even in patients rehabilitated rather early, within 2 months from continuous-flow device implantation [74]. It is not yet known if patients could present different levels of effort tolerance as a consequence of different models of implanted cf-LVADs that could present different adaptation of their output to modifications of preload (different ability to accept the contribution given by the systole of the native heart) and afterload (peripheral resistances) linked to physical effort. In the past, in patients supported by pulsatile LVADs, different exercise performances have been reported for pneumatic versus electrically driven devices [75]. As regards cf-LVADs, only one study performed on a mock circulatory system tested and compared performances of an axial-flow and a centrifugal-flow device: in this experimental model, the axial-flow LVAD reached greater maximal output that – if confirmed on clinical ground – could in theory allow better physical performance; it showed anyway also a greater risk of left-ventricle suck-down, which could be counterproductive [76]. Unfortunately, on the clinical ground, no data are yet available about possible different exercise performances allowed by different models of cf-LVADs; in fact, a single study reported the main clinical differences (survival rate, incidence of perioperative bleeding, gastrointestinal bleeding, stroke, renal dysfunction, liver dysfunction, and infection) between two models of cf-LVADs (an axial-flow and a centrifugal-flow device), but did not collect informations about exercise tolerance [77]. During the initial phases of a physical effort, in patients supported by cf-LVADs, mean arterial blood pressure shows an increase whose amount is correlated to the level of METs achieved [55]. Due to the combination of limited maximum output given by the LVAD, poor function of the native heart, and inadequate autonomic regulation of peripheral vascular resistances, blood pressure could progressively reduce at higher intensities of exercise and eventually drop in case of intense effort. However, a substantial problem exists in cf-LVAD-supported patients that blood pressure is not usually measurable by traditional means in clinical practice. A method combining arm-cuff plus Doppler ultrasound identification of humeral artery opening pressure allows to identify "mean" pressure values. It is obvious that during exercise in gymnasium, it is usually difficult to check blood pressure with such method; it is in any case recommended during a cardiopulmonary exercise test, to properly identify the optimal amount of physical activity sustainable by the individual patient. According to treatment protocols for chronic heart failure patients [78], and in an attempt to maximize the unloading of the left ventricle, improve pulmonary resistances, and eventually obtain reversal remodeling of the failing heart [79], LVAD patients are most often treated with a combination of drugs that include angiotensin-converting enzyme inhibitors or angiotensin II receptor blockers associated with selective beta-blockers and aldosterone receptor antagonists drugs. The target for blood pressure control is often put at levels of mean pressure around or below 80 mmHg [80, 81]. By consequence, hypotension with related symptoms is a frequent finding during CR, as well as during normal life activities. Maintenance of an optimal circulating volume is critical to avoid symptomatic hypotension during physical activities, as well as to avoid suction effects induced by the device on interventricular septum, which modify the geometry of the right ventricle and impair its function. Activation of device alarms during physical activity or during changes of patient's decubitus is most often an indicator of poor "circulating volume," as it may happen, e.g., due to excessive sweating or important vasodilation after strenuous effort. Thus, patients should be stimulated to regularly introduce small amounts of fluids during and after exercise, in order to compensate for perspiration and avoid relative hypovolemia and consequent hypotension. We would suggest that periodical echocardiographic control of dimensions of left ventricle, position and appearance of interventricular septum, and – if possible – calculation of estimated pulmonary systolic pressure should be performed (all controls that are obviously not possible during performance of rehabilitative physical activities) [82]. Besides being linked to volemia and drugs effects, orthostatic hypotension may be present also as a consequence of the already cited profound cardiac dysautonomia. Autonomic imbalance is present during the first months from the beginning of circulatory support [83] and could progressively improve in the following months [84], reaching an almost normal cardiovascular autonomic homeostasis (and baroreflex activity) after 7–32 months [85]. While in chronic heart failure patients, it is known that exercise training reduces sympathetic outflow and leads to an improvement of baroreflex sensitivity and heart rate variability [86], in cf-LVAD-supported patients, it is not yet known if recovery of a normal autonomic activity could be accelerated by endurance exercise. It is usually not recommended to modify LVAD settings during physical exercise. Even though it should seem logical to try and increase rotational speed in order to parallel the device output with the augmented metabolic demand linked to physical activity, it must be remembered that LVAD output seems to be partially adaptive to changes in activities of daily living, allowing at least low levels of physical engagement [87] and supporting near-normal increments in cardiac output and legs perfusion (with constant cerebral perfusion) during even maximal exercise [88]. While it is true that some experiences report positive functional results with an increase of rotational speed of various models of devices (and, conversely, reduced performance with reduction of their operational speed), especially in cases with lower residual left ventricular function [88–91], the results obtained in these small dimension studies need to be evaluated face to the possible negative effects that the increased rotational pump speed may induce on right ventricle function during sustained submaximal exercise. A possible complication during physical exercise in cf-LVAD-supported patients is the appearance or worsening of atrial and ventricular arrhythmias. During the initial phases of an exercise-based rehabilitation, LVAD patients should ideally be controlled by telemetry ECG monitoring, to check for presence or appearance of major atrial or ventricular arrhythmias; it must be remembered, anyway, that ECG monitoring implies application of chest leads and carrying a transmitter that may be disturbing in a patient who is already carrying the device controller and batteries, connected to an abdominal or retroauricular driveline. Ventricular arrhythmias are rather frequent in LVAD-supported patients; it has been reported that ventricular arrhythmias account for 4.66 events per 100 patients/month in the first 12 months after implant of a cf-LVAD [92]. They are a consequence of the underlying heart disease; they may also be linked to hemodynamic modifications induced by the device and to scars around the outflow cannula. During physical exercise in orthostatic position, an even mild dehydration may reduce the diastolic dimensions of the left ventricle and lead to suction events that may cause ventricular irritation and trigger arrhythmic events [93]. This is another reason to stimulate LVAD patients to introduce repeatedly moderate amounts of fluids during and after exercise. If major or life-threatening arrhythmias occur during rehabilitation activities, they usually do not constitute, anyway, an emergency problem:

1. The circulating flow provided by the device is generally sufficient at least for the basic needs of the patient.
2. The majority of patients (at least those assisted by an LVAD as destination therapy) are already implanted with an ICD.
3. It has been reported that even episodes of sustained ventricular tachycardia and ventricular fibrillation are rather well tolerated, with modest hemodynamic deterioration [94–97].

In any case, ventricular arrhythmias, especially if sustained, should be controlled by appropriate pharmacological therapy, as they impact negatively on the function of the right ventricle and lead to reduced effort tolerance during CR [98, 99]. We would like to remember that ventricular fibrillation may be treated as usual by direct current shock, while cardiac massage must be avoided, to avoid detaching or displacing the outflow cannula of the device. Atrial fibrillation may condition some compromise of right ventricular function, due to loss of atrial contribution to ventricular filling and irregular length of diastole; symptoms of right ventricular failure may appear more often in these patients than in patients in sinus rhythm, with consequent reduction of effort tolerance [100, 101]. Patients in atrial fibrillation usually require a level of anticoagulation higher than that of LVAD cases in sinus rhythm [102]; the topic of coagulation monitoring and possible worrisome complications is treated in another chapter of this book. It is not known if the hemorrhagic risk could increase in association with performance of physical exercise. After an intensive period of in-hospital rehabilitation, continuation of a structured out-patient rehabilitative program is advocated [64]. As it is known to happen in chronic heart failure patients that benefit from CR periods as long as 12–52 weeks [103], it is reasonable to suppose that a long-lasting rehabilitative intervention followed by self-maintenance of regular physical activity could help maintaining and improving physical fitness and quality of life also in LVAD-supported patients. Some studies performed on patients supported by pneumatic LVADs reported an increase of exercise capacity over time [36–104], and occasional cases have been reported that patients supported by pulsatile or continuous-flow LVADs continue improving their functional class [105, 106]. By the contrary, a few other observational studies on small groups of patients with continuous-flow devices reported that the improvement in exercise time observed after implant was not accompanied by improvement in peak oxygen uptake, and in evaluations of exercise capacity made after the first 3–6 months, no further significant gain of physical performance was achieved [107–109]. The strategies of prolonging rehabilitative interventions with out-patient rehabilitation, targeting low levels of physical activity in LVAD-supported patients, are, anyway, guided by the aim of giving the best possible improvement of patients' quality of life; they are also supported by the observation that patients who achieve a minimally satisfactory level of physical fitness after CR seem to present better long-term survival, as demonstrated by a study in which patients that walked >300 m at a 6-min walk test conducted >2 months after device implantation presented a significantly lower risk for late all-cause mortality [56]. In general cardiac patients and specifically in chronic heart failure patients, it has recently been demonstrated that home-based long-term maintenance of rehabilitation effects is achievable by adoption of telemedicine applications that may be individually tailored [110–113]; they may also contribute to the achievement of other goals, such as enhanced care for frail patients, home hospitalization and early discharge, and support for remote diagnosis [114]. Although similar experiences applied to patients supported by cf-LVADs are at present ongoing in some centers, to our best knowledge, no results of their efficacy, effectiveness, and sustainability in the specific LVAD population have yet been published.

40.7 LVAD Equipment Wear and Body Posture

Although the models of LVAD that are currently most often implanted in adult patients are regulated by highly portable external controller and fed by rechargeable lightweight batteries, the total weight that must be carried by the patients in a wrist or shoulder bag is usually around 2–2.5 kg. This implies posture changes and a new body balance; often, patients need to change their gait, and this – besides generating earlier fatigue – could lead to easier falls. A practical suggestion for still debilitated patients could be to carry the controller and the batteries in a shoulder bag, instead of in a wrist bag (patients often pull back) or in a bag hanging from a single shoulder (patients lean sideways). Recently it has been argued that body posture may be affected by continuing device wear in LVAD recipients [115]. Further devices' miniaturizing are predictable and very welcome in order to avoid any postural issues in such a class of patient which is, today, strictly dependent on equipment technology size. In LVAD patients, body stability is influenced by the position, size, and weight of the equipment. As the load is always present, and is rather asymmetric, it is possible that a certain degree of postural alteration may develop over time. Comfort issues are important in LVAD patients who must complete daily activities and maintain a correct posture, while wearing a control unit and a power source 24 hours a day. LVAD recipients must wear bags in order to carry the equipment: to this end, a tailored body support can prevent postural alteration and body misalignment. Various LVAD vests are commercially available and may be customized to improve comfort.

Key Points

1. At an early stage, respiratory therapy should be considered in order to prevent postoperative pulmonary complications: device-assisted (i.e., incentive spirometer) and manual (i.e., deep breathings) techniques are suitable as soon as patient is cooperative.
2. Postural passages (in-bed movements, transfer from bed to a chair, and reaching an upright position) should be facilitated as soon as possible during the early postoperative timeframe.
3. Patient should be instructed on making safe movements already during the initial postoperative days and/or when mobility is increasing.
4. Begin exercise-based cardiac rehabilitation as soon as the patient is hemodynamically stable.
5. Evaluate gait and balance of the patient; teach him/her how to correct abnormal gait.
6. Avoid the driveline to be trapped in the handlebars of the cyclette or treadmill; do not leave the connecting cables too long and avoid they swing while the patient is cycling or walking.
7. Choose intensity of exercise activities according to measurable patient's parameters (ideally conduct activities at an effort approximately corresponding to aerobic threshold).
8. Stimulate patients to introduce fluids during and after exercise, in order to avoid relative hypovolemia and hypotension, and possible triggering of ventricular arrhythmias.
9. Telemetry monitoring during the first phases of exercise-based rehabilitation is indicated, to check for atrial and ventricular arrhythmias and possibly guide antiarrhythmic therapy.
10. Aim at reaching a goal of at least 300 m walked at the 6MWT, as it seems linked to better long-term survival.

References

1. Yamakawa M, Kyo S, Yamakawa S, Ono M, Kinugawa K, Nishimura T (2013) Destination therapy: the new gold standard treatment for heart failure patients with left ventricular assist devices. Gen Thorac Cardiovasc Surg 61(3):111–117
2. Potapov EV, Loforte A, Weng Y, Jurmann M, Pasic M, Drews T et al (2008) Experience with over 1000 implanted ventricular assist devices. J Card Surg 23(3):185–194
3. Strüber M, Sander K, Lahpor J, Ahn H, Litzler PY, Drakos SG et al (2008) HeartMate II left ventricular assist device; early European experience. Eur J Cardiothorac Surg 34(2):289–294
4. Lahpor J, Khaghani A, Hetzer R, Pavie A, Friedrich I, Sander K et al (2010) European results with a continuous-flow assist device for advanced heart-failure patients. Eur J Cardiothorac Surg 37(2):357–361
5. Givertz MM (2011) Cardiology patients pages: ventricular assist devices: important information for patients and families. Circulation 124(12):e305–e311
6. Sorensen E (2007) Ventricular-assist devices and total artificial hearts. Biomed Instrum Technol 41(5):385–389
7. Dunlay SM, Park SJ, Joyce LD, Daly RC, Stulak JM, McNallan SM et al (2014) Frailty and outcomes after implantation of left ventricular assist device as destination therapy. J Heart Lung Transplant 33(4): 359–365
8. Emin A, Rogers CA, Parameshwar J, Macgowan G, Taylor R, Yonan N et al (2013) Trends in long-term mechanical circulatory support for advanced heart failure in the UK. Eur J Heart Fail 15(10):1185–1193
9. Neyt M, Van den Bruel A, Smit Y, De Jonge N, Erasmus M, Van Dijk D et al (2013) Cost-effectiveness of continuous-flow ventricular assist devices. Int J Technol Assess Health Care 29(3):254–260
10. Moreno SG, Novielli N, Cooper NJ (2012) Cost-effectiveness of the implantable HeartMate II left ventricular assist device for patients awaiting heart transplantation. J Heart Lung Transplant 31(5):450–458
11. Rogers JG, Bostic RR, Tong KB, Adamson R, Russo M, Slaughter MS (2012) Cost-effectiveness analysis of continuous-flow left ventricular assist devices as destination therapy. Circ Heart Fail 5(1):10–16
12. Maltais S, Jaik NP, Feurer ID, Wigger MA, Disalvo TG, Schlendorf KH et al (2013) Mechanical circulatory support and heart transplantation: donor and recipient factors influencing graft survival. Ann Thorac Surg 96(4):1252–1258
13. Atluri P, Goldstone AB, Fairman AS, Macarthur JW, Shudo Y, Cohen JE et al (2013) Predicting right ventricular failure in the modern, continuous flow left ventricular assist device era. Ann Thorac Surg 96(3):857–863
14. Ammirati E, Oliva F, Colombo T, Botta L, Cipriani M, Cannata A et al (2013) Proposal for updated listing criteria for heart transplantation and indications to implant of left ventricular assist devices. G Ital Cardiol (Rome) 14(2):110–119
15. Carrel T, Englberger L, Martinelli MV, Takala J, Boesch C, Sigurdadottir V et al (2012) Continuous flow left ventricular assist devices: a valid option for heart failure patients. Swiss Med Wkly 142:w13701
16. McDiarmid A, Gordon B, Wrightson N, Robinson-Smith N, Pillay T, Parry G et al (2013) Hemodynamic, echocardiographic, and exercise-related effects of the HeartWare left ventricular assist device in advanced heart failure. Congest Heart Fail 19(1):11–15
17. Nissinoff J, Tian F, Therattil M, Salvarrey RM, Lee SW (2011) Acute inpatient rehabilitation after left ventricular assist device implantation for congestive heart failure. PM R 3(6):586–589
18. Piepoli MF (2013) Exercise training in chronic heart failure: mechanisms and therapies. Neth Heart J 21(2):85–90
19. Taylor RS, Sagar VA, Davies FJ, Briscoe S, Coats AJ, Dalal H et al (2014) Exercise-based rehabilitation for heart failure. Cochrane Database Syst Rev 4:CD003331
20. Arcêncio L, Souza MD, Bortolin BS, Fernandes AC, Rodrigues AJ, Evora PR (2008) Pre-and postoperative care in cardiothoracic surgery: a physiotherapeutic approach. Rev Bras Cir Cardiovasc 23(3):400–410
21. Perme CS, Southard RE, Joyce DL, Noon GP, Loebe M (2006) Early mobilization of LVAD recipients who require prolonged mechanical ventilation. Tex Heart Inst J 33(2):130–133
22. Morrone TM, Buck LA, Catanese KA, Goldsmith RL, Cahalin LP, Oz MC et al (1996) Early progressive mobilization of patients with left ventricular assist devices is safe and optimizes recovery before heart transplantation. J Heart Lung Transplant 15(4):423–429
23. Freeman R, Maley K (2013) Mobilization of intensive care cardiac surgery patients on mechanical circulatory support. Crit Care Nurs Q 36(1):73–88
24. Westerdahl E, Lindmark B, Eriksson T, Friberg O, Hedenstierna G, Tenling A (2005) Deep-breathing exercises reduce atelectasis and improve pulmonary function after coronary artery bypass surgery. Chest 128(5):3482–3488
25. Johnston CL, James R, Mackney JH (2013) The current use of positive expiratory pressure (PEP) therapy by public hospital physiotherapists in New South Wales. New Zealand J Physiother 41(3):88–93
26. Westerdahl E, Lindmark B, Almgren SO, Tenling A (2001) Chest physiotherapy after coronary artery bypass graft surgery: comparison of three different techniques. J Rehabil Med 33(2):79–84
27. D'agrosa-Boiteux MC, Geoffroy E, Dauphin N, Camilleri L, Eschalier R, Cuenin C et al (2014) Left ventricle assist device: rehabilitation and management programmes. Ann Cardiol Angeiol (Paris) 63(4):245–252
28. Corrà U, Pistono M, Mezzani A, Gnemmi M, Tarro Genta F, Caruso R et al (2011) Cardiovascular Prevention and rehabilitation for patients with ventricular assist device. From exercise therapy to long-term therapy. Part I: exercise therapy. Monaldi Arch Chest Dis 76(1):27–32
29. Fattirolli F, Bonacchi M, Burgisser C, Cellai T, Francini S, Valente S et al (2009) Cardiac rehabilitation of patients with left ventricular assist device as "destination therapy". Monaldi Arch Chest Dis 72(4):190–199
30. Hambrecht R, Niebauer J, Fiehn E, Kälberer B, Offner B, Hauer K et al (1995) Physical training in patients with

stable chronic heart failure: effects on cardiorespiratory fitness and ultrastructural abnormalities of leg muscles. J Am Coll Cardiol 25(6):1239–1249
31. Maybaum S, Mancini D, Xydas S, Starling RC, Aaronson K, Pagani FD et al (2007) Cardiac improvement during mechanical circulatory support: a prospective multicenter study of the LVAD Working Group. Circulation 115(19):2497–2505
32. Reedy JE, Swartz MT, Lohmann DP, Moroney DA, Vaca KJ, McBride LR et al (1992) The importance of patient mobility with ventricular assist device support. ASAIO J 38(3):M151–M153
33. Wells CL (2013) Physical therapist management of patients with ventricular assist devices: key considerations for the acute care physical therapist. Phys Ther 93(2):266–278
34. Rogers JG, Aaronson KD, Boyle AJ, Russell SD, Milano CA, Pagani FD et al (2010) Continuous flow left ventricular assist device improves functional capacity and quality of life of advanced heart failure patients. J Am Coll Cardiol 55(17):1826–1834
35. Anagnostakou V, Chatzimichail K, Dimopoulos S, Karatzanos E, Papazachou O, Tasoulis A et al (2011) Effects of interval cycle training with or without strength training on vascular reactivity in heart failure patients. J Card Fail 17(7):585–591
36. de Jonge N, Kirkels H, Lahpor JR, Klöpping C, Hulzebos EJ, de la Rivière AB et al (2001) Exercise performance in patients with end-stage heart failure after implantation of a left ventricular assist device and after heart transplantation: an outlook for permanent assisting? J Am Coll Cardiol 37(7):1794–1799
37. Haft J, Armstrong W, Dyke DB, Aaronson KD, Koelling TM, Farrar DJ et al (2007) Hemodynamic and exercise performance with pulsatile and continuous-flow left ventricular assist devices. Circulation 116(11 Suppl):I8–15
38. Jakovljevic DG, Birks EJ, George RS, Trenell MI, Seferovic PM, Yacoub MH et al (2011) Relationship between peak cardiac pumping capability and selected exercise-derived prognostic indicators in patients treated with left ventricular assist devices. Eur J Heart Fail 13(9):992
39. Laoutaris ID, Dritsas A, Adamopoulos S, Manginas A, Gouziouta A, Kallistratos MS et al (2011) Benefits of physical training on exercise capacity, inspiratory muscle function, and quality of life in patients with ventricular assist devices long-term postimplantation. Eur J Cardiovasc Prev Rehabil 18(1):33–40
40. Marko C, Danzinger G, Käferbäck M, Lackner T, Müller R, Zimpfer D et al (2014) Safety and efficacy of cardiac rehabilitation for patients with continuous flow left ventricular assist devices. Eur J Prev Cardiol 22(11):1378–1384
41. Pruijsten RV, Lok SI, Kirkels HH, Klöpping C, Lahpor JR, de Jonge N (2012) Functional and haemodynamic recovery after implantation of continuous-flow left ventricular assist devices in comparison with pulsatile left ventricular assist devices in patiens with end-stage heart failure. Eur J Heart Fail 14(3):319–325
42. Hayes K, Leet A, Bradley S, Holland A (2012) Effects of exercise training on exercise capacity and quality of life in patients with a left ventricular assist device: a preliminary randomized controlled trial. J Heart Lung Transplant 31(7):729–734
43. Karapolat H, Engin C, Eroglu M, Yagdi T, Zoghi M, Nalbantgil S et al (2013) Efficacy of the cardiac rehabilitation program in patients with end-stage heart failure, heart transplant patients, and left ventricular assist device recipients. Transplant Proc 45(9):3381–3385
44. Kerrigan DJ, Williams CT, Ehrman JK, Bronsteen K, Saval MA, Schairer JR et al (2013) Muscular strength and cardio respiratory fitness are associated with health status in patients with recently implanted continuous-flow LVADs. J Cardiopulm Rehabil Prev 33(6): 396–400
45. Harrington D, Anker SD, Chua TP, Webb-Peploe KM, Ponikowski PP, Poole-Wilson PA et al (1997) Skeletal muscle function and its relation to exercise tolerance in chronic heart failure. J Am Coll Cardiol 30(7):1758–1764
46. Clark AL (2006) Origin and symptoms in chronic heart failure. Heart 92(1):12–16
47. Jaski BE, Lingle RJ, Kim J, Branch KR, Goldsmith R, Johnson MR et al (1999) Comparison of functional capacity in patients with end-stage heart failure following implantation of a left ventricular assist device versus heart transplantation: results of the experience with left ventricular assist device with exercise trial. J Heart Lung Transplant 18(11):1031–1040
48. Compostella L, Russo N, Setzu T, Bottio T, Compostella C, Tarzia V et al (2015) A practical review for cardiac rehabilitation professionals of continuous-flow left ventricular assist devices: historical and current perspectives. J Cardiopulm Rehabil Prev 35(5):301–311
49. Kugler C, Malehsa D, Schrader E, Tegtbur U, Guetzlaff E, Haverich A et al (2012) A multi-modal intervention in management of left ventricular assist device outpatients: dietary counselling, controlled exercise and psychosocial support. Eur J Cardiothorac Surg 42(6):1026–1032
50. Nguyen E, Stein J (2013) Functional outcomes of adults with left ventricular assist devices receiving inpatient rehabilitation. PM R 5(2):99–103
51. Alsara O, Reeves RK, Pyfferoen MD, Trenary TL, Engen DJ, Vitse ML et al (2014) Inpatient rehabilitation outcomes for patients receiving left ventricular assist device. Am J Phys Med Rehabil 93(10):860–868
52. Chu SK, McCormick Z, Hwang S, Sliwa JA, Rydberg L (2014) Outcomes of acute inpatient rehabilitation of patients with left ventricular assist devices. PM R 6(11):1008–1012
53. English ML, Speed J (2013) Effectiveness of acute inpatient rehabilitation after left ventricular assist device placement. Am J Phys Med Rehabil 92(7):621–626
54. Polastri M, Bacchi Reggiani ML, Cefarelli M, Jafrancesco G, Martin-Suarez S (2013) The distance walked daily as a post-operative measure after pulmonary endarterectomy. Int J Ther Rehabil 20(4):195–199
55. Kohli HS, Canada J, Arena R, Tang DG, Peberdy MA, Harton S et al (2011) Exercise blood pressure response during assisted circulatory support: comparison of the total artificial [corrected] heart with a left ventricular assist device during rehabilitation. J Heart Lung Transplant 30(11):1207–1213

56. Hasin T, Topilsky Y, Kremers WK, Boilson BA, Schirger JA, Edwards BS et al (2012) Usefulness of the six-minute walk test after continuous axial flow left ventricular device implantation to predict survival. Am J Cardiol 110(9):1322–1328
57. Busch JC, Lillou D, Wittig G, Bartsch P, Willemsen D, Oldridge N et al (2012) Resistance and balance training improves functional capacity in very old participants attending cardiac rehabilitation after coronary bypass surgery. J Am Geriatr Soc 60(12):2270–2276
58. Podsiadlo D, Richardson S (1991) The timed "Up & Go": a test of basic functional mobility for frail elderly persons. J Am Geriatr Soc 39(2):142–148
59. Mkacher W, Mekki M, Tabka Z, Trabelsi Y (2015) Effect of 6 months of balance training during pulmonary rehabilitation in patients with COPD. J Cardiopulm Rehabil Prev 35(3):207–213
60. Berg KO, Wood-Dauphinee SL, Williams JI, Maki B (1992) Measuring balance in the elderly: validation of an instrument. Can J Public Health 83(suppl 2):S7–11
61. Hurvitz EA, Richardson JK, Werner RA, Ruhl AM, Dixon MR (2000) Unipedal stance testing as an indicator of fall risk among older outpatients. Arch Phys Med Rehabil 81(5):587–591
62. Tinetti M (1986) Performance-oriented assessment of mobility problems in elderly patients. J Am Geriatr Soc 34(2):119–126
63. Myers AM, Fletcher PC, Myers AH, Sherk W (1998) Discriminative and evaluative properties of the Activities-Specific Balance Confidence (ABC) scale. J Gerontol A Biol Sci Med Sci 53(4):M287–M294
64. Pistono M, Corrà U, Gnemmi M, Imparato A, Caruso R, Balestroni G et al (2011) Cardiovascular prevention and rehabilitation for patients with ventricular assist device from exercise therapy to long-term therapy. Part II: long-term therapy. Monaldi Arch Chest Dis 76(3):136–145
65. Ueno A, Tomizawa Y (2009) Cardiac rehabilitation and artificial heart devices. J Artif Organs 12(2):90–97
66. Scheiderer R, Belden C, Schwab D, Haney C, Paz J (2013) Exercise guidelines for inpatients following ventricular assist device placement: a systematic review of the literature. Cardiopulm Phys Ther J 24(2):35–42
67. Compostella L, Russo N, Setzu T, Compostella C, Bellotto F (2014) Exercise performance of chronic heart failure patients in the early period of support by an axial-flow left ventricular assist device as destination therapy. Artif Organs 38(5):366–373
68. Wilson SR, Givertz MM, Stewart GC, Mudge GH (2009) Ventricular assist devices. The challenges of outpatient management. J Am Coll Cardiol 54(18):1647–1659
69. Corrà U, Pistono M, Piepoli MF, Giannuzzi P (2012) Ventricular assist device patients on the horizon of cardiovascular prevention and rehabilitation. Can we convert challenges into opportunities? Eur J Prev Cardiol 19(3):490–493
70. Alsara O, Perez-Terzic C, Squires RW, Dandamudi S, Miranda WR, Park SJ et al (2014) Is exercise training safe and beneficial in patients receiving left ventricular assist device therapy? J Cardiopulm Rehabil Prev 34(4):233–240
71. Wienbergen H, Hambrecht R (2012) Trainingstherapie bei kardiologischen Patienten (Sportkardiologie). Herz 37(5):486–492
72. Matlock DD (2012) Destination unknown: the ventricular assist device and the advance of technology. J Am Geriatr Soc 60(1):154–155
73. Mezzani A, Hamm LF, Jones AM, McBride PE, Moholdt T, Stone JA et al (2012) Aerobic exercise intensity assessment and prescription in cardiac rehabilitation: a joint position statement of the European Association for Cardiovascular Prevention and Rehabilitation, the American Association of Cardiovascular and Pulmonary Rehabilitation, and the Canadian Association of Cardiac Rehabilitation. J Cardiopulm Rehabil Prev 32(6):327–350
74. Compostella L, Russo N, Setzu T, Covolo E, Vettore E, Iliceto S et al (2013) Effects of short-term exercise training at anaerobic threshold in patients with axial-flow left ventricular assist device. Eur J Prev Cardiol 20(Suppl 1):S30
75. Simon MA, Kormos RL, Gorcsan J 3rd, Dohi K, Winowich S, Stanford E et al (2005) Differential exercise performance on ventricular assist device support. J Heart Lung Transplant 24(10):1506–1512
76. Sénage T, Fèvrier D, Michel M, Pichot E, Duveau D, Tsui S et al (2014) A mock circulatory system to assess the performance of continuous-flow left ventricular assist devices (LVADs): does axial flow unload better than centrifugal LVAD? ASAIO J 60(2):140–147
77. Lalonde SD, Alba AC, Rigobon A, Ross HJ, Delgado DH, Billia F et al (2013) Clinical differences between continuous flow ventricular assist devices: a comparison between HeartMate II and HeartWare HVAD. J Card Surg 28(5):604–610
78. Yancy CW, Jessup M, Bozkurt B, Butler J, Casey DE Jr, Drazner MH et al (2013) 2013 ACCF/AHA guideline for the management of heart failure: a report of the American College of Cardiology Foundation/American Heart Association Task Force on practice guidelines. Circulation 128(16):e240–e327
79. Birks EJ, George RS, Hedger M, Bahrami T, Wilton P, Bowles CT et al (2011) Reversal of severe heart failure with a continuous-flow left ventricular assist device and pharmacological therapy: a prospective study. Circulation 123(4):381–390
80. Slaughter MS, Pagani FD, Rogers JG, Miller LW, Sun B, Russell SD et al (2010) Clinical management of continuous-flow left ventricular assist devices in advanced heart failure. J Heart Lung Transplant 29(4 Suppl):S1–39
81. Lampert BC, Eckert C, Weaver S, Scanion A, Lockard K, Allen C et al (2014) Blood pressure control in continuous flow left ventricular assist devices: efficacy and impact on adverse events. Ann Thorac Surg 97(1):139–146
82. Topilsky Y, Oh JK, Shah DK, Boilson BA, Schirger JA, Kushwaha SS et al (2011) Echocardiographic predictors of adverse outcomes after continuous left ventricular assist device implantation. JACC Cardiovasc Imaging 4(3):211–222
83. Compostella L, Russo N, Setzu T, Tursi V, Bottio T, Tarzia V et al (2013) Cardiac autonomic dysfunction in the early phase after left ventricular assist device implant: implications for surgery and follow-up. Int J Artif Organs 36(6):410–418
84. Gardiwal A, Roentgen P, Luesebrink U, Koenig T, Klein G, Oswald H (2010) Left ventricular assist improves

autonomic imbalance in patients with persistent myocardial dysfunction. Int J Artif Organs 33(12): 851–855
85. Tank J, Heusser K, Malehsa D, Hegemann K, Haufe S, Brinkmann J et al (2012) Patients with continuous-flow left ventricular assist devices provide insight in human baroreflex physiology. Hypertension 60(3):849–855
86. Gademan MG, Swenne CA, Verwey HF, van der Laarse A, Maan AC, van de Vooren H et al (2007) Effect of exercise training on autonomic derangement and neurohumoral activation in chronic heart failure. J Card Fail 13(4):294–303
87. Hu SX, Keogh AM, Macdonald PS, Kotlyar E, Robson D, Harkess M et al (2013) Interaction between physical activity and continuous-flow left ventricular assist device function in outpatients. J Card Fail 19(3):169–175
88. Brassard P, Jensen AS, Nordsborg N, Gustafsson F, Møller JE, Hassager C et al (2011) Central and peripheral blood flow during exercise with a continuous-flow left ventricular assist device: constant versus increasing pump speed: a pilot study. Circ Heart Fail 4(5):554–560
89. Jakovljevic DG, George RS, Nunan D, Donovan G, Bougard RS, Yacoub MH et al (2010) The impact of acute reduction of continuous-flow left ventricular assist device support on cardiac and exercise performance. Heart 96(17):1390–1395
90. Noor MR, Bowles C, Banner NR (2012) Relationship between pump speed and exercise capacity during HeartMate II left ventricular assist device support: influence of residual left ventricular function. Eur J Heart Fail 14(6):613–620
91. Jung MH, Hansen PB, Sander K, Olsen PS, Rossing K, Boesgaard S et al (2014) Effect of increasing pump speed during exercise on peak oxygen uptake in heart failure patients supported with a continuous-flow left ventricular assist device. A double-blind randomized study. Eur J Heart Fail 16(4):403–408
92. Kirklin JK, Naftel DC, Kormos RL, Stevenson LW, Pagani FD, Miller MA et al (2013) Fifth INTERMACS annual report: risk factor analysis from more than 6,000 mechanical circulatory support patients. J Heart Lung Transplant 32(2):141–156
93. Vollkron M, Voitl P, Ta J, Wieselthaler G, Schima H (2007) Suction events during left ventricular support and ventricular arrhythmias. J Heart Lung Transplant 26(8):819–825
94. Boilson BA, Durham LA, Park SJ (2012) Ventricular fibrillation in an ambulatory patient supported by a left ventricular assist device: highlighting the ICD controversy. ASAIO J 58(2):170–173
95. Sims DB, Rosner G, Uriel N, González-Costello J, Ehlert FA, Jorde UP (2012) Twelve hours of sustained ventricular fibrillation supported by a continuous-flow left ventricular assist device. Pacing Clin Electrophysiol 35(5):e144–e148
96. Enriquez AD, Calenda B, Miller MA, Anyanwu AC, Pinney SP (2013) The role of implantable cardioverter-defibrillators in patients with continuous flow left ventricular assist devices. Circ Arrhythm Electrophysiol 6(4):668–674
97. Garan AR, Yuzefpolskaya M, Colombo PC, Morrow JP, Te-Frey R, Dano D et al (2013) Ventricular arrhythmias and implantable cardioverter-defibrillator therapy in patients with continuous-flow left ventricular assist devices: need for primary prevention? J Am Coll Cardiol 61(25):2542–2550
98. Raasch H, Jensen BC, Chang PP, Mounsey JP, Gehi AK, Chung EH et al (2012) Epidemiology, management, and outcomes of sustained ventricular arrhythmias after continuous-flow left ventricular assist device implantation. Am Heart J 164(3):373–378
99. Felix SE, Martina JR, Kirkels JH, Klöpping C, Nathoe H, Sukkel E et al (2012) Continuous-flow left ventricular assist device support in patients with advanced heart failure: points of interest for the daily management. Eur J Heart Fail 14(4):351–356
100. Boyle A (2012) Arrhythmias in patients with ventricular assist devices. Curr Opin Cardiol 27(1):13–18
101. Hottigoudar RU, Deam AG, Birks EJ, McCants KC, Slaughter MS, Gopinathannair R (2013) Catheter ablation of atrial flutter in patients with left ventricular assist device improves symptoms of right heart failure. Congest Heart Fail 19(4):165–171
102. Stulak JM, Deo S, Schirger J, Aaronson KD, Park SJ, Joyce LD et al (2013) Preoperative atrial fibrillation increases risk of thromboembolic events after left ventricular assist device implantation. Ann Thorac Surg 96(6):2161–2167
103. Ades PA, Keteyian SJ, Balady GJ, Houston-Miller N, Kitzman DW, Mancini DM et al (2013) Cardiac rehabilitation exercise and self-care for chronic heart failure. JACC Heart Fail 1(6):540–547
104. Nishimura M, Radovancevic B, Odegaard P, Myers T, Springer W, Frazier OH (1996) Exercise capacity recovers slowly but fully in patients with a left ventricular assist device. ASAIO J 42(5):M568–M570
105. Grapow MT, Todorov A, Bernet F, Zerkowski HR (2003) Ambulatory long-term management of a left ventricular assist device. Current modality in terminal heart failure. Swiss Surg 9(1):27–30
106. Park WH, Seo YG, Sung JD (2014) Exercise therapy for an older patient with left ventricular assist device. Ann Rehabil Med 38(3):396–400
107. Leibner ES, Cysyk J, Eleuteri K, El-Banayosy A, Boehmer JP, Pae WE (2013) Changes in the functional status measures of heart failure patients with mechanical assist devices. ASAIO J 59(2):117–122
108. Dunlay SM, Allison TG, Pereira NL (2014) Changes in cardiopulmonary exercise testing parameters following continuous flow left ventricular assist device implantation and heart transplantation. J Card Fail 20(8):548–554
109. Jakovljevic DG, McDiarmid A, Hallsworth K, Seferovic PM, Ninkovic VM, Parry G et al (2014) Effect of left ventricular assist device implantation and heart transplantation on habitual physical activity and quality of life. Am J Cardiol 114(1):88–93
110. Munro J, Angus N, Leslie SJ (2013) Patient focused Internet-based approaches to cardiovascular rehabilitation–a systematic review. J Telemed Telecare 19(6):347–353

111. Antypas K, Wangberg SC (2014) An Internet- and mobile-based tailored intervention to enhance maintenance of physical activity after cardiac rehabilitation: short-term results of a randomized controlled trial. J Med Internet Res 16(3):e77
112. Kraal JJ, Peek N, Van den Akker-Van Marle ME, Kemps HM (2014) Effects of home-based training with telemonitoring guidance in low to moderate risk patients entering cardiac rehabilitation: short-term results of the FIT@Home study. Eur J Prev Cardiol 21(2 Suppl):26–31
113. Corazza I, Bianchini D, Urbinati S, Zannoli R (2014) REHAL©, a telemedicine platform for home cardiac rehabilitation. Minerva Cardioangiol 62(5):399–405
114. Hernández C, Alonso A, Garcia-Aymerich J, Grimsmo A, Vontetsianos T, Garcia Cuyàs F et al (2015) Integrated care services: lessons learned from the deployment of the NEXES project. Int J Integr Care 15:e006
115. Polastri M, Loforte A (2015) Influence of ventricular assist devices equipment wear on body posture. Artif Organs 39(7):640–641

Physiotherapy and Rehabilitation Programs for Pediatric VAD Patients

C. VanderPluym, J. Conway, H. Buchholz, and A. Lorts

© Springer International Publishing Switzerland 2017
A. Montalto et al. (eds.), *Mechanical Circulatory Support in End-Stage Heart Failure*,
DOI 10.1007/978-3-319-43383-7_41

41.1 Introduction

The field of mechanical circulatory support for children has evolved dramatically over the last decade. This is in part attributable to the development of smaller ventricular assist devices (VADs) which has expanded the array of support strategies in pediatrics. Extracorporeal membrane oxygenation (ECMO) was originally the cornerstone of mechanical circulatory support for children. Its ease of implantation, wide accessibility, and applicability to all patient sizes made it the first-line choice for urgent cardiopulmonary support. However, ECMO has significant limitations related to its extracorporeal design (i.e., pump external to the body with cannula inserted either in peripheral vessels or centrally similar to cardiopulmonary bypass), its thrombogenic nature, need for aggressive anticoagulation, and secondary complications. These issues limit the duration of support to weeks, with an exponential rise in complications beyond that time. Additionally, ECMO cannulation prevents easy mobilization of patients. Many patients remain heavily sedated and ventilated for the duration of support, and as such, there is no way to engage patients in active physiotherapy or rehabilitation. The advent of pediatric VADs has changed the way we approach children on mechanical circulatory support. The first pediatric VAD to gain widespread global use was the Berlin Heart EXCOR® (Berlin Heart GmbH, Germany). This paracorporeal pulsatile-flow device can be used for right, left, or biventricular support. A variety of pump sizes are available to accommodate all sized children, infants to adolescent. The more secure central cannulation technique with externalization of the cannula through the upper abdominal wall allows patients to be woken up, extubated, fed, mobilized, reconditioned, and rehabilitated. While the Berlin Heart EXCOR is vastly superior to ECMO in terms of survival to and after transplantation, it still has a high risk of stroke [1]. The largest multicenter prospective study on the Berlin Heart was conducted in North America for the Investigation Device Exemption (IDE) Food and Drug Administration (FDA) trial [1]. This study reported a 29% incidence of stroke despite standardized anticoagulation and antiplatelet therapy. As such, a comprehensive approach to mitigating stroke risk and improving recovery post stroke through rehabilitation has evolved from the Berlin Heart experience.

In recent years, newer-generation continuous-flow (cf) devices designed for adults are now being used to support pediatric heart failure patients. Their smaller size and intracorporeal design have made them preferential alternatives to the Berlin Heart for larger children (sized >15 kg) and adolescents. There is now expanding experience with outpatient management of children on CF-VADs, like the HeartWare HVAD® (HeartWare Inc., Framingham, MA) and HeartMate II® (Thoratec Inc., Pleasanton, CA) [2, 3]. The ability to discharge children home on VAD support is a significant advancement in the field of pediatric mechanical circulatory support, since all previous support strategies including the Berlin Heart were restricted to in-hospital care only. Today, there is a new and growing population of children leaving the hospital with their VADs and reentering their communities and schools [3]. Rehabilitation and physiotherapy are integral parts to making this transition successful.

In this section, we will discuss the role of rehabilitation for children with VADs, focusing on device-specific inpatient and outpatient management strategies.

41.2 Pre-implantation Rehabilitation

In general, children in end-stage heart failure who require mechanical circulatory support are significantly deconditioned. Failure to thrive is a common presentation of heart failure in children, resulting in a clinical picture of poor growth velocity, low weight, low body mass, poor muscle development, and impaired bone density. Additionally, many infants and young children presenting with chronic heart failure have gross and fine motor developmental delays attributable to chronic illness, multiple hospitalizations, and poor nutritional status. In adults, the term *frailty* is used to describe a similar phenotype of patient. Fried et al. defined frailty as a clinical syndrome of individuals of advanced age who meet three out of five functional criteria indicating compromised energetics: low grip strength, low energy, slowed walking speed, low physical activity, and/or unintentional weight loss [4]. In adults, frailty is a significant risk factor for morbidity and mortality in patient with heart failure, with VADs and awaiting heart transplantation. We presume, similar to frail adults, children with decline in functional reserve across multiple physiologic systems due to chronic illness will have a heightened risk associated with VAD implantation and/or transplantation. As such, many pediatric VAD programs have dedicated teams to thoroughly evaluate all children prior to VAD implantation. This comprehensive evaluation examines all organ systems (neurologic, pulmonary, renal, hepatic, gastrointestinal, musculoskeletal, infectious, immunologic and hematologic) for risk factors that may complicate VAD implantation and long term VAD support. In addition, children are evaluated by physiotherapist, occupational therapist, speech-language pathologist and neurodevelopmental specialists to establish the child's functional baseline prior to any further surgical procedures. These comprehensive evaluations help identify deficits that need focused attention by the care team. Since children may present for VAD implantation at any age, from infants to adolescents, there is a wide spectrum of developmental abilities that need to be assessed. Evaluation of gross motor, fine motor, language, social skills, and cognition needs to be tailored to the age of the child. Tools for evaluation can be limited for very young children, since infants and neonates do not have a large repertoire of developmental capabilities that can be easily quantified. As such, in the youngest children, the assessment is primarily focusing on motor abilities and global neurological physical examination including symmetry of movement, muscle tone, and reflexes. With older children, a wider battery of tests can be performed to obtain a more objective measure including but not limited to the DENVER II Developmental Screening Test (DDST), Bayley Scale of Infant and Toddler Development (Bayley-III), Kaufman Assessment Battery for Children (KABC-II) (ages 3–18 years), Stanford-Benet Intelligence Scale (SB-5) (ages 2–85+ years), Wechsler Intelligence Scale for Children (WISC-IV) (ages 6–16 years), Wechsler Preschool and Primary Scale of Intelligence (WPPSI-III), (ages 2.5–7 years), and Beery-Buktenica Developmental Test of Visual-Motor Integration, 6th Edition (VMI) (ages 2–18 years).

41.3 Post-implantation Rehabilitation

Early mobilization post VAD implantation is paramount. Regardless of the type of VAD, the sooner the patient can be woken up, extubated, and fed, the less likely they will acquire complications and morbidities. Regardless of the type of VAD used (paracorporeal, LVAD, or BiVAD), early extubation followed by aggressive chest physiotherapy and age-appropriate incentive spirometry is vital. Prolonged intubation is associated with more pronounced deconditioning of respiratory and skeletal muscles and may lead to ventilator-associated pneumonia. As such, optimization of pulmonary function through diuresis and chest physiotherapy to recruit lung space is a top priority in the early postoperative period. Involvement of physiotherapy and occupational therapy should begin in the intensive care unit as soon as patient is clinically stable. Even if the patient is sedated, passive range of motion activities can be completed by physiotherapists or parents to help prevent pressure sores and muscle contractures. Once patients are extubated, mobilization by sitting up in bed, encouraging play and ambulation, should be a key priority. Identifying activities that are age appropriate is important. Hollander et al. described the benefits of a structured inpatient rehabilitation program for children on paracorporeal devices such as the Berlin Heart EXCOR [5]. Between 2010 and 2013, they enrolled 14 patients aged 0.5–14 years for a standardized care pathway (SCP) for physical rehabilitation. Of the 14 patients, eight participated in the infant SCP, and six participated in the children SCP. There were no adverse events related to any of the therapies. Twelve of the 14 patients survived to transplantation, and 11 patients achieved all the goals of the SCP. Barriers to participation included cannula infection ($n = 1$), repeated respiratory infection ($n = 1$), and intolerance to being handled ($n = 1$). Their study demonstrated that most children and infants could complete many of the activities including riding the adaptive bicycle with hand and foot pedals for older children and tolerate physiotherapy in the prone position for infants. Most notable was that several patients exceeded the expectations of the SCP without complications, completing activities such as playing on

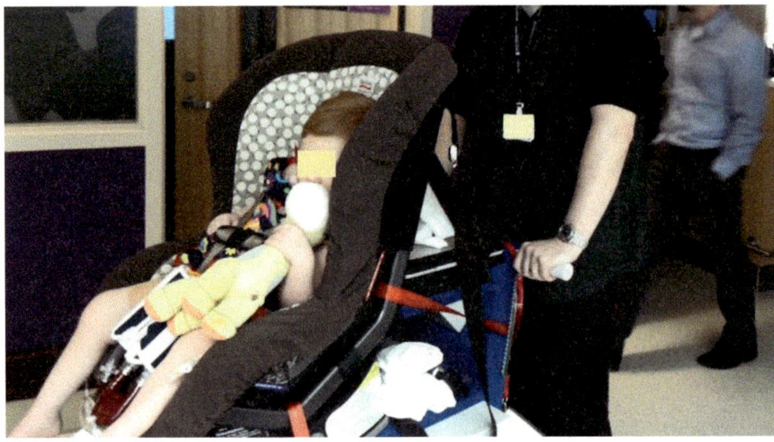

Fig. 41.1 Child supported on Berlin Heart BiVAD seated in car seat mounted on IKUS driving unit

swings and slides. Despite these patients' complex care needs, challenges with paracorporeal VAD equipment, and need for intense anticoagulation, no adverse events were noted during any physiotherapy. The investigators concluded that intensive rehabilitation and facilitation of age-appropriate activities is safe when supervised by expert personnel.

Mobilization with the Berlin Heart EXCOR® driving unit (IKUS) can be a challenge. Trying to coordinate the patient, the IKUS, and any other pumps (IV or feeding pumps) can require multiple caregivers which can limit the number and duration of time to move around. As such, centers have devised ways to facilitate ambulation by attaching car seats to the IKUS unit (Fig. 41.1).

For larger children and adolescents, ambulation is much easier because of the use of intracorporeal VADs such as the HeartWare® and HeartMate II/III®. The goal of postoperative care should be early extubation (ideally <12–24 h), with ambulation and mobilization immediately thereafter. Daily physiotherapy should commence as soon as possible to ensure that patients achieve functional status that is back to or exceeds their pre-implantation baseline. Many centers advocate quantitative assessment of exercise ability through 6 min walk test (6MWT) and/or exercise stress test with spirometry and metabolic testing. Most ambulatory children can perform a 6MWT, and older children and adolescents can navigate an exercise stress test on a treadmill or bicycle. This can be completed prior to discharge home for baseline assessment of exercise capacity in order to identify and follow outpatient rehabilitation needs.

41.4 Outpatient Cardiac Rehabilitation

It is well established that cardiac rehabilitation (CR) improves survival, functional ability, and quality of life in adults on LVAD support [6, 7]. Hayes et al. investigated whether supervised exercise training improved maximal exercise capacity (peak VO_2), submaximal exercise capacity (6 min walk distance, 6MWD), and quality of life (QoL) scores in 14 adult LVAD patients, through a prospective, assessor-blinded randomized controlled trial [8]. They demonstrated no adverse events, with a trend toward improved peak VO_2, 6MWD, and QoL in the exercise group ($n = 7$) as compared with the control group. However, the difference was not statistically significant and warranted further evaluation with a larger cohort. In a larger study completed by Kerrigan et al., improved indicators of functional capacity and health status were demonstrated among 26 adults with LVADs who attended CR. Functional capacity was determined by peak oxygen uptake, treadmill time, 6MWD, and leg strength. They concluded that CR was well tolerated by LVAD patients, and when all metrics of functional capacity were assessed in their entirety, CR was favorably associated with increased exercise tolerance [9]. In contrast, little is known regarding the utility of formal outpatient CR in children on VAD support. The goal of all CR therapy is to improve patient's functional abilities, exercise endurance, and most importantly QoL. Outpatient CR may be of variable benefit depending on the patient's age, developmental abilities, underlying cardiac disease, comorbidities, and duration of illness prior to device support. Facilitating a return back to school and participation in extracurricular activities should be the primary goal of CR program. Many children and adolescents may benefit from a tailored CR program that is focused on activities that interest the pediatric population, such as sports and games. Assessment by a comprehensive team of physiotherapists, occupational therapists, and rehabilitation physicians will help delineate deficiencies in functional abilities and areas for improvement. The level of deconditioning prior to VAD support will likely dictate the potential for functional improvement post VAD support. Most children on dischargeable VAD support (HeartWare®, HeartMate II®, and Syncardia®) are of ages and developmental abilities to participate in many exercise regimes. Additionally, exercise testing including 6MWD, treadmill, and bicycle exercise tests is generally feasible in most ambulatory children and adolescents, allowing metrics to measure improvement. Pediatric centers are learning from the experiences garnered by adult cardiovascular facilities in terms of evaluation and availability of rehabilitation services. We expect that with the growing population of complex cardiac children transitioning to outpatient facilities, CR for children will be an area of tremendous potential for evaluation and development.

References

1. Fraser CD Jr, Jaquiss RD, Rosenthal DN, Humpl T, Canter CE, Blackstone EH et al (2012) Prospective trial of a pediatric ventricular assist device. N Engl J Med 367(6):532–541
2. Conway J, VanderPluym C, Jeewa A, Sinnadurai S, Schubert A, Lorts A (2016) Now how do we get them home? Outpatient care of pediatric patients on mechanical circulatory support. Pediatr Transplant 20(2):194–202. doi:10.1111/petr.12674
3. Schweiger M, Vanderpluym C, Jeewa A, Canter CE, Jansz P, Parrino PE et al (2015) Outpatient management of intra-corporeal left ventricular assist device system in children: a multi-center experience. Am J Transplant 15(2):453–460
4. Fried LP, Xue QL, Cappola AR, Ferrucci L, Chaves P, Varadhan R et al (2009) Nonlinear multisystem physiological dysregulation associated with frailty in older women: implications for etiology and treatment. J Gerontol A Biol Sci Med Sci 64(10):1049–1057
5. Hollander SA, Hollander AJ, Rizzuto S, Reinhartz O, Maeda K, Rosenthal DN (2014) An inpatient rehabilitation program utilizing standardized care pathways after paracorporeal ventricular assist device placement in children. J Heart Lung Transplant 33(6):587–592
6. Dugmore LD, Tipson RJ, Phillips MH, Flint EJ, Stentiford NH, Bone MF et al (1999) Changes in cardiorespiratory fitness, psychological wellbeing, quality of life, and vocational status following a 12 month cardiac exercise rehabilitation programme. Heart 81(4):359–366
7. Karapolat H, Engin C, Eroglu M, Yagdi T, Zoghi M, Nalbantgil S et al (2013) Efficacy of the cardiac rehabilitation program in patients with end-stage heart failure, heart transplant patients, and left ventricular assist device recipients. Transplant Proc 45(9):3381–3385
8. Hayes K, Leet AS, Bradley SJ, Holland AE (2012) Effects of exercise training on exercise capacity and quality of life in patients with a left ventricular assist device: a preliminary randomized controlled trial. J Heart Lung Transplant 31(7):729–734
9. Kerrigan DJ, Williams CT, Ehrman JK, Saval MA, Bronsteen K, Schairer JR et al (2014) Cardiac rehabilitation improves functional capacity and patient-reported health status in patients with continuous-flow left ventricular assist devices: the rehab-vad randomized controlled trial. JACC Heart Fail 2(6):653–659

Patient- and Device-Tailored Antithrombotic Treatment

Vincenzo Tarzia, Giacomo Bortolussi, Jonida Bejko, Tomaso Bottio, and Gino Gerosa

© Springer International Publishing Switzerland 2017
A. Montalto et al. (eds.), *Mechanical Circulatory Support in End-Stage Heart Failure*,
DOI 10.1007/978-3-319-43383-7_42

Hemorrhagic and thrombotic complications largely contribute to the morbidity and mortality associated with VADs [1].

Thrombotic complications are attributed to nonphysiological flow patterns resulting in shear stress and platelet activation as well as the interaction of blood with the artificial surfaces of the VAD system [2].

Efforts to minimize these complications include lifelong treatment with anticoagulant and antiplatelet agents. Although vital for preventing catastrophic thrombotic complications, this therapy leads to the risk of iatrogenic hemorrhage, which starts in the early postoperative period and continues for the duration of support [3].

Balancing the risk of thrombosis and hemorrhage is a major challenge, and there are two key interactions, which must be understood: the one between different VAD designs and the coagulation system and the individual patient's response to the VAD and antithrombotic therapy.

42.1 Individual Effect of Different VADs on Hemorrhagic and Thrombotic Risk

The fifth INTERMACS annual report, comparing the adverse event rate of pulsatile and continuous-flow VAD technology, demonstrated a significantly lower risk of bleeding and thrombotic events in patients treated with the newer-generation continuous-flow VADs [4].

This decreased risk of thrombotic and hemorrhagic events has been one of the drivers behind the marked increase in the use of continuous-flow devices in recent times. However, continuous devices are not a homogenous group, as they include both axial-flow and centrifugal-flow pumps, which differ significantly in their characteristics and would be expected to have different effects on the coagulation and hematological systems [5].

Indeed, patients with HeartWare HVAD®, a centrifugal-flow pump, show higher levels of D-dimer, MCF in ROTEM tests, platelet count, and activation at the aggregometer. On the other hand, axial-flow pumps, namely, Thoratec HeartMate II® and Jarvik 2000 FlowMaker®, are associated with signs of hemolysis, as suggested by elevated LDH [6, 7].

Beyond the theoretical interest in understanding the effects of various VAD designs on the coagulation and hematological systems, there is also significant potential for clinical application of this knowledge.

For example, in 2011 HeartWare noticed an unexpectedly high rate of pump thrombosis, which was associated with subtherapeutic INR and low aspirin dose (81 mg or less). The implementation of a stricter INR protocol, together with ASA adjustment to 325 mg, resulted in a drop of pump exchange and ischemic strokes. Interestingly, the more aggressive antithrombotic treatment was not associated with higher incidence of bleeding or hemorrhagic strokes [8].

However, these results were also due to technical improvements, as the introduction of an enhanced coring tool and sintered inflow cannula. Yet another example of a specific VAD model enhancement having a clinical impact is the one of Jarvik 2000, where the shift of the bearing mechanism from pin to cone design resulted in improved survival and reduced incidence of stroke [9].

Lastly, in the USA, an abrupt increase in pump thrombosis was also observed with HeartMate II, starting in mid-2011 [10]. The precise causes still remain unknown, but it has been hypothesized that the level of anticoagulation was insufficient.

According to the aforementioned findings, it is possible to outline a rational antithrombotic therapy from the outset. In fact, HeartWare patients are usually treated with both anticoagulant and antiplatelet drugs, and HeartMate II alike, while Jarvik patients are kept only on anticoagulation.

42.2 Variation in Patient's Coagulation Status

Another factor to bear in mind is that the patient's coagulation system, and subsequently its interaction with the VAD, changes over time. This occurs either per se, and following several physiological and pathological processes, which are not always evident or predictable. Examples include infections, hemorrhages, right ventricular failure, and other medications.

As a result, it is essential to constantly monitor coagulation with both quantitative and qualitative tests and tailor the antithrombotic therapy accordingly.

Generally, MCS patients are treated with a modified version of the multitargeted antithrombotic approach (MTA) originally proposed for total artificial heart management [11]. Protocols consist of anticoagulation with unfractionated heparin and warfarin, eventually bridged with fondaparinux, and antiplatelet therapy with aspirin, and clopidogrel when appropriate.

MTA is best calibrated with a multimonitoring system (MMS) using conventional laboratory markers such as complete blood count, prothrombin time, aPTT, D-dimer, and fibrinogen and ATIII levels, together with thromboelastometry and aggregometry.

Rotational thromboelastometry (ROTEM®, Tem International GmbH, München, Germany) is a whole blood coagulation method that provides information about clot strength and stability and indirectly about platelet function. The clot forming in an oscillating cuvette transmits its movement onto a suspended piston, which is recorded continuously and given a graphic representation [12]. Various tests, performed with specific reagents, allow to evaluate the different contributions to coagulation cascade: Intem® activates the contact phase of hemostasis, evaluating intrinsic pathway; Extem® screens extrinsic pathway via tissue factor activation; and Fibtem® eliminates platelet contribution, allowing evaluation of fibrinogen activity. Briefly, the measured parameters are clotting time (CT), which is the time until initiation of clotting, affected by coagulation factors; clot formation time (CFT), which is the time from CT until a clot firmness of 20 mm is reached; and maximum clot firmness (MCF), which is the greatest amplitude reached by the clot. Both CFT and MCF correlate with platelet number and function, fibrin polymerization disorders, and fibrinogen function, but MCF is usually considered in that it best describes the clot quality.

Platelet aggregation can be measured with the Multiplate® analyzer (Roche Diagnostics, Mannheim, Germany), a whole-blood impedance aggregometer (which measures the change of resistance between two platinum electrodes, proportional to the amount of platelets attached to them) [13]. Again, several tests are available to evaluate platelet aggregation induced by different agonists:

TRAPtest®: TRAP-6 stimulates the thrombin surface receptor
COLtest®: collagen leads to a release of endogenous arachidonic acid
ASPItest®: arachidonic acid is transformed into thromboxane A2
ADPtest®: adenosine diphosphate stimulates ADP receptor.

The parameter expressing platelet activation in each of the tests is the area under the aggregation curve (AUC), derived from total height of aggregation measured in arbitrary aggregation units (AU) over time (in minutes). TRAPtest and COLtest evaluate overall platelet activity, but are not reliable in vivo, being both largely influenced by platelet count. ASPItest and ADPtest measure the effect of therapy with aspirin and clopidogrel, respectively.

42.3 Practical Therapeutic Algorithms

Traditionally, antithrombotic prophylaxis has been adjusted based on aPTT, INR, and platelet count.

What the MMS further achieves is to give clues on whether the patient is normo-coagulant, thus allowing the prearranged therapy, or is unbalanced toward a hypo- or hypercoagulant status, prompting, respectively, a decrease or increase in antithrombotic therapy, which still is calibrated according to the classical tests.

In this sense, the single most meaningful parameter is the MCF in ROTEM Intem and Extem tests.

In the range between 50 and 70 mm, it reflects an overall normo-coagulant status.

When it drops below 50 mm, the target aPTT or INR (with heparin or warfarin, respectively) should be lowered. If this is associated with a decrease in platelet count, and the fibrinogen level is correct, then antiplatelet therapy can be reduced.

On the other hand, when MCF exceeds 70 mm, and this is usually related to elevated levels of platelet or fibrinogen, it is advised to increase antiaggregation, by inhibiting one or both the arachidonic acid and ADP pathways.

42.3.1 ECMO and Paracorporeal VADs

Before implant, a heparin intravenous bolus of 70 U/Kg (usually 5000 units) is administered, to obtain an activated clotting time (ACT) of 180 s.

At arrival in the ICU, heparin infusion is started, to maintain activated partial thromboplastin time (aPTT) between 50 and 60 s.

Normally, international normalized ratio (INR), aPTT, and antithrombin III (ATIII) assays are to be performed 4 times per day and platelet counts, fibrinogen, and D-dimer assays once daily.

Antithrombin is supplemented with 1000 IU when ATIII activity is <80%.

In cases of hemorrhagic or thrombotic complications, or unexpectedly elevated D-dimer, thromboelastometry can help to rule out coagulation disorders [14].

42.3.2 Implantable VADs

Prior to ventricular apex coring, and subsequent VAD implant, 5000 IU of heparin is given.

After 2–3 h since the transfer to the ICU, in the absence of ongoing bleeding, antithrombin III is corrected. Heparin infusion is commenced at 500 IU/hour and then adjusted based on aPTT: between 45 and 50 s on first postoperative day and 50–60 s thereafter.

In the following days, bridging to therapeutic INR of 2–3 is achieved with fondaparinux.

Regarding antiplatelet therapy, a differentiated approach is adopted, according to the implanted device.

With HeartMateII, aspirin dose has varied greatly between reports, ranging from none to 325 mg daily [15].

In patients with Jarvik 2000, ROTEM tests express a reduced platelet and fibrinogen activity, a situation reflected by platelet count, which rarely exceeds normal limits. Therefore, unless indicated for other comorbidities (e.g., ischemic heart disease, recent stents, severe peripheral vasculopathy), antiplatelet therapy is not necessary in that it would increase hemorrhagic risk, without reducing the already low thrombotic risk.

Conversely, HVAD demands 320 mg of aspirin daily, usually split in 2 administrations. The effect of therapy should be checked with aggregometric essays, to verify that the arachidonic pathway is blocked. If not, aspirin dose can be increased to 480 mg (160 mg three times a day), or dual therapy with clopidogrel can be initiated. This is especially important in the first month post-implant, when the hypercoagulant reaction is often more pronounced. On the other hand, to avoid the opposite issue of hemorrhage, strict follow-up is warranted, to enable prompt reduction of antiaggregation when the coagulative status gets back to normality.

42.3.3 Total Artificial Heart (CardioWest)

The perioperative management is similar to that of implantable VADs, except for a slightly higher target INR of 3 (2.5–3.5), due to the presence of multiple mechanical valves.

However, in light of studies demonstrating that the risk of hemorrhage is greater than thrombosis, the once very aggressive antithrombotic protocol (dipyridamole, pentoxifylline, ASA) [11] has been recently simplified to ASA 100 mg.

In conclusion, the protocols described above should provide a general guidance for setting up therapy. However, this ought to be calibrated on the patient, to follow the changes taking place over time.

References

1. Kirklin JK, Naftel DC, Pagani FD, Kormos RL, Stevenson LW, Blume ED, Myers SL, Miller MA, Baldwin JT, Young JB (2015) Seventh INTERMACS annual report: 15,000 patients and counting. J Heart Lung Transplant 34:1495–1504
2. Bluestein D (2004) Research approaches for studying flow-induced thromboembolic complications in blood recirculating devices. Expert Rev Med Devices 1:65–80
3. Schaffer JM, Arnaoutakis GJ, Allen JG, Weiss ES, Patel ND, Russell SD et al (2011) Bleeding complications and blood product utilization with left ventricular assist device implantation. Ann Thorac Surg 91:740–747
4. Kirklin JK, Naftel DC, Kormos RL, Stevenson LW, Pagani FD, Miller MA et al (2013) Fifth INTERMACS annual report: risk factor analysis from more than 6,000 mechanical circulatory support patients. J Heart Lung Transplant. 32:141–156
5. Tarzia V, Buratto E, Bortolussi G, Gallo M, Bejko J, Bianco R, Bottio T, Gerosa G (2014) Haemorrhage and thrombosis with different LVAD technologies: a matter of flow? Ann Cardiothorac Surg 3:582–584
6. Birschmann I, Dittrich M, Eller T, Wiegmann B, Reininger AJ, Budde U et al (2014) Ambient hemolysis and activation of coagulation is different between HeartMate II and HeartWare left ventricular assist devices. J Heart Lung Transplant. 33:80–87
7. Tarzia V, Bortolussi G, Penzo V, Bejko J, Gallo M, Bianco R, Bottio T, Gerosa G (2014) Are all continuous flow left ventricular assist devices equal on platelet activation and inflammatory response? A comparison of

centrifugal versus axial flow pump. Interact Cardiovasc Thorac Surg 19(suppl 1):S7–S8

8. Slaughter MS, Pagani FD, McGee EC, Birks EJ, Cotts WG, Gregoric I, Howard Frazier O, Icenogle T, Najjar SS, Boyce SW, Acker MA, John R, Hathaway DR, Najarian KB, Aaronson KD (2013) HeartWare Bridge to Transplant ADVANCE Trial Investigators. HeartWare ventricular assist system for bridge to transplant: combined results of the bridge to transplant and continued access protocol trial. J Heart Lung Transplant 32:675–683
9. Tarzia V, Di Giammarco G, Di Mauro M, Bortolussi G, Maccherini M, Tursi V, Maiani M, Bernazzali S, Marinelli D, Foschi M, Buratto E, Bejko J, Gregori D, Scuri S, Livi U, Sani G, Bottio T, Gerosa G (2016) From bench to bedside: Can the improvements in left ventricular assist device design mitigate adverse events and increase survival? J Thorac Cardiovasc Surg 151:213–217
10. Starling RC, Moazami N, Silvestry SC, Ewald G, Rogers JG, Milano CA, Rame JE, Acker MA, Blackstone EH, Ehrlinger J, Thuita L, Mountis MM, Soltesz EG, Lytle BW, Smedira NG (2014) Unexpected abrupt increase in left ventricular assist device thrombosis. N Engl J Med 370:33–40
11. Ensor CR, Cahoon WD, Crouch MA, Katlaps GJ, Hess ML, Cooke RH et al (2010) Antithrombotic therapy for the CardioWest temporary total artificial heart. Tex Heart Inst J 37:149–158
12. Calatzis A, Leiter M, Panzer S (2009) Monitoring anticoagulation of primary haemostasis – Estimation of platelet function in whole blood assays. Hamostaseologie 29:279–284
13. Tóth O, Calatzis A, Penz S, Losonczy H, Siess W (2006) Multiple electrode aggregometry: a new device to measure platelet aggregation in whole blood. Thromb Haemost 96:781–788
14. Tarzia V, Bortolussi G, Bianco R, Buratto E, Bejko J, Carrozzini M, De Franceschi M, Gregori D, Fichera D, Zanella F, Bottio T, Gerosa G (2015) Extracorporeal life support in cardiogenic shock: impact of acute versus chronic etiology on outcome. J Thorac Cardiovasc Surg 150:333–340
15. Baumann Kreuziger LM, Kim B, Wieselthaler GM (2015) Antithrombotic therapy for left ventricular assist devices in adults: a systematic review. J Thromb Haemost 13:946–955

Coagulation Monitoring

Alexander Stepanenko and Ivan Netuka

© Springer International Publishing Switzerland 2017
A. Montalto et al. (eds.), *Mechanical Circulatory Support in End-Stage Heart Failure*,
DOI 10.1007/978-3-319-43383-7_43

43.1 Introduction

43.1.1 Cell-Based Model of Coagulation and Its Application to MCS Systems

In the 1960s two groups independently proposed a model of coagulation as a sequential series of steps in which activation of one clotting factor leads to the activation of another, finally leading to a burst of thrombin generation [1, 2].

Evolution of thinking on process of hemostasis in cell-based model of coagulation has moved the field from focusing primarily on the protein components to putting the cellular participants in a central role. Hoffman and Monroe proposed in 2001 a so-called "cell-based" model of hemostasis.

Briefly, the goal of hemostasis is to produce a platelet and fibrin plug to seal a site of injury in the blood vessel wall. Hemostasis is initiated when tissue factor bearing cells are exposed to the blood at a site of injury. Extrinsic pathway operates on the TF-bearing cell to initiate and amplify coagulation. By contrast, the "intrinsic" pathway operates on the activated platelet surface to produce the burst of thrombin that causes formation and stabilization of the fibrin clot. Platelets play a crucial role in localizing clotting reactions to the site of injury because they adhere and aggregate at sites where TF is also exposed. Platelets provide the primary surface for generation of the burst of thrombin needed for effective hemostasis during propagation phase of coagulation. This model allows us to see the extrinsic and intrinsic pathways of coagulation as having distinct and nonredundant role, as they act on different cell surfaces at different stages of hemostatic process [3].

Bleeding and thromboembolism are serious adverse events that have been associated with the use of mechanical circulatory support and were medical devices being connected to patient circulation via artificial grafts and interacting with patients' organism. This kind of interaction occurs on systems ("pulseless circulation," AV malformation, blood exposure to shear stress), tissue (integration of inflow connection site, "neointima" growth; cellular (RBC, PLT)), and molecular (fibrinogen, von Willebrand factor protein, PF4 receptor protein) levels. Hematological interactions between end-stage heart failure patient and ventricular assist device became clinically "visible" through onset of bleeding and thrombotic complication during support time.

Historically antithrombotic therapy was recommended in the treatment protocol and included the early postoperative use of IV heparin as a transition to warfarin and aspirin therapy [4–6].

Hence, anticoagulation therapy is by itself an additional risk factor for onset of hematological complications: hypercoagulable blood status with consequent arterial and venous thrombosis, as in heparin-induced thrombocytopenia syndrome, and intracerebral or GI bleeding due to overanticoagulation. Some groups performed reduced protocol with aim to eliminate related to heparin complication and start directly warfarin and aspirin after LVAD placement [7]. But it is still a subject of debate.

All our struggles of postoperative anticoagulation (IV and later oral therapy) are targeting to overcome persisting activation of contact-phase proteins and platelets, to turn down intrinsic pathway of thrombin production during blood-VAD interaction (▫ Figs. 43.1, 43.2, and 43.3). In this way, we are inhibiting excessive thrombin generation and clotting at surface of VAD and at the same time permitting thrombus formation at site of vessel injury to avoid excessive or/and lethal bleeding. It is important to keep balanced another part of coagulation system – fibrinolysis.

Important is to recognize other factors contributing to onset of thrombosis/bleeding event. Fibrin deposition which is almost persistent around intracardiac inflow part of all types of LVAD cannula may be mobilized by sudden ICD shocks, electrical cardioversion. Its degree may be promoted by suboptimal inflow cannula position in left ventricle cavity triggering suction events and related thrombus ingestion. This all may lead to thromboembolic event despite optimal level of given anticoagulant. At the same time preexisting coagulopathy as sequela of cardiogenic shock or chronic liver congestion will pronounce postoperative bleeding.

43.2 Assessment of Coagulopathy

(a) Heparin monitoring: aPTT versus ACT, TEG overanticoagulation control
(b) Argatroban monitoring
(c) PLT function assessment (LTA, PFA-100, Multiplate)

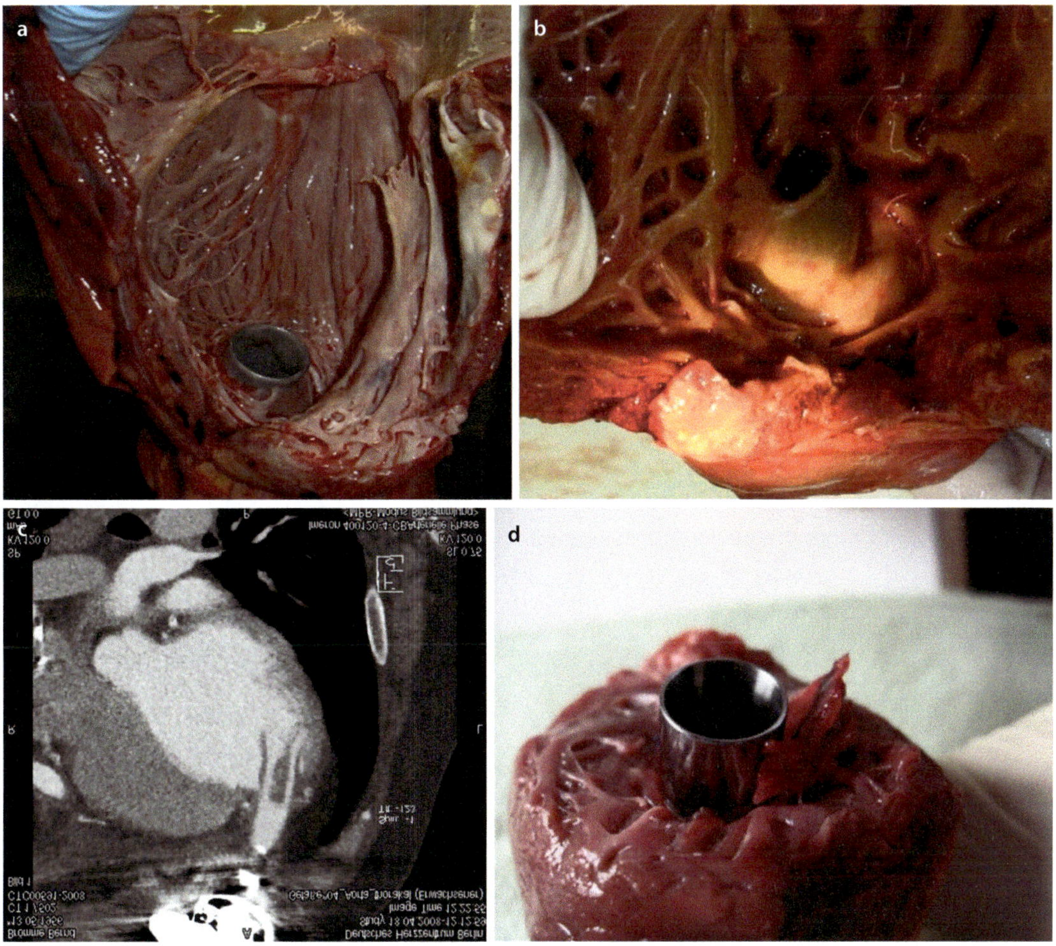

Fig. 43.1 Virchow-Triad in MCS setting: Flow stagnation areas (around VAD inflow, aortic root, prosthetic valves). (**a**) A large LV cavity and HM II inflow; (**b**) malposition of HM II inflow/partial integration into the LV wall; (**c**) inflow malposition with thrombus ingestion/CT scan of Ventracor pts.; (**d**) fibrin deposition at stasis area/DuraHeart inflow

(a) Identification of the level of anticoagulation is the key of VAD management. In the initial years of cardiac surgery with CPB, a fixed dose of heparin was administered without monitoring for level of anticoagulation. The introduction of anticoagulation monitoring was a great advancement to improve care in postoperative period.

The earliest and most popular test to monitor anticoagulation for extracorporeal circuits was the activated clotting time (ACT).

It measures the integrity of the intrinsic coagulation and common pathways. To perform an ACT, whole blood is placed in a test tube with 1 of 2 activators of the contact pathway, celite (diatomaceous earth) or kaolin (clay). The celite ACT forms clot that will disrupt the magnetic field of the magnetic detector by pulling iron away from it, thereby halting the timer. The kaolin ACT has a plunger that actively rises and falls in whole blood until the rate of the falling plunger is slowed by clot formation and an optical sensor detects the change halting the timer.

ACT remains the one of the predominant test to manage heparin anticoagulation during ECMO. However, the ACT's capability to correctly measure the level of anticoagulation has been questioned.

Concern about the ACT's ability to provide adequate anticoagulation is because the test results are affected by patient characteristics, such as coagulopathy, platelet dysfunction, hypothermia, AT level, age, and hemodilution, as well as

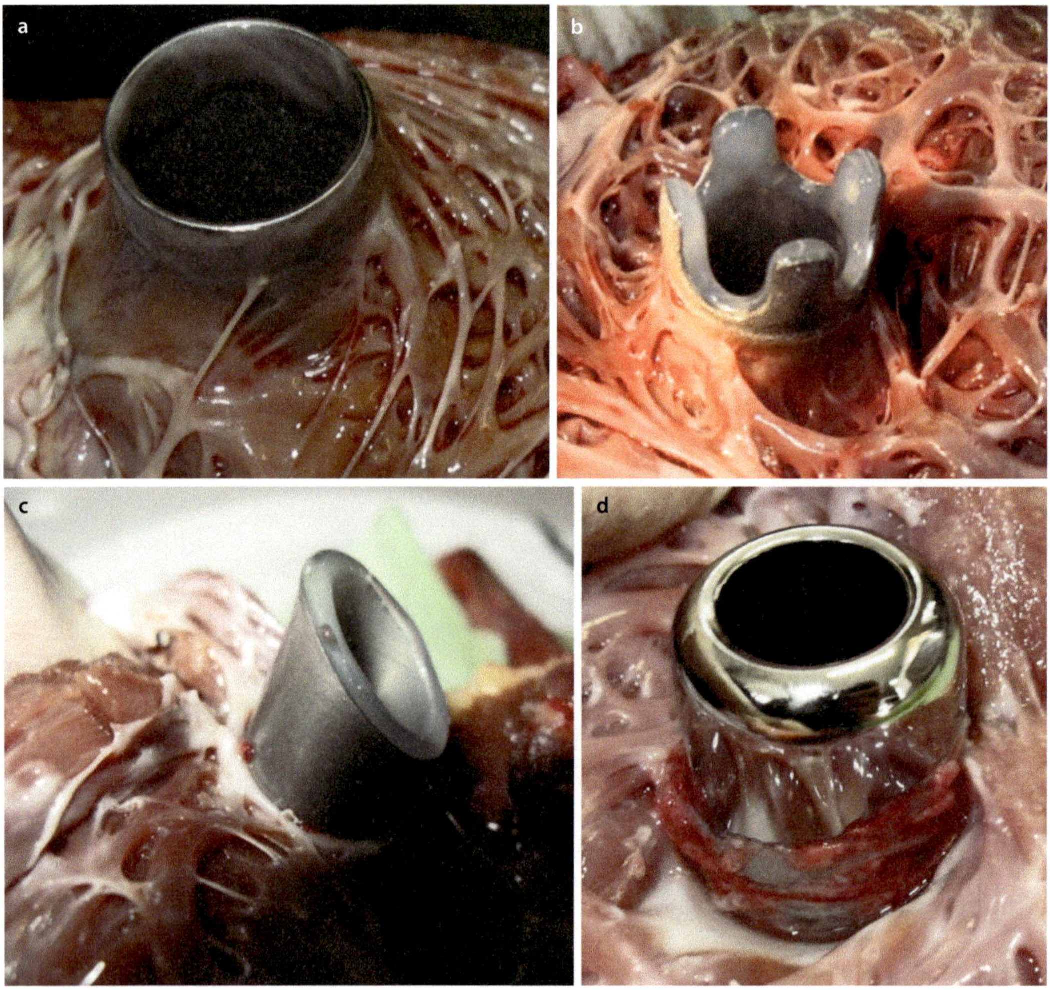

Fig. 43.2 Virchow-Triad in MCS setting: Exposure to foreign surface/healing at inflow insertion site. "Neointima" or scar tissue formation at (**a**) HM II, (**b**) INCOR, (**c**) EXCOR, (**d**) HVAD inflows

technical factors, such as sample size, venous or arterial blood, and temperature.

In very ill patients requiring continuous infusions of heparin, the ACT could not delineate between low and moderate levels of anticoagulation compared with the aPTT. This may result in unrecognized inadequate anticoagulation [8, 9].

Recent study of Atallah confirmed again this discrepancy: The heparin dose correlated better with aPTT relative to ACT and, thus, may be considered a more effective tool for the dosing of heparin in adult ECMO patients [10].

We observed the same phenomenon in our MSC patient population and modified our therapy through the years to use aPTT for heparin or argatroban dose guidance.

The activated partial thromboplastin time (aPTT) is universally recognized as a standard monitor for heparin therapy except when high heparin dosing is required as in CPB. The aPTT is performed on recalcified citrated plasma and represents the intrinsic and common pathways. Its reagent contains phospholipids that act as platelets for clotting to occur [8].

aPTT level reflects not only status of intrinsic and common thrombin generation pathways but also existing (preoperative measured without anticoagulants) or produced (iatrogenic via heparin or argatroban) degree of coagulopathy. Not only intrinsic factors deficit, but first fibrinogen consumption, platelet dysfunction, and hemodilution may significantly impact on and may prolong aPTT in the first phase after VAD insertion.

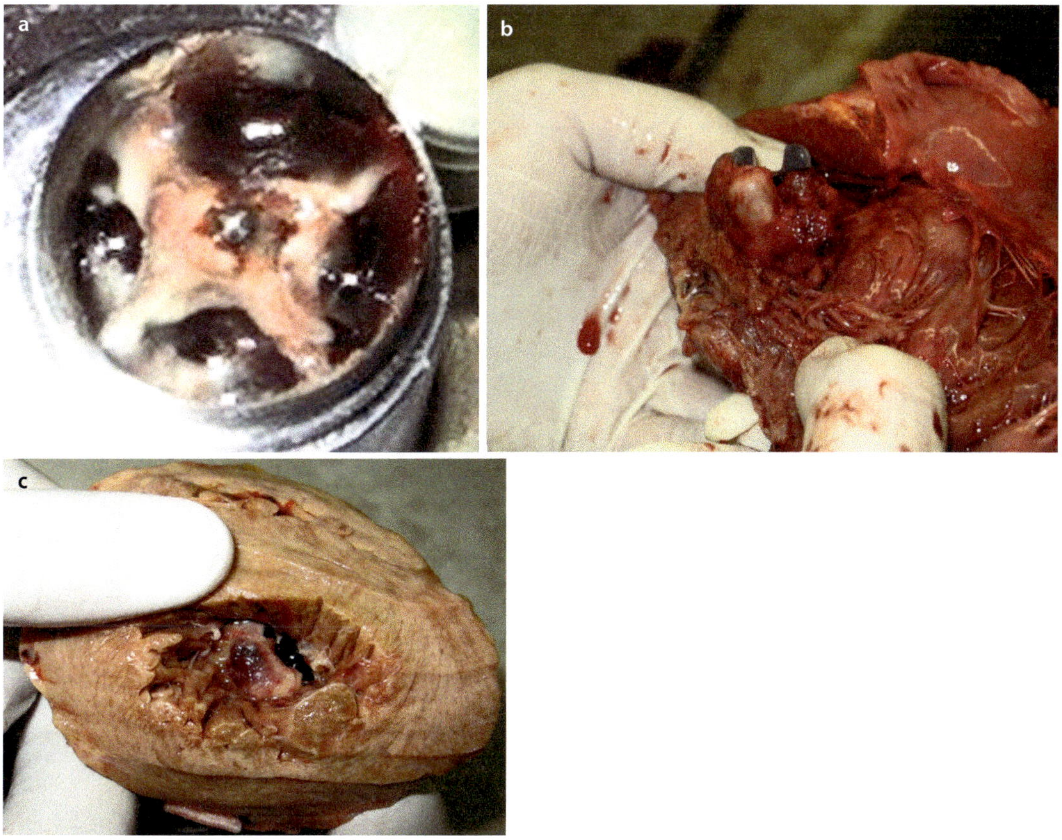

Fig. 43.3 Virchow-Triad in MCS setting: Acute changes of blood coagulation balance (sepsis, HIT syndrome, liver failure). (**a**) Thrombus at rotor f HM II in MRSA sepsis pts. who died due to lethal ICB; (**b**) sever thrombus formation at INCOR inflow in sepsis pts.; (**c**) thrombosed inflow in HVAD pts. with cardiac amyloidosis and sepsis

There are also situations where aPTT guidance is limited due to patient factors – lupus coagulant and antiphospholipid syndrome. Both disorders present clinically prolonged aPTT with increased thromboembolic risk. IV anticoagulation guidance using aPTT in this case is challenging. In most cases as early as possible anti vitamin K and antiplatelet agent's start may be one of the safe solutions.

Looking on aPTT level together with performed kaolin-thromboelastogram is useful to prevent overanticoagulation with consequently increased risk for bleeding. This backup control of heparin therapy is failing in case of postoperative use of IV direct thrombin inhibitors.

(b) From all direct thrombin inhibitors available for clinical use, argatroban is the most proven and safe agent for postoperative anticoagulation after VAD implantation in HIT setting [11–13].

Manufacturer recommends argatroban IV therapy: anticoagulation in adult patients with heparin-induced thrombocytopenia type II who require parenteral antithrombotic therapy. Therapy monitoring is performed using aPTT. Initial infusion rate is 2 mcg/kg/min and for hepatically impaired or critically ill pts. 0.5 mcg/kg/min.

The target range for steady-state aPTT is 1.5–3.0 times the initial baseline value, but not exceeding 100 seconds. In dose range at aPTT levels over 100 s, there is no direct dose/aPTT correlation. Agent cumulation with overanticoagulation is then possible. Ecarin-TEG or modified thrombin time may be of value, but is still at present time an subject of investigation.

The maximum recommended dose is 10 mcg/kg/min. The maximum recommended duration of treatment is 14 days [14].

Liver congestion due to right ventricular failure may interact with argatroban elimination. In

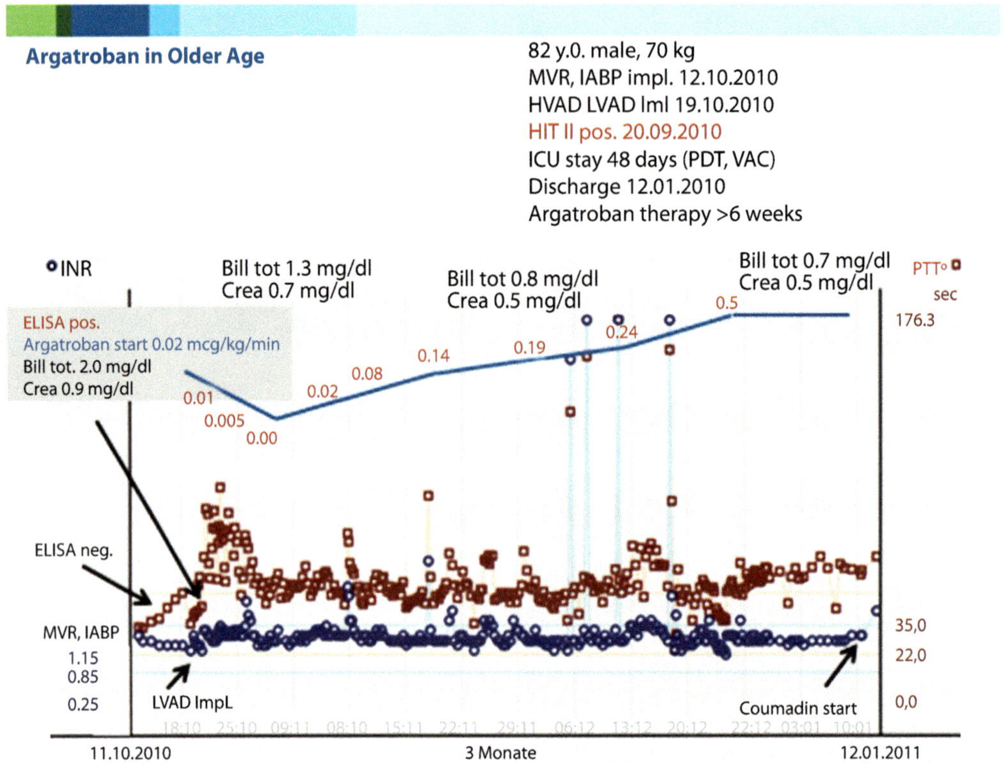

Fig. 43.4 Argatroban in elderly LVAD recipients

this case, pts. require significantly lower dose to prolong aPTT to 1.5–2 times. Also elderly destination therapy recipient had to be treated with careful dose adjustment (Fig. 43.4) [15].

We recommend lower starting dose (as recommended by manufacturer) in critically ill patient and after VAD insertion (0.1 mcg/kg/min). Argatroban bolusing (1–10 mg) allows rapid achievement of target anticoagulation level for each specific clinical situation (VAD weaning/exchange) without increased bleeding risk. During switch to warfarin, it is important to recognize some kind of interaction between argatroban and INR measurements. INR is prolonged approximately for 0.3–0.5. At the moment of argatroban discontinuation at time of target INR, additional measurements of INR 4–6 h after shall be performed. In case of drop-off of INR level due to argatroban clearance, some additional warfarin dose adjustment may be of value.

(c) Platelet function assessment and antiplatelet therapy.

At present time, three platelet function tests are widely used for assessment of PLT aggregation by adding different reagents. It mimics in vivo PLT activation and helps to quantify effect of antiplatelet therapy and identify nonresponders.

PFA 100 was introduced as POC device and measures the time needed to form a platelet plug that occludes a given aperture (coated with collagen and epinephrine or ADP) during high shear stress of whole blood probe (Fig. 43.5a). PFA is suitable for monitoring therapy with aspirin and as a screening test for detection of von Willebrand syndrome. In our single-center study, we found PFA 100 membrane closure time already after 1 week after insertion of a rotary LVAD doubled and has been kept so prolonged until follow-up of 1 year. That reflects that all our rotary LVAD recipients suffers in some kind from acquired von Willebrand syndrome, described elsewhere [19–23]. Based on this fact, clinical value of PFA-100 test in MCS pts. is limited. We do not use this test for platelet therapy timing and dose adjustment.

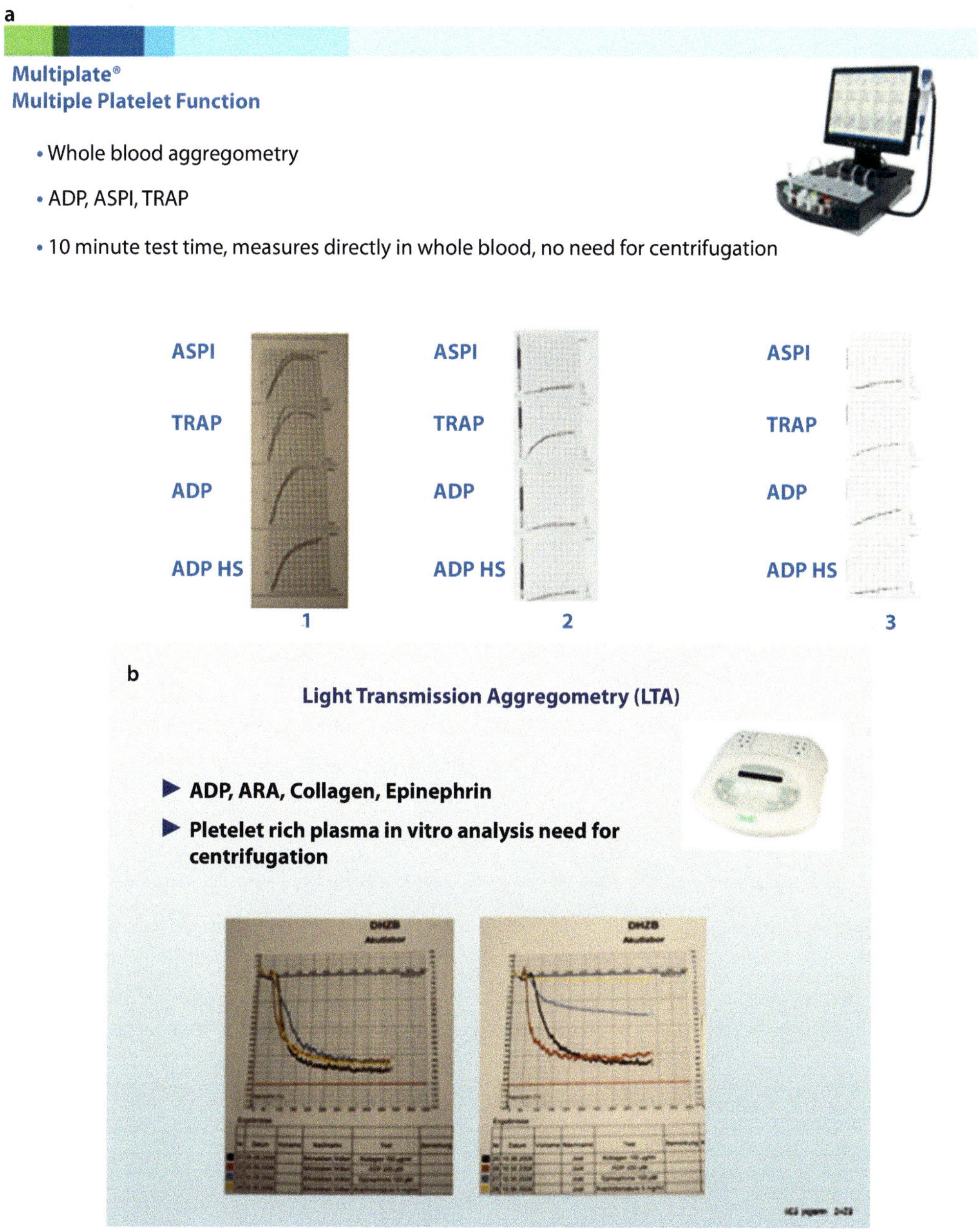

Fig. 43.5 (**a**) Multiplate: *column 1* represents patient without antiplatelet therapy, *column 2* represents sufficient platelet suppression in patient with dual therapy (aspirin and clopidogrel), and *column 3* represents patient with IV Aggrastat therapy for thrombotic LVAD dysfunction (all pathways of PLT activation are suppressed). (**b**) Light transmission aggregometry test: *right* – ARA, ADP, collagen, and epinephrine are not suppressed; *left* – ARA is suppressed in patient with aspirin therapy

Light transmission aggregometry assesses effects of aspirin and Plavix. Historically this test has been used in the last two decades to define platelet suppression. Hence, test has some disadvantages (Fig. 43.5b).

Another newly introduced POC instrument, the Multiplate, measures PLT aggregation after adding commonly used agonist by detecting changes in electrical resistance in whole blood. This eliminates the need for centrifugation of plasma or adjustment of PLT concentration as requires for classical aggregometry. Agonists were used according to laboratory routine to perform LTA assay and induced with collagen, epinephrine, ADP, and arachidonic acid. Agonists used for Multiplate assay are arachidonic acid (ASPI), ADP, and TRAP (thrombin receptor-activating peptide).

We start on POD 3–7 antiplatelet agents after recovery of PLT number and function with low dose of 50–81 mg per day (Multiplate test) [18, 24].

43.2.1 Treatment at ICU, ROTEM TEG for Therapy Guidance, Assessment of All Factors (Pts., Hemolysis, Technical Data)

After admission at ICU, hemodynamic monitoring and clinical monitoring for post-implant bleeding are performed. Maintenance of adequate end organs and body perfusion and standard values as pH, body temperature, and Ca++ plasma level may be of great value to keep coagulation system in a balance. In the presence of continuing drainage blood loss, optimization of plasmatic coagulation system (coagulation factors concentrate (PPSB or Cofact), fibrinogen, tranexamic acid) and platelet function is performed (see ◘ Table 43.1).

Dynamic assessment of clot formation via both pathways (extrinsic and intrinsic) is possible by thromboelastography performed by ROTEM devices (EXTEM, INTEM, HEPTEM, FIBTEM, APTEM). POC ROTEM analysis has been shown as important guide of targeted hematological therapy. Our unpublished data, same as recently published experience from USA showed effective and safe management of coagulation bleeding disorders using prothrombin complex concentrate without increase of thrombotic event rate [16].

◘ **Table 43.1** Anticoagulation protocols (Dr. Netuka)

LVAD	Postoperative	Antiplatelet therapy	Target INR
HeartMate II	Heparin when chest tube drainage is less than 50 ml/h. Titrate to a PTT of 45–50 for 24 h. After 24 h, titrate to PTT 50–60. After another 24 h, titrate to PTT 55–65	On POD 2–3, initiate aspirin 81–100 mg QD and dipyridamole 75 mg TID	On POD 3–5, no bleeding, and the chest tubes removed, begin warfarin (overlapping with the heparin) Maintain INR 2.0–3.0
HeartMate III	Heparin to achieve PTT 45–65 s once chest tube drainage is <50 ml/h for 3 h. Heparin titrated up over 2 days to PTT of 55–65	Aspirin 81–100 mg daily and dipyridamole 75 mg TID	On POD 3–5, no bleeding, and the chest tubes removed, begin warfarin (overlapping with the heparin) Maintain INR 2.0–3.0.
HeartWare HVAD	Heparin at 10 units/kg/h to a target PTT of 40–50 s. Maintain the PTT in a range of 50–60 s	Aspirin 325 mg/day within 24 h after implant, or clopidogrel at doses of 75–150 mg/day	Warfarin started within 4 days post-op and titrated to maintain an INR of 2.0–3.0
Berlin Heart INCOR	Heparin 5–7 U/kg/hr. to PTT 60–80 s. AT III to achieve activity >70%	Aspirin 100 mg daily and dipyridamole	Target INR 2.5–3.0
Berlin Heart EXCOR	After 12 h, heparin to a PTT of 50–60, then PTT 60–80	Aspirin 75–500 mg daily	Target INR 3.0–3.5
Jarvik 2000	Heparin to PTT of 40–45 s	Aspirin 100 mg daily and dipyridamole	Warfarin to INR 2.0–3.0

There are seldom reports of use of recombinant factor VII to control postoperative bleeding. Bruckner et al. reported that, in most patients with "off-label" indications for rFVIIa administration, a low dose (10–20 g/kg) of this drug is sufficient to control bleeding and that higher doses are associated with a significant risk of thromboembolic complications [17].

In case of ongoing surgical bleeding, indication for revision has to be evaluated.

It is important to control all the time hemolysis parameters and technical data of power consumption, especially if aggressive intervention using coagulation factors or derivatives is performing. In any case of gradual or sudden increase of free plasma hemoglobin and LDH plasma levels together with increase of energy consumption or presence of its spikes in LVAD data history, decision for start of IV anticoagulation shall be evaluated despite presence of bleeding.

Drainage blood loss less than 50 ml per hour within consecutive 4 h together with stable hemoglobin level, absence of tamponade, or pleural effusion is accepted at our hospital as cessation of bleeding IV anticoagulation [18]

43.2.2 Initiation of IV Anticoagulation

Most of published protocols for postoperative anticoagulation do not specify differences between individuals regarding bleeding and thromboembolic risk factors. Hence, it may play a great role to define starting dose for IV anticoagulants and avoid early manifestation of hematological adverse events.

We suggest to check before the start of anticoagulation all exiting factors – pro-thrombotic and pro-bleeding. Pro-thrombotic factors are as follows: known thrombophilia, atrial fibrillation, IABP, large myocardial infarction, ongoing infection, and tumor disease. Pro-bleeding factors are as follows: liver failure, low PLT count and dysfunction in test, antiplatelet therapy immediately before surgery, CVVHDF therapy, or dialysis (◘ Figs. 43.6a and b).

Dividing patients into 2 groups according their risk may help by choosing starting dose of anticoagulants and aggressivity of dose escalation. Those with higher thrombotic risk are requiring anticoagulant start with higher dose (heparin 5 U/kg/h or argatroban 0.1 mcg/kg/min) after 6–8 h (exceptionally immediately after ICU arrival). Others with higher bleeding risk may be evaluated every 4–6 h up to 24 h postoperatively and require start with low dose (heparin 2 U/kg/h or argatroban 0.05 mcg/kg/min).

Older recipients and subjects with liver congestion may require even lower dose of argatroban.

43.2.3 Oral Anti-vitamin K, Self-Measurements of INR

International normalized ration (INR) is the standard parameter for hospital or self-monitoring during therapy with anti-vitamin K agents (Coumadin, Phenprocoumon). It gives information about extrinsic and common hemostasis pathway. INR level differs from hospital to hospital depending on reagents used. However, INR level 2,0–3,0 is accepted in the community for outpatient anticoagulation for almost all rotary pumps. Extracorporeal devices with mechanical valves of total artificial heart (CardioWest) require INR level of 2,5–3,5.

There is described interaction between argatroban and anti-vitamin K agents in the form of slightly increased INR level. This is important at the moment of discontinuation of IV argatroban during switch to Coumadin. INR shall be measured 4 h after argatroban stop, and Coumadin dose has to be readjusted – INR drop-off due to this interaction is expected.

After recovery of hepatic and renal function and after improvement in nutritional status (albumin), free of systemic infection, we start oral anticoagulants (Coumadin or Marcumar) and carefully titrate doses to achieve VAD-specific INR range. We facilitate the education of patients for INR self-measurement – patients keep INR level within given target being at home [18].

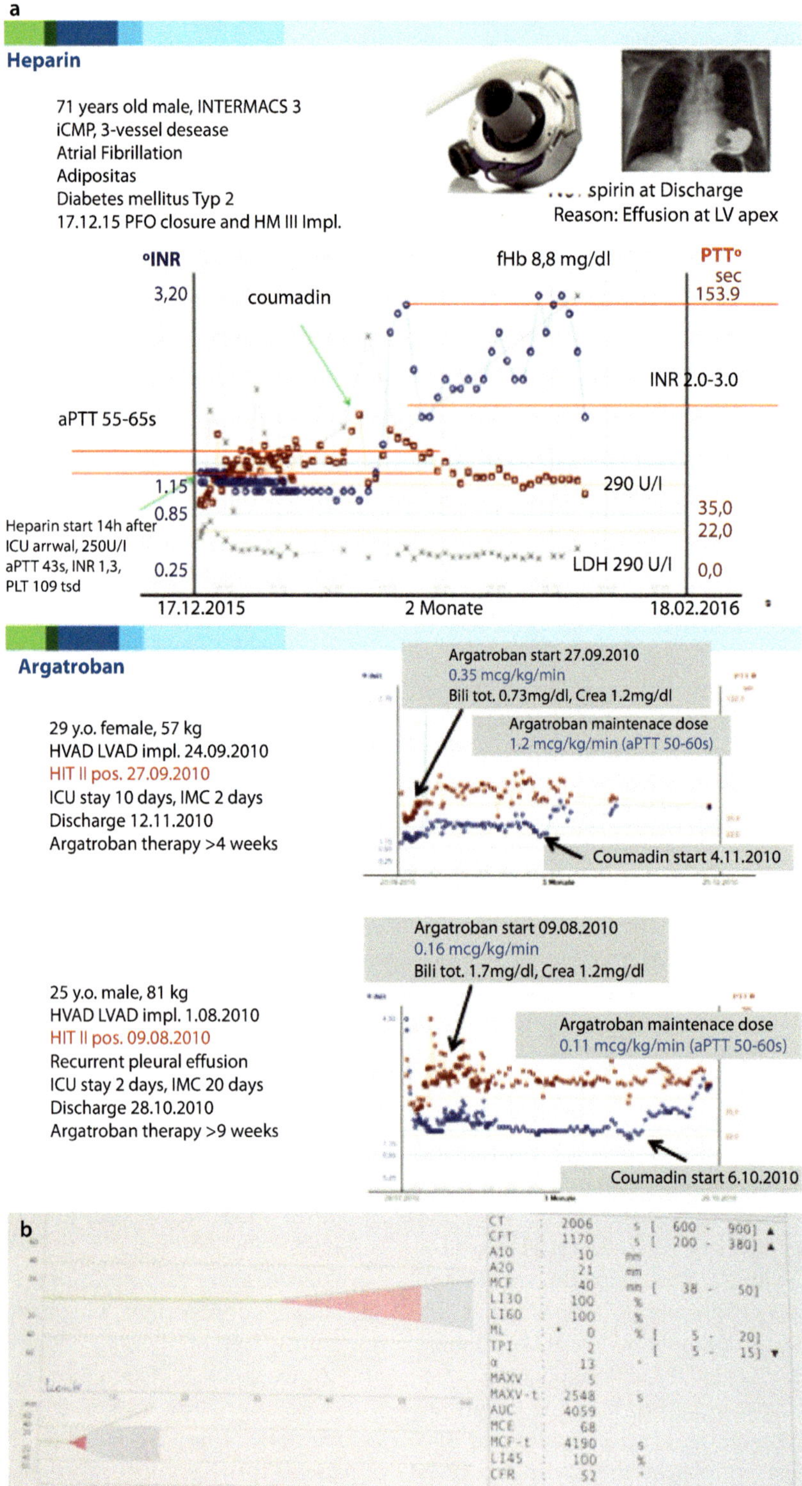

Fig. 43.6 (**a**) aPTT-guided IV anticoagulation in HVAD, HM II, and HM III pts. (**b**) Overanticoagulation due to heparin: backup control using kaolin-TEG, aPTT 60 s, INR 1,3, quick 65%, PLT 50 tsd. Kaolin-TEG: significantly prolonged initiation and kinetic of clot formation during IV heparin therapy. TEG indicates risk for bleeding – heparin dose shall be adjusted (reduced)

43.3 Conclusion

Despite continuing progress in rotary blood pump technology, anticoagulation using IV agents and later warfarin therapy together with antiplatelet are still obligatory.

Modern VADs and improvements in understanding of complex interaction processes between VAD and patient have resulted in low incidence of bleeding/thromboembolic events. Optimal anticoagulation regime leads to balance between bleeding and thromboembolism. Initially higher anticoagulation level with subsequent de-escalation in outpatient department may lead to long-term stroke/bleeding-free support. Antiplatelet therapy plays an important role and is applied in almost all types of rotary VADs.

Tailored regime involving all risk factors in decision-making process (infection, HIT, avWF disease, age, sex, comorbidities, inflow cannula-related factors, etc.) is crucial to avoid serious thrombotic and/or bleeding adverse events.

References

1. Macfarlane RG (1964) An enzyme cascade in the blood clotting mechanism, and its function as a biochemical amplifier. Nature 202:498–499
2. Davie EW, Ratnoff OD (1964) Waterfall sequence for intrinsic blood clotting. Science 145(3638):1310–1312
3. Hoffman M, Monroe DM 3rd (2001) A cell-based model of hemostasis. Thromb Haemost 85(6):958–965
4. Szefner J (1995) Control and treatment of hemostasis in cardiovascular surgery. The experience of La Pitie Hospital with patients on total artificial heart. Int J Artif Organs 18(10):633–648
5. Himmelreich G, Ullmann H, Riess H, Rosch R, Loebe M, Schiessler A et al (1995) Pathophysiologic role of contact activation in bleeding followed by thromboembolic complications after implantation of a ventricular assist device. ASAIO J 41(3):M790–M794
6. Koster A, Loebe M, Hansen R, Potapov EV, Noon GP, Kuppe H et al (2000) Alterations in coagulation after implantation of a pulsatile Novacor LVAD and the axial flow MicroMed DeBakey LVAD. Ann Thorac Surg 70(2):533–537
7. Slaughter MS, Naka Y, John R, Boyle A, Conte JV, Russell SD et al (2010) Post-operative heparin may not be required for transitioning patients with a HeartMate II left ventricular assist system to long-term warfarin therapy. J Heart Lung Transplant 29(6):616–624
8. Oliver WC (2009) Anticoagulation and coagulation management for ECMO. Semin Cardiothorac Vasc Anesth 13(3):154–175
9. De Waele JJ, Van Cauwenberghe S, Hoste E, Benoit D, Colardyn F (2003) The use of the activated clotting time for monitoring heparin therapy in critically ill patients. Intensive Care Med 29(2):325–328
10. Atallah S, Liebl M, Fitousis K, Bostan F, Masud F (2014) Evaluation of the activated clotting time and activated partial thromboplastin time for the monitoring of heparin in adult extracorporeal membrane oxygenation patients. Perfusion 29(5):456–461
11. Koster A, Huebler S, Potapov E, Meyer O, Jurmann M, Weng Y et al (2007) Impact of heparin-induced thrombocytopenia on outcome in patients with ventricular assist device support: single-institution experience in 358 consecutive patients. Ann Thorac Surg 83(1):72–76
12. Warkentin TE, Greinacher A, Koster A (2009) Heparin-induced thrombocytopenia in patients with ventricular assist devices: are new prevention strategies required? Ann Thorac Surg 87(5):1633–1640
13. Pappalardo F, Scandroglio AM, Potapov E, Stepanenko A, Maj G, Krabatsch T et al (2012) Argatroban anticoagulation for heparin induced thrombocytopenia in patients with ventricular assist devices. Minerva Anestesiol 78(3):330–335
14. [cited 2015 31 December]; http://www.mt-pharma-eu.com/products/argatroban
15. Levine RL, Hursting MJ, McCollum D (2006) Argatroban therapy in heparin-induced thrombocytopenia with hepatic dysfunction. Chest 129(5):1167–1175
16. Bradford CD, Stahovich MJ, Dembitsky WP, Adamson RM, Engelbert JJ, Perreiter AS (2015) Safety of prothrombin complex concentrate to control excess bleeding during continuous flow LVAD insertion. ASAIO J 61(5):509–513
17. Bruckner BA, DiBardino DJ, Ning Q, Adeboygeun A, Mahmoud K, Valdes J et al (2009) High incidence of thromboembolic events in left ventricular assist device patients treated with recombinant activated factor VII. J Heart Lung Transplant 28(8):785–790
18. Stepanenko A, Potapov EV, Weng Y, Pasic M, Krabatsch T, Hetzer R (2014) Anticoagulation assessment. Ann Cardiothorac Surg 3(5):538–540
19. Geisen U, Heilmann C, Beyersdorf F, Benk C, Berchtold-Herz M, Schlensak C et al (2008) Non-surgical bleeding in patients with ventricular assist devices could be explained by acquired von Willebrand disease. Eur J Cardiothorac Surg 33(4):679–684
20. Meyer AL, Malehsa D, Bara C, Budde U, Slaughter MS, Haverich A et al (2010) Acquired von Willebrand syndrome in patients with an axial flow left ventricular assist device. Circ Heart Fail 3(6):675–681
21. Klovaite J, Gustafsson F, Mortensen SA, Sander K, Nielsen LB (2009) Severely impaired von Willebrand factor-dependent platelet aggregation in patients with a continuous-flow left ventricular assist device (HeartMate II). J Am Coll Cardiol 53(23):2162–2167
22. Birschmann I, Dittrich M, Eller T, Wiegmann B, Reininger AJ, Budde U et al (2014) Ambient hemolysis and activation of coagulation is different between HeartMate II and HeartWare left ventricular assist devices. J Heart Lung Transplant 33(1):80–87
23. Dranishnikov NSA, Frumkin A, Vierecke J, Potapov EV, Krabatsch T (2012) Hetzer R von Willebrand factor in recipients of different VAD systems and its clinical relevance. J Heart Lung Transplant 31(4 Suppl):34
24. Stepanenko ADN, Canteli A, Vierecke J, Jurmann B, Lehmkuhl H, Drews T, Potapov EV, Krabatsch T, Hetzer R (2012) Outpatient antiplatelet therapy in rotary blood pump recipients: single-center experience. J Heart Lung Transplant 31(4 Suppl):S197

Outpatient Management: The Role of the VAD Coordinator and Remote Monitoring

Dawn M. Christensen, Christina VanderPluym, Jennifer Conway, Angela Lorts, Holger Buchholz, Thomas Schlöglhofer, Juliane Vierické, Alexander Stepanenko, Friedrich Kauffman, and Gro Sorenson

© Springer International Publishing Switzerland 2017
A. Montalto et al. (eds.), *Mechanical Circulatory Support in End-Stage Heart Failure*,
DOI 10.1007/978-3-319-43383-7_44

Abbreviations

ACC	American College of Cardiology
ASAIO	American Society for Artificial Internal Organs
CMS	Centers for Medicare and Medicaid Services
ESAO	European Society for Artificial Organs
ESC	European Society of Cardiology
GP	General practitioner
HTx	Heart transplant
ICCAC	International Consortium for Circulatory Assist Clinicians
INR	International normalized ratio
ISHLT	International Society for Heart and Lung Transplantation
LDH	Lactate dehydrogenase
LVAD	Left ventricular assist device
MCS	Mechanical circulatory support
PFHb	Plasma free hemoglobin
PT	Prothrombin time
VAD	Ventricular assist device

44.1 The VAD Coordinator

The VAD coordinator is an integral part of any successful VAD program. The role of the VAD coordinator is to help to bridge the medical and mechanical aspects of the field. They are tasked with providing direct patient care as well as ensuring that all aspects of a VAD patient's care are provided. The VAD coordinator also serves as a central organizational point for the entire VAD team overseeing regulatory and organizational requirements as well as facilitating communication among team members.

Historically the role of the VAD coordinator originated in the early to mid 1990s when the first devices became commercially available. At that time the transition from the lab to clinical use demonstrated a need for a practitioner to bridge the technical and clinical requirements of this new type of patient, one that relied on a machine to provide continuous and long-term circulatory support outside of the operating room. Background education of a VAD coordinator varies and includes practitioners with background fields such as nursing, medicine, perfusion, and biomedical engineering.

Table 44.1 Reported VAD coordinator responsibilities 2009 and 2015 [1, 2]

VAD coordinator responsibilities	% reporting responsibility for task 2009	% reporting responsibility for task 2015
Patient evaluation	95.5	85
Financial clearance	31.8	23
Pre-op	100	83
Intra-op	81.8	44
Post-op	100	79
Patient education	100	91
Staff education	97.7	88
Data collection	93.2	74
Regulatory compliance	81.8	65
Outpatient management	97.7	90
Inventory	70.5	51
Billing	36.4%	22
Other	25%	24

Day-to-day responsibilities of a VAD coordinator vary depending on program structure and personnel. In a survey designed to try to help characterize the role of the VAD coordinator, the International Consortium of Circulatory Clinicians (ICCAC), the professional group for VAD Coordinators and MCS professionals, has identified areas of VAD coordinator responsibility that are consistent across VAD programs (Table 44.1).

44.1.1 VAD Program Structure

Basic VAD program structure is something that has evolved over the past several years. As the technology changes and use increases, identifying the key members of a VAD team has become fairly straightforward. Institutional variations

Table 44.2 VAD program recommended personnel [2–6]

	ISHLT	CMS	JC	DNV-GL	ICCAC
Cardiac surgeon (with implant requirements)	X	X	X	X	X
HF cardiologist	X	X	X	X	X
VAD coordinator	X	X	X	X	X
Palliative care	X	X	X	X	X
Psychiatry	X				X
Social worker	X	X	X	X	X
Psychologist	X				
Pharmacist	X				
Dietitian	X		X		
Physical therapist	X				X
Occupational therapist	X				
Rehabilitation services			X		
Financial coordinator			X		X
Research coordinator					X
Equipment specialist					X

exist but each successful program has consistent key personnel. Several groups have described their recommendations for essential programmatic personnel (Table 44.2).

44.1.2 VAD Program Organization

Basic program organization requires that attention be applied to all aspects of patient contact, from identification to discharge from the program. Breaking down care of the patient into the individual points of contact and optimizing each point of contact can aid in maximizing outcomes of patient care [7].

44.1.3 Pediatric VAD Programs

In the last 10 years, we have seen significant improvements in the outcomes of children supported on VADs, and this in turn has led to a growing interest in improving quality of life in children on long-term VAD support. Learning from the expansive experience accumulated from the field of adult VAD support, dedicated pediatric VAD programs are becoming more common across North America and Europe. Most pediatric VAD programs are connected academically, administratively, and clinically to pediatric heart transplant programs, since the most common indication currently for pediatric VAD support is a bridge to transplantation. Key components of a successful pediatric VAD team have yet to be defined but in many setting consist of physicians, dedicated nurses or nurse practitioners, dieticians, social workers, and pharmacists. Each of these individuals plays an important role in the inpatient and outpatient setting where the primary goals are to prevent complications, ensure adequate growth and development, and allow for integration back into community life. Pediatric VAD programs mirror many adult programs except for some unique additional and vital personnel – namely, the role of child life specialist (CLS). Child life specialists, otherwise named "play therapists," are specially trained individuals who help make inpatient and outpatient life for children with complex medical needs more bearable through child-centric activities. This may

Table 44.3 VAD program outreach: key components for referring providers

Component	Discussion	Special considerations
Introduction	Introduction to VAD technology Purpose for use	Display device models Manufacturer information
Overview of program	Key team members Program Capabilities Outcomes	Photo directory of each team member with individual direct contact information
Referral	Appropriate patients for referral Appropriate timing of referral Referral process	Provide "cheat sheet" of minimum data requirements needed for referral (i.e., echo, meds, VS, etc.)
Contact information	How to contact program members routinely Emergency contact information for key team members	Direct physician to physician contact for consultation if necessary

include music therapy, play therapy, video games, or any other activities that are identified by the child or adolescent to be important to their quality of life. Many of CLS providers have additional VAD training so that they can accompany the child and their family around the hospital or on outings out of the hospital before they are ready for discharge. For younger and smaller patients, VAD options are limited to paracorporeal devices such as the Berlin Heart EXOCR® that does not allow outpatient care. As such, with long wait list times for transplantation, children and their families are required to remain in the hospital for weeks, months, and possibly even years. The role of CLS, as well as other allied health team members such as physiotherapist, occupational therapist, neurodevelopmental specialists, and teachers, becomes of paramount importance to "normalize" inpatient stay as best possible and strive to improve quality of life for the patient and their family.

44.1.4 Access to the Program

Access to a VAD program is key to success. Unless people know about your program, you won't have patients to care for. There are two ways that a potential VAD candidate can access any VAD program through identification within the program's institutional boundaries or through referral from an outside source (either medical or not). To maximize referrals from any source, some amount of outreach is necessary (i.e., face to face interactions, information seminars, educational offerings, advertising). Table 44.3 outlines key components of a successful medical provider outreach offering [8].

44.1.5 Program Process

Optimization of program efficiency requires that each stage of patient contact and decision making have a standardized process or procedure with outlined roles for all team members. Table 44.4 outlines typical points of contact within a VAD program and issues to be considered. Table 44.5 suggests useful resources for VAD programs.

44.1.6 Discharging Patients with Ventricular Assist Devices

The overall goals for VAD therapy include patient survival and improved quality of life. For this population, improved quality of life encompasses, among other things, absence of pump-related complications, such as thrombotic complications or infection, and discharge from the implanting center with absence of re-hospitalizations. Since the introduction of implantable ventricular assist devices (VADs), routine discharge of patients has become feasible. For most patients this is a desired goal for both therapeutic

Table 44.4 Program components with considerations

Patient evaluation	
Identify: Information necessary for patient evaluation Contact points associated with each source of information (scheduling secretaries, etc.) Personnel responsible for arranging/completing evaluation	*Develop:* Internal educational plan for contact points Process to streamline scheduling Process to document evaluation progress and completion
Evaluation review and decision making	
Identify: Core and other relevant participating team members	*Develop:* Team "code of conduct" concerning evaluation procedure discussions Standardized process for patient review Process for emergency patient implant Process for notifying patient of decision (positive and negative with written and verbal explanation)
Pre-implant *(Time from patient approval to arrival in the operating room)*	
Identify: Team member responsibilities Floor personnel educational plan	*Develop:* Pre-implant educational processes (patient and staff) Consent forms and process for completion Process to ensure that all testing and procedures are complete prior to surgery (i.e., checklist including pre-op day or time tasks should be completed) Criteria and process to initiate postoperative educational plan and discharge planning when appropriate
Implant *(Time from when patient arrives in operating room to discharge from ICU)*	
Identify: Team member roles and responsibilities Specific knowledge, skills, tasks associated with device implant, and operation Personnel responsibilities once the patient is in the ICU (i.e., intensivist, coordinator, surgeon, cardiologist, nursing)	*Develop:* A list of qualified personnel who can perform device-specific tasks (i.e., device setup, device start-up, device adjustments, echo interpretation, etc.) Protocols of practice for routine treatment scenarios
Post-implant *(From transfer out of ICU to discharge from hospital)*	
Identify: Team member roles and responsibilities	*Develop:* Standardized educational plans for each device Emergency team contact system Process for dispensing equipment and supplies Process for notification and education of community providers and resources

Table 44.4 (continued)

Identify	Develop
Discharge	
Identify: Team outpatient follow-up philosophy (see surveillance of the patient at home) Personnel responsible for outpatient visits both scheduled and urgent Equipment necessary in the outpatient area and who is responsible for maintenance Routine tasks required for outpatients (i.e., INR, labs, studies, preventative maintenance)	*Develop:* A schedule for routine visits, follow-up testing, INR and lab monitoring, preventative maintenance schedule, and any other routinely scheduled tasks that are identified Process for outpatient scheduling and where outpatient visits will be completed Process to communicate outpatient condition to the entire VAD team
Readmission	
Identify: Standard scenarios that require patient readmission (i.e., infection, device complications, bleeding)	*Develop:* Standardized admission practice guidelines Process for urgent/emergent contact of VAD team
Discharge from the program	
Identify: Possible scenarios for patient discharge from the program (i.e., death, transplant, transfer to another center, loss to follow-up) Personnel responsibilities	*Develop:* Procedures for retrieval of external equipment if it is hospital owned Process for device retrieval if indicated Develop debriefing process for unexpected patient discharge
Education and competency documentation Hospital staff and VAD team members *(individual process for each)*	
Identify: Appropriate levels of training for different levels of hospital personnel Who is responsible for staff education Identify where records are kept and who is responsible for maintaining	*Develop:* Institutional competency requirements Process for documentation of staff education and competency
Quality control	
Identify: Institutional quality team and contacts Personnel responsible for quality review Personnel responsible for maintaining and enforcing certification required practices	*Develop:* Quality parameters for program Program quality plan for and process for review Program certification plan and process for review
Program Records and Data Collection	
Identify: Program data that needs to be collected; Personnel responsible for data collection and submission;	*Develop:* Plan for regular review of program data

Table 44.5 Useful resources for VAD programs

ISHLT – International Society for Heart and Lung Transplantation	www.ishlt.org
ICCAC – International Consortium for Circulatory Assist Clinicians	www.vadcoordinator.org
Centers for Medicare and Medicaid Services Coverage Determinations	https://www.cms.gov/Regulations-and-Guidance/Guidance/Manuals/downloads/ncd103c1_part1.pdf
Joint Commission – Disease Specific Care Resources	http://www.jointcommission.org/certification/dsc_resources.aspx
DNV GL Guidelines	http://cms.ipressroom.com.s3.amazonaws.com/107/files/20154/VAD+Standards-v4.pdf
MyLVAD	www.mylvad.com
ACC – American College of Cardiology	www.acc.org
ESC – European Society of Cardiology	www.escardio.org
ASAIO – American Society for Artificial Internal Organs	www.asaio.com
ESAO – European Society for Artificial Organs	www.esao.org

and financial reasons. The increasing number of patients supported by VAD as well as the increasing length of wait time for a donor organ, hospitalization of a patient not requiring any special therapy cannot be justified. Discharge should be achieved despite any barriers, including geographic concerns, as long as the patient's condition allows for safe discharge.

Home discharge with a VAD as well as long-term support while at home requires that a patient be in stable condition and be comfortable with the performance of their care, whether it is provided by the implanting institution or a local facility. In order to maintain this state, extensive patient and caregiver training, local community caregiver training, and regular outpatient department visits at the implanting center are required. It is not unusual for a VAD center to be following patients located in another geographic area, several hours, by car, boat, or airplane, away. Increasing numbers of outpatients on VAD support has necessitated that outpatient department clinics associated with VAD implant centers make adjustments in the way patients are followed. Subsequently, many implanting centers must rely on the resources located in the patient's community and have increased the interval between routine outpatient visits.

44.1.7 Special Considerations for Discharging the Pediatric VAD Patient

With the introduction of implantable continuous-flow ventricular assist devices (VADs) into pediatric practice, discharge has now become a reality for children with end-stage heart failure. The number of children discharged is still relatively small compared to the adult VAD population, but there is a growing body of literature in this expanding patient population.

Complication prevention starts in the inpatient setting with comprehensive education of the families and patient, including how to recognize complications, how and when to contact the VAD team, and how to deal with emergency situations. Booklets or handouts describing potential complications as well as the number where the VAD team can be reached are important tools in the outpatient setting. While avoiding complications is an important goal, the reality is that many of these patients are likely to be readmitted to hospital. The INTERMACS has shown that in the adult population by 1-year post-VAD implant, at least 70% percentage of patients had experienced major complications, with even a higher percentage requiring readmission at this time point [9]. In the largest series of continuous-flow pumps in children from the PediMACS Registry (*n* =72), 53% were discharged with over half requiring readmission [10]. In a smaller multicenter experience, examining the outpatient experience of 12 patients with cardiomyopathy, readmission was not uncommon with an average of 2.5 readmissions per person [11]. The most frequent cause of readmission was driveline infection, followed by subtherapeutic INRs and VAD alarms. In this patient cohort none of the patients required the use of emergency services. Lastly, it has been shown that it is possible to manage even smaller patients (<25 kg) in the in community with 45% of the patient cohort discharged after implantation [12]. Preparing for these readmissions is important and not only includes family education but also education and effective lines of communication with the community healthcare providers, transportation plans, and determining the appropriate place for readmission. While it is not possible to educate all people that come into contact with a child that has been discharged home, there are some groups that may benefit from education. This education can be patient specific or more general and targeted toward emergency response personnel, local emergency departments, primary care providers, and school administration. The type of education that occurs can be in the form of lectures, webinars, or simulation with the additional of written educational material. In some settings education is not possible given the number of first responders and the areas in which the family lives or travels; therefore, providing families with the necessary documentation to give to first responders and empowering the families to be an expert on the device is an alternative solution.

Integration back into school is an important milestone for discharged patients, and this has been reported to be possible in the pediatric patients discharged with a VAD [13]. Providing education to an aide or identified person at the school will provide some respite for the family and normalize the child's experience as much as possible.

While we presume that management in the outpatient setting and integration back to school is beneficial for this patient population and their families, this must be balanced against the responsibilities placed on care givers in this complex patient population. Further understanding of the balance of quality of life as an outpatient with caregiver burden is needed as we move forward with this unique group of patients.

44.1.8 Coordinating the Patient Discharge from the VAD Center

Discharge planning starts before implantation by collecting information about patient support systems as well as local resources. If the patient has already been followed by a local general practitioner (GP) or heart failure team, contact should be made as soon as possible to obtain any outlying information about the patient, such as former history of psychiatric illness, coping skills, adherence to medical therapy and social support/network (G1), and local resources as well as starting to prepare them for care of the patient after discharge.

The local medical providers who will be involved in the patient's care should be invited to the VAD center for training. Ideally there should be a local team created that is responsible for VAD patient follow-up. Training should be provided and include written documentation outlining the care of the VAD patient. Topics that should be included at the very minimum are:

- Theory and operation of the pump and all supporting equipment
- Practice guidelines for ongoing care of the patient including goals of outpatient therapy, testing procedures, and procedures for outpatient visits
- Device troubleshooting including identifying conditions indicating suspected pump thrombus and pump related infection [3]
- Emergency procedures and protocols with implanting center team emergency contact information

At the time of discharge, every effort should be made for a member of the VAD team to accompany the patient to their local community. Sessions should be scheduled for the patient and family as well as the local team to meet with local hospital and emergency department providers. The purpose of the meeting is to provide a common understanding of expectations, follow-up visits (regularity, continuity), and review handling of potential emergency situations. It should also include training on dressing change procedures as well as the measurement of blood pressure with a Doppler. Additionally, notification should be given to the local ambulance service including abbreviated instruction about the pump and the emergency phone number at the VAD center to call for instructions if an emergency transport is needed. If the patient lives more than 2 h away from the implanting center, it is imperative that everyone caring for the patient "speaks the same language" so that safe and effective care can be provided within the patient's community.

Assumptions necessary for a successful long distance patient discharge:

- The implanting center and the patient must have trust in the local health system: Long distance follow-up demands that the local health system be the first line of contact in the patient's "chain of care." The provider may be the home care nurse, the general practitioner, the heart failure nurse, or the cardiologist in the local hospital. The chain might consist of several parts or only a few. Independent of this, the "chain" has to be strong in every link.
- The local team has to trust the implanting center: The VAD team should offer 24/7 emergency phone contact that is staffed by trained professionals. The implanting team should also be available for regular discussions by phone or video conference.
- Both the patient and his/her support system have to trust the entire medical team. Lines of communication must be freely open, and cooperation must occur between the patient, the local providers, and the VAD center for the patient to feel safe in their home community.
- The VAD team has to trust the patient: Both patient and his/her relatives have undergone oral and written instruction and have been tested to show their understanding of their expectations, the device, and its operation, precautions, and troubleshooting. They have been instructed to identify situations that require VAD team notification, and they have been instructed in how to perform self-monitoring of pump parameters and INR.
- You have to streamline the treatment in the patient care pathway from preoperative assessment to the end of treatment (HTx or dead). A care plan should be present, including the patient's decision concerning a surrogate decision maker if he/she is not able to make decisions for themselves [14].
- The patient must understand that he/she is in charge of his/her life. He/she must understand the lifestyle adjustments that are necessary to live with a VAD [15].

Long distance follow-up of LVAD patients may be successful when you build a strong triage between the patient/family, the local health service (shared care center/heart failure clinic), and the VAD center. Dedicated and trained professionals involved in each link of the chain in combination with a good system for cooperation are success factors (see ◘ Table 44.6).

44.1.9 Ongoing Outpatient Care

Ongoing care of the VAD outpatients is mainly focused on medical issues, specifically, anticoagulation, maintaining the percutaneous driveline exit site, and dressing along with blood pressure management. The VAD therapy should be perceived as a specific treatment (most patients have left VADs) of the pumping function of the (left) ventricle. Sometimes secondary disease patterns evolving from left heart failure may worsen or ameliorate despite LVAD support (dyspnea, arrhythmia, kidney failure, ascites). Other comorbidities such as diabetes, chronic obstructive pulmonary disease, or thyroid disease cannot be cured by LVAD therapy. This can lead to an unclear understanding of the scope of responsibility that the VAD team has for the treatment of non-VAD-related conditions. Interpretations vary among the VAD implant teams/centers. Some teams/centers assume responsibility for implanting the VAD and for providing supplies and necessary equipment related specifically to the VAD. On the opposite end of the spectrum are teams/centers that take responsibility for everything that happens to the VAD patient including treatment of routine illness such as influenza.

Ideally, regardless of distance from the implanting center, the VAD outpatient should regularly visit his/her general practitioner (GP) for routine care as well as management of any non-VAD-related health issues. Consultation of a

Table 44.6 Considerations for patient discharge

Topic	Considerations
Patient demographics	Age/time of advanced heart failure Is this a patient that is supposed to go back to school? Back to work? Who else in the patient's community will need to be trained in addition to the local team?
Support system	Does the patient have adequate support at home? Who are they? Are the patient's loved ones willing and prepared to share responsibility for the VAD with the patient and medical team?
Geographic considerations	Does the patient live in an area that is sparsely populated, have challenging topography, and/or challenging weather conditions? Does the patient live in an area that has frequent loss of electricity, closed roads, or closed airports? What are the options for communication? Long distances may challenge the implanting center to create other ways of communicating with the patient and also with the local health team. Photos, face time, and video conferences may be helpful in identifying possible issues.
Local medical services	How long does it take emergency services to get to the patient's home? How far is the closest hospital? Does a local GP need to be involved? Where is the closest home health nursing service? Do they need to be involved? How far is it to the local physiotherapist? Is contact established between VAD center physiotherapist and local?
Emergency planning	How far is the VAD center from the patient's home or closest hospital? What options are available for transport if necessary? It is an advantage and a contribution to the patient safety to have a travel plan in case of emergency and an alternative plan in case of bad weather conditions, in cooperation with the local hospital and ambulance service

specialist should be initiated, if necessary, as patient diagnosis and condition require. If a cardiologist had previously treated the patient, this should be resumed. The VAD does not abolish the need for maintenance and monitoring of pacemakers and ICDs, and local cardiologists can assist in management of the patient if circumstances allow. In all of these situations, as well as any additional medical treatment, it is imperative that the VAD implanting center is informed about any diagnoses, treatment, or changes in medication.

Reality is that caring for the patient supported by a VAD can lead to some uncertainty for the GP or staff of the patient's local community hospital who are not familiar with the knowledge and financial implications of the VAD therapy. Unclear reimbursement rules as well as lack of knowledge related to management of a VAD patient (e.g., to never use vitamin K for a high INR or the presence of pulsatility indicating poor ventricular unloading suggesting impaired function of the VAD when nonpulsatile blood pressure usually indicates proper pump function and adequate unloading the left ventricle). In some cases, the GP or the local community hospital may refuse to care for a VAD patient to avoid added responsibility, cost, and liability issues.

Increased support times at home also increase possibility that the patient will experience a problem or deterioration of their condition while at home. Any deterioration in patient condition may necessitate admission to a hospital. This does not necessarily have to be the implanting VAD center. The implanting VAD team should be contacted first in case any technical problems or emergency situations with the VAD arise. The decision surrounding the best option for transport and treatment for the VAD patient can then be made collaboratively.

44.1.10 Surveillance of the Patient at Home

Home monitoring of the VAD patient is an important aspect of a successful outpatient program. Determining how a program monitors outpatients depends on the infrastructure and resources dedicated to the VAD team as well as characteristics of the patient cohort.

The opposite ends of the spectrum concerning a program's approach to home monitoring of their VAD patients include:

- Empowerment of the patient and caregiver to contact the VAD center with concerns or questions surrounding their condition (i.e., emergency situations, developing issues such as fever or exit site concerns, or ongoing support to avoid complications)
- Routine contact, initiated by the VAD team to question the patient about their status in an effort to detect issues at an early state

The first requires rigorous patient education as well as the ability to instill confidence in the patient that they can provide safely care for themselves and the device. This requires infrastructure to educate and evaluate patient knowledge. The latter requires an infrastructure within the VAD team to provide personnel with time dedicated to patient follow-up outside of the outpatient clinic. Many centers choose one philosophy or the other. Others use a blended approach. The success of either approach ultimately relies on program organization and on consistency of care within the system.

Regardless of the philosophy of home surveillance, all VAD programs must provide 24 h emergency contact procedure to outpatients. Use of the emergency contact system should at the very least be able to address issues related to VAD system alarms or emergency medical conditions related to VAD support and a way to initiate further hospital evaluation if indicated. Emergency contact personnel must have the knowledge and understanding of the patient and device in order to determine whether immediate evaluation (emergency visit either through an outlying hospital or directly to the implanting center) or urgent evaluation (scheduled outpatient department visit as soon as possible) is required. Technical hotlines provided by device manufacturers are not appropriate for use in the case of a patient requiring advice during an emergency use should be limited to provider use only.

44.1.11 Outpatient Monitoring Specific to VAD Patients

In the routine outpatient scenario, normal VAD operation should be assumed. Teaching the patient how to monitor and report any changes gives the VAD patient and VAD team the best chance at detecting an issue, either technical or medical, early. Regular documentation of VAD technical data by the patient is the cornerstone of home monitoring. Patients should be provided with a documentation sheet and instructed in the desired frequency of recording technical data from the pump as well as basic clinical data. They should also be taught what each parameter represents as well as the importance of monitoring and reporting any changes in those values. Home documentation is also key during an acute or alarm situation (see "challenges of remote pump monitoring"). Current MCS devices do not have an extended data storage capability. Because of this, patient documentation may be the only way to determine trends as well as sudden changes in pump performance that led to the alarm situation.

44.1.12 Outpatient Follow-Up

Multidisciplinary Team Approach

Ongoing follow-up is a key part of effective care for outpatients supported by VADs. "Management of the patient with an VAD should be performed by a multidisciplinary team that includes cardiovascular surgeons, advanced heart failure cardiologists, and specialized MCS coordinators and/or nurses. Other healthcare providers may collaborate with the primary MCS team when additional expertise is required" [3].

Frequency

The frequency of outpatient clinic visits varies among MCS centers. It largely depends on center protocol and patient characteristics (clinical stability, concomitant medical conditions, and distance from the implanting center).

After discharge, patients should typically return to the outpatient clinic weekly until their condition improves and all immediate medical concerns have been resolved. Frequency of outpatient visits can then be decreased at increasing increments as long as the patient remains stable. For some centers the time between follow-up visits for stable patients can be up to 12 months.

Routine Outpatient Evaluation

The components of a routine outpatient evaluation of a VAD patient should include the following components:

- Laboratory studies
- Routine testing
- Technical check
- Medication review
- History and physical
- Vital signs
- Driveline check
- Device adjustment
- Adjustment of medical regimen, review of device function, and future plan

Laboratory Studies

Laboratory studies should be obtained at regular intervals initially to establish a baseline for comparison and then for monitoring while the patient is at home. They should also be performed prior to upcoming clinic visits to allow for device updates and to aid in medical decision making at the time of the visit.

Routine testing typically includes coagulation evaluation (PT/INR) and hemolysis markers, specifically lactate dehydrogenase (LDH), and plasma-free hemoglobin (PFHb) may provide early indication of pump thrombosis or abnormal shear stress. Blood chemistry and blood cell counts are also routinely followed with additional tests performed as patient condition indicates.

Routine Testing

Routine testing at each outpatient clinic visit relies heavily on center protocols as well as patient condition. Typical testing includes (see Table 44.7):

44.1.13 Technical Check

The technical check involves inspection of external device components, documentation of all system parameters, and downloading of data.

Inspection of External Device Components

All external device components should undergo a comprehensive visual inspection to exclude damage to any part of the system. Preventative maintenance

Table 44.7 Typical components of routine testing

Test	Interval	Purpose
ECG	Every clinic visit	Detect presence of arrhythmia Monitor for changes over time
Chest X-ray (modified)	Every clinic visit	Monitor patient fluid status and ventricular unloading Detect changes in pump position Monitor and detect issues with proximal driveline integrity
Transthoracic echocardiogram	Routinely per team protocol (with or without ramp studies) With clinical signs of circulatory dysfunction	Assessment of RV/LV function Assessment of valve status Assessment of unloading of the heart chambers Assessment of myocardial recovery To aid in making pump speed adjustments
Cardiopulmonary stress testing	Routinely per team protocol	Objective assessment of patient's functional capacity
Quality of life questionnaires	Routinely per team protocol	Objective measurement of patient's quality of life

procedures, as outlined by the device manufacturer, should be completed or scheduled to be completed by an external service.

The Controller

Visual inspection should be done on the controller to identify any physical damage (i.e., broken housing or damaged insulation of any cables). Special attention should be paid to the components of the power connectors since they tend to be fragile and are damaged easily. Visible wear on the sockets may indicate impending problems.

Batteries

Batteries should be visually inspected for any physical damage to the casing as well as condition of the electrical connectors. They should further be evaluated for lifetime and charging cycles. If batteries are approaching the end of their maximum charge cycles or any physical damage is noted, they should be exchanged to avoid alarms or failure [16].

Driveline

Visual, tactile, and X-ray (when indicated) inspection of the driveline should be performed to detect any breaches in integrity (Table 44.8) [3]. The

Table 44.8 Driveline evaluation

Methods of driveline inspection	Description
Visual	Comprehensive visual inspection of the external portion of the driveline from the exit site to controller connection including gentle manipulation along the entire length to identify any breaches in the silicone sleeve
Tactile	Tactile assessment of the driveline using palpation to determine if there are any irregularities (kinks, sharp areas, or internal texture changes) in the external driveline indicating internal insulation breaches, slippery movement of the external sheath (leakage of body fluids into the driveline), or crackling sensation under the sheath (presence of dried blood)
X-ray	Modified 2 view thoracoabdominal projection (Images 44.1, 44.2, and 44.3); mapping and evaluation for: Changes in position of the pump or inflow cannula Visualization of internal wires and shielding for irregularities or breaches

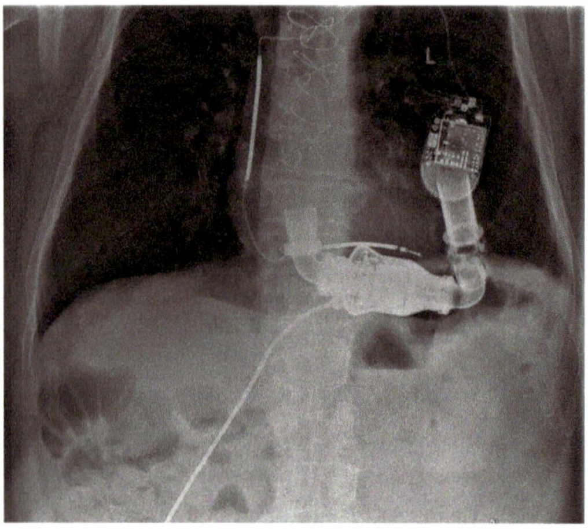

Image 44.1 Modified AP view of patient to evaluate pump position and proximal driveline

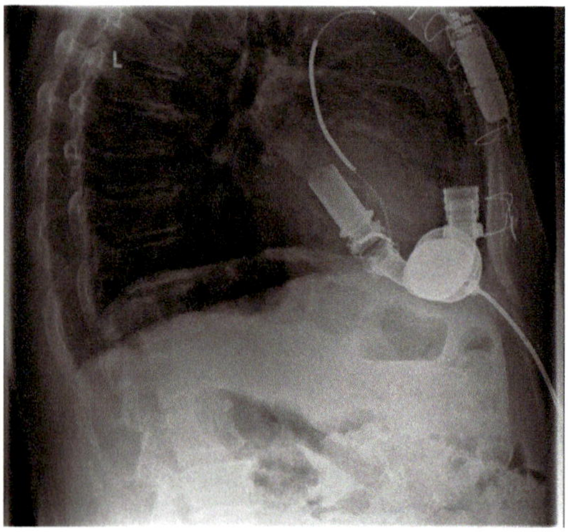

Image 44.2 Modified lateral view of patient to evaluate pump position and proximal driveline

driveline is the most sensitive part of any device and must remain intact for the internal components of the VAD to function correctly. Patients should be instructed to handle it with care. Current devices do not allow for driveline exchange and the ability to repair a driveline is limited.

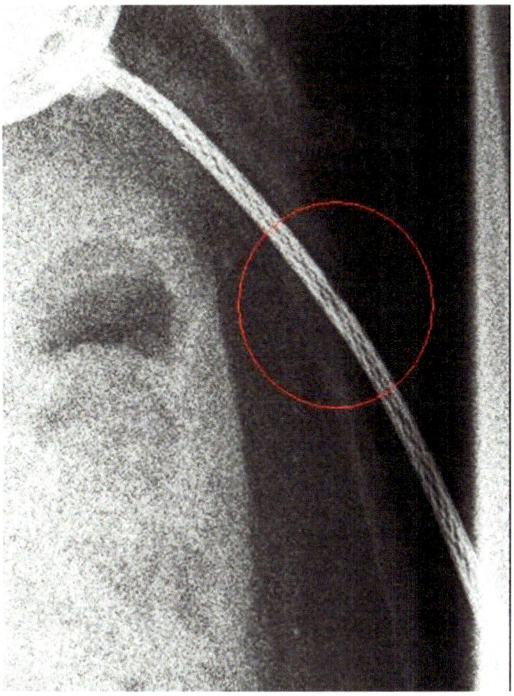

Image 44.3 Detailed view of irregularity in driveline indicating proximal driveline

Review of Log

Review of the alarm log should be performed at every visit and history download performed. Alarm thresholds should be reviewed and adjusted to appropriate parameters, and hematocrit settings should be reviewed and updated. Any changes in "normal" patient patterns should prompt additional history taking and questioning of the patient to determine the reason for the change (see Table 44.9) [3].

44.1.14 Medication Review

Review of medication is important to determine if the patient is taking medications as prescribed. It is also necessary to determine whether any other medications have been started or stopped by an outside provider in the time since the patient was last seen by the VAD team.

Heart Failure Medications

Most VAD patients should be started on a full heart failure medication regimen if it can be tolerated. This is necessary to support the right ventricle and to provide the most optimal potential for myocardial recovery [3].

Anticoagulation

Anticoagulation and antiplatelet therapy are central components of outpatient management of the patient receiving VAD therapy. It must be carefully

Table 44.9 Device-specific technical considerations

HeartWare HVAD® (HeartWare Inc., Framingham, MA, USA)	
Item to review	Considerations
Power alarm threshold settings	Maximum setting should be set 1 W above the highest power consumption reading over the previous 30 days
Flow/power curve analysis	Evaluation for aortic valve opening and arrhythmias Presence of circadian variation (indicating patient's daily activity); sudden circadian variation changes (indicating changes in patient patterns of activity)
Trend curve analysis	Evaluation for signs of suction, low flow situations, power elevations, changes in flow trends
Date range record	If <30 days, can be indicative of power loss to the system
Thoratec HeartMate II® (Thoratec Inc., Pleasanton, CA, USA)	
Event history	Review previous 120 events; evaluate unscheduled event recordings; evaluate for "clock reset" messages indicating loss of power to the controller

Table 44.10 Common medications used in VAD patients

Medication class	Use
Diuretics	Management of volume overload
Angiotensin-converting enzyme inhibitor or angiotensin receptor blocker	Hypertension Risk reduction in patient with vascular disease and diabetes
Beta blockers	Hypertension Rate control in patients with tachyarrhythmias
Mineral corticoid receptor antagonists	Help to limit the need for potassium repletion in patients with normal renal function Potential beneficial antifibrotic effects on the myocardium
Antiarrhythmic therapy	Prevention of arrhythmias

monitored to avoid large variations in the PT/INR and to minimize the chances of anticoagulation related complications. All current devices are associated with complications involving bleeding, stroke, and pump thrombosis. Some hospitals provide INR self-measurement (e.g., COAGU-CHECK) for their patients (see *Remote Monitoring*), while others require patients to go to the outpatient laboratory for INR measurement. Platelet function tests can also help to determine the time point to restart, adapt, or de-escalate antiplatelet therapy.

Patients supported by VAD therapy typically anticoagulation use a vitamin K antagonist such as warfarin. The therapeutic goal is to maintain an INR within a range as specified by each device manufacturer (e.g., HeartMate II 2–2.5, HeartWare 2.5–3). Additionally, antiplatelet therapy with aspirin (USA 81–325 mg daily, EUROPE 100 mg daily) or clopidogrel may be used. Exceptionally, some patients take dual antiplatelet agents (in the presence of known congenital or acquired thrombophilia, drug-eluting coronary stents or aortic valve prostheses or recurrent thrombotic pump dysfunction, etc.) (see Table 44.10).

44.1.15 History and Physical

History and Review of Systems

A thorough history as well as a thorough review of systems can help to identify any issues that may need to be addressed. Specific areas of interest include:

- Occurrence of any VAD alarms
- Neurological issues (i.e., headache, weakness, dizziness, changes in vision, etc.)
- Symptoms of right heart failure (i.e., weight gain, edema, abdominal fullness, etc.)
- Symptoms of hemolysis (i.e., dark urine, yellow skin or eyes)
- Changes in exercise tolerance
- Appearance of driveline exit site

Physical Examination

A comprehensive head to toe physical examination should be performed and documented. Special attention should be paid to any signs of VAD (e.g., pleural effusion, SOB, etc.) or right heart failure (e.g., increased JVD, edema, abdominal distention, etc.). Patients in the early postoperative period (<3 months after implant) should be evaluated for chest stability.

44.1.16 Driveline Exit Wound Site

The potential for infection of the exit site is high making visual inspection of the wound at every outpatient visit essential. Visual inspection can also give insight into the diligence a patient may have in regard to the wound dressing. Attention should be paid to proper driveline position and use of binder or driveline immobilization devices. Additional teaching and corrective measures can be initiated if issues are identified. If any signs of infection (pain, redness, drainage, etc.) are present, wound culture and initiation of antibiotic therapy may be necessary. Systemic signs of infection (i.e., fever, elevated WBC count) necessitate patient admission to the hospital and appropriate infectious disease consultation. A photographic record of the driveline exit site may also be helpful in assessing its appearance over time.

44.1.17 Vital Signs

As with any outpatient clinic visit, vital signs are essential to care. Patient weight should be monitored to assess for fluid retention. Apical heart rate should be measured to detect arrhythmias. Respiration rate and effort should be noted to indicate any issues with low flow states producing respiratory symptoms. Blood pressure measurement is also essential but can be difficult in patients who are nonpulsatile.

Blood Pressure Measurement

Blood pressure measurement can be performed utilizing a Doppler probe when necessary. In patients with low or nonpulsatile blood flow, blood pressure measurement with a standard cuff pressure monitor is not possible because very little or no pressure difference within the arteries is present. When this is the case monitoring and maintaining a moderate mean pressure is important to avoid low flow situations due to a high afterload on the VAD. Typically patients with nonpulsatile VADs should have a mean blood pressure goal of below 80 mmHg. Studies have been shown that VAD patients with a high RR are at high risk for ICB and stroke.

44.1.18 Discussion, Decision Making, and Disposition [15, 17]

The visit ends with the decision as to the disposition of the patient (home or hospital). Adjustments to medical regimen are made and discussed with the patient, and transplant listing status (if applicable) should be discussed. Any referrals to specialists should be made and explained. Future follow-up visits should be scheduled along with routine outpatient testing. The decision to hospitalize the patient should be made if severe problems have been identified or with admission being arranged for necessary additional tests or interventions (e.g., pacemaker exchange).

44.1.19 Shared Care and Additional Surgery

Even with long distance follow-up, the VAD patient should either come to the VAD center for additional surgery if needed; or the VAD team must be aware of the surgery taking place [3]. If geographical issues make it more practical to perform additional surgery at the patient's the local hospital, it is important that the surgeon and anesthetist stay in contact with the thoracic anesthetist and surgeon at the VAD center for guidance if necessary.

44.1.20 Shared Care and End of Life Treatment

Long distance follow-up and close cooperation with the local health team should also include cooperation about a care plan for palliative treatment (comfort care). Together they can help the patient and family realistically to understand the time to change from active treatment to a comfort care plan [14]. When the change of treatment takes place in the local hospital, it is important that the VAD team is in close contact and give support if needed.

44.2 Remote Monitoring

Mechanical circulatory support (MCS) devices are an established therapeutic option for patients with severe heart failure as bridge to transplant (BTT) or destination therapy (DT) [18]. Left ventricular assist devices (VADs) improve the quality of life, functional capacity, as well as survival rates of the recipients [19, 20].

44.2.1 Why Monitor?

Over the last decade, continuous-flow rotary blood pumps have become more commonly used and have less adverse events than pulsatile extracorporeal VADs [18]. There are still adverse events related to MCS therapy such as device thrombosis [21, 22], bleeding, or infection [20]. The highest risk of death while supported by a continuous-flow VAD is in the perioperative phase [18].

After initial discharge from the implanting hospital, patients and their caregivers need to know how to maintain and use their VAD equipment. This includes how to monitor and assess significant changes in their pump parameters, anticoagulation, blood pressure, or other symptoms and to consider them as potential adverse events. They must also recognize when to contact the VAD coordinator to avoid complications. Teaching patients to record this information daily on a home monitoring worksheet may help them to know what is normal and help them to detect complications early.

To prevent readmission of VAD patients to the hospital, optimization of VAD speed, strict management of hypertension, and mandatory follow-up visits in the clinic are essential [23]. A frequency of outpatient follow-up visits varies from center to center depending on the number of patients on device and the distance between patient and the implanting center.

44.2.2 What to Monitor?

Traditional heart failure monitoring measurements are also feasible for VAD outpatients. These include body weight, temperature, and blood pressure (mean arterial pressure or *MAP* for the VAD patient) as well as clinical signs of worsening heart failure such as peripheral edema and or shortness of breath. Additionally the VAD patient must monitor pump parameters to detect issues with pump function as well as INR measurements to maintain an adequate state of anticoagulation.

Follow-up using telephone calls [24] may also be useful in maintaining frequent communication with patients, especially with those patients who do not live near the VAD center. Weekly phone calls by specialized nurses [25] lead to a significant reduction in mortality and earlier identification of potential adverse events. One has to keep in mind that telephone calls are time consuming to assess VAD outpatient data and cannot be considered as real-time monitoring.

Recent studies [22] have demonstrated that subtherapeutic INR and elevated mean arterial blood pressure (>90 mmHg) are independent risk factors for pump thrombosis

and strokes. Therefore, incorporating remote monitoring in VAD patient management has become of special interest in order to improve patients' quality of life and independence, to prevent adverse events, and to minimize readmission and personal costs during MCS support.

44.2.3 PT/INR Monitoring

VAD support therapy requires anticoagulation. Commonly used are anti-vitamin K substances like warfarin. Therapeutic dosage usually is set to a target INR between 2.0 and 3.5, depending on the used device. Dietary habits as well as other factors can have an effect on INR level, and medication dosage is frequently changed to maintain a therapeutic range. For this reason frequent INR measurement must be undergone to prevent pump-related thrombotic events.

INR surveillance and management is organized differently according to regional refunding options, cost aspects, and established procedures. In some centers the majority of VAD patients have to visit their GP, the VAD center, or specialized monitoring centers for INR measurements. Other centers routinely follow INR levels using specialized home monitoring devices.

For successful INR self-management using a home monitoring device, the patient must receive extensive training. Patients need to have an understanding of how to use the home monitoring device and, more importantly, how to calculate the appropriate anticoagulant dosage. Most importantly the patient must be trained how to handle emergency situations with extremely high or low INR levels. Although this method may be beneficial [35], depending on the patient, it may not be reliable and at worst can be dangerous.

Surveillance of successful self-management is important to avoid hazardous situations, which may even not recognized by the patient, may be neglected by patients, or are treated wrongly by the patient. Some centers provide active surveillance for patients by initiating regular contact. This method is time consuming.

Several telemetric systems have been developed, to transmit PT/INR test results from the patient's home to the VAD hospital. These include:

- AlereINRatio®2 PT/INR Monitoring Systems: Handheld blood coagulation system for monitoring patients taking warfarin. Used by healthcare professionals and patients at home, the system consists of a small monitor and disposable test strips. It provides an accurate and convenient measurement of blood clotting time or PT/INR values. Test results can be transferred via AlereVADWatch™ Telemonitoring program to the hospital.
- Roche CoaguChek XS mPOC Kit: This mobile point-of-care solution (mPOC) is specifically designed to work together with

the CoaguChek XS meter to wirelessly transmit PT/INR test results from home to CoaguChek Link and the hospital or company. Several third-party products exist – e.g., ClotFree, Genesis Advanced Technologies, USA – which may allow online transfer of PT/INR measured with Roche CoaguChek to the hospital.

Future aspects include integration of telemetric functionality directly into the INR measuring device or integration of the INR meter into a telemetric interface and transmitter.

44.2.4 Blood Pressure Monitoring

Due to the continuous blood flow in currently used VADs and the resulting absence of a palpable peripheral pulse, assessing noninvasive MAP at home can be rather challenging for VAD patients and caregivers. The recommended noninvasive gold standard for MAP measurement in LVAD patients without a palpable pulse is obtained through the use of Doppler signals [26]. Expense coupled with limited financial resources make the use of portable Doppler devices to measure MAP at home is rather uncommon. If available, the *AlereVADWatch*™ Telemonitoring Program is designed to assist participating hospitals (for US hospitals) and VAD coordinators to meet the demands of the VAD patient in the outpatient setting. *VADWatch*™ is a wireless telehealth monitoring service, provided exclusively for VAD outpatients, and is designed to assist hospital staff in dealing with issues that might lead to readmissions. It consists of a wireless scale, wireless blood pressure meter and cuff or Doppler, AlereDayLink® monitor, thermometer, and an optional INR meter and glucometer. The VAD coordinator is able to see the metrics online – input by a visiting nurse or the patient – of pump parameters, MAP and pulse, temperature, and body weight. They are then able to make any changes, conduct patient interviews, and adjust medications based on also INR and/or glucose results, if applicable. The disadvantage of these systems is the delayed and noncontinuous monitoring.

The key for effective remote VAD patient monitoring is the automated, real-time monitoring of pump speed, power consumption, and pump flow. These three VAD parameters could be used to alert the VAD center to abnormalities via the Internet. Despite the fact that the technical prerequisites are available for such a remote data transfer, currently the manufacturers of the most commonly used VAD systems (Thoratec/St. Jude Medical, Inc. and HeartWare, Inc.) have not introduced this capability into their current generation pumps/controllers.

44.2.5 Challenges of (Remote) Pump Parameter Monitoring?

Almost all available VADs display several pump-specific parameters that could be reported to healthcare providers to assist in the remote management of these patients. Each VAD manufacturer has different peripheral designs, but most of the patient controllers display the three key pump parameters (speed, power, flow), and many products – e.g., Thoratec/St. Jude Medical HeartMate II and HeartMate 3 pocket controller or the HeartWare MVAD Pal™ controller – also provide the alarm history of a certain number of alarms. If patients are equipped with home monitors (not routinely available in any VAD system), historical data – called log files – can be downloaded and sent via email or social media to the VAD coordinator or implanting hospital. This way of remote monitoring is limited, as especially in the elderly DT population as many patients are not familiar with information technology or do not have Internet access at home.

Remote monitoring of trends of the key pump parameters is of major importance as they can assist VAD coordinators in the management of these patients. Log files are useful tools to detect possible pump malfunction or significant problems such as inflow/outflow obstruction or pump thrombus. In situ clot formation results in gradual or sudden increases in power which patterns [27] are well known. But what are the limitations of currently available log files? Overall, the interval between two stored pump parameter data points is too big and allows for the investigation of trends, but as the beat-by-beat pump flow waveform is not available, these pump data do not have enough sensitivity to detect worsening heart failure or hemodynamic changes leading to severe clinical problems such as suction, arrhythmia, or hypovolemia. Thus, even if current generation controllers would be equipped with remote monitoring access by the manufacturer, the available pump data is still limited, and it is difficult to determine whether this would allow for sufficient remote monitoring. Axial flow pumps, such as the Thoratec/St. Jude Medical HeartMate II, provide an estimation of pump flow and pulsatility but no flow waveform [16]. Because there is a nonlinear behavior between motor current and speed in these pumps, certain ranges without estimated pump flow exist which may lead to problems during remote monitoring. The current configuration of the HeartMate II pocket controller is not optimized for remote monitoring in the current state since pump parameters (flow, power, speed, and pulsatility index) are recorded at the maximum of every 30 min – additionally these log files are encrypted and have to be sent to the company for decryption, thus not allowing for real-time monitoring. The pocket controller has a limited storage capacity of approximately 240 entries – with a 30 min sampling rate, no more than 5 days of pump history can be stored – and in the case of alarms or suction events, even less regular data entries are available. St Jude Medical's newest generation centrifugal pump – the HeartMate 3 – has an increased record interval of pump parameters (up to 10 min), but still limited data storage.

The HeartWare HVAD is a miniaturized, continuous-flow, centrifugal blood pump and has a unique controller log file that records the pump power, impeller speed, and VAD flow every 15 min [28, 29] with a maximum controller storage capacity of approximately 30 days. If the controller is connected to the patient monitor, real-time flow waveforms are available but are not stored on the controller and cannot be transferred to the hospital. Such log files are useful for trending but do not have enough sensitivity to assess, e.g., suction events, arrhythmias, or aortic valve status with remote monitoring of approx. 250 entries and do not provide flow waveforms or support remote monitoring.

Currently, the *ReliantHeart HeartAssist5®* is the only commercially available VAD that provides secure access to real-time and historical VAD parameters (measured by an ultrasonic flow probe) and alarms from any computer or smartphone. The VAD coordinator can view current flow waveforms and graphic historical data for 4 h, 24 h, 7 days, and 30 days and receive text and email of alarms with links directly to the live data [30]. In a published case series of 5 HeartAssist5® patients, the remote monitoring program showed satisfactory performance [31].

Another remote monitoring system, the *TeCNeT Telematics Module* for the *BerlinHeart INCOR®*, is still undergoing testing and not yet approved for clinical use [32]. The system provides secure data transfer between patient controller and the hospital including log file transfer and remote monitoring.

44.2.6 Outlook

Next-generation controllers (log files) must not only provide average pump parameters but must also provide real-time pump flow waveforms. Additionally larger data storage capacity and the possibility of remote 24/7 transfer of this data to the VAD centers would help to facilitate patient management. The implementation of flow estimators with a higher-frequency content [32] of the signal in the controller would allow more detailed analysis – without any additional flow sensors – including heart rate and its variability, suction events, aortic valve status, etc. and be the first step for optimal remote VAD patient monitoring.

The ongoing risk of recurrent heart failure after VAD implantation will open the door to other strategies for VAD patient management by remote hemodynamic monitoring. At least in theory, trends in pulmonary artery pressure (PAP) can predict heart failure events in patients supported with MCS. Therefore, devices like the *CardioMEMS™ HF* system – a wireless, implantable PAP monitoring system with external electronics and secure website – could transmit PAP information to the hospital in the future and, for example, in combination with hemolysis parameters, identify pump thrombus formation or right heart failure [34].

References

1. Christensen D, Petty M (2011) MCS coordinator role and program structure recommendations. Paper presented at: GRC 2011. Assisted circulation, Waterville Valley
2. Christensen D, Petty M, Bollen H (2015) Role of the mcs coordinator; an update. Paper presented at: GRC 2015. Assisted circulation, Barga
3. Feldman D, Pamboukian SV, Teuteberg JJ, Birks E, Lietz K, Moore SA, Morgan JA, Arabia F, Bauman ME, Buchholz HW, Deng M, Dickstein ML, El-Banayosy A, Elliot T, Goldstein DJ, Grady KL, Jones K, Hryniewicz K, John R, Kaan A, Kusne S, Loebe M, Massicotte P, Moazami N, Mohacsi P, Mooney M, Nelson T, Pagani F,

Perry W, Potapov EV, Rame JE, Russell SD, Sorensen EN, Sun B, Strueber M (2013) The 2013 international society for heart and lung transplantation guidelines for mechanical circulatory support: executive summary. J Heart Lung Transplant 32:157–187
4. Centers for Medicare & Medicaid Services (2015) Decision memo for ventricular assist devices for bridge-to-transplant and destination therapy (CAG-00432R). Medicare National Coverage Determinations Manual. 10:42–46
5. Joint Commission (2014) Disease-specific care certification manual. Oak Brook Terrace: Joint Commission Resources; VAD p 1–5
6. DNV GL-Healthcare (2014) Vad facility credentialing program requirements 4.0. Milford: DNV GL Healthcare USA, Inc; p 9–10
7. Wagner EH, Austin BT, Davis C, Hindmarsh M, Shaefer J, Bonomi A (2001) Medicine & chronic illness: improving chronic illness care; translating evidence into action. Health Aff 20:664–678
8. Soumerai SB, Avorn J (1990) Principles of educational outreach ('academic detailing') to improve clinical decision making. JAMA 263(4):549–556
9. Kirklin JK, Naftel DC, Pagani FD, Kormos RL, Stevenson LW, Blume ED, Miller MA, Timothy Baldwin J, Young JB (2014) Sixth intermacs annual report: a 10,000-patient database. J Heart Lung Transplant 33:555–564
10. Rossano JW, Lorts A, VanderPluym CJ, Jeewa A, Guleserian K, Bleiweis MS, Reinhartz O, Blume ED, Rosenthal D, Naftel D, Cantor RS, Kirklin JK (2016) Utilization and outcomes of continuous-flow ventricular assist devices in pediatric: patients: a report from the pediatric interagency registry for mechanical circulatory support (PediMACS). J Heart Lung Transplant 34:S102 Epub
11. Schweiger M, VanderPluym C, Jeewa A, Canter CE, Jansz P, Parrino PE, Miera O, Schmitto J, Mehegan M, Adachi I, Hubler M, Zimpfer D (2015) Outpatient management of intra-corporeal left ventricular assist device system in children: a multi-center experience. Am J Transplant 15:453–460
12. Miera O, Kirk R, Buchholz H, Schmitt KRL, VanderPlym C, Rebeyka IM, Wrightson N, Berger F, Criselli M, Conway J (2016) A multicenter study of the HeartWare HVAD® ventricular assist device in small children. J Heart Lung Transplant 34:S328. doi:10.1016/j.healun.2016.01.019
13. Conway J, VanderPlugm C, Jeewa A, Sinna durai S, Shubert A, Lorts A (2016) Now how do we get them home? Outpatient care of pediatric patients on mechanical circulatery support. Pediatr Transplant 20(2):194–202
14. Dudzienski M (2006) Ethics guidelines for destination therapy. Ann Thorac Surg 81:1185–1188
15. Casida JM et al (2011) Lifestyle adjustments of adults with long-term implantable left ventricular assist devices: a phenomenologic inquery. Heart Lung 40:511–520
16. HeartMate II LVAS Operating Manual. Available online: http://www.fda.gov/ohrms/dockets/ac/07/briefing/2007-4333b2-18%209_2%20HM%20II%20Operating%20 Manual.pdf
17. Mancini D (2014) Practical management of long-term circulatory support devices. UpToDate
18. Kirklin JK, Naftel DC, Pagani FD et al (2014) Sixth INTERMACS annual report: a 10,000-patient database. J Heart Lung Transplant 33:555–564
19. Rogers JG, Aaronson KD, Boyle AJ et al (2010) Continuous flow left ventricular assist device improves functional capacity and quality of life of advanced heart failure patients. J Am Coll Cardiol 55:1826–1834
20. Slaughter MS, Pagani FD, McGee EC et al (2013) HeartWare® ventricular assist system for bridge to transplant: combined results of the bridge to transplant and continued access protocol trial. J Heart Lung Transplant 32:675–683
21. Uriel N, Han J, Morrison KA et al (2014) Device thrombosis in HeartMate II continuous-flow left ventricular assist devices: a multifactorial phenomenon. J Heart Lung Transplant 33:51–59
22. Najjar SS, Slaughter MS, Pagani FD et al (2014) An analysis of pump thrombus events in patients in the HeartWare ADVANCE bridge to transplant and continued access protocol trial. J Heart Lung Transplant 33:23–34
23. Haglund NA, Davis ME, Tricarico NM et al (2015) Readmissions after continuous flow left ventricular assist device implantation: differences observed between two contemporary device types. ASAIO J 61:410–416
24. Slaughter MS, Pagani FD, Rogers JG et al (2010) Clinical management of continuous-flow left ventricular assist devices in advanced heart failure. J Heart Lung Transplant 29:1–39
25. Pamboukian SV, Tallaj JA, Brown RN et al (2011) Improvement in 2-year survival for ventricular assist device patients after implementation of an intensive surveillance protocol. J Heart Lung Transplant 30:879–887
26. Bennett MK, Roberts CA, Dordunoo D et al (2010) Ideal methodology to assess systemic blood pressure in patients with continuous-flow left ventricular assist devices. J Heart Lung Transplant 29:593–594
27. Jorde UP, Aaronson KD, Najjar SS et al (2015) Identification and management of pump thrombus in the heartware left ventricular assist device system: a novel approach using log file analysis. JACC Heart Fail 3(11):849–856
28. HeartWare Ventricular Assist System Instructions for use. Available online: http://www.heartware.com/sites/default/files/uploads/docs/ifu00001_rev_15.pdf
29. Chorpenning K, Brown MC, Voskoboynikov N et al (2014) HeartWare controller logs a diagnostic tool and clinical management aid for the HVAD pump. ASAIO J 60:115–118
30. ReliantHeart HeartAssist-5 Technology. Available online: http://reliantheart.com/international/
31. Pektok E, Demirozu ZT, Arat N et al (2013) Remote monitoring of left ventricular assist device parameters after HeartAssist-5 implantation. Artif Organs 37:820–825
32. TeCNeTTelematikModul. Available online: http://www.tecnet.de/index.php?option=com_content&task=view&id=78&Itemid=95&lang=en
33. Granegger M, Moscato F, Casas F et al (2012) Development of a pump flow estimator for rotary blood pumps to enhance monitoring of ventricular function. Artif Organs 36(8):691–699
34. Lampert BC, Emani S (2015) Remote hemodynamic monitoring for ambulatory left ventricular assist device patients. J Thorac Dis 7(12):2165–2171
35. Bishop MA, Streiff MB, Ensor CR et al (2014) Pharmacist-managed international normalized ratio patient self-testing is associated with increased time in therapeutic range in patients with left ventricular assist devices at an academic medical center. ASAIO J 60:193–198

Psychosocial Considerations of Mechanical Circulatory Support: Decision Making, Behavioral Evaluation, Quality of Life, Caregivers, and End of Life

Kathleen L. Grady, Larry A. Allen, and Paul W. Goetz

© Springer International Publishing Switzerland 2017
A. Montalto et al. (eds.), *Mechanical Circulatory Support in End-Stage Heart Failure*,
DOI 10.1007/978-3-319-43383-7_45

Abbreviations

BTT	Bridge to transplant
DT	Destination therapy
HRQOL	Health-related quality of life
INTERMACS	Interagency Registry for Mechanically Assisted Circulatory Support
MCS	Mechanical circulatory support
NYHA	New York Heart Association

Patients with advanced heart failure who may be candidates for surgical treatment options, including mechanical circulatory support (MCS) and heart transplantation (HT), engage in a process of shared decision making, considering the benefits, risks, alternatives to these therapies, and preferences within the context of their deteriorating health and prognosis. Adverse events, postoperative outcomes including survival and health-related quality of life (HRQOL), and the potential burden imposed on caregivers are important topics for discussion. Surgical options offered to advanced heart failure patients are tailored, based on an evaluation of the patient's clinical, psychosocial, and behavioral benefits and risks. The purpose of this chapter is to discuss decision making and informed consent, psychosocial/behavioral evaluation prior to surgery, HRQOL outcomes (i.e., overall HRQOL and physical, psychological, and social domains), caregiver burden, and palliative care/end-of-life care for patients who undergo long-term MCS implantation. An understanding of the tenets of medical ethics and related fundamentals of medical decision making and communication is critical to the optimal implantation, maintenance, and discontinuation of long-term MCS devices.

45.1 Decision Making

45.1.1 Autonomy

Healthcare providers have an ethical and legal mandate to involve patients in their medical decisions and healthcare delivery. The presence of life-threatening cardiac disease and the highly invasive option of MCS only heighten the importance of patient autonomy. Adults are presumed to have capacity, but may have impaired decision-making abilities under certain circumstances, including sedation, delirium, and dementia. Therefore, assessment of capacity is necessary to determine whether and to what extent a patient can participate in decisions involving MCS. In most cases, any clinician should be able to assess decision-making capacity as long as the clinician is familiar with its elements. Asking patients to express key ideas in their own words is central to assessing capacity. Patients with capacity have the right to determine how their decisions are made and may choose to involve others in the process or delegate decision making to a friend or family member.

45.1.2 Informed Consent

The process of informed consent prior to surgical interventions is an important formal application of the ethical principle of autonomy. The elements of informed consent are disclosure, decision-making capacity, and voluntariness [1]. Disclosure underscores the clinician's obligation to ensure that the patient is aware of the diagnosis and prognosis, the nature of the proposed intervention, the risks and benefits of that intervention, and all the reasonable alternatives and their associated risks and benefits. A patient with decision-making capacity around MCS is able to (1) understand the relevant information presented about diagnosis, prognosis, MCS, and non-MCS treatment options, risks, and benefits of each option, (2) reason about the options in the context of personal values and goals, and (3) make and communicate a choice. Voluntariness means that the patient makes a decision free from manipulation or coercion. The signed informed consent document is a record that a discussion took place between the clinician and the patient or appropriate surrogate decision-maker.

45.1.3 Shared Decision Making

Shared decision making builds upon the principles that guide informed consent. It asks that clinicians and patients share information with each other and work toward patient-centered decisions about treatment [2]. Shared decision making incorporates the perspective of the patient, who is responsible for articulating values, goals, and preferences as they relate to his or her healthcare. Thus, shared decision making puts into practice the principle of "patient-centered care," which the Institute of Medicine has identified as one of the six pillars of healthcare quality [3]. Shared decision making also incorporates the perspective of the clinician, who is responsible for narrowing the diagnostic and treatment options to those that are medically reasonable and seem to fit within the patient's values framework. Notably, MCS may be considered unreasonable above a certain age and comorbidity burden and therefore may not be included as a treatment option.

The shared decision making model is particularly appropriate for value-laden decisions with uncertain outcomes like MCS. Shared decision making grounds such discussions in the ideal that patients' values, goals, and preferences should guide the medical decision-making process. It should be assumed that discussions and decision making with patients also include, when appropriate, the family and other individuals involved, such as caregivers and companions. Due to the high stakes and complex nature of MCS, detailed and iterative discussions between patients of varying degrees of capacity, multiple family members, and healthcare providers are the standard.

The shared decision to proceed with long-term MCS therapy is a complex one. Although durable MCS offers a higher probability of survival and enhanced HRQOL for populations of carefully selected patients with stage D heart failure, it also comes with the short-term risk of major surgery and involves relatively high rates of complications over time (◘ Fig. 45.1) [4]. Lifestyle considerations and everyday burdens for LVAD patients are much greater than for other cardiac therapies, and patients conceptualize these burdens separately from risks.

Inherent to the ethical considerations of shared decision making regarding MCS as a treatment option are a discussion about discontinuing MCS and alternatives to MCS. Although the legal construct of patient autonomy does not recognize different degrees of dependence on therapies to be withdrawn, individuals may view proactive withdrawal that leads to direct patient demise as unique and emotionally difficult. Thus, a discussion about discontinuing MCS therapy should be part of the consent process prior to implantation.

Regarding alternatives to MCS, patients often do not see declining MCS as an option [5]. Few existing MCS educational materials even recognize other options or acknowledge that there needs to be a decision [6]. Therefore, it becomes even more important for clinicians to provide a parallel comparison of life with and life without MCS, a choice between two imperfect options, which can then contribute to a more engaged and realistic decision-making process. Importantly, MCS decision making may occur, while patients with progressive heart failure are actively dying and have heightened emotions with mortality salience pushed to the front of consciousness. Thus, clinicians need to attend to patients' fear of dying. Studies have shown that patients with end-stage illness find it helpful to discuss death, and retrospectively, many prefer direct and honest communication [7].

Finally, advanced heart failure and long-term MCS – with its high degree of prognostic uncertainty and complex trade-offs between choices of medical care – demand high-quality communication. Most patients and families want accurate and honest conversations with their clinicians. These interactions require time for assessment and planning in order to determine how much information patients desire and create a supportive environment for effective communication. These discussions also require attention to both cognitive and emotional needs, as well as concerns related to health literacy.

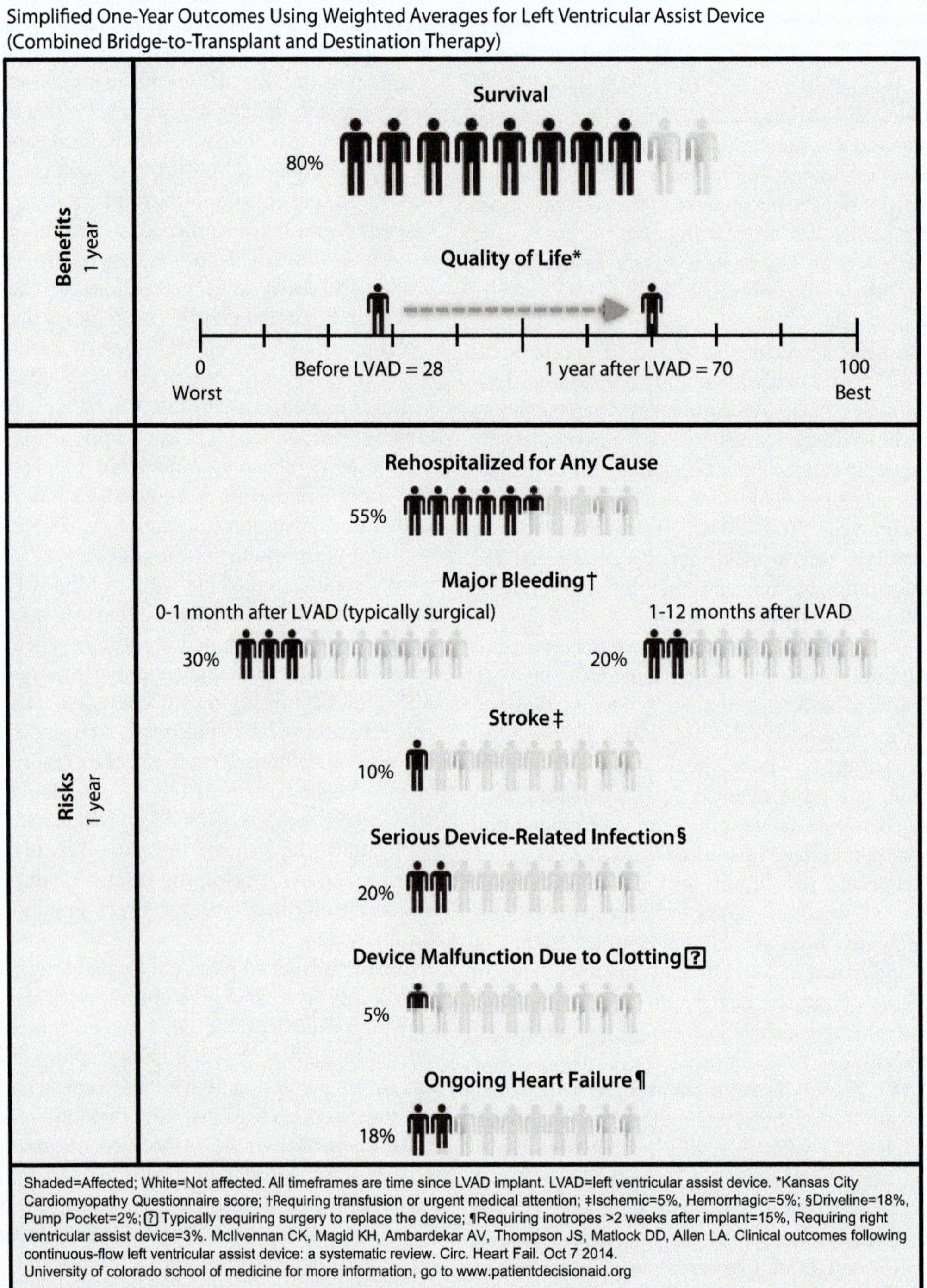

Fig. 45.1 Depiction of benefits and risks through 1 year after mechanical circulatory support

45.2 Behavioral Evaluation

The behavioral and psychosocial evaluation is a critical component of determining whether a patient is an appropriate candidate for MCS implantation. A great deal of self-care and responsibility are required to live successfully with MCS. Patients who are not fully engaged in self-care after MCS may suffer from disastrous outcomes. Patients being evaluated for advanced therapies should evidence willingness and capacity to engage in required health behaviors, compliance with medical recommendations, sufficient social support, and cognitive and psychological stability. All of these elements should be considered when determining whether MCS will be helpful, or potentially harmful, to someone with advanced heart failure. There are two scenarios when conducting a psychosocial evaluation for MCS candidacy: bridge to transplant and destination therapy. While the evaluation is typically the same for both scenarios, MCS centers may modify criteria for patients who are being implanted for destination therapy [8, 9].

There is a dearth of research examining the standardization of psychosocial assessment criteria for MCS, especially for destination therapy MCS [8, 9]. There has been some attempt at creating standardized assessment tools [8, 9], but studies are limited by small sample sizes and single-center designs. Nonetheless, a number of consistent variables emerge that are important to consider in the psychosocial assessment of an MCS candidate.

A psychologist on a MCS team will interview the patient about his or her psychosocial history, health behaviors, compliance, social support, and psychiatric functioning. ◘ Table 45.1 provides

◘ Table 45.1 Psychosocial assessment domains and questions

Domain	Example question topics
Social history	With whom the patient resides Employment or disability Life stressors Family and/or friends who could provide social support Occupation and health of the possible caregivers Transportation method to medical appointments
Health behaviors	Exercise Diet (e.g., sodium and fat intake) Amount of fluids consumed per day, especially if on a fluid restriction Medical follow-up ETOH, tobacco, illicit drug use (frequency, amount, duration of use) Motivation and self-efficacy to change behaviors
Medical adherence	Symptom reporting Medication compliance, system for medication (e.g., pillbox) Patient's knowledge about his/her medications Medical appointment follow-up
Psychiatric	Level of alertness and orientation Speech rhythm, rate, volume Notable cognitive deficits (e.g., difficulties with concentration or memory) History of depression, anxiety, or other psychiatric issues Current depressive or anxiety symptoms (follow diagnostic criteria) History of or current suicidal ideation Family psychiatric history Recent changes in weight Change in sleep Panic symptoms Current psychotropic medications History of therapy Typical methods of coping with stress Current understanding of their cardiac/medical status Patient's thoughts about MCS

domains of assessment topics, along with examples of specific content to assess. First, social support (practical support and emotional support) assessment is a critical part of the psychosocial assessment. The criterion for having a caregiver present 24/7 is variable among device programs and includes consideration of the patient's functional capacity, frailty, and cognitive functioning. Meeting with caregivers can provide an understanding of their willingness and ability to provide sufficient support and care for that particular patient's needs.

While it is important to assess and reinforce adaptive health behaviors (e.g., exercise and a healthy diet), there are certain health behaviors that may be considered relative contraindications for device implantation [9]. For example, smoking tobacco may be a relative contraindication, or the patient may be strongly encouraged to quit if they are being considered for destination therapy. However, complete abstinence is typically required for someone who is a bridge-to-transplant candidate.

It is especially important to assess history and current symptoms of clinical depression and anxiety, as presence of these symptoms interact with other areas of assessment. For example, depression is associated with poorer self-care behaviors, a generally more unhealthy lifestyle, such as smoking and minimal physical activity [10], and poorer compliance with medications [11], all of which are necessary for maintaining good health with MCS. Assessing the patient's cognitive status is also important, given that even mild cognitive impairment is a risk factor for increased mortality following surgery [12]. In addition to informally assessing the patient's cognitive status via interview, a brief screening tool (e.g., the Montreal Cognitive Assessment [MoCA]), validated in cardiac populations [13, 14], may also be utilized to provide objective data.

Following assessment, the data should be used to formulate impressions about each of the assessment domains, and from those impressions, concrete and specific recommendations should be communicated to the MCS team. For example, if the patient is a poor historian, tangential, and seems to have difficulty processing questions, it may be recommended that the patient undergo comprehensive neuropsychological testing. If clinical depressive symptoms are present, it may be recommended that the patient continues to follow up with a health psychologist or another mental health professional, including a psychiatric consult, if psychotropic medication seems warranted.

45.3 Health-Related Quality of Life

During the period of shared decision making and evaluation for MCS, advanced heart failure patients need to be informed about postimplant outcomes. HRQOL, both before and after implant, is an important patient-centric outcome to discuss with patients and their families who are considering MCS as a treatment option (Fig. 45.2). Patients with advanced heart failure have very poor HRQOL [15]. They have frequent and distressing symptoms, including fatigue, shortness of breath, paroxysmal nocturnal dyspnea, lack of energy, difficulty sleeping, daytime drowsiness, and weakness [15]. Poor HRQOL in advanced heart failure patients is associated with symptom distress [15].

Patients need to be informed that overall HRQOL improves from before to as long as 2 years after continuous-flow MCS [16], including destination therapy [17]. Findings from the Risk Assessment and Comparative Effectiveness of Left Ventricular Assist Device and Medical Management (ROADMAP) study, a prospective, nonrandomized observational study of outcomes in ambulatory NYHA class IIIB/IV non-inotrope

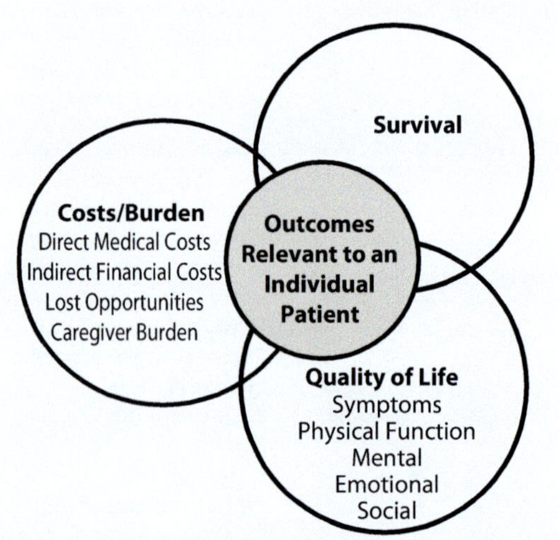

Fig. 45.2 Outcomes of importance to patients

patients, demonstrated greater improvement in HRQOL in MCS patients, as compared to optimal medical management patients through 12 months [18]. Furthermore, while patients with lower INTERMACS profiles (i.e., higher severity of heart failure) had worse HRQOL prior to implant, by 12 months after implant, HRQOL improved significantly for all profiles and did not differ significantly among profiles at 6 and 12 months after implant [19]. Lastly, while patients who undergo destination therapy implantation are typically older, may have comorbidities that preclude heart transplantation, and have a higher risk for post-implant adverse events (especially if older) and lower survival, than those who are bridge to transplant, destination therapy MCS patient HRQOL nonetheless significantly improves from before to after surgery [17].

Early substantial improvement also occurs in heart failure symptomatology and domains of HRQOL. Patients report that most symptoms of heart failure (e.g., shortness of breath and peripheral edema) abate relatively soon after implant, while other symptoms (e.g., fatigue and decreased energy level) persist for several weeks to months [20]. New symptoms emerge after MCS implant (e.g., dizziness/syncope and gastrointestinal bleeding) [20]. Most patients also report significantly fewer problems with mobility, usual activities, and self-care from before to 12 months after implant [16, 19]. Patients often returned to home management, work, and leisure activities [20]. Reports of decreased anxiety/depression [18] and pain/discomfort from before to after implant were also noted, which varied somewhat by preimplant INTERMACS profile [19]. Anxiety and depression often decreased later after implant when patients had adjusted to living with MCS [20].

45.3.1 Risk Factors for Poor HRQOL After MCS

Patients and their families also need to be informed of risk factors for poor HRQOL after MCS implantation. From before to 6 months after implant, adverse events (i.e., renal dysfunction, respiratory failure, neurological dysfunction, and infection), comorbidities (i.e., chronic obstructive pulmonary disease and ascites), and having a moderate or lower likelihood of undergoing heart transplantation are significantly related to decreased HRQOL [21]. Unplanned hospital readmission is a marker of morbidity, reflecting disease and treatment-related adverse events (e.g., gastrointestinal bleeding and cardiac-related causes). From before to 1 year after MCS implant, re-hospitalization is associated with poor HRQOL after destination therapy MCS [17].

45.3.2 Differences in HRQOL by Demographics

Differences in MCS HRQOL exist based on gender and age. Both male and female patients, as well as younger and older patients, experience improved HRQOL from before to early after implant, overall and by HRQOL domain [22]. Improvement from before to 6 months after implant is similar by gender and age for mobility, self-care, usual activities, anxiety/depression, and pain/discomfort [22]. However, at 6 months post-implant, female patients report significantly more problems with usual activities, pain/discomfort, and anxiety/depression than male patients, and younger patients report significantly more problems with pain/discomfort and anxiety/depression than older patients [22]. The age-related findings at 6 months are similar to findings at 1 year after destination therapy MCS implant, wherein improvement among all age groups was demonstrated from before to 1 year postimplant, but younger patients reported lower overall HRQOL, more pain/discomfort, and more anxiety/depression than older patients at 1 year [17].

45.4 Caregiver Burden

MCS has significant implications that extend beyond the individual patient. Caregiver involvement is central to the longitudinal success of MCS. This is especially notable for patients with long-term MCS. Caregivers, as critical members of the MCS team, spend much of their time with MCS patients and often assist with medications, transportation, and providing emotional support. Thus, understanding the burden and emotional toll of the caregiver role and providing resources and support are beneficial and may ultimately improve outcomes for both caregivers and patients.

Caregivers are often greatly affected by MCS. MCS caregivers devote significant amounts of time to nursing care and caregiving in general, often experiencing worsening of health themselves. Moreover, caregivers of MCS patients are more likely than MCS patients to develop symptoms of post-traumatic stress disorder (PTSD) related to MCS issues [23]. Early after implant, MCS caregivers may be quite overwhelmed given their sense of responsibility for equipment/supplies and care of the patient. In a qualitative study of 13 MCS caregivers [24], participants also reported fear and anxiety, related to the medical urgency of MCS implantation. A feeling of loss, related to their usual family or career role, was also a common experience. Relatedly, the potential loss of their loved one was frequently reported. Two types of caregiver burden were identified: the burden of making the decision to move forward with implantation if patients were not able to make the decision themselves and the burden of time and effort required to care for their loved one. Other common caregiver burden themes that have emerged in the literature include hypervigilance regarding the MCS patient's well-being, having less personal time, and financial strain [25].

Caregivers of long-term MCS patients may need to acquire skills of self-preservation (e.g., coping skills) to sustain their role as a caregiver. Common coping strategies that MCS caregivers report are developing a routine, acceptance of the new lifestyle as a caregiver, positive self-talk, and faith and religiosity [25]. The patient's medical team can be instrumental in facilitating and acquiring coping skills for those caregivers who need more formal skills acquisition training.

Caregivers of long-term MCS patients may also benefit from monthly or bimonthly "check-ins" to assess the social support dynamics and the environment not only to ensure that sufficient patient support is in place but also to assess the emotional and physical status of the caregiver. Important components of a caregiver assessment include: confidence and competence regarding assessing the patient's medical condition and providing treatment, willingness to accept assistance themselves, methods used to cope with stress, personal health status, the current nature and health of their relationship with the patient, and the status of their own QOL [26].

Respite from caregiving and having access to a support network is essential for being an effective caregiver. During check-ins with the caregiver, clinicians should help primary caregivers identify other family members and/or friends who may be able to assist with caregiving and provide training for those individuals. Family meetings can be held to facilitate identification of specific roles and responsibilities of each caregiver. Providing the caregiver with counseling resources may also be warranted. Local support groups [26] or credible, well-established, online caregiver support groups may also be a method to obtain practical and emotional support from other caregivers. Overall, the value, role, and burden of MCS caregivers are important components of MCS patient care, in order to enhance patient and caregiver health and well-being.

45.5 Palliative Care and End-of-Life Care

While MCS can prolong survival, reduce symptom burden, and improve HRQOL for patients with advanced heart failure, MCS is associated with risks (e.g., adverse events and re-hospitalization). MCS patients must also face the inevitability of death and the dying process, which they will approach with a pump in place. Several guidelines and reviews recommend integration of palliative care for all patients with advanced heart failure, including MCS patients [2, 27, 28]. Palliative care goals of care include relief of suffering, enhancement of HRQOL, and provision of psychosocial and spiritual support to MCS patients and their families and caregivers. These goals can be addressed by multidisciplinary MCS teams and palliative care specialists. MCS teams can provide primary palliative care (e.g., basic management of symptoms, depression, and anxiety and basic discussions on current health status, prognosis, uncertainty, suffering, and code status) [28, 29]. Palliative care consultation is indicated for patients (e.g., MCS patients) with more challenging issues (e.g., complicated advance care planning, disabling adverse events post-MCS, complex and/or refractory symptom control, and conflict of resolution regarding goals or treatment strategies) [29].

As MCS patients approach end of life, burden and suffering may outweigh benefits of MCS, and patients with decision-making capacity or their surrogates may request that the device be turned off, an ethically and legally permissible action allowing patients to simply succumb to their underlying condition (i.e., heart failure) [30]. Advance care planning is important to facilitate end-of-life care, with participation by patients and loved ones, as well as the MCS team and palliative care/hospice specialists.

Withdrawal of MCS can be done in the hospital setting or at home, depending on patient and family preferences [30]. Patient comfort is of utmost importance. Administration of anesthetics, analgesics, and anxiolytics, at appropriate doses, can relieve symptoms and reduce suffering. Additionally, loved ones need support during this difficult time. Device deactivation is typically done by an MCS team member, with expertise in MCS management, who can properly disconnect the device, without initiating alarms, which can cause distress for all present. Protocols and checklists for discontinuing device support facilitate this process [30]. Following MCS patient death, bereavement support for family and friends should be offered.

45.6 Conclusions

Patients with advanced heart failure, who have an option of MCS, and their families, simultaneously engage in the process of shared decision making while being evaluated for MCS, either as BTT or DT. Important components of decision making include understanding the risks, benefits, alternatives, and outcomes (i.e., survival and HRQOL), as well as changes in lifestyle, potential for withdrawal of MCS, and caregiver burden, within the context of patient values, preferences, and goals. An ethical process fully engages patients, their families, and the advanced heart failure/MCS team and supports the objective of successful decision making and enhanced outcomes.

References

1. Hall DE, Prochazka AV, Fink AS (2012) Informed consent for clinical treatment. Can Med Assoc J 184:533–540
2. Allen LA, Stevenson LW, Grady KL, Goldstein NE, Matlock DD, Arnold RM, Cook NR, Felker GM, Francis GS, Hauptman PJ, Havranek EP, Krumholz HM, Mancini D, Riegel B, Spertus JA (2012) Decision making in advanced heart failure: a scientific statement from the American Heart Association. Circulation 125:1928–1952
3. Institute of Medicine Committee on Quality of Health Care in America (2001) Crossing the quality chasm: a new health system for the 21st century. National Acadamy Press, Washington, DC
4. McIlvennan CK, Magid KH, Ambardekar AV, Thompson JS, Matlock DD, Allen LA (2014) Clinical outcomes after continuous-flow left ventricular assist device: a systematic review. Circ Heart Fail 7:1003–1013
5. McIlvennan CK, Allen LA, Nowels C, Brieke A, Cleveland JC, Matlock DD (2014) Decision making for destination therapy left ventricular assist devices: "there was no choice" versus "I thought about it an awful lot.". Circ Cardiovasc Qual Outcomes 7:374–380
6. Iacovetto MC, Matlock DD, McIlvennan CK et al (2014) Educational resources for patients considering a left ventricular assist device: a cross-sectional review of Internet, print, and multimedia materials. Circ Cardiovasc Qual Outcomes 7:905–911
7. Curtis JR, Engelberg RA, Nielsen EL, Au DH, Patrick DL (2004) Patient-physician communication about end-of-life care for patients with severe COPD. Eur Respir J 24:200–205
8. Bruce CR, Delgado E, Kostick K, Grogan S, Ashrith G, Trachtenberg B, Blumenthal-Barby JS (2014) Ventricular assist devices: A review of psychosocial risk factors and their impact on outcomes. J Card Fail 20:996–1003
9. Maltby M, Flattery MP, Burns B, Salyer J, Weinland S, Shah KB (2014) Psychosocial assessment of candidates and risk classification of patients considered for durable mechanical circulatory support. J Heart Lung Transplant 33:836–841
10. Bonnet F, Irving K, Terra JL, Nony P, Berthezene F, Moulin P (2005) Anxiety and depression are associated with unhealthy lifestyle in patients at risk of cardiovascular disease. Atherosclerosis 178:339–344
11. Grenard JL, Munjas BA, Adams JL, Suttorp M, Maglinone M, McGlynn EA, Gellad MF (2011) Depression and medication adherence in the treatment of chronic diseases in the United States: a meta-analysis. J Gen Intern Med 26:1175–1182
12. Tully PJ, Baune BT, Baker RA (2013) Cognitive impairment before and six months after cardiac surgery increase mortality risk at median 11 year follow-up: a cohort study. Int J Cardiol 168:2796–2802
13. Cameron J, Worrall-Carter L, Page K, Riegel B, Kai Lo S, Stewart S (2010) Does cognitive impairment predict poor self-care in patients with heart failure. Eur J Heart Fail 12:508–515
14. Nasreddine ZS, Phillips NA, Bedirian V, Charbonneau S, Whitehead V, Collin I, Chertkow H (2005) The montreal cognitive assessment, MoCA: a brief screening tool for mild cognitive impairment. J Am Geriatr Soc 53:695–699
15. Blinderman C, Homel P, Billings A, Portenoy R, Tennstedt S (2008) Symptom distress and quality of life in patients with advanced congestive heart failure. J Pain Symptom Manage 35:594–603
16. Kirklin JK, Naftel DN, Pagani FD, Kormos RL, Stevenson LW, Blume ED, Miller MA, Baldwin JT, Young JB (2014) Sixth INTERMACS annual report: a 10,000-patient database. J Heart Lung Transplant 33:555–564

17. Grady KL, Naftel D, Myers S et al (2015) Change in health-related quality of life from before to after destination therapy mechanical circulatory support is similar for older and younger patients: analyses from INTERMACS. J Heart Lung Transplant 34:213–221
18. Estep JD, Starling RC, Horstmanshof DA et al (2015) Risk assessment and comparative effectiveness of left ventricular assist device and medical management in ambulatory heart failure patients. J Am Coll Cardiol 66(16):1747–1761
19. Grady KL, Naftel D, Stevenson L et al (2014) Overall quality of life improves to similar levels after mechanical circulatory support regardless of severity of heart failure before implantation. J Heart Lung Transplant 33(4):412–421
20. Grady KL, Magasi S, Hahn E et al (2015) Health-related quality of life in mechanical circulatory support: Development of a new conceptual model and items for self-administration. J Heart Lung Transplant 34:1292–1304
21. Grady KL, Naftel DC, Myers SL et al (2015) Pre and post operative factors related to change in HRQOL from before to 6 months following LVAD implantation: an INTERMACS analysis. J Heart Lung Transplant 34(4S):S75
22. Wissman S, Naftel DC, Myers SL et al (2015) Health-related quality of life improves dramatically from pre implant to post implant (6 months) for continuous flow LVAD patients in INTERMACS. J Heart Lung Transplant 34(4S):S75–S76
23. Bunzel B, Laederach-Hofmann K, Wieselthaler G, Roethy W, Wolner E (2010) Mechanical circulatory support as a bridge to heart transplantation: what remains? Long-term emotional sequelae in patients and spouses. J Heart Lung Transplant 26:384–389
24. Kaan A, Young QR, Cockell S, Mackay M (2010) Emotional experiences of caregivers of patients with a ventricular assist device. Prog Transplant 20:142–147
25. Marcuccilli L, Casida JM (2011) From insiders' perspectives: adjusting to caregiving for patients with left ventricular assist devices. Prog Transplant 21:137–143
26. Adelman RD, Tmanova L, Delgado D, Dion S, Lachs MS (2014) Caregiver Burden. A clinical review. JAMA 311:1052–1059
27. Fang JC, Ewald GA, Allen LA, Butler J, Westlake Canary CA, Colvin-Adams M, Dickinson MG, Levy P, Stough WG, Sweitzer NK, Teerlink JR, Whellan DJ, Albert NM, Krishnamani R, Rich MW, Walsh MN, Bonnell MR, Carson PE, Chan MC, Dries DL, Hernandez AF, Hershberger RE, Katz SD, Moore S, Rodgers JE, Rogers JG, Vest AR, Givertz MM (2015 Jun) Advanced (stage D) heart failure: a statement from the Heart Failure Society of America Guidelines Committee. J Card Fail 21(6): 519–534
28. Fendler TJ, Swetz KM, Allen LA (2015) Team-based palliative and end-of-life care for heart failure. Heart Fail Clin 11(3):479–498
29. Quill TE, Abernethy AP (2013) Generalist plus specialist palliative care-creating a more sustainable model. N Engl J Med 368(13):1173–1175
30. Swetz K, Ottenberg AL, Freeman MR, Mueller PS (2011) Palliative care and end-of-life issues in patients treated with left ventricular assist devices as destination therapy. Curr Heart Fail Rep 8:212–218

Adverse Events Management

Contents

Ischemic and Hemorrhagic Stroke

Rachel A. Beaupré and Jeffrey A. Morgan

© Springer International Publishing Switzerland 2017

A. Montalto et al. (eds.), *Mechanical Circulatory Support in End-Stage Heart Failure*,
DOI 10.1007/978-3-319-43383-7_46

46.1 Introduction

One of the most potentially devastating complications in the period following ventricular assist device (VAD) implantation is the incidence of stroke or major thromboembolic events. Patients on mechanical circulatory support, as with the general population, may be afflicted by either embolic or hemorrhagic strokes. In the postimplantation period, different circumstances may make the individual patient more susceptible to either form of stroke. The inherent thrombogenicity of the mechanical support device surfaces; patient comorbidities, such as diabetes, prior history of stroke, and hypertension; and secondary complications that may develop in relation to implantation and the need for and use of anticoagulation in the postsurgical period all have the potential to increase an individual's proclivity toward suffering an adverse neurological event.

The physician, clinician, and other members of the medical team contributing to and advancing the care of the patient on mechanical circulatory support must be ever aware of the incidence of stroke, its effects on the long-term patient care goals, and prognostic value, as well as the possible prophylactic strategy and points of intervention in order to minimize the occurrence and effects of stroke in the preoperative and postoperative period.

46.2 Incidence

The overall incidence of stroke in patients on mechanical circulatory support ranges from 8–17%. The Backes et al. review showed a stroke and transient ischemic attack rate of 20% across nearly 2000 patients with either HeartMate II (HMII) or and Novacor devices [1]. As the HeartMate II is the most commonly implanted device, most of the larger research series are focused on this particular subpopulation. Morgan et al. and Tsiouris et al. have both reported overall stroke incidence rate of 12% in their overall study populations [2, 3], while Kato et al. and Trachtenberg et al. have reported similar rates of 12.9% and 13% [4, 5]; this is compared to 17% reported in the Harvey et al. series of 230 HMII patients [6]. These rates of stroke represent a greater risk for adverse neurological events than when compared with heart failure patients in the medical management arm of head-to-head studies [7]. A stroke risk of 6.4% per patient-year was significantly elevated when compared to patients with advanced heart failure who were treated with medical management [6]. As such, physicians and practitioners working with the mechanical circulatory support patient population must be in tune with the unique risk profile of patients in the vigilant attempt to prevent patients from experiencing this devastating complication.

Stroke risk on mechanical circulatory support can further be broken down between bridge-to-transplant (BTT) and destination therapy (DT) patients. Owing to the fact that the destination therapy population is more sick and thus less likely to be a candidate for future transplantation, one might expect this group to not only suffer from more advanced heart failure but also more extensive comorbidities. It would be expected that destination therapy patients may suffer from a greater number of adverse neurological events. This has been recorded in the literature as such. When overall stroke incidence is investigated between these two cohorts, it is demonstrated that this is the case. In the study by Morgan et al. (2014) reporting an overall 12% stroke rate, the incidence of stroke in BTT patients was 10.8% versus 14.3% for DT [2]. In larger BTT studies, stroke rates have been recorded as 8% in series conducted by Pagani et al. and by Miller et al. [2–8] and 11% in the Starling series which investigated 281, 133, and 169 enrolled HeartMate II patients, respectively. Katz et al. (2015) report a stroke rate of 4% for BTT patients and 6% for DT patients [9]. Lushaj et al. report a nearly 2.5× increased risk of stroke for DT patients as compared to BTT [10]. The 14.3% stroke incidence in destination therapy patients reported by Morgan et al. is similar to other DT series, 4 with an 18% incidence of stroke (8% embolic and 11% hemorrhagic) in 134 patients who underwent HMII implantation as DT [2].

Komoda et al. report higher body surface area (BSA) as a protective variable; a patient with a larger BSA had a 1-year mortality freedom from death due to stroke or bleeding of 82.7% as opposed to 49.1% for those of a lower BSA [11]. Women whose heart failure was treated with LVAD implantation were at a twofold risk for ischemic and hemorrhagic strokes than men after controlling for these differences in body size [12]. Morris et al. found a threefold increased risk in women but no differences in patient mortality [13]. Boyle et al., in an analysis of 900 HMII patients, supported this higher stroke rate for women while also finding younger women at higher risk for hemorrhagic stroke with older women experiencing ischemic stroke [14]. The propensity for women to suffer stroke events in significantly greater numbers than men warrants a greater investigation to elucidate what mechanisms increase the proclivity for cohort-matched women on MCS to experience this adverse postimplantation effect as it may indicate lower quality of life and perhaps less future opportunity to receive cardiac transplantation in this subset of patients.

In the Morgan et al. study, the median duration of support until time of stroke was 340.5 days with embolic strokes occurring earlier than hemorrhagic (281 versus 380.5 days) [2]. This was similar in the Harvey et al. study where embolic strokes occurred at median 146 days versus 240 days for hemorrhagic [6]. Time from implantation to stroke can show a predilection for one stroke subtype over another and may potentially be useful in understanding the mechanisms behind these subsets in the MCS population.

46.2.1 Embolic Versus Hemorrhagic Stroke

Some studies have found a relatively balanced percentage of ischemic and hemorrhagic strokes [5, 6, 14]. Both Kato et al. and Katz et al. had an ischemic stroke occurrence in 80% of their study population [4, 9, 15]. In contrast, Morgan et al. and Tsiouris et al. reported a greater percentage of patients suffering from hemorrhagic stroke [2, 3]. These differences in stroke etiology may reflect the individual patient cohort and preoperative risk factors. Each patient and their individual risk profiles should be considered preoperatively in order to gear management strategy toward their inherent proclivity toward hemorrhagic or ischemic stroke as best as possible.

46.2.2 Pathogenesis of Hemorrhagic Stroke in the LVAD Population

The incidence of embolic strokes has many possible causes. As blood travels through the artificial circulatory system, it can be expected that upon contact with foreign surface material platelets and the coagulation cascade may become activated. Goldstein et al. (2013) describe blood-surface contact, platelet activation due to shear stress, and thrombus formation at cannulation or migrated cannula sites as potential causes for thrombus formation [16]. Endothelial cell adherence and activation of coagulation system (such as tissue factor VII) also can contribute to the development of coagulopathy. These factors as a function of the unique VAD position and its inherent functionality and interaction with blood cells and tissue sites can all predispose the VAD patient to development of thrombus and ischemic stroke.

Thus, the inherent thrombogenicity of the device will have an independent effect on the risk profile of a particular patient. The HMII is reported to be less thrombogenic than the previous generation HMI. Thromboembolic events may occur in 25% of patients on LVAD support [17]. Each available device would carry its own set of thrombogenic risk due to the nature of the materials used in its manufacture. However, as most large trials are conducted with the use of the HMII, not enough studies are available to compare adequately due to the large differences in patient enrollment numbers and power of the studies. Several emulation methods and models are being design to test and evaluate the thrombogenic potential and thromboresistance of devices [18–20]. The ability to calculate or accurately numerically quantify the thrombogenicity of any one device remains theoretical as such effects would present an enormous challenge that would require not only a superb ability to control for confounding factors but would also remain a qualitative assessment of one device in comparison to its peers, and it may therefore be impossible to isolate the intrinsic thrombogenic effect and stroke risk profile of any one particular device in a quantitative, predictive manner.

In comparing pulsatile flow devices with continuous flow devices, Yuan et al. demonstrated that the incidence of stroke was not significantly higher for one patient cohort in comparison with the other; however, comparing the pulsatile HMI with the continuous flow HMII, the median postoperative day of stroke occurrence was 19 days compared to 363 days for the HMII device [21]. In demonstrating a better outcome for later-occurring strokes with the HMII device, one can predict that the time frame in which the stroke occurs is likely to have a significant influence on patient recovery and long-term prognosis rather than only the device flow itself.

46.2.3 Pathogenesis of Hemorrhagic Stroke in the LVAD Population

Many factors may play a role in the development of hemorrhagic stroke in LVAD patients. In addition to the inherent risks of bleeding secondary to cardiopulmonary bypass for on-pump VAD placement, VAD physiology itself can pose increased risk for bleeding and as such stroke. Acquired von Willebrand syndrome can develop in the post-implant period due to the shearing forces created on platelets as they pass through the pump structure; these forces can cause the platelet surfaces to be disrupted, destroy cells, and lead to a decreased amount of available von Willebrand factor, a platelet factor that contributes to the adherence of platelets to disrupted endothelial surfaces. Reduced von Willebrand factor leads to pathologic bleeding and may play a role in the development of hemorrhagic strokes.

The pathogenesis of hemorrhagic stroke in the LVAD patient has not been fully elucidated. Of course, the occurrence of supratherapeutic anticoagulation leading to adverse cerebral bleeding events is a readily discernible cause; however, other cases of its etiology may not be as clear. Aggarwal et al. (2012) describe the rate of intracranial hemorrhage in LVAD patients to 13–14% and describe the current hypotheses to be broken down into three categories. In the first category, hemorrhagic transformation from angiogenesis and reperfusion at the site of a previous infarct is attributed to the migration of prior emboli fragments [22]. The second hypothesis relates to the advent of rupture and bleeding from bloodstream infection seeding that leads to formation of cerebral mycotic aneurysms. Trachtenberg et al. describes the incidence of mycotic aneurysm formation in patient who suffered from hemorrhagic stroke and bacteremia likening the pathology to that of cererbrovascular accidents (CVA) related to embolization and bacterial seeding that occur in patients with infective endocarditis [5]. Aggarwal et al. also purports that infectious vasculitis can also weaken microvasculature in the brain leading to bleeding [22]. Hence, the main themes surrounding the postulations as to the mechanism of hemorrhagic stroke development can be divided into etiologies based on anticoagulation level abnormalities, consequences of pump characteristics, hemorrhagic transformation of ischemic stroke, and the predisposition of infection to increase susceptibility to intracranial hemorrhage.

46.2.4 Sidedness of Strokes

LVAD studies that have examined the sidedness of strokes suffered by LVAD study participants have showed a greater incidence of right-sided over left-sided strokes. In the Kato et al. study, 58.7% of strokes occurred in the right hemisphere as compared to 28.2% in the left [4]. With no difference in patient anticoagulation profiles, 59.3% of right-sided strokes occurred in patients with either sepsis or LVAD-related infections as compared to 23.1% of those who suffered left-sided strokes. Harvey et al. study concurs with this analysis and gives support to the increased incidence of right-sided strokes and its correlation with patients afflicted by concurrent infection at the time of stroke [6]. The introduction of an LVAD and its related postoperative position of the outflow cannula works along with anatomical positioning of the innominate such that embolic fragments are more frequently directed into the right-sided cerebral vasculature.

46.2.5 Effect of Stroke on Mortality and Morbidity

Adverse neurological events can have a significant effect on patient mortality, future ability to receive cardiac transplant, and prolong the patient recovery period.

Mortality after stroke is increased twofold and is reported to be as high as 20–25% within 30 days and 30–43% at 1 year. [2, 6, 23] Survival rate at 24 months is reported to be 53.9% in contrast to 74.7% in stroke-free patients [6]. Of those surviving after stroke, 67% remained on ongoing mechanical support [2]. In particular, hemorrhagic stroke and the need for tracheostomy are significant predictors of patient survival [3]. Although some studies have found no significant differences in mortality related to ischemic versus hemorrhagic stroke [6], the mortality rate is reported to be increased 1.5× after hemorrhagic stroke and has been reported with 100% mortality [5–22]. Patient mortality is significantly augmented after the advent of a stroke with evidence for an even more devastating patient course after occurrence of a hemorrhagic subtype.

Aside from effects on patient survival and mortality, patients suffering from strokes on mechanical circulatory support can experience significant quality of life changes or rehabilitation setbacks. In addition, strokes are responsible for upward of 8% of hospital readmissions after implantation [24]. Nearly 56% of patients surviving stroke spend time in a skilled nursing or rehabilitation facility [23]. Stroke is associated with significant decreased rate of nearly threefold less cardiac transplantations per person-year [6].

46.2.6 Significant Contributing Factors to Stroke Susceptibility

Issues with Anticoagulation

Secondary to the inherent thrombogenicity of an implanted device or foreign circulatory system, all patients must be placed on anticoagulation therapy in order to decrease the risks of subsequent thromboembolic events and their complications. While anticoagulation therapy aids in safeguarding patients from the risks of embolic events and therefore decreases the risks of embolic strokes, this same prophylactic measure can also increase the chances of patients experiencing a bleeding event, including increasing the risks for hemorrhagic stroke. Therefore, a delicate balance must be struck and maintained for optimal minimization of adverse neurological events.

The therapeutic INR levels at the time of a stroke may reflect a patient's proclivity toward developing one type of stroke versus another. However, the presenting INR level of the patient suffering from a stroke may serve as only a single pinpoint in time, whereas the overall therapeutic level history of each patient very well may be a better indicator of the patient's current clinical scenario and hence serve in painting a more holistic picture and offer some insight into seemingly paradoxical situations such as the case of a patient with a supratherapeutic INR (and normal aPPT and platelet function) and embolic stroke event if other risk factors for embolic stroke are absent. At the time of stroke, all patients with embolic strokes had mean subtherapeutic INRs, whereas 50% of the patients suffering from hemorrhagic strokes had supratherapeutic mean INR values [2]. Proper patient education programs and establishing further measures for adequate tracking of levels with deeper patient involvement may be useful in promoting appropriate therapeutic levels. The ability to observe nuances in patients' individual responses to dosages and setting stricter control INR value range may be of additional benefit. The control of postoperative anticoagulation to avoid INR values <1.7 IU or >3.0 IU may significantly impact the incidence of this postoperative complication [2]. It is possible that the patient's mean INR levels can serve a predictive factor for adverse neurological events; therefore, investigation into its predictive value and development of universal range guidelines may be useful in future stroke prevention after VAD implantation.

46.2.7 Diabetes

Diabetes as a disease process and the long-term complications associated with suboptimal control lead to a higher incidence of stroke. Thus, one would naturally expect that diabetic patients on LVAD support are at a higher for stroke than their non-diabetic peers. Using diabetes as an independent risk factor, after controlling all other variables, it has been shown that patients with diabetes are at a 76% higher risk of mortality after LVAD placement [25]. Morgan et al. showed a significantly higher incidence of diabetes (66.7% versus 40.9%) in the cohort of patients suffering from stroke. However, there appears to be no significant in-group survival difference between insulin- and non-insulin-dependent diabetics [25]. It is possible that the increased stroke risk in diabetics may reflect the severity of disease and individual history of diabetic control and may not represent an opportunity to prevent or reduce the pre-existing micro- and macro-vascular complications of diabetes. However, lowering the potential risk of diabetes-related stroke in LVAD patients should begin with modifying the diabetic risk factors and stressing the importance of adherence to diabetic diet and appropriate medical management whether this be through the means of insulin or other non-insulin alternatives.

46.2.8 History of Prior Stroke

Kato et al. and Morgan et al. have established previous history of stroke and as an independent risk factors associated with postimplantation cerebrovascular accidents (CVAs), associated with a nearly 3.5× higher risk for subsequent stroke [2, 9, 15].

46.2.9 Elevated Blood Pressure

Elevated blood pressure postimplantation is an additional risk factor for stroke in LVAD patients. Patients with elevated median systolic blood pressure (SBP) as compared to those below the median SBP (16% versus 7% risk); this risk is increased stepwise for every 5 mmHg (19%) and every 1 mmHg (3.5%) increase in patient blood pressure and represented 2.5× risk for stroke when blood pressure remains high at discharge [23]. These risks can be lowered for patients placed on antihypertensives, and risk is not dependent on the number of medications required to control blood pressure [23–26].

46.2.10 Atrial Fibrillation

As atrial fibrillation increases the risk of thromboembolic stroke in the general population, it is reasonable to believe that heart failure patients with preoperative atrial fibrillation would be at a similarly increased risk for stroke status post placement of mechanical support devices when compared with patients without preoperative atrial fibrillation. Patients with preoperative atrial fibrillation are at a 24% risk of thromboembolic events as compared to a 17% risk with no preoperative history [27]. This incidence increases to 45% when patients have a comorbid GI bleeding which necessitated the cessation of anticoagulation [27]. The anticoagulation efforts to avoid atrial fibrillation related or other causes of stroke can lead to adverse bleeding events; cessation of anticoagulation for such an event can therefore put the patient at an increase for stroke. This points to the importance of properly anticoagulating the patient while keeping in mind their additional risk factors for stroke.

46.2.11 Aortic Cross Clamping with Cardioplegic Arrest During LVAD Implantation

Complete aortic cross clamping is a significant operative factor leading to increased risk for stroke that has not been widely isolated in mechanical circulatory support research. Outside of the VAD literature, the use of cross clamp has been found to increase the risk of stroke; in CABG patients who had experienced three period of intraoperative cross clamping, the stroke risk was raised from 1.5% risk to 3.3% [28]. Half of all patients suffering stroke had undergone complete cross clamping in the Morgan et al. series, establishing this operative practice as an independent predictor of stroke; these patients also presented with stroke much earlier in their postoperative course (median 131 days). However, the same effect was not found for partial aortic clamping with a side-biting clamp. As opposed to the complete clamping, partial clamping refrains from compressing the posterior aorta. It is possible, therefore, that complete clamping may cause greater endothelial damage, creating a surface area amenable to the formation of thrombus and, subsequently, create an environment for future embolization. Further investigation into cross-clamp time, positioning, and the level of aortic compression during implantation surgery would be beneficial to elucidate the wider significance of the elevated risks and mechanisms that lead complete cross clamping to increase postoperative stroke incidence in the VAD population.

46.2.12 Bloodstream Infections

Infection has been found to be an independent risk factor for postimplantation stroke [4]. Aggarwal et al. reported a stroke incidence of 10% in the post-LVAD implantation patient population with no concurrent bloodstream infection in contrast to a quadrupled 44% risk for patients experiencing systemic infection [22]. The median time to hemorrhagic stroke was 12 days compared to 49 days for ischemic strokes, while infection was not associated with higher risk of ischemic stroke [22]. A study in which 30% of CF-LVAD patients developed bloodstream infections in the postimplantation period, 11% of which were persistent, demonstrated not only a sevenfold increase in all cause stroke incidence, but significant differences in the etiology of stroke, and 60% of strokes being hemorrhagic in the infection cohort and 100% ischemic stroke etiology in control population [5], and 73% of deaths in the infection group were secondary to stroke [5]. In addition, 27% of the adverse neurologic events were associated with preceding infection [29]. This stresses the importance of taking strict prophylactic measures to avoid the postoperative complication of device and implantation-related infection as it can have a significant effect on patient risk for stroke and stroke-related mortality in addition minimizing the adverse effects of postoperative infection itself.

46.3 Conclusion

Stroke in the patient population on mechanical circulatory support is a devastating event that not only quality of life but has the potential to end the life of a patient or ruin their eligibility to undergo future cardiac transplantation. Ischemic and hemorrhagic strokes have unique pathogenic mechanisms. Anticoagulation monitoring and delicately balancing the risk of bleeding with the risk of thrombosis is an important factor in guarding a patient's disposition to develop opposing types of cerebrovascular accidents. Aspects unique to the care of patients with assist devices such as the inherent device thrombogenicity, surgical techniques, and secondary complications of implantation, especially the development of bloodstream infections and bleeding, and the need for anticoagulation all contribute to the greater incidence of stroke than their cohort-match peers on medical management. The effects of immutable factors such as gender, age, and bridge-to-transplant or destination therapy indications, along with patient comorbidities and preexisting disease processes, all play a significant role in influencing individual stroke risk. It is our hope that this text has further elucidated the incidence, pathogenesis, development, and risks of ischemic and hemorrhagic stroke in this unique and growing patient population.

References

1. Backes D, van den Bergh WM, van Duijn AL, Lahpor JR, van Dijk D, Slooter AJ (2012) Cerebrovascular complications of left ventricular assist devices. Eur J Cardiothorac Surg 42(4):612–620. doi:10.1093/ejcts/ezs320 . Epub 2012 Jun 1. Review. PubMed PMID: 2659892
2. Morgan JA, Brewer RJ, Nemeh HW, Gerlach B, Lanfear DE, Williams CT, Paone G (2014) Stroke while on long-term left ventricular assist device support: incidence, outcome, and predictors. ASAIO J 60(3):284–289. doi:10.1097/MAT.0000000000000074 . PubMedPMID: 24625532
3. Tsiouris A, Paone G, Nemeh HW, Brewer RJ, Borgi J, Hodari A, Morgan JA (2015) Lessons learned from 150 continuous-flow left ventricular assist devices: a single institutional 7 year experience. ASAIO J 61(3):266–273. doi:10.1097/MAT.0000000000000191 . PubMed PMID: 25485563
4. Kato TS, Ota T, Schulze PC, Farr M, Jorde U, Takayama H, Naka Y, Yamashita T, Mancini DM (2012) Asymmetric pattern of cerebrovascular lesions in patients after left ventricular assist device implantation. Stroke 43(3):872–874. doi:10.1161/STROKEAHA.111.639682 . Epub 2011 Dec 29. PubMed PMID: 22207509
5. Trachtenberg BH, Cordero-Reyes AM, Aldeiri M, Alvarez P, Bhimaraj A, Ashrith G, Elias B, Suarez EE, Bruckner B, Loebe M, Harris RL, Zhang JY, Torre-Amione G, Estep JD (2015) Persistent blood stream infection in patients supported with a continuous-flow left ventricular assist device is associated with an increased risk of cerebrovascular accidents. J Card Fail 21(2):119–125. doi:10.1016/j.cardfail.2014.10.019 . Epub 2014 Nov 6. PubMed PMID: 22207509
6. Harvey L, Holley C, Roy SS, Eckman P, Cogswell R, Liao K, John R (2015) Stroke after left ventricular assist device implantation: outcomes in the continuous-flow era. Ann Thorac Surg 100(2):535–541. doi:10.1016/j.athoracsur.2015.02.094 . Epub 2015 Jun 9. PubMed PMID: 26070599
7. Lazar RM, Shapiro PA, Jaski BE, Parides MK, Bourge RC, Watson JT, Damme L, Dembitsky W, Hosenpud JD, Gupta L, Tierney A, Kraus T, Naka Y (2004) Neurological events during long-term mechanical circulatory support for heart failure: the Randomized Evaluation of Mechanical Assistance for the Treatment of Congestive Heart Failure (REMATCH) experience. Circulation 109(20):2423–2427 . Epub 2004 May 3. PubMed PMID: 15123534
8. Pagani FD, Miller LW, Russell SD et al (2009) HeartMate II Investigators: Extended mechanical circulatory support with a continuous-flow rotary left ventricular assist device. J Am Coll Cardiol 54:312–321
9. Katz MR, Dickinson MG, Raval NY, Slater JP, Dean DA, Zeevi GR, Horn EM, Salemi A (2015) Outcomes of patients implanted with a left ventricular assist device at nontransplant mechanical circulatory support

centers. Am J Cardiol 115(9):1254–1259. doi:10.1016/j.amjcard.2015.02.010 . Epub 2015 Feb 12. PubMed PMID: 25772738

10. Lushaj EB, Badami A, Osaki S, Murray M, Leverson G, Lozonschi L, Akhter S, Kohmoto T et al (2015) Impact of age on outcomes following continuous-flow left ventricular assist device implantation. Interact Cardiovasc Thorac Surg 20(6):743–748. doi:10.1093/icvts/ivv051. Epub 2015 Mar 13. PubMed PMID:25770085
11. Komoda T, Drews T, Hetzer R, Lehmkuhl HB (2013) Lower body surface area is highly related to mortality due to stroke or systemic bleeding in patients receiving an axial flow blood pump as a left ventricular assist device. Eur J Cardiothorac Surg 43(5):1036–1042. doi:10.1093/ejcts/ezs483 . Epub 2012 Sep 4. PubMed PMID: 22952143
12. Najjar SS (2014) Late bleeding and neurological sequelae after HeartMate II left ventricular assist device: risk factors from the prequel. J Am Coll Cardiol 63(9):889–890. doi:10.1016/j.jacc.2013.11.018 . Epub 2013 Dec 11. PubMed PMID: 24333495
13. Morris AA, Pekarek A, Wittersheim K, Cole RT, Gupta D, Nguyen D, Laskar SR, Butler J, Smith A, Vega JD (2015) Gender differences in the risk of stroke during support with continuous-flow left ventricular assist device. J Heart Lung Transplant 34(12):1570–1577. doi:10.1016/j.healun.2015.08.013 . Epub 2015 Sep 3. PubMed PMID: 26508726
14. Boyle AJ, Jorde UP, Sun B, Park SJ, Milano CA, Frazier OH, Sundareswaran KS, Farrar DJ, Russell SD (2014) HeartMate II Clinical Investigators. Pre-operative risk factors of bleeding and stroke during left ventricular assist device support: an analysis of more than 900 HeartMate II outpatients. J Am Coll Cardiol 63(9):880–888. doi:10.1016/j.jacc.2013.08.1656 . Epub 2013 Dec 11. PubMed PMID: 24316083
15. Miller LW, Pagani FD, Russell SD et al (2007) HeartMate II Clinical Investigators: use of a continuous-flow device in patients awaiting heart transplantation. N Engl J Med 357:885–896
16. Goldstein DJ, John R, Salerno C, Silvestry S, Moazami N, Horstmanshof D, Adamson R, Boyle A, Zucker M, Rogers J, Russell S, Long J, Pagani F, Jorde U (2013) Algorithm for the diagnosis and management of suspected pump thrombus. J Heart Lung Transplant 32(7):667–670. doi:10.1016/j.healun.2013.05.002. PubMedPMID: 23796150
17. Stulak JM, Lee D, Haft JW, Romano MA, Cowger JA, Park SJ, Aaronson KD, Pagani FD (2014) Gastrointestinal bleeding and subsequent risk of thromboembolic events during support with a left ventricular assist device. J Heart Lung Transplant 33(1):60–64. doi:10.1016/j.healun.2013.07.020 . Epub 2013 Sep 7. PubMed PMID: 24021944
18. Arjunon S, Ardana PH, Saikrishnan N, Madhani S, Foster B, Glezer A, Yoganathan AP (2015) Design of a pulsatile flow facility to evaluate thrombogenic potential of implantable cardiac devices. J Biomech Eng 137(4):045001. doi:10.1115/1.4029579 . Epub 2015 Feb 11. PubMed PMID: 25587891; PubMed Central PMCID:PMC4347304
19. Chiu WC, Girdhar G, Xenos M, Alemu Y, Soares JS, Einav S, Slepian M, Bluestein D (2014) Thromboresistance comparison of the HeartMate II ventricular assist device with the device thrombogenicity emulation-optimized HeartAssist 5 VAD. J Biomech Eng 136(2):021014 . PubMed PMID: 24337144; PubMed Central PMCID: PMC4023653
20. Girdhar G, Xenos M, Alemu Y, Chiu WC, Lynch BE, Jesty J, Einav S, Slepian MJ, Bluestein D (2012) Device thrombogenicity emulation: a novel method for optimizing mechanical circulatory support device thromboresistance. PLoS One 7(3):e32463. doi:10.1371/journal.pone.0032463. . Epub 2012 Mar 2. PubMed PMID: 22396768; PubMed Central PMCID: PMC3292570
21. Yuan N, Arnaoutakis GJ, George TJ, Allen JG, Ju DG, Schaffer JM, Russell SD, Shah AS, Conte JV (2012) The spectrum of complications following left ventricular assist device placement. J Card Surg 27(5):630–638. doi:10.1111/j.1540-8191.2012.01504.x. PubMed PMID: 22978843
22. Aggarwal A, Gupta A, Kumar S, Baumblatt JA, Pauwaa S, Gallagher C, Treitman A, Pappas P, Tatooles A, Bhat G (2012) Are bloodstream infections associated with an increased risk of hemorrhagic stroke in patients with a left ventricular assist device? ASAIO J 58(5):509–513. doi:10.1097/MAT.0b013e318260c6a6. . PubMed PMID: 22820918
23. Nassif ME, Tibrewala A, Raymer DS, Andruska A, Novak E, Vader JM, Itoh A, Silvestry SC, Ewald GA, LaRue SJ (2015) Systolic blood pressure on discharge after left ventricular assist device insertion is associated with subsequent stroke. J Heart Lung Transplant 34(4):503–508. doi:10.1016/j.healun.2014.09.042 . Epub 2014 Oct 23. PubMed PMID: 25540881; PubMed Central PMCID: PMC4402112.
24. Akhter SA, Badami A, Murray M, Kohmoto T, Lozonschi L, Osaki S, Lushaj EB (2015) Hospital readmissions after continuous-flow left ventricular assist device implantation: incidence, causes, and cost analysis. Ann Thorac Surg 100(3):884–889. doi:10.1016/j.athoracsur.2015.03.010 . Epub 2015 Jun 19. PubMed PMID: 26095106
25. Butler J, Howser R, Portner PM, Pierson RN 3rd (2005) Diabetes and outcomes after left ventricular assist device placement. J Card Fail 11(7):510–515 . PubMed PMID: 16198246
26. Lampert BC, Eckert C, Weaver S, Scanlon A, Lockard K, Allen C, Kunz N, Bermudez C, Bhama JK, Shullo MA, Kormos RL, Dew MA, Teuteberg JJ et al (2014) Blood pressure control in continuous flow left ventricular assist devices: efficacy and impact on adverse events. Ann Thorac Surg 97(1):139–146. doi:10.1016/j.athoracsur.2013.07.069. Epub 2013 Sep 25. PubMed PMID: 24075484
27. Stulak JM, Deo S, Schirger J, Aaronson KD, Park SJ, Joyce LD, Daly RC, Pagani FD (2013) Preoperative

atrial fibrillation increases risk of thromboembolic events after left ventricular assist device implantation. Ann Thorac Surg 96(6):2161–2167. doi:10.1016/j.athoracsur.2013.07.004. Epub 2013 Sep 12. PubMedPMID: 24035302

28. Antunes PE, de Oliveira JF, Antunes MJ et al (2003) Predictors of cerebrovascular events in patients subjected to isolated coronary surgery. The importance of aortic cross-clamping. Eur J Cardiothorac Surg 23(3):328–333 . PubMed PMID: 12614802

29. Whitson BA, Eckman P, Kamdar F, Lacey A, Shumway SJ, Liao KK, John R (2014) Hemolysis, pump thrombus, and neurologic events in continuous-flow left ventricular assist device recipients. Ann Thorac Surg 97(6):2097–2103. doi:10.1016/j.athoracsur.2014.02.041. Epub 2014 Apr 26. PubMed PMID: 24775803

Gastrointestinal Bleeding

Anna L. Meyer and Ivan Netuka

© Springer International Publishing Switzerland 2017
A. Montalto et al. (eds.), *Mechanical Circulatory Support in End-Stage Heart Failure*,
DOI 10.1007/978-3-319-43383-7_47

Gastrointestinal bleeding (GIB) is a common and severe complication after continuous-flow left ventricular assist device (LVAD) implantation. The incidence is described between 15 and 30% with an incidence per patient year between 0.27 and 0.45 [1–4]. Differences between LVAD pumps are presumably of small importance. Results of the ENDURANCE destination therapy clinical trial, a multicenter study between the HeartMate II® (HM II, Thoratec, Pleasanton, CA) and HeartWare® Ventricular Assist Device (HVAD, HeartWare, Inc., Framingham, MA), with 445 patients showed in this respect no significant differences within 2-year postoperative follow-up. In both groups around 34% of the patients showed a GIB with frequency of events per patient year of 0.44 EPPY (HM II) and 0.55 EPPY (HVAD), respectively. Uncontroversial is the fact that patients with a continuous-flow assist device, which implicates anticoagulation with vitamin K antagonist in combination with inhibitor of platelet aggregation, have a higher incidence of GIB in contrast to patients with a pulsatile assist device of the first generation with single anticoagulation with a platelet aggregation inhibitor [5]. Interestingly, the rate of GIB in patients with a continuous-flow LVAD is also higher than in patients without an LVAD with the same anticoagulation. The duration until the first episode of GIB occurred after LVAD implantation is reported in mean after 73 days [6].

The definition of a GI bleeding is different; some studies count every event with a positive fecal occult blood test. Most of the studies use the INTERMACS definition. This definition for gastrointestinal bleeding as an adverse event is encompassed within major bleeding. Events are registered, if the GIB results in death, reoperation, hospitalization, or transfusion of red blood cells.

Locations of the GIB are presented in ◘ Fig. 47.1 [1]. Most frequently the bleeding is located in the upper gastrointestinal tract 48% (until Treitz band) and in 22% in the lower gastrointestinal tract [4]. The source of a GIB is offered in ◘ Table 47.1 [1]. Notably, a high percentage is caused by angiodysplasias.

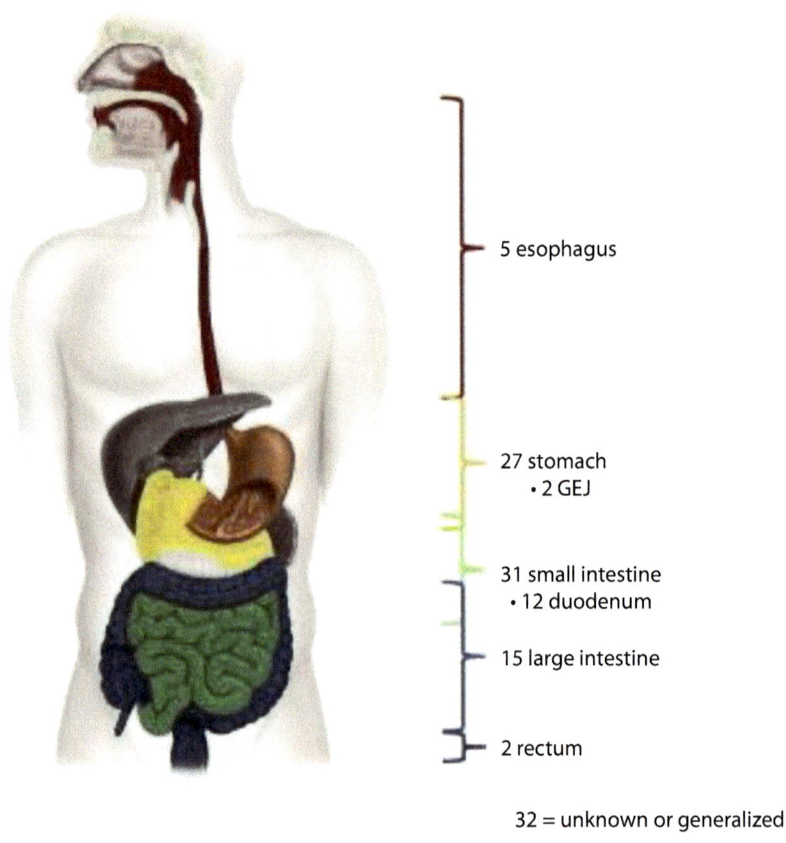

◘ **Fig. 47.1** Localization of gastrointestinal bleeding events in patients after LVAD implantation [1]

Table 47.1 Lesions identified as source of lower gastrointestinal bleeding in patients after LVAD implantation, modified from Draper et al. [4]

Source	Frequency (%)
Angiodysplasia	29
Gastritis	22
Ulcer	13
Diverticulitis	6
Polyp	5
Colitis	3
Other/unkown	22

47.1 Diagnostics

The cause of bleeding is found in approximately 75% of the patients. In case of a suspicious upper GIB, the best diagnostic tool is an upper endoscopy, for lower GIB a colonoscopy. If the upper or lower endoscopy is not successful, a capsule endoscopy is a less traumatic method. The diagnostic yield of capsule endoscopy has been superior in the diagnosis of small bowel disease compared to small bowel series, computerized tomography, or push enteroscopy. The results of the capsule study may indicate the further need for therapeutic intervention by a double balloon endoscopy [7]. To detect the source of GIB by angiography, the bleeding has to be more than 0.5 ml/min and for tagged red blood cell scan for more than 0.1 ml/min. The yield of different diagnostic tools is evaluated by Kushnir et al. in 44 episodes of GIB in LVAD patients, Fig. 47.2 [8].

47.2 Risk Factors

One reason for the high rate of GIB in patients after continuous-flow LVAD implantation is a dual therapy with vitamin K antagonist and a platelet aggregation inhibitor. However, the higher rate of GIB in LVAD patients than in comparable anticoagulated patients without an LVAD can be explained by additional coagulation disorder in LVAD patients. Importantly, patients with a continuous-flow LVAD develop an acquired von Willebrand syndrome due to the shear stress of the pump and thus show a dysfunction of the primary hemostasis [9, 10]. Additionally, an impaired platelet function was detected in these patients by Klovaite et al. [11]. Furthermore several risk factors were identified to influence the GIB. In majority of the studies, age represents in a multivariate analysis a significant risk factor for GIB [1, 12]. Therefore older patients with an age > 65 years show a 1.5-fold higher risk for bleeding [3]. Other studies identified a history of GIB before LVAD implantation as a significant risk factor [2, 13].

Decreased pulsatility in continuous-flow LVADs may also contribute to GIB as lower tertiles of pulsatility index subsets demonstrated in a study from Wever-Pizon et al. as a significant risk factor for GIB [2]. Renal dysfunction reflected in elevated creatinine impairs platelet function; therefore an elevated creatinine was observed in the group of patients with GIB [1].

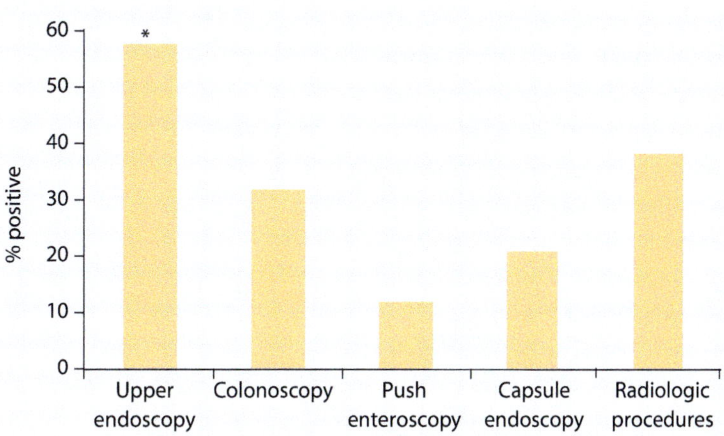

Fig. 47.2 Diagnostic yield of endoscopic and radiologic procedures performed for the evaluation of gastrointestinal bleeding in patients with LVADs. Upper endoscopy had the highest yield for a source of bleeding, significantly higher than that seen with colonoscopy or enteroscopy. The number of capsule endoscopy (5) and radiologic procedures (8) performed was limited [8]

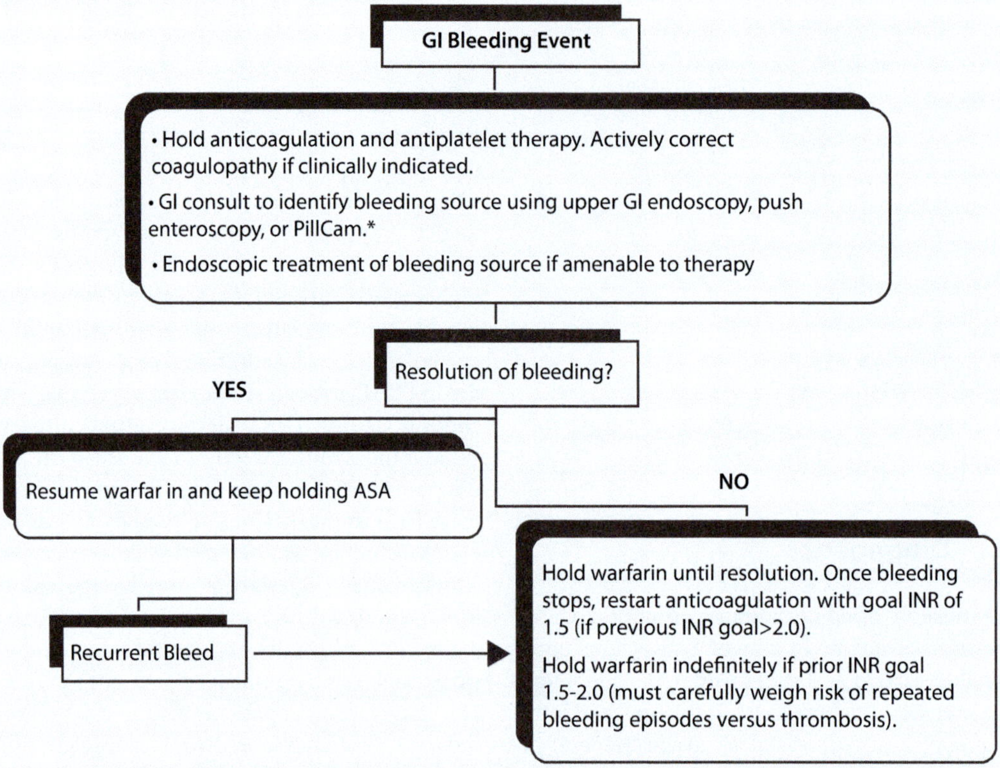

Fig. 47.3 Algorithm for gastrointestinal bleeding in LVAD patients by Suarez et al. *There are no data indicating that endoscopy or the PillCam are beneficial in management of GIB early after LVAD implantation when pre-LVAD endoscopy showed no bleeding source [17]

Goldstein found that patients with GIB after LVAD implantation had a significant higher body mass index, more frequently diabetes and ischemic etiology of heart failure which were further confirmed in other series [1, 12]. Adipose tissue is a complex highly secretory endocrine organ that can regulate insulin sensitivity and inflammation and releases among others vascular endothelial growth factor (VEGT), TNF-α, and inflammatory cytokines leading to impaired vasoregulation [14–16]. However, the correlation of the development of vascular changes in terms of angiodysplasia and the different flow pattern in continuous-flow LVADs are not completely defined.

47.3 Therapy

The therapy of a GIB primarily consists of the analysis of blood and coagulation parameter with subsequent correction of anemia and potential excessive anticoagulation. The minimal hemoglobin level should be more than 6 g/dL. The transfusion of one unit of packed red blood cell concentrate increases the hemoglobin level of 1.0–1.5 g/dL. The administration of fresh frozen plasma and coagulation factors is recommended. Due to the chronic antiplatelet therapy, application of platelet concentrates should be considered. Secondly, detection of the source of bleeding with its possible elimination is of a paramount importance. An algorithm for the evaluation and treatment of GIB is provided by Suarez et al., Fig. 47.3 [17].

The anticoagulation should resume with vitamin K antagonist. A platelet inhibitor may be paused. In recurrent GIB, high urgency or UNOS 1A listing for heart transplantation should be considered. A surgical solution with partial resection of the intestine is a high-risk procedure in these patients and should be reserved as the last resort. The recurrence of a GIB was described in up to 43% of the patients with a GIB [2, 13, 18, 19]. Aggarwal et al. found that 60% of the patients had a recurrence of bleeding from the same anatomic site [18].

Reports on pharmacological therapy of GIB are typically isolated case reports or case series. The effectiveness of estrogen and progesterone is not clarified [20], and a multicenter, randomized, placebo-controlled study failed to show an effect of hormonal therapy in the prevention of rebleeding from gastrointestinal angiodysplasia [21]. Medical treatment with subcutaneous octreotide of 50 μg twice a day is described by Junquera et al. as a potential treatment in preventing rebleeding from gastrointestinal angiodysplasia. The somatostatin analogue reduces the portal venous pressure and decreases the splanchnic blood flow. The side effects were diarrhea and abdominal pain [21]. Thalidomide was used due to the anti-angiogenetic effect in patients with GIB. To date, a randomized study supporting this approach is missing [22].

Another future therapeutic strategy represents a prevention of excessive degradation of HMW-VWF multimers by partial inhibition of VWF-ADAMTS13 interactions with a use of an anti-VWF monoclonal antibody published by Rauch et al. [23]. Recently, a novel approach to ADAMTS13 inhibition was proposed in experimental model by administration of doxycycline [24].

47.4 Outcome

The total mortality in patients with GIB is not significantly increased [18]. Nevertheless, GIB may lead to fatal consequences as described in the literature. Importantly, the patients with GIB on LVAD typically receive multiple blood product transfusions which can increase the development of autoantibodies. Consequently, immunosensitization appears to have a negative effect on mortality [25]. These patients have a decreased donor pool and a longer duration of support with increased inherent morbidity such as infections and thromboembolic complications [26, 27].

References

1. Goldstein DJ, Aaronson KD, Tatooles AJ, Silvestry SC, Jeevanandam V, Gordon R, Hathaway DR, Najarian KB, Slaughter MS (2015) Gastrointestinal bleeding in recipients of the HeartWare Ventricular Assist System. JACC Heart Fail 3(4):303–313
2. Wever-Pinzon O, Selzman CH, Drakos SG, Saidi A, Stoddard GJ, Gilbert EM, Labedi M, Reid BB, Davis ES, Kfoury AG et al (2013) Pulsatility and the risk of nonsurgical bleeding in patients supported with the continuous-flow left ventricular assist device HeartMate II. Circ Heart Fail 6(3):517–526
3. Boyle AJ, Jorde UP, Sun B, Park SJ, Milano CA, Frazier OH, Sundareswaran KS, Farrar DJ, Russell SD (2014) Pre-operative risk factors of bleeding and stroke during left ventricular assist device support: an analysis of more than 900 HeartMate II outpatients. J Am Coll Cardiol 63(9):880–888
4. Draper KV, Huang RJ, Gerson LB (2014) GI bleeding in patients with continuous-flow left ventricular assist devices: a systematic review and meta-analysis. Gastrointest Endosc 80(3):435–446 e431
5. Crow S, John R, Boyle A, Shumway S, Liao K, Colvin-Adams M, Toninato C, Missov E, Pritzker M, Martin C et al (2009) Gastrointestinal bleeding rates in recipients of nonpulsatile and pulsatile left ventricular assist devices. J Thorac Cardiovasc Surg 137(1):208–215
6. Lopilato AC, Doligalski CT, Caldeira C (2015) Incidence and risk factor analysis for gastrointestinal bleeding and pump thrombosis in left ventricular assist device recipients. Artif Organs 39(11):939–944
7. Adler SN, Bjarnason I (2012) What we have learned and what to expect from capsule endoscopy. World J Gastrointest Endosc 4(10):448–452
8. Kushnir VM, Sharma S, Ewald GA, Seccombe J, Novak E, Wang IW, Joseph SM, Gyawali CP (2012) Evaluation of GI bleeding after implantation of left ventricular assist device. Gastrointest Endosc 75(5):973–979
9. Meyer AL, Malehsa D, Bara C, Budde U, Slaughter MS, Haverich A, Strueber M (2010) Acquired von Willebrand syndrome in patients with an axial flow left ventricular assist device. Circ Heart Fail 3(6):675–681
10. Meyer AL, Malehsa D, Budde U, Bara C, Haverich A, Strueber M (2014) Acquired von Willebrand syndrome in patients with a centrifugal or axial continuous flow left ventricular assist device. JACC Heart Fail 2(2):141–145
11. Klovaite J, Gustafsson F, Mortensen SA, Sander K, Nielsen LB (2009) Severely impaired von Willebrand factor-dependent platelet aggregation in patients with a continuous-flow left ventricular assist device (HeartMate II). J Am Coll Cardiol 53(23):2162–2167
12. Demirozu ZT, Radovancevic R, Hochman LF, Gregoric ID, Letsou GV, Kar B, Bogaev RC, Frazier OH (2011) Arteriovenous malformation and gastrointestinal bleeding in patients with the HeartMate II left ventricular assist device. J Heart Lung Transplant 30(8):849–853
13. Morgan JA, Paone G, Nemeh HW, Henry SE, Patel R, Vavra J, Williams CT, Lanfear DE, Tita C, Brewer RJ (2012) Gastrointestinal bleeding with the HeartMate II left ventricular assist device. J Heart Lung Transplant 31(7):715–718
14. Farb MG, Gokce N (2015) Visceral adiposopathy: a vascular perspective. Horm Mol Biol Clin Investig 21(2):125–136
15. Fain JN, Madan AK, Hiler ML, Cheema P, Bahouth SW (2004) Comparison of the release of adipokines by adipose tissue, adipose tissue matrix, and adipocytes from visceral and subcutaneous abdominal adipose tissues of obese humans. Endocrinology 145(5):2273–2282

16. Farb MG, Tiwari S, Karki S, Ngo DT, Carmine B, Hess DT, Zuriaga MA, Walsh K, Fetterman JL, Hamburg NM et al (2014) Cyclooxygenase inhibition improves endothelial vasomotor dysfunction of visceral adipose arterioles in human obesity. Obesity (Silver Spring) 22(2): 349–355
17. Suarez J, Patel CB, Felker GM, Becker R, Hernandez AF, Rogers JG (2011) Mechanisms of bleeding and approach to patients with axial-flow left ventricular assist devices. Circ Heart Fail 4(6):779–784
18. Aggarwal A, Pant R, Kumar S, Sharma P, Gallagher C, Tatooles AJ, Pappas PS, Bhat G (2012) Incidence and management of gastrointestinal bleeding with continuous flow assist devices. Ann Thorac Surg 93(5): 1534–1540
19. Jabbar HR, Abbas A, Ahmed M, Klodell CT Jr, Chang M, Dai Y, Draganov PV (2015) The incidence, predictors and outcomes of gastrointestinal bleeding in patients with Left Ventricular Assist Device (LVAD). Dig Dis Sci 60(12):3697–3706
20. Szilagyi A, Ghali MP (2006) Pharmacological therapy of vascular malformations of the gastrointestinal tract. Can J Gastroenterol 20(3):171–178
21. Junquera F, Saperas E, Videla S, Feu F, Vilaseca J, Armengol JR, Bordas JM, Pique JM, Malagelada JR (2007) Long-term efficacy of octreotide in the prevention of recurrent bleeding from gastrointestinal angiodysplasia. Am J Gastroenterol 102(2):254–260
22. Dray X, Camus M, Coelho J, Ozenne V, Pocard M, Marteau P (2011) Treatment of gastrointestinal angiodysplasia and unmet needs. Dig Liver Dis 43(7): 515–522
23. Rauch A, Legendre P, Christophe OD, Goudemand J, van Belle E, Vincentelli A, Denis CV, Susen S, Lenting PJ (2014) Antibody-based prevention of von Willebrand factor degradation mediated by circulatory assist devices. Thromb Haemost 112(5):1014–1023
24. Bartoli CR, Kang J, Restle DJ, Zhang DM, Shabahang C, Acker MA, Atluri P (2015) Inhibition of ADAMTS-13 by Doxycycline reduces von Willebrand factor degradation during supraphysiological shear stress: therapeutic implications for left ventricular assist device-associated bleeding. JACC Heart Fail 3(11):860–869
25. Kidambi S, Mohamedali B, Bhat G (2015) Clinical outcomes in sensitized heart transplant patients bridged with ventricular assist devices. Clin Transplant 29(6): 499–505
26. Urban M, Gazdic T, Slimackova E, Pirk J, Szarszoi O, Maly J, Netuka I (2012) Alloimmunosensitization in left ventricular assist device recipients and impact on posttransplantation outcome. ASAIO J 58(6):554–561
27. Holley CT, Harvey L, Roy S, Cogswell R, Eckman P, Liao K, John R (2015) Gastrointestinal bleeding during continuous-flow left ventricular assist device support is associated with lower rates of cardiac transplantation. ASAIO J 61(6):635–639

Pump Thrombosis

E. Potapov, F. Kaufmann, A.M. Scandroglio, and M. Pieri

© Springer International Publishing Switzerland 2017
A. Montalto et al. (eds.), *Mechanical Circulatory Support in End-Stage Heart Failure*,
DOI 10.1007/978-3-319-43383-7_48

48.1 Introduction/Pathogenesis

Pump thrombosis is one of the most severe adverse events in the use of ventricular assist device (VAD) systems. The blood coagulation system is activated by all VAD systems via several mechanisms. The blood contact to the artificial materials of VAD pumps and cannulas triggers the coagulation cascade as well as high shear stress due to high flow velocities, small gaps, or high-speed moving parts (the impeller of rotary blood pumps) [1]. Areas of flow stagnation represent preferred thrombus developing sites as well as areas with recirculation vortices. Heat spots, e.g., produced by mechanical bearings, often are subjected to thrombus buildup when low-flow situations impair washout and thus the necessary cooling. To prevent thrombosis careful consideration of the three following factors in the use of VAD is important:

- Low activation of the coagulation system by a good hydrodynamic design. This also applies to running the device in the specified optimal range of operation.
- A good washout. Kinks and other causes obstructing the flow path like cannula malposition have to be avoided. A small clearance of the apical inflow cannula to the ventricle wall will likely promote the risk of wedge thrombus genesis.
- Sufficient anticoagulation and anti-aggregation therapy are most important [2].

Ideally the inflow cannula of the LVAD, implanted in the apex of the left ventricle, is directed to the mitral valve. This ensures good drainage of the left ventricle, low risk of suction, e.g., of the septal wall to the inflow cannula, optimal washout of the area around the cannula protruding into the cavum, and no obstruction of the inlet by myocardial structures such as trabeculae, papillary muscle, or the walls of the left ventricle [3].

Low flow also can be caused by an angled outflow-graft bend relief, a shifted position of the pump with resulting kinks in the outflow graft or a position of the inflow opening close to the lateral or the septal wall causing narrowing of the lumen.

Thrombus formation can be located at different parts of the VAD system:

(a) In the inflow section – which thus can be described as pre-pump thrombosis.
(b) In the pump itself – accordingly named pump thrombosis, which does not necessarily mean total thrombotic occlusion of the pump.
(c) In the graft connecting the pump to the arterial vessel of the patient – usually the ascending aorta, sometimes the descending aorta in the case of less-invasive implantation procedures, in rare cases also the brachial artery. This would be called post-pump thrombosis or graft thrombosis.

There may be added a fourth location, which does not directly impair the function of the system but seems to be the main source of occluding inflow thrombosis and most probably of in-pump thrombosis: thrombus development around the apical inflow section of the pump or the inflow cannula anchored at either the apical myocardial wound or the textured part of the inflow cannula, most often seen at the transition from a structured section (titanium sintered) to the smooth, polished section toward the tip of the inflow.

According to the different locations, dissimilar effects are generated. Detection of VAD thrombosis has to rely on a variety of methods and parameters. According to the appearance of indicating effects, the diagnosis of which type of thrombosis is present can be made, which then will lead to the appropriate treatment.

In para- or extracorporeal pulsatile pneumatically powered VADs, thrombus formation can immediately and best be detected by visual examination of the transparent pump and cannula. A daily visual check is important with the pediatric Berlin Heart EXCOR device, which is straightforward and easy to perform with a good flashlight. There is almost no way of thrombus detection in pulsatile implanted pumps (e.g., SynCardia total artificial heart, TAH) apart from the recognition of clinically apparent thromboembolism episodes like TIA or stroke. In the following, the detection of pump thrombosis is focused on implantable rotary blood pumps supporting the vast majority of today's patients.

48.2 Effects of Thrombus Formation in the Various Parts of a Ventricular Assist Device

48.2.1 Hydrodynamic Effects of Thrombus Material in a VAD

If the thrombotic material is of considerable size and thus is narrowing the flow path in one or more sections of the device, the pumping capacity is diminished by the higher flow resistance. Clinically this would lead to low pump flow, thus reducing unloading of the left ventricle, and as a consequence the patient will show signs of heart failure. Dyspnea, weakness, or dizziness may occur, and ultimately, if there is no sufficient residual capacity of the patient's heart, it would lead to signs of cardiogenic shock.

Thrombi adhering to the impeller of a rotary blood pump may change the hydrodynamic properties of the pump. The flow path may not be greatly affected, but the deviation from the optimized geometry will reduce the hydrodynamic efficiency also with the consequence of decreased pump output.

48.2.2 Mechanical Effects

If thrombus material is filling the gap between the rotating impeller and the pump housing, friction will result. To overcome this energy loss, more power is required in order to keep the preset rotational speed. Most rotary blood pumps of today calculate or rather estimate the flow created by the pump from power consumption (exceptions are the Berlin Heart INCOR where the flow is calculated out of the created pressure head, whose level is retrieved from rotor displacement data provided by the magnetic levitation sensors, and the ReliantHeart HeartAssist5, in which flow is directly and independently measured using ultrasound Doppler technology in a sensor attached to the outflow graft). In-pump thrombosis thus is likely to create false high flow readings. To complicate the situation, these two effects of flow decrease and power increase may compensate for each other, resulting in unsuspicious flow readings despite thrombotic material causing both flow reduction and power increase.

With extremely high friction and power consumption, the heat generated by and in the pump will increase significantly: firstly by the energy conversion into heat by the friction and secondly by the necessary electric current to produce the power to overcome the friction. Heat effects in extreme pump thrombosis situations requiring driving power of up to or more than 20 W so far have not been investigated but may very well be existent.

With magnetic or hydrodynamic bearings, thrombus on the impeller may cause substantial rotor displacement resulting in contact of the rotor with the housing producing scratch marks. At these no longer highly polished surfaces of the rotor secondary thrombus formation is likely, aggravating the situation.

48.2.3 Effects on the Corpuscular Blood Components

Thrombus material at sensitive areas like regions of high flow velocities or high shear stress often increases the shear rate and thus hemolysis. Sometimes hemolysis is the most impressive result and thus an indicator of pump thrombosis even with only small changes of system parameters like flow or power consumption. Dark urine output may be the first sign to be recognized in an outpatient and requires immediate reaction: hospitalization for a thorough investigation of the situation. On the other hand, severe pump thrombosis may produce no or only very slight hemolysis when a big thrombus is reducing the pumping capacity and the blood volume passing through the system to small amounts or zero. If no blood is passing through the pump, it cannot be damaged by high shear rates.

48.2.4 Acoustic Effects and Changes of the Sound of the Running Pump

Thrombotic material adhering to the impeller of a rotary blood pump will cause an imbalance. Like an imbalanced tire on a car, high rotational speeds will excite vibration of the whole system, causing an alteration of the sound produced by the running pump. One effect is an intensified volume of the sound. Another effect is the excitation of a different acoustic spectrum or pattern. These effects may be small if the rotor is forced to rotate stably by means of mechanical bearings. If the bearings allow deviation from the ideal rotation axis (which is possible with magnetic radial bearings), the changes are profound and thus can be measured and accordingly analyzed.

Turbulences created or intensified by obstructions like occluding inflow thrombi may create specific noise. If measured and compared to existing acoustic spectra of a specific pump (acoustic footprint), this was indicative of thrombus formation in an in vitro setting as well. However, clinical application of this method so far was not possible but it could be promising if obstacles like a poor signal-to-noise ratio could be improved [4, 5].

48.3 Methods to Detect Thrombus Formation - System Specific Aspects (Table 48.1)

Table 48.1 Methods to detect thrombus formation

Method	Advantage	Disadvantage	Problem	Device	Remarks
Angiography (ventriculography)	Flow visualization, diagnosis plus treatment of outflow-graft thrombosis	Needs catheter lab Contrast fluid necessary Arterial puncture	Outflow-graft thrombosis	All	Use Cerebral Protection System (e.g., Sentinel TAVR) in case of mobilization of thrombus material
CT scan/CT angiography	Less invasive	High radiation exposure Strong artifacts esp. at the site of the pump, contrast fluid required	Inflow position/ occlusion by myocardial structures, inflow-/ outflow-graft stenosis, kinking	All	Contrast fluid necessary for reliable thrombus detection
Echo	Noninvasive	Obscured view by anatomy, shadowing by pump, interference of Doppler signals by motor current impulses	Pump thrombosis (ramp test, unloading of LV, AV opening) Floating structures at inflow cannula	All	High interobserver dependency, always plausibility check required
Acoustic spectrum analysis	Noninvasive, highly specific	Noncommercial special equipment	Pump thrombosis	HVAD	Thrombus adhering to rotor detectable, applicable as screening method

The methods which can be applied to detect pump thrombosis depend on the respective system or pump technology. The most common parameter indicating thrombus formation at the moving part of the pump is an increased power consumption caused by friction.

48.3.1 Berlin Heart INCOR

Only with the Berlin Heart INCOR is motor power consumption a rather unspecific parameter. There is a big gap between the magnetic field created in the stator coils and the magnet of the rotor. To create the necessary magnetic flux, the magnetic fields have to be strong and thus the additional effect of friction is less distinctive. Thrombus adherence with the INCOR is very sensitively and securely detected by changes in the accurate pressure head signal derived from magnetic levitation sensor signals. Thrombus material captured by the rotor blades of the INCOR impeller causes a severely diminished pressure buildup which is reflected in an abruptly diminished pressure head causing respective alarms. Thrombus material adhering to the impeller circumference will cause an imbalance of the magnetically levitated impeller. To compensate this and stabilize the rotation, the magnetic levitation requires stronger magnetic fields. An increased power consumption of the levitation circuit – which is displayed on the patient monitor – or activation of the respective alarm if the levitation power is exceeding 3.5 W is indicative of a thrombus particle on the impeller. Occlusion of the flow path (including the pump impeller) will result in a zero or low flow reading.

Because of a comparatively low implant frequency and low number of patients on device, the specific aspects of thrombus detection, explanation of the effects, and treatment options are not elaborated. However, although the technical aspects are quite different compared to those of the other mainly used systems (Thoratec HeartMate and HeartWare HVAD), the clinical effects are similar.

48.3.2 Thoratec HeartMate

Data logging in the Thoratec HeartMate II is restricted to 256 data sets. Usually the log file extends only over some days and has irregular sample points. Creating a trend line in order to locate the onset of changes in the system parameters usually is not successful in capturing the whole event. Even though the HeartMate II also has a regular pump data file, this also is restricted to 256 entries which limits high resolution trendlines to a few days or, if it is required to cover prolonged periods of months, the sample rate has to be as low as once or twice a day.

The effect of a reduced pump output caused by pump thrombosis can be investigated by ultrasound echo, mainly by determining signs of poor unloading of the left ventricle. Because the hemodynamics of individual patients can differ a lot, an independent test protocol is necessary to evaluate the actual state of the pump functionality, the so-called ramp test.

Performing a ramp test – "ramping up" rotary speed over a wide range – dimensions of the left ventricle, aortic valve opening, and flow into the pump inflow at systole and diastole are measured and opposed to the calculated flow. If these dimensional properties of the heart do not meet the expected changes when the rotational speed is increased, pump thrombosis is likely [6].

High flow readings caused by increased power consumption compensating friction, which may lead to the assumption of good unloading of the left ventricle, together with opening of the aortic valve or large size of the left ventricle at the same time are suspicious. Good contraction of the left ventricle but low pulsatility of the pump flow (displayed pulsatility index [PI] or analysis of wave form samples) is also highly implausible. Doppler measurements indicating low flow velocities in the left ventricle toward the pump inflow which do not correlate with a high pump flow also have to be scrutinized.

However, high power transitions are noticed frequently with the HeartMate II VAD. Though up to now there is no plausible and clinically confirmed explanation of these power spikes, they do not qualify as indicative for thrombus formation. Only together with signs of flow impairment and hemolysis, respective treatment is advisable. The HeartMate III fully magnetically levitated radial flow pump also logs technical parameters of the levitation circuit. Single experiences indicate that changes in these parameters will very likely indicate thrombus formation or passage through the pump comparable to other magnetically levitated devices such as the INCOR. However, no such case has been published so far. Analysis and interpretation of these levitation log files is not feasible by the clinical user. Thus this data up to now may be used rather for confirmation of suspected pump thrombosis than for its detection.

HeartWare HVAD

Retrospective analysis of the motor power consumption trends stored in the HeartWare HVAD controller data logs over 30 days with a sample period of 15 min provides good trend line information. Onset of changes caused by thrombotic effects is accurately determinable [7]. Awareness of such changes usually is triggered by respective alarms like high power consumption or low flow.

48.3.3 Elevated Power Consumption

Thrombus formation in the pump chamber, touching both the impeller and the housing, causes friction. Higher motor power is required to compensate this power loss in order to keep the set rotor speed. Slightly elevated power consumption (usually not more than 0.5 W) can also be explained by increased hematocrit – sometimes noticed in patients after discharge, influenced by healthy nutrition. Regaining physical activity or myocardial recovery can also cause an increased flow level producing higher Watt readings. Power elevations of more than 1 W are highly suspicious and always should be investigated thoroughly. To be aware of them, setting of the alarm thresholds should be close to this demarcation so that the patient will be sensitized by the triggered alarm and is forced to contact the clinic. The pattern of power elevations stored in the log files of the device can differ substantially. Analysis of the time constant of the power increase may predict the success of thrombolysis [8].

48.3.4 Changes of the Acoustic Spectrum of the HVAD

With the HeartWare HVAD, the acoustic spectrum emitted by the running pump can be used to detect and confirm thrombus material adhering to the impeller of the pump. Because the hybrid bearing of the rotor is a combination of a hydrodynamic bearing for the axial component and a passive magnetic radial bearing, it allows the impeller to rotate slightly off the geometric center. Additional mass, usually a fibrin layer on the hydrodynamic bearing planes, causes an imbalance, deflecting the rotation to an eccentric movement. The three symmetrically placed pairs of driving solenoids not only accelerate the rotor tangentially to produce the rotation but also pull the impeller back toward the center, while the outwardly deflected section of the impeller sweeps over each solenoid, therefore forming a triangular-shaped movement of the rotor axis. Thus, the rotor vibrates with the so-called *3rd harmonic*, a frequency three times the rotational speed of the pump. If this frequency peak in the acoustic spectrum is existent, it points very specifically to pump thrombosis or thrombus mass on the rotor. It is not present with a completely balanced rotor, that is, a clean rotor [9].

48.3.5 Flow Decrease

An unexpected or unexplained decrease of flow (not related to hypovolemia, hypertonia, or decreasing hematocrit, e.g., due to bleeding) may point to a constricted flow path, likewise by thrombus formation. This hydrodynamic resistance in the flow path also will cause dampening of the flow pulsatility which can be registered on the clinical monitor. Flow pulsatility also is logged in the controller memory.

A *slow decrease*, sometimes over several days or even weeks, indicates thrombus buildup. Successive growing of thrombus in the inflow section has never been reported and is extremely unlikely because of the polished inner lumen of the cannula. It is more likely in the outflow section with its flow path discontinuities like the step at the outflow-graft fixation or if a kink or constriction may have developed, causing flow disturbances.

An *abrupt decrease* of flow most likely points to congestion of the inflow caused by ingestion of thrombotic material and thus would be diagnosed as pre-pump thrombosis.

The presence of a 3rd harmonic in the acoustic spectrum together with a sudden decrease of flow confirms the diagnosis of inflow thrombus ingestion. In this case the thrombus reaches down to the impeller. Being caught by blood channels of the impeller, it will rotate and thus cause an imbalance.

Obviously a growing thrombus in the outflow graft cannot adhere to the impeller and will not excite a 3rd harmonic.

Low flow due to a constricted flow path resulting in lower power consumption (remember:

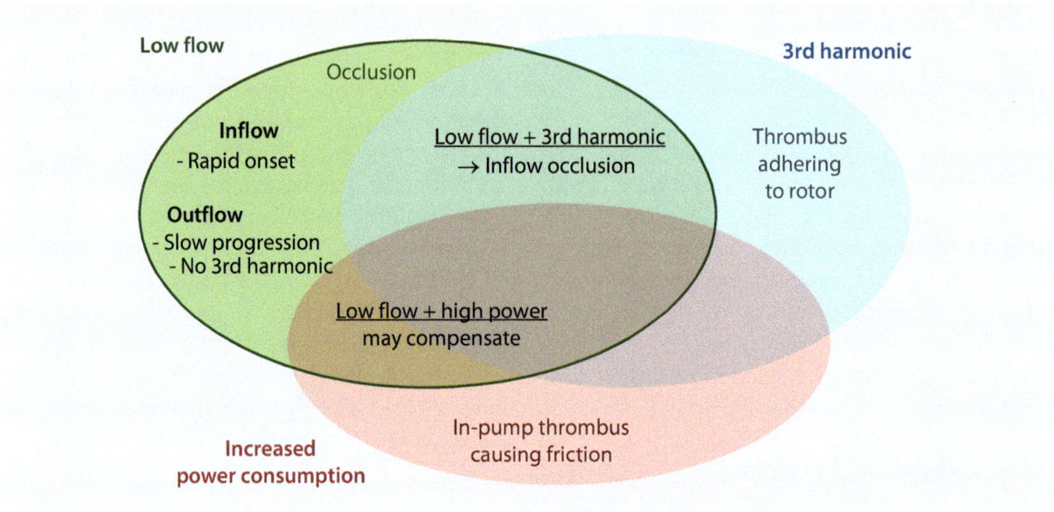

Fig. 48.1 HVAD thrombosis scenarios

flow calculation is directly coupled to power consumption) may be compensated if thrombus components being wedged between impeller and housing additionally cause friction. In this case the existence of a 3rd harmonic will prove the suspicion of pump thrombosis, and a sudden reduction of pulsatility may reveal clogging by thrombus material (Fig. 48.1).

48.4 Trends in LVAD Thrombosis and Design Improvements

Device thrombosis is an uncommon but potentially catastrophic complication of continuous flow LVAD. The most common cf devices implanted operate according to different principles and cause and react to thrombosis in different ways. Many factors are involved regarding device dynamics, flow dynamics, and nevertheless platelet activation. In the last years three main reports documented a spike in thrombosis rate for HMII [10, 11] and HVAD as well [12], beginning in 2011. More recent reports observe a decrease in risk in the first half of 2014, even if a plateau has occurred in pump thrombosis incidence; its rates have not returned to pre-2011 levels: the risk of thrombosis is between 65 and 12% at 6 months after implant and has remained 10% at 1 year, threefold higher than in the registration trials. From the first reports regarding pump thrombosis, awareness of the phenomenon has grown, and nowadays the diagnosis is based on the integration of clinical and device parameters, improved echocardiographic data, and "enforced" interpretation of hemolysis. INTERMACS definition of hemolysis has been changed to a lower threshold, reflecting interest in this topic. Some factors are generally involved in the development of pump thrombosis:

Patient management

- Inadequate anticoagulation: during the past years, many centers began to gradually decrease the target INR levels for long-term management and to use low-dose aspirin or no antiplatelet drug, due to the risk of intracerebral hemorrhage and gastrointestinal bleeding. Moreover, some centers have no longer bridged patients to oral anticoagulation with intravenous heparin.
- Pump speed reduction: reduction of pump speed has become frequent to allow intermittent opening of the native aortic valve for greater pulsatility.
- Condition of general hypercoagulability due to associated comorbidities and precipitating factor, such as systemic or driveline infections.

Surgical issue

- Suboptimal positioning of the device: the position of the inflow cannula and the dislodgement of the bend relief or kinking of the outflow tract may play a role.

Pump design [13]

- The incidence of pump thrombosis increased from 0.02 EPPY to 0.14 EPPY for HMII after 2010 when sealed inflow connector and outflow graft (gelatin-sealed grafts) for HMII were introduced.
- After the introduction of the sintered inflow cannula for HVAD in 2011, the incidence of pump thrombosis decreased from 0.15 to 0.05 EPPY.

Moreover, new knowledge arrived about innovations in the treatment, according to location of thrombosis along the device.

48.5 Clinical Methods to Detect Thrombus Formation

48.5.1 Hemolysis

Hemolysis is one of the most common complications of MCS, particularly among patients requiring short-term assist devices.

Two mechanisms are involved in the process of destruction of circulating red blood cells (RBCs): the death of aging (senescent) red blood cells and age-independent RBC destruction (random hemolysis). Both of them cause anemia, during MCS, the damage to the RBC membrane is severe enough to cause destruction of RBC within the intravascular space, causing intravascular hemolysis. Mechanical trauma and hypercoagulability typical of these patients are responsible for the destruction of RBCs: direct trauma, artificial surfaces, shear stress, and heat damage alter the RBC membrane and cause immediate lysis within the circulation. During this process, free Hgb appears in the plasma and binds to haptoglobin into a complex that is rapidly removed by the liver, leading to a reduction in plasma haptoglobin. If the plasmatic concentration of free Hgb is high, however, free Hgb is filtered by the glomerulus, appearing in the urine as hemoglobinuria. Lactate dehydrogenase (LDH) is released from hemolyzed RBCs into the plasma as well. The typical picture of hemolytic anemia includes increased level of LDH, free Hgb and indirect bilirubin, decreased haptoglobin values, increased reticulocyte count, and abnormalities on the peripheral smear.

Given these explanations, the definition of hemolysis in MCS recipients is nevertheless not thorough, lacking a univocal quantification of the degree of the phenomenon which may appear in different moments during the time on support and may reflect alterations in device operation, clinical conditions (hypertension, arrhythmia, hypercoagulable state), and, ultimately, thrombosis. Consensus diagnostic criteria are currently not available. However, monitoring of LDH, free Hgb, and haptoglobin has become a worldwide routine. As a general rule, the presence of hemolysis mandates hospital admission and further diagnostic testing. The range of values above which asymptomatic intravascular hemolysis should be considered clinically significant and suggestive of thrombus has not been clearly defined. Previous reports have shown a clinical effect of hemolysis during LVAD support, with the risk of having an adverse event being 8-fold to 15-fold higher in patients with hemolysis than in those without elevated hemolysis markers.

Patients presenting with isolated LDH elevations in the late clinical course should be evaluated and, if hemolysis is confirmed, they should be admitted to the hospital for further diagnostic testing. Thresholds have been defined for LDH, and values are considered pathologic if 2.5-fold higher than the upper limit of normal for each laboratory. Furthermore, a fivefold increase in LDH level is highly specific (92.5%) and sensitive (100%) for the diagnosis of pump thrombosis [14].

In accordance with these findings, INTERMACS definition of hemolysis has been updated to be more accurate, as the previous definition included values that may already represent an indication for surgical device exchange. However, all of these data were obtained in a population implanted with HMII (axial flow, bearings), whereas few data exist about centrifugal devices, which by their nature should have lower hemolysis rate.

Chronic elevation in LDH as a marker of hemolysis does not occur often in the HVAD. Clinically, it is not likely to see an HVAD patient with chronic elevation of LDH. The occurrence of hemolysis in centrifugal pumps is more indicative of thrombosis and could be delayed: certainly the presence of hemoglobinuria is a sign of overt hemolysis and triggers emergency treatment.

Hemolysis is detected in ambulatory VAD patients as a precursor of adverse event, but the scenario of hemolysis as a leading symptom of pump thrombosis is completely different: it appears later after alteration of pump parameters, and the course after treatment is crucial because the recovery of end-organ function from hemolysis is the key to clinical success.

LVAD elements potentially contributing to hemolysis are inflow cannula positioning, pump speed, and concomitant aortic valve insufficiency. However, other possible causes of hemolysis should be ruled out. Causes of elevated LDH are multiple: lymphoproliferative diseases, tissue necrosis, use of statins, and chemotherapy. Other relevant medical conditions are bacterial infections and drug-induced or transfusion-induced reactions.

A. *Types of pump thrombosis – pre/intra/post*
   Hemolysis is the leading symptom of intra-pump thrombosis. In this case the part of the pump involved in the process is the pump itself. Other types of blood flow obstructions through the pump are not likely to generate intravascular hemolysis.
B. *Most used pumps as LVAD*
   Although hemolysis has been described with the HVAD device, the preponderance of data comes from the HMII population.
   HeartWare HVAD
   Hemolysis is typically acute in presentation, and abnormalities in pump parameters are often present at the time of diagnosis. Data about long-term outcomes after hemolysis episodes are not well characterized.
   HeartMate II
   Actual thresholds for hemolysis definitions come from the study on HMII patients. It is clear that hemolysis is a hallmark sign of thrombosis and is associated with adverse outcome, increased risk for cerebrovascular accident, or death. An LDH level >2.5× normal is considered clinically relevant and should be intervened on. The traditional plasma-free hemoglobin 40 definition will underestimate the incidence of hemolysis.
C. *Other pumps*
   No reliable data are available.
   The new centrifugal continuous-flow LVAD HM III is designed to minimize shear stress and blood trauma. During pivotal clinical trial in Europe, no episodes of hemolysis were reported, but clinical data out of approval study are not available but clinical data out of approval studies are preliminary: the phenomenon of in-pump thrombosis is uncommon, but thrombosis of the outflow graft has been observed and cases of pre-pump thrombosis have already been reported.

48.5.2 Low Output Symptoms and Shock

Low cardiac output syndrome will be the result of pump malfunction, worsened by the consequences of intravascular hemolysis on end-organ function.

Symptoms of low cardiac output are common in the case of intra-pump thrombosis despite high power and high flow displayed by the pump (except HeartAssist5). The patient should be transferred to an intensive care unit for close monitoring and intravenous therapy. Hemodynamic monitoring and echocardiographic parameters are useful to ascribe low cardiac output syndrome to pump thrombosis. The typical picture is an uncoupling between hemodynamics, echo, and pump parameters. Right-heart catheterization can confirm elevated right-sided pressures, and two-dimensional echocardiographic parameters are essential to confirm pump malfunction, evaluating the status of LV which will present signs of suboptimal unloading such as frequent opening of the aortic valve, recurrent MR, and rightward shift of the interventricular septum.

The optimization of LVAD patients' hemodynamic profile is currently made with echocardiographic ramp study developed for speed optimization and useful for the diagnosis of device thrombosis in continuous-flow LVAD (cf-LVAD) [14]. This method, as it was published, shows limitations in the study of HVAD due to the characteristics of centrifugal pump and acoustic artifacts [15]. On the contrary, it is standardized for HMII with analysis of the slope of LVEDD, PI, and power combined with clinical parameters (LDH levels) during ramping of the speeds to detect obstruction of flow through the pump. LVEDD slopes are the most accurate measure in the diagnosis of thrombosis because impediment to flow leads to an uncoupling of the relationship between device speed and LVEDD. Blunted reduction in LVEDD in response to an increase in pump speed indicates an obstruction to flow through the device. In a short non-standardized version, this test is very reliable for diagnosis of pre-/post-pump thrombosis of HW HVAD. Increasing the revolutions per minute from 2200 to up to 3200–3500 rpm, unlike with the HeartMate II system, the blood flow signal on the monitor of the HeartWare HVAD provides important information. If the amplitude and morphology of the blood flow curve do not change despite the increase in rpm, it is a sign of blood flow obstruction. In this case the rpm increase produces an increase in power consumption caused by increased fluid friction inside the pump leading to shift of the blood flow curve without a change in amplitude and morphology. In the opposite case, a change in the amplitude and morphology of the curve from pulsatile form to a flat line suggests absence or insignificance of pre-pump or post-pump blood flow obstruction, making additional echocardiographic assessment of size changes of the left ventricle unnecessary.

For intra-pump thrombosis, early intervention is key for success. The clinical presentation may vary from mild to severe symptoms, but if not promptly treated, low cardiac output syndrome will progress into irreversible impairment of organ function. Restoring of normal pump flow is not always enough to reverse organ dysfunction and guarantee survival.

With centrifugal pumps, pump stop is a possibility with dreadful results.

Severe hemodynamic instability is the leading symptom of pre-pump thrombosis where the wedge thrombus occluding the inflow cannula causes abrupt decrease in pump flow and clinical emergency. In every case of pump low flow, echocardiography is crucial in the diagnostic procedure to rule out other causes of low flow status (right ventricular failure) and to examine the outflow tract. Low flow status with a slow decrease of flow is typical of post-pump thrombosis where symptoms of heart failure and congestion are mainly recognized in this case. Echocardiography evaluation of patient-device interface is dynamic and integrated with hemodynamic parameters to test a peak continuous wave Doppler velocity of the LVAD outflow tract in different clinical conditions of volume, inotropic status, and pump speeds. As recently reported, the range of outflow cannula velocity for patients supported with the HMII is <2.7 m/s and for HVAD <3.4 m/s [16].

48.6 Treatment of VAD System Thrombosis

Our algorithms for diagnosis and treatment of the different types of flow obstructions in HVAD and HeartMate II LVAD are presented in ◘ Figs. 48.2 and 48.3, respectively.

48.6.1 Pre-pump Thrombosis

HVAD: Backwash Maneuver with Carotid Protection (Claret Medical Sentinel CPS)

The "backwash maneuver" is a recently developed, noninvasive technique to "wash out" the occlusive thrombus under catheter-based protection of the carotid arteries by the Sentinel Cerebral Protection System (Claret Medical, Inc., Santa Rosa, CA), whose specific indication is HVAD pre-pump thrombosis.

When the inflow cannula of the HeartWare HVAD is occluded by a wedge thrombus that has been sucked into it, indeed, this procedure is a good alternative to more invasive strategies, namely, pump exchange [17, 18].

However, this maneuver carries a major risk of peripheral thromboembolism, above all thromboembolic occlusion of the carotid artery, which would be a disastrous complication.

With the aim to avoid thromboembolism into the carotid arteries, the routine use of a cerebral protection device, such as the Sentinel device, is recommended.

As a general rule, the washout procedure should be carried out in the hybrid operating room with the patient either awake or under general anesthesia according to the clinical situation and with standby for pump exchange or for thrombectomy, in case of unsuccessful washout maneuver.

The first step of the procedure is the positioning of the cerebral protection device. The Sentinel is inserted into the right brachial artery or the right radial artery under fluoroscopic guidance: the first proximal filter is positioned within the brachiocephalic artery, and the second distal filter is deployed in the left common carotid artery.

Once the correct positioning of the Sentinel has been confirmed with angiography, the pump

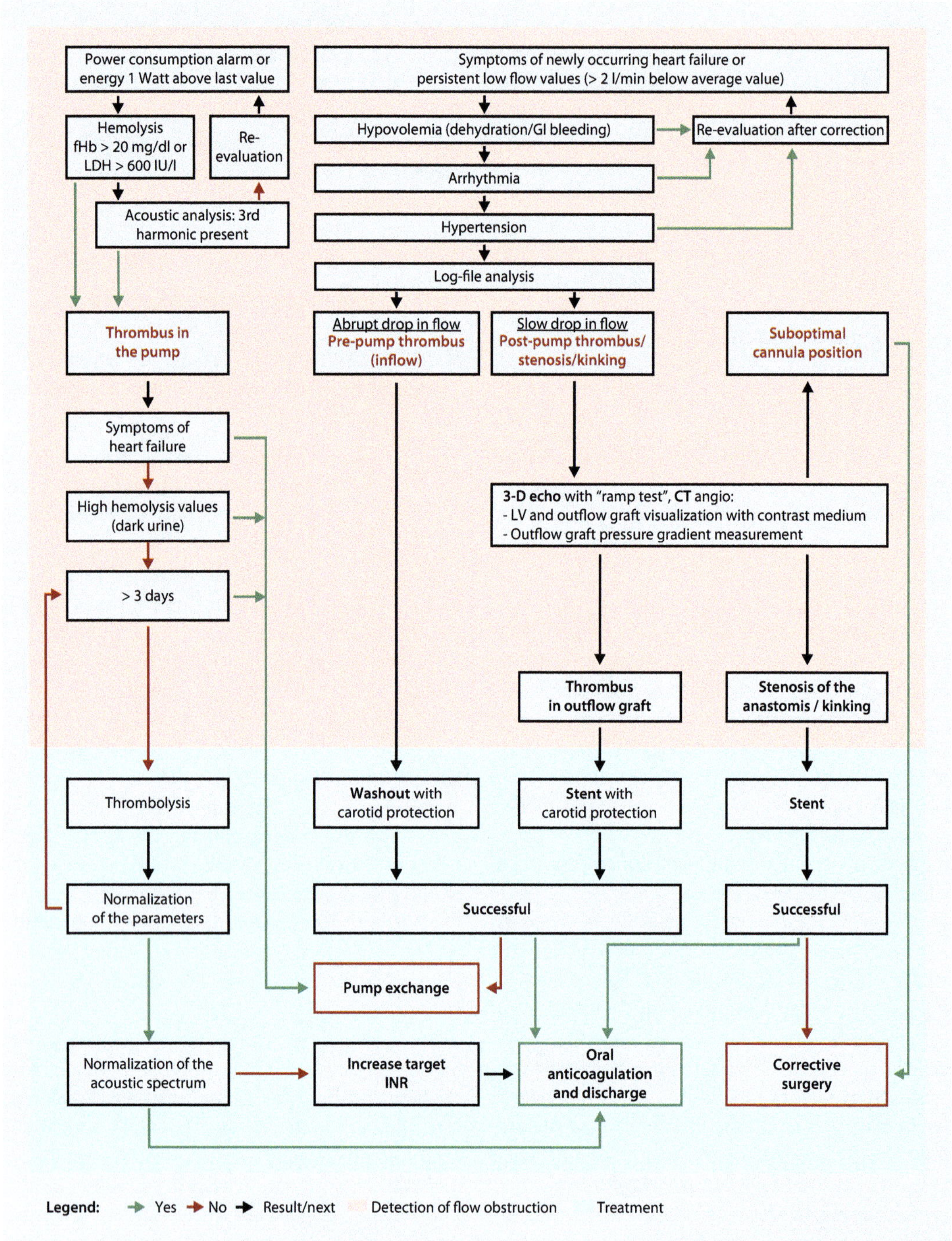

Fig. 48.2 Algorithm for the detection and treatment of flow obstruction in the HeartWare HVAD system

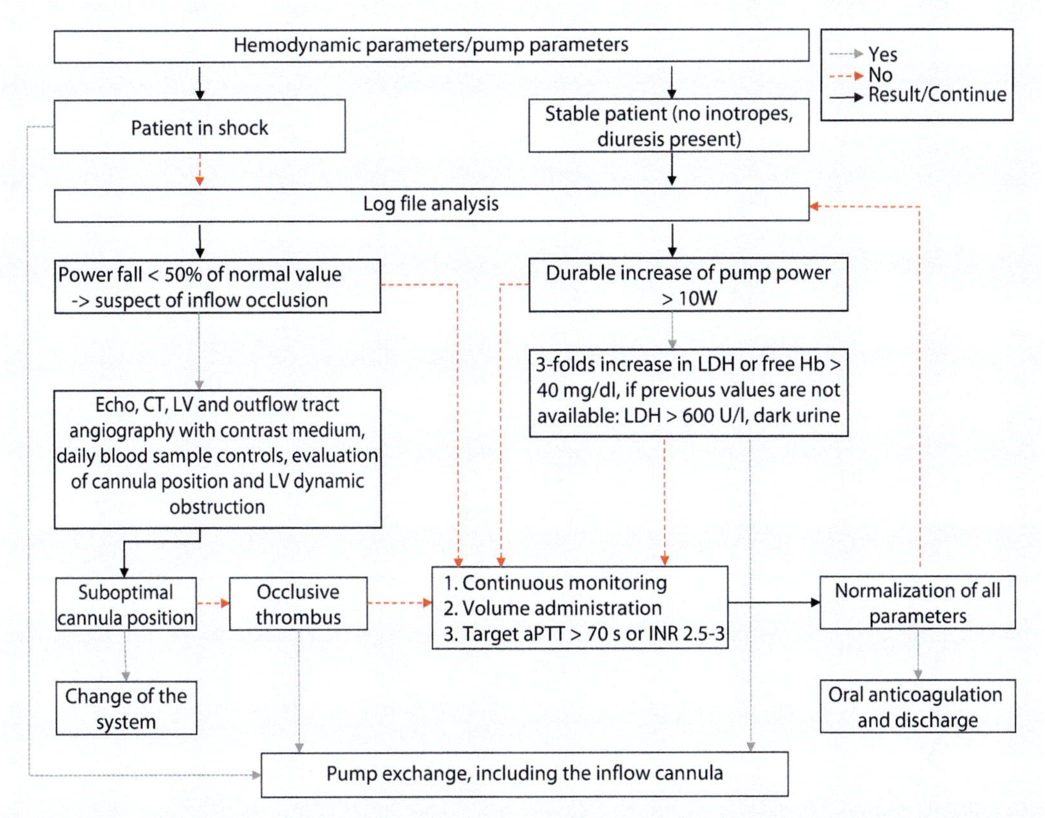

Fig. 48.3 Algorithm for the detection and treatment of flow obstruction in the HeartWare HeartMate II system

is stopped for approximately 10 s and then restarted.

The success of the maneuver in washing out the thrombus is assessed with the screenshot from the log file of the HeartWare HVAD and with the invasive arterial pressure monitoring.

The log file of a successful backwash maneuver is shown in Fig. 48.4 where the pump flow and power consumption before and during obstruction of the pump inflow, during the washout maneuver with pump stop, and after normalization of the flow and power consumption of the pump can be clearly identified. Similarly, the invasive arterial blood pressure will show: first, low blood flow and full left ventricular ejection at the time of pre-pump obstruction, then retrograde flow indicated by low diastolic arterial blood pressure, caused by retrograde blood flow through the pump during diastole during pump stop, and finally increase in blood pressure and unloading of the left ventricle after washout of the occlusive thrombus from the inflow cannula.

The last step of the washout maneuver is angiography of the peripheral arteries to detect possible distal thromboembolization of the clot and act immediately with surgical thrombectomy. No neurologic complication has been recorded with this strategy, as far as reported in literature. In a small percentage of patients, the thrombus cannot be found after the procedure (neither in the Sentinel device nor in the peripheral arteries).

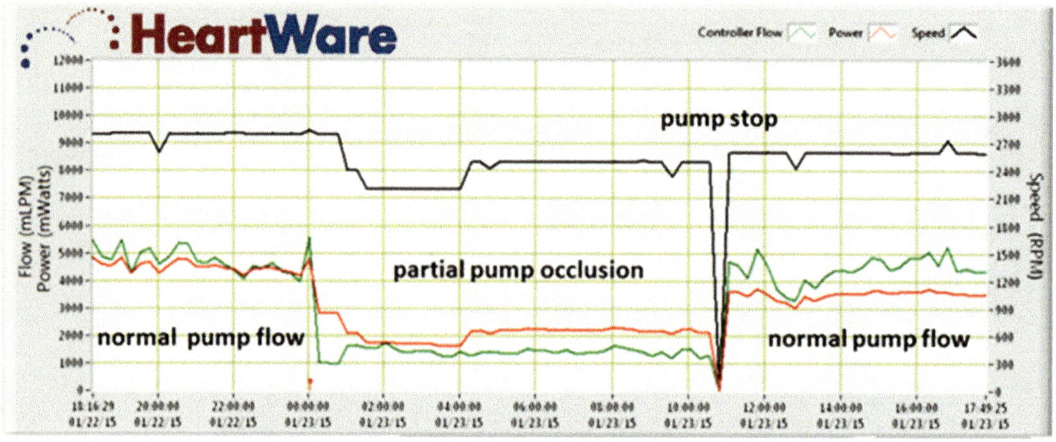

Fig. 48.4 Changes in flow curves before, during and after successful backwash maneuver

48.6.2 In-pump Thrombosis

Pump Exchange

Pump exchange is the definitive treatment for intra-pump thrombosis. However, it represents a major cardiac operation, which is performed in an acute setting on a compromised and hemodynamically instable patient. Furthermore, it represents the rescue treatment for all cases of unsuccessful lysis. Some clinical signs, for example, hemoglobinuria with dark urine, may suggest that severe hemolysis has occurred as a consequence of intra-pump thrombosis and should trigger the decision for pump exchange instead of a thrombolysis attempt. Early pump exchange indeed may prevent imminent renal failure in such cases [18].

Once the decision to perform pump exchange is undertaken, the appropriate strategy should be identified, according to each patient's characteristics. Indeed, several surgical approaches to pump exchange have been described, each presenting unique advantages and disadvantages [19].

The traditional approach to pump exchange includes median sternotomy and use of the heart-lung machine.

A "minimally invasive" approach has been recently reported in clinical practice and may be precious in patients in whom median sternotomy and the use of heart-lung machine would pose a significant risk for postoperative morbidity, as both of them are avoided. In more detail, two thoracotomy incisions are performed: the first in the sixth left intercostal space to access the LV apex and the second in the third right intercostal space to approach the ascending aorta.

A "lateral implantation" to the descending aorta can be also performed and represents a suitable solution for patients with a history of complex cardiac operations, where a redo-sternotomy would bear a significant risk of damage to the grafts or other cardiac structures.

Finally, venoarterial extracorporeal membrane oxygenation can be considered for mechanical circulatory support during pump exchange, as it is a closed circuit, not exposed to air, and allows a lower degree of heparinization compared to the traditional heart-lung machine.

Several series have documented outcomes after LVAD device exchange, and, although initially considered a highly morbid procedure, improvements of periprocedural care and surgical approach have resulted in lower mortality and complication rates.

48.6.3 Lysis

Thrombolysis is present in every algorithm for treatment of pump thrombosis, as a less-invasive therapy compared to surgical pump exchange, but recent data suggest a burden of complications that questions this role. Medical options in the therapy of LVAD thrombosis include intensification of anticoagulation with intravenous unfractionated heparin and systemic administration of GpIIb/IIIa inhibitor as an antiplatelet drug or administration of intravenous or

■ **Table 48.2** Example of soft lysis protocol with tirofiban

	Continuous infusion, µg/kg/min	Continuous infusion, µg/kg/min (if severe renal failure)	Bolus (INR<3)	Bolus (INR>3)	Bolus (INR<3, if severe renal failure)
Tirofiban	0.4	0.2	25 µg/kg	0	12 µg/kg

intraventricular thrombolytics. Intensification of anticoagulation is recommended in the presence of isolated LDH elevation adding iv unfractionated heparin to chronic therapy with warfarin and aspirin. Up-titration of antithrombotic therapy to a higher INR target is recommended after normalization of parameters with medical therapy. Use of direct thrombin inhibitor is described in this context, but is theoretically not useful to treat a clot already formed and indicated only in specific circumstances such as postoperative heparin-induced thrombocytopenia. Efficacy of lysis is limited by the composition of the thrombus (fibrin-laden thrombus is theoretically less responsive) and the location of thrombosis. Conservative therapy has high recurrence rate of thrombosis, because by measuring only indirect parameters it is hard to determine whether the thrombus was fully resolved or just reduced. Besides, high mortality is reported for medical therapy, ranging from 17% to 52%.

48.6.4 Soft Lysis

Lysis with antiplatelet drugs is an interesting option because the rate of bleeding is low, it is safer than thrombolysis, and does not preclude a following surgical pump exchange. The key for success is the timing of treatment compared to the onset of pump thrombosis. Soft lysis is a viable option to treat intra-pump thrombosis as an early approach, when the event started <3 days before; however, in the presence of overt hemolysis, it is not effective, and surgical treatment is indicated before clinical evolution into renal failure. Small case series reported successful use of eptifibatide (Merck & Co., Inc., Whitehouse Station, NJ) as continuous infusion (1–2 µg/kg/min) after a bolus (180 µg/kg) in the treatment of HMII thrombosis, but with a substantial rate of bleeding [20, 21]. An alternative strategy is tirofiban (Aggrastat, Merck & Co., Inc., West Point, Pennsylvania) as tirofiban as continuous infusion of 0.4 µ/kg/min for at least 48 h to a maximum of 72 h [18].

In ■ Table 48.2 an example of soft lysis protocol with tirofiban [18]

48.6.5 rTPA Lysis

The use of tissue plasminogen activator (rTPA) has been shown to have a 50–70% chance of successfully resolving a device thrombus in an HVAD cohort [12], and following studies confirm this rate of success, pointing out further recurrence of thrombosis which lowered the percentage of success to 21% [22]. However, serious adverse events were observed in the treated cases [23]: stroke from 10% to 15%, bleeding complications at 65%, and intracranial bleeding at 24%. Furthermore, the use of thrombolysis with rTPA complicates a staged approach with successive surgical treatment.

No standardized protocol exists; therefore, dosage and time of administration may greatly vary among different institutions [12], and different protocols may be applied according to the local experience [24, 25]. Furthermore, high dosages of drug are commonly infused (up to 100 mg) [12], as it is administered systemically.

No consensus exists however, concerning the administration route of thrombolytic agents and intraventricular administration of recombinant tissue plasminogen activator (rtPA) has also been reported [12], although in the absence of validated protocol. Some authors reported their experience with rTPA continuous infusion into the left ventricle through a pigtail catheter (rate of 1 mg/min for a total dose ranging from 30 to 50 mg) [26], via either the femoral or the radial artery.

An advantage of the intraventricular route is the direct suctioning of the drug from the LVAD, which is expected to result in an improved local effect within the pump, and reduced dosage of thrombolytic administered (30–50 mg) [26, 27], thus reducing the risk of intracranial hemorrhage and noncerebral bleeding [26, 27].

48.6.6 Outflow-Graft Thrombosis: Stenting

Although uncommon, outflow-graft obstruction represents a severe complication after LVAD implantation [28–31].

There are three main reasons for blood flow obstruction in the outflow graft: kinking of the graft, stenosis of the aortic anastomosis by ingrowth of an intimal flap, or graft thrombosis.

Regular follow-up with transthoracic echocardiography is crucial, but can provide only indirect information about the outflow cannula. On the other hand, imaging of the LVAD itself is complex by definition due to the presence of its metal parts. The CT scan has limited accuracy in picturing the outflow, beyond cases of thrombotic obstruction and kinking. Fluoroscopy, with intubation of the outflow graft and contrast medium, should be regarded as the gold standard in assessing stenosis of the aortic anastomosis. Additionally, measurements of the pressure gradient along the outflow graft further support the diagnosis and may be the unique sign of outflow-graft obstruction. If the aortic anastomosis is found to be stenosed (anatomically or functionally), stenting should be performed immediately. Kinking of the outflow tract can be treated by stenting alone and thrombosis of the outflow tract by stenting with a covered stent while using cerebral endovascular protection [32, 33].

48.7 Other Options for Treatment

48.7.1 Acute Weaning

"Acute weaning" for pump thrombosis should not be routinely recommended, with few exceptions. Indeed, it can be successfully performed in patients previously evaluated as having myocardial recovery in whom intra-pump thrombosis occurs after they have been evaluated or already scheduled for pump explantation. However, they represent a minority of cases.

48.7.2 HU Listing/Heart Transplantation

Cardiac transplantation may be a strategy for some patients, but this therapy is limited by donor availability.

Urgent listing for transplantation can be pursued if the estimated waiting time is no more than a few days, and symptoms can be managed readily. In the presence of low output state and progressive heart failure, device exchange is mandatory. Awareness of the effect of pump thrombosis on patient outcomes prompted the United Network of Organ Sharing in 2013 to allow emergency priority listing for patients with impending or manifest pump thrombosis. No bailout strategy is available for destination therapy patients.

48.8 Conclusions and Outlook

Certainly over the years, growing knowledge of the problem has improved approaches to pump malfunction due to pump thrombosis, from recognition and diagnosis to treatment. Many centers worldwide faced pump thrombosis and nowadays have gained extensive experience. The device industry focused on this type of adverse event in developing new devices. Results from the HM III European pivotal trial are promising; however, new biosurfaces are needed tending toward full hemocompatibility. At the same time, effort by clinicians should be placed on novel management strategies since outpatient care is crucial in this topic and every opportunity of telemonitoring is welcomed to start the treatment at an early stage.

References

1. van Oeveren W (1995) Biomaterials for rotary blood pumps. Artif Organs 19(7):603–607
2. Adatya S, Bennett MK (2015) Anticoagulation management in mechanical circulatory support. J Thorac Dis 7(12):2129–2138
3. Adamson RM, Mangi AA, Kormos RL, Farrar DJ, Dembitsky WP (2015) Principles of HeartMate II implantation to avoid pump malposition and migration. J Card Surg 30(3):296–299
4. Hubbert L, Sundbom P, Loebe M, Peterzen B, Granfeldt H, Ahn H (2014) Acoustic analysis of a mechanical circulatory support. Artif Organs 38(7):593–598

5. Yost GL, Royston TJ, Bhat G, Tatooles AJ (2016) Acoustic characterization of axial flow left ventricular assist device operation in vitro and in vivo. ASAIO J 62(1):46–55
6. Uriel N, Morrison KA, Garan AR, Kato TS, Yuzefpolskaya M, Latif F et al (2012) Development of a novel echocardiography ramp test for speed optimization and diagnosis of device thrombosis in continuous-flow left ventricular assist devices: the Columbia ramp study. J Am Coll Cardiol 60(18):1764–1775
7. Chorpenning K, Brown MC, Voskoboynikov N, Reyes C, Dierlam AE, Tamez D (2014) HeartWare controller logs a diagnostic tool and clinical management aid for the HVAD pump. ASAIO J 60(1):115–118
8. Jorde UP, Aaronson KD, Najjar SS, Pagani FD, Hayward C, Zimpfer D et al (2015) Identification and management of pump thrombus in the heartware left ventricular assist device system: a novel approach using log file analysis. JACC Heart Fail 3(11):849–856
9. Kaufmann F, Hormandinger C, Stepanenko A, Kretzschmar A, Soltani S, Krabatsch T et al (2014) Acoustic spectral analysis for determining pump thrombosis in rotary blood pumps. ASAIO J 60(5):502–507
10. Starling RC, Moazami N, Silvestry SC et al (2014) Unexpected abrupt increase in left ventricular assist device thrombosis. N Engl J Med 370:33–40
11. Kirklin JK, Naftel DC, Kormos RL et al (2014) Interagency Registry for Mechanically Assisted Circulatory Support (INTERMACS) analysis of pump thrombosis in the HeartMate II left ventricular assist device. J Heart Lung Transplant 33:12–22
12. Najjar SS, Slaughter MS, Pagani FD et al (2014) An analysis of pump thrombus events in patients in the HeartWare ADVANCE bridge to transplant and continued access protocol trial. J Heart Lung Transplant 33:23–34
13. Soltani S, Kaufmann F et al (2015) Design changes in continuous-flow left ventricular assist devices and life threatening pump malfunctions. Eur J Cardiothoracic Surg 47(6):984–989
14. Uriel N, Morrison KA et al (2012) Development of a novel echocardiograph ramp test for speed optimization and diagnosis of device thrombosis in continuous-flow left ventricular assist device. The Columbia Ramp study. JACC 60(18):1764–1775
15. Uriel N, Levin AP et al (2015) Left ventricular decompression during speed optimization ramps in patients supported by continuous-flow left ventricular assist device: device-specific performance characteristics and impact on diagnostic algorithms. J Card Fail 21(10):785–791
16. Grinstein J, Kruse E et al (2016) Screening for outflow cannula malfunction of left ventricular assist devices (LVADs) with the use of Doppler Echocardiography: new LVAD-specific reference values for contemporary devices. J Card Fail 22(10):808–814
17. Potapov EV, Krabatsch T, Buz S, Falk V, Kempfert J (2015) Cerebral protection system applied during washout of thrombus occluding inflow cannula of HeartWare HVAD left ventricular assist device. J Heart Lung Transplant 34(12):1640–1641. doi:10.1016/j.healun.2015.10.017
18. Scandroglio AM, Kaufmann F, Pieri M, Kretzschmar A, Müller M, Pergantis P, Dreysse S, Falk V, Krabatsch T, Potapov EV (2016) Diagnosis and treatment algorithm for blood flow obstructions in patients with left ventricular assist device. J Am Coll Cardiol 67(23):2758–2768. doi:10.1016/j.jacc.2016.03.573
19. Krabatsch T, Drews T, Potapov E, Weng Y, Pasic M, Hetzer R (2014) Different surgical strategies for implantation of continuous-flow VADs-Experience from Deutsches Herzzentrum Berlin. Ann Cardiothorac Surg 3(5):472–474. doi:10.3978/j.issn.2225-319X.2014.09.06
20. Tellor B, Smith J et al (2014) the use of eptifibatide for suspected pump thrombus or thrombosis in patients with left ventricular assist devices. J Heart Lung Transplant 33:94–101
21. Al-Quthami A, Jumean M et al (2012) Eptifibatide for the treatment of HeartMate II left ventricular assist device thrombosis. Circ Heart Fail 5:68–70
22. Jorde U, Aaronson K, Najjar S et al (2015) Identification and management of pump thrombus in the HeartWare left ventricular assist device system. A novel approach using log-file analysis. JACC Heart Failure 3(11):849–856
23. Stulak J, Dunlay S, Sharma S et al (2015) Treatment of device thrombus in the HeartWare HVAD: Success and outcome depend significantly on the initial treatment strategy. J Heart Lung Transplant 34:1535–1541
24. Maria Schürner A, Wilhelm MJ, Falk V, Ruschitzka F, Bettex D, Rudiger A (2015) Recurrent clotting of a continuous-flow right ventricular assist device--repeated thrombolysis with two different protocols. J Cardiothorac Vasc Anesth 29(6):1614–1617
25. Webber BT, Panos AL, Rodriguez-Blanco YF (2016) Intravenous thrombolytic therapy for patients with ventricular assist device thrombosis: an attempt to avoid reoperation. Ann Card Anaesth 19(1): 192–196
26. Raffa GM, D'Ancona G, Sciacca S, Pietrosi A, Hernandez Baravoglia CM, Turrisi M et al (2015) Systemic or endoventricular thrombolysis to treat HeartWare left ventricle assist device thrombosis: a clinical dilemma. Artif Organs 39:526–529
27. Raffa GM, D'Ancona G, Romano G, Falletta C, Sciacca S, Todaro C et al (2015) Should device replacement be the first choice strategy in continuous-flow left ventricular device thrombosis? Analysis of 9 events and results after endoventricular thrombolysis. Int J Cardiol 178:159–161
28. Abraham J, Remick JD, Caulfield T et al (2015) Left ventricular assist device outflow cannula obstruction treated with percutaneous endovascular stenting. Circ Heart Fail 8(1):229–230
29. Pham DT, Kapur NK, Dermody M, Halin N (2015) Stenting of an outflow graft obstruction after implantation of a continuous-flow, axial-flow left ventricular assist device. J Thorac Cardiovasc Surg 150(1): 11–12
30. Pieri M, Scandroglio AM, Kukucka M, et al (2016) Heart failure after five years on left ventricular assist device: diagnosis and treatment of out-flow graft obstruction. ASAIO J 2017 Jan/Feb;63(1):e1-e2. doi: 10.1097/MAT.0000000000000370

31. Hanke JS, El Sherbini A, Rojas SV, Avsar M, Shrestha M, Schmitto JD (2016) Aortic outflow graft stenting in patient with left ventricular assist device outflow graft thrombosis. Artif Organs 40(4):414–6. doi: 10.1111/aor.12569
32. Naber CK, Ghanem A, Abizaid AA et al (2012) First-in-man use of a novel embolic protection device for patients undergoing transcatheter aortic valve implantation. EuroIntervention 8:43–50
33. Lansky AJ, Schofer J, Tchetche D et al (2015) A prospective randomized evaluation of the TriGuard HDH embolic DEFLECTion device during transcatheter aortic valve implantation: results from the DEFLECT III trial. Eur Heart J 36:2070–2207

Infectious Complications

Ezin Deniz, Christina Feldmann, Jan D. Schmitto, and Margaret M. Hannan

© Springer International Publishing Switzerland 2017
A. Montalto et al. (eds.), *Mechanical Circulatory Support in End-Stage Heart Failure*,
DOI 10.1007/978-3-319-43383-7_49

49.1 Introduction

One of the major challenges and limits to the successful use of VADs is infection. VAD-specific and VAD-related infections are difficult to treat and remain a major cause of death in these patients [1]. The impact of VAD-specific and VAD-related infections depends on the site and the severity of the infection, with high infection mortality rates associated with VAD-related infective endocarditis (IE) and mediastinitis.

The Infectious Diseases (ID) Council of ISHLT in 2011 published much needed novel definitions of infection in these patients which were subdivided into three sections, VAD-specific, VAD-related, and non-VAD infections (▣ Table 49.1) [2].

▣ **Table 49.1** Classification of infections in patients using ventricular assist devices

VAD-specific infections
Pump and/or cannula infections
Pocket infections
Percutaneous driveline infections
Superficial infection
Deep infection
VAD-related infections
Infective endocarditis
Bloodstream infections (including CVC-associated BSIs)
CVC present
Bloodstream infection presumed VAD-related
Bloodstream infection presumed CVC-related
No CVC present
Bloodstream infection VAD-related
Bloodstream infection non VAD-related
Mediastinitis
VAD related
Sternal wound infection SSI-organ space
Pocket infection (continuous with mediastinum or already situated in the mediastinum depending on the device used)
Non-VAD related
Other causes of mediastinitis, perforation of the esophagus
Non-VAD infections
Lower respiratory tract infection
Cholecystitis
Clostridium difficile infection
Urinary tract infection

49.2 Definition of Infection in Patients Using Ventricular Assist Devices

When investigating any case of suspected VAD infection, prompt investigation is required, and testing as outlined below should be pursued (▣ Table 49.2) [2]. VAD-specific infections include infections that are specific to patients with VADs, are related to the device hardware, and do not occur in non-VAD patients, e.g., pump and cannula infections, pocket infections, and percutaneous driveline infections [3–6]. VAD-related infections refer to those that can also occur in patients who do not have VADs; however, in patients with VADs, there may be unique considerations with respect to making the correct diagnosis or determining the cause-effect relationship, e.g., mediastinitis and IE. Non-VAD infections are essentially not affected by the presence of the VAD and are unlikely related to the VAD presence but are included to encourage comprehensive and comparable data recording of all infections in this patient population to facilitate multicenter review.

49.3 VAD-Specific Infections

VAD-specific infections may be of the hardware itself or the body surfaces that contain them and include pump, cannula, and anastomotic infections, pocket infections, and percutaneous driveline or tunnel infections. Accurate VAD-specific infections required new definitions to be constructed to reflect the specifics of such infection to enable study of the potential sources or risk factors for these infections. Guidelines on the diagnosis of prosthetic joint infection (PJI) [7], IE [8], cardiovascular device infections [5, 9], intra-abdominal infections [10], catheter-related bloodstream

Table 49.2 Investigations for suspected infection in a patient using a ventricular assist device

All patients:
White blood cell count, serial C-reactive protein, or erythrocyte sedimentation rate
Sterile aspirate for Gram stain, KOH, routine bacterial and fungal culture of driveline at exit site if pus present
Echocardiogram (a TEE, if a TTE is negative)
Blood cultures: At least 3 sets of cultures taken at different times over 24 h; 2 sets from peripheral sites preferably. At least 1 central and 1 peripheral set of blood cultures should be taken at the same time if there is a CVC in situ. Each set including aerobic and anaerobic bottles with at least 10 ml of blood per bottle in adult cases or 1 ml/kg of blood per bottle for pediatric patients (up to a max of 10 kg)b
Chest X-ray If VAD removed: samples to be obtained at the time of explantation
Aspirate from external aspect of VAD (anterior) for culture
Aspirate from external aspect of VAD (posterior) for culture
Aspirate from outflow cannula part of VAD (internal aspect) for culture
Aspirate from inflow cannula part of VAD (internal aspect) for culture
Culture of saline instilled into VAD (internal aspect)
Sample of pus from for Gram stain, KOH, bacterial and fungal culture
Two tissue samples from suspicious tissue surrounding VAD, driveline or anastomoses sent for histology, Gram stain, KOH, bacterial and fungal culture
When clinically indicated:
Nasal, throat, and groin aspirate for *Staphylococcus aureus* carriage
If suspicious of a pocket infection, obtain an abdominal US, CT abdomen/thorax, nuclear imaging study
Image-guided aspiration or brush of pocket/driveline
Rule out all other possible causes of the septic episode (e.g., sputum culture, urine for microscopy and culture, etc.)

CT computed tomography, *US* ultrasound, *TEE* transesophageal echocardiogram, *TTE* transthoracic echocardiogram

(CRBS) [11], and skin and soft tissue infections [12] have provided the basis on which the definitions were constructed. These infections share many features of VAD-specific infections as they are often difficult to diagnose conclusively and difficult to treat due to the presence of biofilms on prosthetic surfaces that markedly reduce the likelihood of successful treatment with anti-infectives alone.

The first group of VAD-specific infections is hardware related (e.g., pump and/or cannula infections); see Fig. 49.1. The "pump" or "VAD" refers to that part of the device that is involved in the propulsion of blood and includes both continuous-flow (cf) and/or pulsatile (intracorporeal and paracorporeal)-flow devices, though the majority of implants today are CF pumps, >90% [1]. The term "inflow cannula" refers to that part of the device connecting the ventricle to the pump device. The term "outflow cannula" refers to that part of the device connecting the pump device to the patient's cardiovascular system. Suture lines refer to the surgical anastomoses between pump and patients' cardiovascular system. These generic terms have been chosen to allow as many VAD devices (including LVADs and RVADs) as possible to be incorporated into this definition framework.

A patient must have at least one of the microbiological, histopathological, radiological, or clinical criteria to achieve a firm diagnosis as outlined in

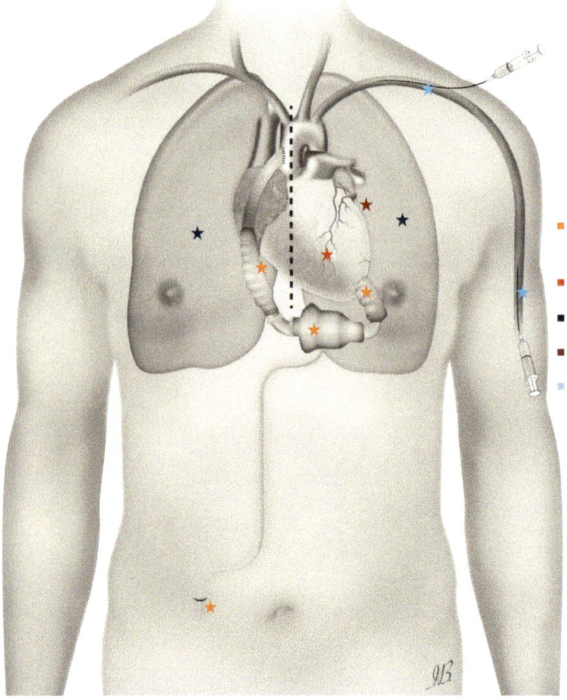

Fig. 49.1 Illustration of ventricular assist device VAD-specific, VAD-related, and non-VAD infection. *CVC* central venous catheter, *PVC* peripheral vascular catheter (Illustration by Ilaria Bondi's Peppermint Advertising)

Tables 49.3 and 49.4. The retrieval of a pathogen or an indistinguishable organism from more than one site is critical for validating the microbiological criterion.

The term "pocket" in these definitions is used to describe infections that occur in the body space or pocket that holds the pump inside the body of the patient. Classically the pocket may be newly created within the abdominal wall or within proximity to the pericardium and the diaphragm. The most recent devices use natural body cavities and are placed entirely within the left ventricle or within the pericardial sack (Tables 49.5 and 49.6). Pocket infections in those devices still requiring a surgical pocket may be diagnosed without removing the VAD at the time of surgery if samples from the inner surface of the pocket and the exterior surface of the VAD are taken (Table 49.2, Fig. 49.1). Cardiothoracic surgeons, cardiologists, and, in specialized centers, interventional radiologists working closely with microbiology teams may be able to aspirate diagnostic fluid surrounding devices by imaging guidance.

Percutaneous driveline infections (PDIs) are important but challenging to define. Objectively they lie between existing standards for tunneled central lines and implantable intraports [5, 9, 11]. It is difficult to strike a balance between fully comprehensive definitions and definitions that are practical and useful for clinicians. Consequently, PDI definitions have been adapted from CDC/NHSN surveillance definitions of healthcare-associated infection and classified as superficial or deep, based on the depth of the infection [13], and subclassified into proven, probable, and possible superficial and deep infections. Each subclassification is described under the following four categories, general appearance, microbiology, surgical/histology, or clinical criteria (Table 49.7), and should allow for detailed analysis of the etiology and risk factors for both superficial and deep PDI. This is considered the

Table 49.3 Definition of terms used for the diagnosis of ventricular assist device-specific pump and/or cannula infection

Major clinical criteria

If the VAD is not removed, then an indistinguishable organism (genus, species, and antimicrobial susceptibility pattern) recovered from 2 or more peripheral blood cultures taken >12 h apart with no other focus of infection or

All of 3 or a majority of ≥4 separate positive blood cultures (with the first and last sample drawn at least 1 h apart) with no other focus of infection

When 2 or more positive blood cultures are taken from the CVC and peripherally at the same time, and defined by criteria in Table 49.5 as either BSI-VAD-related or presumed VAD-related

Echocardiogram positive for VAD-related IE (TEE recommended for patients with prosthetic valves, rated at least "possible IE" by clinical criteria, or complicated IE [paravalvular abscess] and in any patient in whom VAD-related infection is suspected and TTE is nondiagnostic, TTE as first test in other patients) defined as follows: intracardiac mass suspected to be vegetation adjacent to or in the outflow cannula, or in an area of turbulent flow such as regurgitant jets, or consistent with a vegetation on implanted material, or abscess, or new partial dehiscence of outflow cannula

Minor clinical criteria

Fever 38 °C

Vascular phenomena, major arterial emboli, septic pulmonary infarcts, mycotic aneurysm, intracerebral or visceral, conjunctival hemorrhage, and Janeway's lesions

Immunologic phenomena: glomerulonephritis, Osler's nodes, Roth spot

Microbiologic evidence: positive blood culture that does not meet criteria as noted above (excluding single positive culture for coagulase-negative staphylococci excluding *Staphylococcus lugdunensis*)

Adapted from the Modified Duke's Criteria
CVC central venous cannula, *BSI* bloodstream infection, *IE* infective endocarditis, *TEE* transesophageal echocardiogram, *TTE* transthoracic echocardiogram, *VAD* ventricular assist device.

Table 49.4 Definitions of ventricular assist device-specific pump infections and/or cannula infection

Proven

Microbiology. Isolation of indistinguishable organism (genus, species, antimicrobial susceptibility pattern) at explantation or intraoperatively from:

- ≥ 2 positive internal aspect culture samples from pump and/or cannula
- 1 positive peripheral blood culture and 1 positive culture from VAD internal aspect aspirate or endovascular brushings (internal aspect refers to the inner lumen of the cannula)
- In the case of coagulase-negative staphylococci excluding *Staphylococcus lugdunensis*; 2 or more positive sets of peripheral blood cultures and a positive internal aspect culture of pump and/or cannula

Histologic features of infection from heart tissue samples from around the VAD pump and/or cannula at explantation or intraoperatively

Clinical criteria (see Table 49.3)

- 2 major criteria

(continued)

Table 49.4 (continued)

Probable
1 major criterion and 3 minor criteria or
4 minor criteria
Possible
1 major and 1 minor or
3 minor
Rejected
Firm alternative diagnosis explaining the clinical findings
Resolution of evidence of pump and/or cannula infection with antibiotic therapy for ≤ 4 days or
No pathologic evidence of pump and/or cannula infection at surgery or autopsy with antibiotic therapy for ≤4 days or
Does not meet criteria for possible pump and/or cannula

Table 49.5 Definition of terms used for the diagnosis of ventricular assist device-specific pocket infection

Major clinical criteria
Microbiologic: aspirated fluid culture positive or fluid/pus diagnostic of infection[a]
Radiologic: new fluid collection by radiologic criteria-CT/US/indium (enhancement or gas or sinus tract or leukocyte migration)
Minor clinical criteria
Fever _ 38 °C with no other recognized cause
New local erythema over the pocket site
Local pain and tenderness
Induration or swelling
Radiologic evidence: lymphangitis seen radiologically
New fluid collection without major criteria (above) and without diagnostic culture but not explained by other clinical conditions such as failure/anasarca/seroma

CT computed tomography, *US* ultrasound
[a]Image-guided aspiration

most useful way to define driveline infections as management of driveline infections typically depends upon the depth of the infection, which likely correlates with the source of the infection (Table 49.7) [12]. All percutaneous drivelines should be surgically examined at time of removal or replacement, and where infection involves both superficial and deep incision will be classified as a deep infection. PDI are the most commonly occurring infections in VAD patients and may reflect the presence of a deeper infection of the pocket space or pump and/or cannula. This

Table 49.6 Definition of ventricular assist device-specific pocket infection

Proven
Pathologic/microbiologic criteria
Patient has organisms cultured from the pocket space obtained during a surgical operation or needle sampling, taken intraoperatively or with radiologic guidance
Isolation of indistinguishable organism (genus, species, antimicrobial susceptibility pattern) from aspirate taken intraoperatively
2 exterior aspect culture positive samples from VAD
1 exterior aspect culture-positive sample from the VAD and 1 culture from pocket space surrounding VAD obtained intraoperatively
Abscess or other evidence of infection seen in the pocket area during a surgical operation/imaging or histopathology examination
Clinical criteria (Table 49.5)
2 major criteria
Probable
1 major criteria and 3 minor criteria
4 minor criteria
Possible
1 major and 1 minor
3 minor
Rejected
Firm alternative diagnosis explaining clinical findings
Resolution of evidence of VAD pocket infection with antibiotic therapy for 4 days
No pathologic evidence of VAD pocket infection at surgery or autopsy with antibiotic therapy for 4 days
Does not meet criteria for possible VAD pocket infection
Rejected microbiology evidence; negative culture or scanty growth of coagulase-negative staphylococcus excluding *Staphylococcus lugdunensis* and non-purulence aspirated fluid or tissue obtained during surgical operation or needle aspiration from the pocket area

VAD ventricular assist device

infection may be the result of local trauma at the exit site during device implantation, which may act as a cutaneous source of infection at a later date [14]. Sonography and CT angiography can reveal cuffs of fluid around the drivelines, cannula, and pump. Indium-labeled WBC scanning may also be helpful but, as yet, has not been validated for diagnosing these infections. The intraoperative exploration of the percutaneous driveline exit site (PDL-ES) at explantation or revision is required to satisfy these definitions, making them more useful for epidemiologic study than for clinical diagnosis. More recently different types of clinical grading systems as illustrated in Table 49.9 are used in combination with this ISHLT classification to aid diagnosis and management of infection.

Table 49.7 Definitions of ventricular assist device-specific percutaneous driveline infection

	Surgical/histology	Microbiology	Clinical	General wound appearance
A. Superficial VAD-specific percutaneous driveline infection				
Proven = Surgical/ histology criteria ± other criteria	Involvement of tissues superficial to the fascia and muscle layers of the incision documented	Aseptic skin culture positive or not cultured	Local increase in temperature around the exit site	Purulent discharge from the incision but not involving fascia or muscle layers or Erythema spreading around the exit sitea
Probable = No surgical/ histology criteria with purulent discharge ± other criteria	Surgical debridement not performed No histology	Aseptic skin culture positive or negative but patient already on antibiotic or had antiseptic used to clean wound	Local increase in temperature around the exit site and Treated as superficial infection with clinical response	Purulent discharge from the incision but not involving fascia or muscle layers or Erythema spreading around the exit site[a]
Possible = No surgical/ histology or purulent discharge ± other criteria	Surgical debridement not performed No histology	Aseptic skin culture positive or negative and patient not on antibiotics or had antiseptic used to clean the wound	Local increase in temperature around the exit site and Treated as superficial infection with clinical response	No discharge Erythema spreading around the exit site[a]
B. Deep VAD-specific percutaneous driveline infection				
Proven = Surgical/ histology criteria ± other criteria	Involves deep soft tissue (e.g., fascial and muscle layers) on direct examination or on direct examination during reoperation An abscess is found on direct examination during reoperation	Culture positive or histology puncture positive for infection	Temperature >38 °C Localized pain or tenderness	A deep incision spontaneous dehiscence Abscess deep to the incision around the driveline
Probable = No surgical/histology criteria with spontaneous dehiscence ± other criteria	No surgical debridement No histology	Culture negative but patients already on antibiotics or had antiseptic used on exit site	Temperature >38 °C Localized pain or tenderness or Treated as a deep infection	An incision spontaneous dehiscence
Possible = No surgical/ histology criteria with positive ultrasound ± other clinical criteria	No surgical debridement No histology	Cultures not reserved	Localized pain or tenderness and Treated as a deep infection with clinical response	Positive ultrasound

VAD ventricular assist device
[a]Erythema excluding stitch abscess (minimal inflammation and discharge confined to the points of suture penetration)

49.4 VAD-Related Infections

VAD-related infections include IE, bloodstream infections (BSIs), mediastinitis, and sternal wound infection and are outlined in ◘ Table 49.8. Imaging has a particular role in revealing new inflammatory change in the mediastinum, and newer cardiac CT can show large valve vegetations and cannula insertion infections. It has been reported that CT may have a role in sternal wound infection characterization though we would mainly use it today to define the extent of deep-seated infection or collection and occasionally to guide tissue sampling by core biopsy for culture if swabs have not yielded a specific diagnosis [15, 16].

Diagnosing VAD-related BSI in the presence of a CVC may be particularly difficult. The technique of "differential time to positivity" (DTP) as a method of determining which infections are due to the VAD and which are due to the CVC is recommended, consistent with recent IDSA guidelines [11]. This method uses a 2 h time to positivity differential to determine the source of infection when a CVC is present. This method, though not 100% accurate, may implicate the CVC as the source of the bacteremia if the CVC blood cultures become positive >2 h before peripheral blood cultures become positive. Efforts can be made to avoid secondary seeding of the infection to the VAD by prompt removal

◘ **Table 49.8** Definition of ventricular assist device-related infections

Clinical condition	Classification of disease
Endocarditis	
All cases (default)	VAD-related endocarditis
Vegetation seen on native valves and not on VAD (Define native valve IE using modified Duke's criteria)	VAD-related endocarditis
Bloodstream infection CVC present:	
Central culture positive ≤2 h before peripheral	BSI *presumed* VAD-related
Central culture positive ≥ 2 h before peripheral culture (Definitions made using the IDSA guidelines when CVC present)	BSI *presumed* CVC-related
No CVC present:	
BSI due to VAD infection or cause unclear	Bloodstream infection VAD-related
BSI due to cause other than VAD infection (e.g., UTI, pneumonia) (Definitions made using CDC/NHSN definitions when no CVC present)	Bloodstream infection non-VAD-related
Mediastinitis VAD-related: This is when mediastinitis is due to the VAD device	
(1) Sternal wound infection-related, SSI-organ space	Mediastinitis VAD-related
(2) Pocket infection (continuous with mediastinum or already situated in the mediastinum depending on the device used) Classify as (1) and (2) per "surgical site infection-organ space" in CDC/NHSN surveillance definitions for healthcare-associated infection	
Non-VAD mediastinitis: This is when mediastinitis is definitely due to another cause (e.g., esophageal perforation during endoscopy). Classify as "CVS infections-mediastinitis" in CDC/NHSN surveillance definitions for healthcare-associated infection	Mediastinitis non- VAD-related
CDC/NHSN	

of the CVC. If the DTP of CVC and peripheral blood cultures are less than 2 h, it is possible the VAD is the source of infection. Other causes such as non-VAD infection should also be considered, as the VAD may not always be the source of the BSI [17]. Mycotic aneurysms have also been reported in patients using VADs and associated with persistent or relapsing BSI [18]. Mycotic aneurysms may be visceral or intracerebral (usually presenting as an intracranial hemorrhage).

49.5 Non-VAD Infections

Non-VAD infections are essentially "independent" or not directly related to the presence of the VAD but infections occurring in a "cardiac sick" population of immunocompromised hosts with underlying comorbidities such as diabetes, prolonged hospitalization, multiple drug regimens, and renal impairment. The purpose of including non-VAD infection is to provide a comprehensive overview of all infections in this "cardiac sick" population (▫ Table 49.9).

▫ **Table 49.9** Recommended international definitions for non-VAD infections for registry data gathering

Lower respiratory tract infections[a]
Cholecystitis[a]
Clostridium difficile infection[b]
Urinary tract infection[a]
Urinary tract infection[a]

[a]Defined as per Centers for Disease Control and Prevention/National Healthcare Safety Network definition
[b]Defined as per Health Protection Agency, UK definitions and Infectious Disease Society of America definition

49.6 Diagnostic Tests Used for Investigating Suspected Infection in a Patient Using a VAD

Patients with VAD infections may present in a variety of ways making definitive diagnosis difficult. Patients often present with non-specific symptoms such as lethargy, fatigue, fever, or anorexia as well as a wide spectrum of ailments ranging from minor erythema at the PDL-ES to severe sepsis and clinical shock. All clinicians must be alert to the possibility of infection in VAD patients and should be educated regarding the clinical symptoms and signs, which ensure early detection and guide the most efficient diagnostic algorithm.

The initial evaluation should include a careful history and review of symptoms. Physical examination, review of the VAD function, surgical wounds, and PDL-ES are essential as early detection and treatment of a localized process may prevent progression to more serious VAD infections. It can also help to direct the clinician to non-VAD infections that may be present such as a UTI or CDI. Laboratory studies including a full blood count [19–21], serial erythrocyte sedimentation rate (ESR) [19], or C-reactive protein (CRP) are recommended in all patients [19–21, 23]. If there is pus visible at the PDL-ES, then an aspirate of this pus should be sent for bacterial and fungal cultures. Routine surveillance cultures of exit sites may be considered as colonization often precedes infection and can serve as valuable information for subsequent infection. Initial imaging should include a standard chest radiograph; an echocardiogram will be needed if there is suspicion of native valve infective endocarditis (IE) or concomitant cardiac implantable electrical device infective endocarditis (CDIE). At least three sets [24] of blood cultures should be obtained and at least two sets taken from a peripheral site at times consistent with modified Duke's criteria [8] (outlined in ◘ Table 49.3) before commencing anti-infectives and where a CVC is present one set from the line concurrent with one of peripheral blood cultures [11]. Difficulty in obtaining blood samples from children and concerns about drawing large volumes may result in lower volumes of blood being submitted for culture and may reduce the negative predictive value of the culture [11]. When clinical, laboratory, and microbiology culture data point to a particular VAD or non-VAD infection, imaging can play a role in supporting such suspicions or directing tissue samples. Further when infection source eludes standard evaluation, imaging can have a role in primary diagnosis.

Sonography is a useful tool to visualize fluid around percutaneous and tunneled drivelines and in pump pockets and can be used to direct tissue samples or lavage. HIDA scanning was the gold standard for diagnosing cystic duct obstruction and remains a first-line test in many centers. Due to ease of access, widespread practice and rapid diagnosis and ultrasound have become the first-line study for infections such as cholecystitis [10]. Various CT protocols beyond the scope of this chapter can be used to evaluate the lungs, pleura, and mediastinum as well as other organ structures. They are clearly of value in investigating suspected infection in a patient using a VAD [15, 16, 25]. Since MRI is largely precluded, CT and digital subtraction angiography are the tests of choice for mycotic pseudoaneurysm assessment and treatment. The ability of modern scanners to provide whole-body assessment is very helpful. We have also found it of value to assess cannulae, thrombi, and vegetations. Sternal wound infections have been assessed by CT, or bone/indium-labeled leukocyte [26] scan with specific protocols may have a role in characterization of infection but in the surgically "damaged" sternum may have limited value [15].

In selected patients, the VAD may need to be removed due to uncontrolled infection or for technical reasons. When this happens, the VAD should always be sent to the laboratory for processing. Sterile aspirates or sterile syringe aspirates (from surgery) should be taken for Gram stain, KOH and Calcofluor white stain, bacterial and fungal cultures, and broad-range PCR at the time of explantation from the internal and external aspect of the inflow cannula and from the internal and external aspect of the outflow cannula when a VAD is removed. A small volume of sterile water (<5 ml) should be instilled into the explanted VAD and then aspirated and sent for bacterial and fungal culture. Defining the optimal method of culture of VADs is beyond the scope of these guidelines; however in the future, it would be beneficial to devise a standardized culture process for VADs so that the microbiology laboratory practice can be standardized across all centers (e.g., VAD sonication or even scraping of the biofilm) [26]. In particular, the use of broth cultures for the retrieval of organisms (currently used for explanted heart valves) including broad-range PCR should be considered where possible. Cardiothoracic surgeons, cardiologists, and, in specialized centers, interventional radiologists working closely with microbiology teams may be able to aspirate diagnostic fluid surrounding devices by imaging guidance [10]. Risk of introducing infection into a sterile fluid collection using this technique should be considered and performance of such procedures must have direct oversight for specimen handling by those involved in the infection management.

Any purulence present in the pocket area should also be sent for Gram stain, KOH, and Calcofluor white stain, bacterial and fungal culture, broad-range PCR, and a further two swabs processed in the same way taken from the external surface of the VAD, anterior and posterior. Finally at least two samples of tissue from the pocket area and insertion site of the cannulas into the heart should be sent for histology and tissue stains for bacteria and for microbiology, Gram stain, KOH and Calcofluor white stain, bacterial and fungal cultures, and broad-range PCR.

It may also be necessary to send additional samples to the microbiology laboratory if non-VAD infections are suspected (e.g., urine, stool for *C. difficile* toxins A and B, sputum, and wound swabs). The investigation of suspected VAD infections should be done in consultation with an infectious disease physician or clinical microbiologist, a cardiologist, and a cardiothoracic surgeon to optimize both the diagnosis and management of the potential infection. The anti-infective regimen must be carefully chosen since prolonged, even lifelong, therapy may be required (■ Table 49.10).

■ Table 49.10 Management of percutaneous driveline infection. Photograph: Thoratec corporation

	1	2	3
	Possible	**Probable**	**Proven**
Definition	No surgical/histology or purulent discharge ± other criteria	No surgical/histology criteria with purulent discharge ± other criteria	Surgical/histology criteria ± other criteria
Surgical or histopathological	Surgical debridement not performed No histopathology	Surgical debridement not performed No histopathology	Involvement of tissues superficial to fascia or muscle layer = superficial infection Involvement of tissues deep to fascia or muscle layer = deep infection.
Microbiological	Skin culture positive or negative and patient not on antibiotics or had antiseptic used to clean the wound	Skin culture positive or negative but patient already on antibiotic or had antiseptic used to clean wound	Skin culture positive or not cultured or Blood cultures positive and no other source for bloodstream infection = deep infection
Clinical	Local increase in temperature around the PDL exit site Treated as superficial infection with clinical response	Local increase in temperature around the PDL exit site Treated as superficial infection with clinical response	Local increase in temperature around the PDL exit site
General wound appearance	No discharge Erythema spreading around the exit site Dry wound	Purulent discharge from the incision but not involving fascia or muscle layers Erythema spreading around the PDL exit site Wet wound	Purulent discharge from the incision but not involving fascia or muscle layers Erythema spreading around the exit site Wet wound
Example	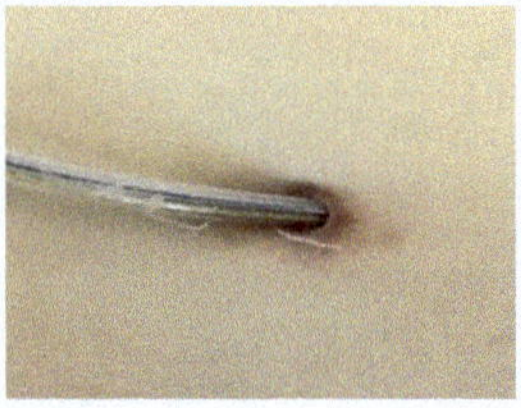	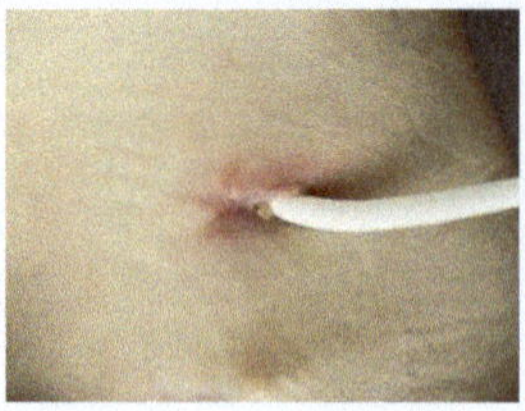	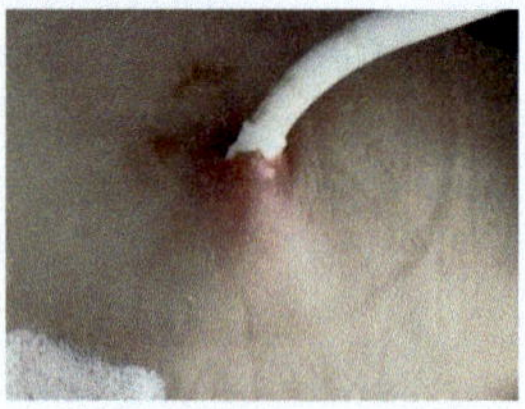

Table 49.10 (continued)

	1	2	3
	Possible	Probable	Proven
Management	Driveline exit site dry Take a photograph and save Clean using wound antiseptic Allow 5 min to dry before applying new dressing Change dressing daily Check driveline-fixation device is secure	Take a photograph and save Take microbiological swab if wound discharge present Use wound antiseptic hydrochloride 0.1% and 2.0% ethanol Change dressing 2–3 times a week Use oral antibiotics guided by cultures If no response, then wound should be managed as per → 3	Attend hospital Take a photograph and save Take microbiological swab if wound discharge present Use hydrochloride 0.1% and 2.0% ethanol Change dressing daily Use antibiotics 2/52 for superficial or 6/52 for deep infection. Commence with iv antibiotics and then switch to po. Choose antibiotic based on cultures and consult microbiology team/ID Commence individualized surgical wound management with repositioning and/or vacuum therapy if necessary

49.7 Infection Prevention and Control

49.7.1 Preoperative Screening, Skin Preparation, and Antiseptic

All patients should undergo the same preoperative investigation and theater preparation for cardiac surgery. All patients should be screened in a similar way to a heart transplant candidate as many VAD implant candidates are stratified as bridge to transplantation or following VAD implant for other strategies may be escalated to urgent cardiac transplant candidate if they develop a major infection. All patients should be screened for colonization with methicillin-resistant *Staphylococcus aureus* (MRSA), carbapenem-resistant Enterobacteriaceae (CRE), vancomycin-resistant enterococci (VRE), and extended-spectrum beta-lactamases (ESBL). Patients should also be screened serologically for prior infection and latent infectious diseases such as HIV; hepatitis A, B, C, E; and syphilis. Interferon gamma release assay (IGRA) tests should be used to screen for patients for latent tuberculosis. In countries where endemic infection is prevalent such as Latin America and Southwestern USA, patients should be screened serologically for Chagas disease and coccidioidal infection, respectively.

Preoperative skin preparation should include three chlorhexidine 4% aqueous solution showers. These should be timed as follows: the day before surgery, the evening before surgery, and the morning of surgery. Prior to showering, the patient should be instructed to use chlorhexidine 4% aqueous solution to scrub chest (from chin to umbilicus), arms, and legs using a clean sterile dressing pad for each shower. The patient should then be dressed in his/her theater gown or fresh

Table 49.11 Prevention of VAD infection: preoperatively, intraoperatively, and postoperatively

	Preoperative stage	Intraoperative stage	Postoperative stage
Patient-related prevention	Reduce risk factors for development infection by carefully reviewing Immune status Weight Active or occult infection Nutritional status	Patient preparing IV infusion 1 h before incision Careful selection of broad spectrum antimicrobials Alcohol iodophor antiseptic allow to dry to maximize effect Sterile drapes	Reduce risk factors for developing infection Avoid immunosuppressant due to malnutrition, diabetes, and drugs, monitored for signs and symptoms of VAD- and non-VAD-related infections Avoid situations that could place them at a greater risk (contact with sick individuals, poor hygiene and poor living conditions)
Not-patient-related prevention	Reduce risk factors for development infection Careful pump-device selection CVC change where possible preoperatively	Clean implantation technique Sterile operating-room conditions with limited traffic Sterile procedure Appropriate hand and arm washing with an antimicrobial agent for a minimum of 3 min Device opening under sterile conditions and only immediately before use Use minimal-implantation-technique Avoid pump pocket Maximized tunneling of driveline Secure driveline fixation	Reduce risk for developing infection PDL exit site should be carefully managed postoperatively in order to prevent the introduction of pathogens Dressings should be changed starting 24–48 h after surgery Dressings should be changed under sterile conditions Use of various anchoring devices to help stabilize the driveline to minimize the risk of trauma to the exit site Patient training on dressing change, showering technique and hand hygiene PDL exit sites should be documented with photographs

nightwear. As near as possible to the time of surgery, male patients should have arm and chest hair clipped where necessary. Where patient was unable to shower due to clinical limitations, a healthcare worker should apply chlorhexidine 4% aqueous solution to the chest (chin to umbilicus), arms, using sterile pads. This must be then allowed to dry on the skin (Table 49.11).

49.7.2 Intraoperative Antiseptic and Antibiotic Prophylaxis

Several studies comparing alcoholic povidone iodine (API) with 2% chlorhexidine in 70% alcohol (CHG) have been published in general surgery. A recently published study using CHG as preoperative antiseptic in cardiothoracic surgery in a risk-adjusted cohort with education of the surgical team found significantly lower SSI infection rates when compared with API [27].

In addition to the preoperative skin preparation and surgical antiseptic, the antibiotic prophylaxis (AP) is an important component of infection prevention. While there is no randomized study that clearly favors a particular preoperative antibiotic protocol, local cardiothoracic surgical site infection (SSI) surveillance data should be used to guide choice of antibiotic prophylaxis regimen for VAD implantation. Therefore, the use of antibiotic prophylaxis regimen may vary from one institution to another and be changed based on local SSI epidemiological data but should be based on the following principles.

The AP regimen should always target staphylococcal infection with coverage for MRSA recommended in colonized patients or at centers where MRSA prevalence is high. The most widely used regimen is vancomycin with a first- or second-generation broad-spectrum cephalosporin (e.g., cefazolin or cefuroxime) for 24–48 h with nasal mupirocin on the night of surgery. Based on lower rates of surgical site infections, antibiotics should be infused within one hour of skin incision with the exception of vancomycin that requires 1 h infusion [28, 29]. When used, vancomycin should be started up to 2 h prior to VAD surgery. The duration of AP should not exceed 24–48 h [30]. The routine use of antifungal medications is not recommended [31].

49.8 Management of Infection in General in the VAD Patient

There are no randomized controlled studies regarding the management of LVAD infections. The principles in the management of MCS infections are guided by small observational studies and expert opinion and based on the following factors: identification of the responsible microorganism, device-related infection type (driveline, pocket, pump/cannula), presence or absence of bloodstream infection (BSI), and transplant candidacy status. All patients should be carefully assessed as outlined above under the diagnosis of infection section. In patients with driveline infections but without BSI or systemic illness, empiric antibiotics can be deferred pending culture results. Oral antibiotics targeting the identified pathogens should be initiated when feasible. In the presence of systemic illness and/or sepsis, empiric IV antibiotics targeting staphylococcal, pseudomonal, and Enterobacteriaceae infections should be initiated as soon as cultures have been taken. The choice of empiric therapy should also be influenced by local hospital epidemiology and antibiotic stewardship program. Once culture results are available, treatment should be adjusted to target the identified pathogens. Further use of antibiotics should be judiciously guided by infection experts on daily multidisciplinary (MDT) rounds with the surgical team and be based on early microbiology laboratory data from each VAD patient and used to guide changes and choices of appropriate antibiotics or antifungals when needed. Regular monitoring of the safety and efficacy of antimicrobial therapy is essential. Therapeutic drug monitoring should be considered for specific antimicrobial therapies (e.g., vancomycin, aminoglycosides, voriconazole, and posaconazole). In addition, since both infection and antimicrobial therapy may affect the international normalized ratio (INR), close monitoring of the INR is warranted to adjust anticoagulation therapy (◘ Table 49.12).

49.8.1 Surveillance of Infection

As with all cardiothoracic surgery, each center should have an active surgical site surveillance program in place to monitor infection and trends and use this data to guide AP and prevention strategy [32]. The new CDC guidelines

Table 49.12 Management of VAD-specific and VAD-related infection

	Driveline treatment	Pump-pocket treatment	Pump and/or cannula treatment
Step 1	Take prompt culture and Gram stain if discharge is present and blood cultures prior to commencing broad-spectrum antibiotics	Take prompt cultures and Gram stain of any wound discharge present and several sets of blood cultures ideally over 24 h prior to commencing broad-spectrum antibiotics. Perform radiology-guided aspiration of collections where possible	Take prompt cultures and Gram stain of any wound discharge present and several sets of blood cultures ideally over 24 h prior to commencing broad-spectrum antibiotics. Perform radiology-guided aspiration of collections where possible
Step 2	Start empiric broad-spectrum antibiotics targeting Gram-positive organisms and consult an infection expert	Start empiric broad-spectrum antibiotics targeting Gram-positive organisms and consult an infection expert	Start broad-spectrum antibiotics targeting Gram-positive organisms and consult an infection expert
Step 3	Start targeted therapy after reviewing blood cultures and drainage cultures, and organisms identification and susceptibility results	Start targeted therapy after reviewing blood cultures and drainage cultures, and organism identification and susceptibility results.	Start targeted therapy after reviewing blood cultures and drainage cultures, and organisms identification and susceptibility results
Step 4	*Mild infection* Treat as an outpatient using oral antibiotics Perform aggressive wound care increasing the frequency of dressing changes Review dressing change protocols to ensure compliance and close monitoring Keep driveline exit site and dressing clean Immobilize driveline to prevent disruption of the area surrounding the driveline itself *Moderate infection* Treat on an outpatient basis using oral antibiotics Perform inpatient treatment if patient has systemic infection such as fever or leukocytosis Perform aggressive wound care with increasing the frequency of dressing changes Reviewing dressing change protocols to ensure compliance and close monitoring Keep driveline exit site and dressing clean Immobilize driveline to prevent disruption of the area surrounding the driveline itself Perform local debridement if necessary	*For all pump-pocket infection* Treat as an inpatient with systemic antibiotic Perform percutaneous or surgical drainage Perform device pocket revision: debride infectious tissue and send 3–5 specimens for bacterial and fungal culture, Gram stain, KOH/Calcofluor white stain, and broad-range PCR to diagnose bacterial or fungal infection Clean pump pocket and the place around it with several saline lavages and use vacuum-assisted closure (V.A.C., KCI USA, Inc. San Antonio, TX, USA) of a pocket wound if necessary Presence of Gram-negative bacteria or yeast requires more invasive management and complete revision of the driveline tract or a pump exchange Consider alternative therapy with less systemic side effects of the use of antibiotic-impregnated beads applied locally to the pump pocket in select cases	*For all pump and/or cannula infection* Treat as an inpatient with systemic antibiotics Perform device replacement If VAD replacement is not an option, perform aggressive IV antibiotic therapy for a prolonged period of time Persistent pump or cannula infection requires lifelong IV or oral suppressive therapy Escalate to urgent heart transplant list in patients with chronic pump and/or cannula infection If all of these fail, escalate to urgent heart transplant list

Table 49.12 (continued)

	Driveline treatment	Pump-pocket treatment	Pump and/or cannula treatment
	Severe infection Treat as an inpatient with systemic antibiotic Perform aggressive wound care with increasing the frequency of dressing changes Reviewing dressing change protocols to ensure compliance and close monitoring Keep driveline exit site and dressing clean Immobilize driveline to prevent disruption of the area surrounding the driveline itself Perform surgical drainage and incision of driveline site with driveline revision to remove dead tissue and allow for faster wound healing and recovery under sterile conditions in the operating room Use negative-pressure wound therapy (NPWT, vacuum therapy) to accelerate the healing of the wound if necessary Consider additional methods: debride infected tissue and cover the driveline with well-perfused tissue such as rectus muscle or use antimicrobial beads and novel therapies such as Mepilex™ or Aquacel® dressing changes If all of these fail, move the driveline into the intraperitoneal space, wherein a completely new exit site is created and the driveline is covered with omentum. Perform device exchange for unsuccessful cases *Recurrent or chronic infection* Use intravenous antibiotics and long-term oral antibiotic therapy to suppress and prevent recurrence of infection Perform device exchange or Perform wide debridement of the pump pocket and driveline with the institution of antibiotic beads and negative pressure dressing therapy If all of these fail, escalate to urgent heart transplant list	Use muscle or omental transposition flaps in severe cases of pump pocket or VAD-related mediastinitis infection with tissue defects If all of these fail, exchange the full pump particularly in the presence of VAD-related infective endocarditis.	

Table 49.13 Preparing patient for VAD surgery

Time of VAD implant surgery	Procedure
Day before surgery	Allergies should be documented Risk factors such as old age, obesity, malnutrition, other comorbidities, and in situ cannulas should be documented (e.g., periphery vein or central vein cannulae) Old cannulas (e.g., periphery vein or central vein cannulae) should be removed or exchanged Jewelry should be removed where possible, although local policy may allow tape to be applied around jewelry that is difficult to remove Patients should wash or shower using soap and water the evening before surgery or with preoperative antiseptic shower wash, chlorhexidine 4% Prescribed medication should be reviewed preoperatively and only essential medicines given – those taken orally should be swallowed with the smallest amount of water possible Medicines that will cause drowsiness should be administered once the patient has been prepared for theatre and the patient should be advised to stay on the bed with a call bell Laboratory results, chest X-ray, midstream urine, or clinical infection signs (fever, etc.) should be checked, and operation should be canceled if there are positive signs of infection
Day of surgery	Patients' comfort and dignity should be maintained when they are changing into their theatre gown Patients should remove bras and pants before surgery Anti-embolism stockings should be measured and fitted before transfer to theatre, depending on VTE risk Dentures and hearing aids should be removed Loose teeth, caps, or crowns should be identified as a safety precaution to prevent choking during anesthesia Wristband details should be checked with patients and to ensure they match those on patient records, medicine records, X-rays, and test results Vital signs should be recorded and abnormal readings reported The site of surgery should be marked on the ward before patients go to theater or receive premedications. This should be checked by the nurse on the ward who is completing the preoperative checklist Patients head hair should be covered with a cap Hair around the incision site should be removed, using electric clippers with a single-use disposable head, not longer than 24 h prior to surgery Use of alcohol skin preparation fluids Perform patient skin preparation in the operating room with antiseptics: iodine/iodophor, 2% chlorhexidine, and alcohol-based preparations

recommend 30-day and 90-day surveillance for all surgery. Where possible MCS patients should also have ongoing infection surveillance throughout the duration of the device implant and record all infections in MCS ISHLT databases.

49.9 Surgical Prevention

VAD-specific and VAD-related infections negatively impact patient's mortality and morbidity. Therefore, numerous prevention strategies have been attempted to reduce the growing number of infections associated with VADs. The incidence of infection after VAD implantation depends on patient-related risk factors, e.g., diabetes [33], obesity [34], malnutrition [35], and device-related risk factors such as driveline position [36], pump pocket [37], long duration support [38], as well as pump design [39]. For this reason pre-, peri-, and postoperative management strategies should be developed in all VAD centers to limit the risk of VAD-specific infection and to improve patient outcomes (Table 49.13).

49.9.1 Preoperative Stage

As was discussed earlier in infection control, the prevention of infection during the preoperative period is very important. The prevention of VAD-specific infection begins even before surgical implantation of the device with appropriate patient selection, which is best performed by a multidisciplinary team of surgeons and cardiologists [40]. To improve the success of surgical outcome, previously developed VAD scoring systems and screening criteria may be particularly useful in this selection process [41].The screening process includes that physicians should consider optimizing modifiable risk factors for development of infection such as immune status [33], weight [34], and nutritional status [35]. Patients on immunosuppression for comorbid conditions should be thoroughly evaluated prior to surgery. Comorbid conditions that may themselves alter a patient's immune status such as hyperglycemia in diabetes should also be optimized and routinely monitored prior to proceeding for VAD to decrease infectious risk [33]. Nutritional status also contributes to a patient's overall immune status, and a thorough nutritional evaluation should be undertaken in any patient being considered for a VAD [35]. Assessment by a nutritionist with appropriate supplementation may be indicated in patients with signs and symptoms of nutritional imbalance prior to VAD implantation. Studies suggest that obesity and associated metabolic syndrome may predispose VAD recipients to device-related infections [34]. In nonemergency cases, physician should evaluate patient's habitus and consider weight reduction with the patient prior VAD implantation. In addition to intrinsic patient characteristics, a thorough evaluation for active or asymptomatic subclinical infection should also be undertaken in every candidate, including a chest X-ray; urine, blood, and sputum culture (where available); and cardiac echo and dental evaluation.

Next to the appropriate patient selection, the choice of an appropriate device design remains a very important determinant of device-related infections. As smaller continuous-flow left ventricular assist devices (CF-LVADs) have replaced bulkier pulsatile-flow devices, the rate of infections has decreased by as much as 50%, and survival rates for patients with end-stage heart failure have dramatically improved [39]. These new-generation devices are smaller in size, require less surgical dissection, are easier to implant in extra-abdominal position with no need of pump pocket and more durable compared with older-generation devices.

49.9.2 Intraoperative Stage

Different implantation techniques were developed, and the physician should make the right choice depending on patient's status and pump design to reduce the infection rate. Technique-related infection is lower in the minimally invasive implanted VAD-patients [42]. As described above, using minimally invasive implantation technique avoids sternotomy, big incisions, and pump pocket and results in reduced potential wound infection and instability of sternum, which also can induce infection [43, 44].

Pump-pocket infection can occur within the recess that is developed within the abdominal cavity to house the VAD device. The choice of pump design decides whether a pump pocket is needed. The recent studies show the use of a third-generation centrifugal LVAD implanted in the pericardial cavity eliminating the need for pump pocket (HeartWare® device, HeartWare International, Inc.) which has been associated with lower rates of device-related infection compared with historical controls [37]. In cases where a pump pocket is needed, the use of tissue layer or GORE-TEX between the device and the intrathoracic or intra-abdominal organs should be considered because this has two positive effects: first, it compartmentalizes the device from organs protecting the organs from injury due to the device and, second, it fills any cavities around the pump which may reduce pocket infections.

The PDL is among the most important channels for VAD-related infection. Proper tunneling and positioning are therefore imperative for infection prevention. To decrease the incidence of driveline infections, the distance between the exit site and pump pocket should be maximized, and the driveline tunnel should be as long as possible to prevent the transmission of infection from the exit site to the pocket itself. Therefore, surgical techniques such as increasing interfacial tunneling of the driveline may help reduce infections [36, 45]. Additionally, the velour portion of the PDL should not extend more than 1–2 cm outside the body [46, 47]. Some centers have even begun to implant the velour portion on the skin level or completely inside the skin (as opposed to the velour portion) also decreasing infections [48]. The driveline should begin at the VAD and be tunneled to the right or left upper abdominal quadrant where it should exit near the midclavicular line. Some centers use a right midaxillary subcostal exit; however, this has not yet been supported with any long-term studies.

Careful attention is taken to ensure that the driveline site is completely isolated from the chest tubes, other dressings, or scars. Immediately after tunneling, the percutaneous lead should be stabilized with occlusive dressing, a Hollister clip, Montgomery strap, or a Secutape to reduce trauma at the driveline exit site as independent predictor of driveline infection [14].

49.9.3 Postoperative Stage

Prevention and control of VAD-related infections are essential in the management of VAD patients. These strategies are not only to prevent infection during the pre- and intraoperative period but also in the postoperative period [49]. Prophylactic antibiotics are usually discontinued after 24–48 h postoperatively. Prolonged prophylactic systemic antibiotic use may actually be harmful to patients and significantly increase risk of subsequent antimicrobial resistance infection and *Clostridium difficile* infection. Also it is not recommended to use topical antibiotics such as silver sulfadiazine or polymyxin-neomycin-bacitracin due to the risk of tissue maceration [50]. Postoperative prevention of infection depends primarily on continuous wound care and prevention of catheter-related bloodstream infection and proper exit site management and reduction of patient-related risk factors such as immunosuppression, e.g., due to malnutrition, diabetes, and drugs.

In the early post-implantation period, patients should be closely monitored for signs and symptoms of VAD-specific, VAD-related, and non-VAD infections. The PDL-ES should be carefully managed postoperatively in order to prevent the introduction of pathogens. Dressings should be changed starting 24–48 h after surgery and earlier if the dressing becomes saturated with blood or drainage. Strict attention to driveline cleanliness is ensured from postoperative day zero. Although there are no current clinical trials delineating the best regimen for the care of driveline infections, exit-site care with a persistent antiseptic cleansing agent is recommended [50] . Dressings should be changed under sterile conditions using sterile technique with a sterile drape, and sterile gown and gloves as well as cap and mask. Using sterile gloves, the old dressing should be removed and discarded. At this point, a new set of sterile gloves should be put on, and the exit site should be inspected for signs of infection, tissue breakdown, and drainage. Deep probing should generally be avoided. Any drainage should be swabbed and sent for culture. The driveline wound should be cleaned with a sterile diluted hydrogen peroxide and covered with an antimicrobial occlusive dressing. Dressing changes should be performed once per day [49]. It is very essential to keep the driveline exit site dry. After completion of all these steps, the abdominal binder should be reapplied.

One of the most important factors in preventing the morbidity of infections is the use of various anchoring devices to help stabilize the driveline to minimize the risk of trauma to the exit site [2, 51]. Concomitantly, significant efforts are made to standardize postoperative patient education related to the driveline care. The patients should receive 2–3 weeks of in-house training of driveline care with family members before their discharge home. Following hospital discharge, patients and/or their caregivers should strictly adhere to proper sterile technique. It is imperative that good hygiene and sterile technique be exercised at all times. A driveline management pack should be given to the patient that contains all of the necessary equipment for a sterile dressing change. Education about driveline care includes topical management as well as careful attention to manipulation of the controller. Careful instructions are also provided to the patient in the event of trauma to the driveline. Dropping the controller and subsequent traction injury is one of the more common injuries to the driveline exit site in the immediate postoperative period. Patients should also receive monitored training on showering technique to ensure that the driveline remains protected. It is generally advised that patients avoid showering until after adequate tissue in-growth into the velour has occurred and until there is no drainage or signs of infection at the exit site. Even when sponge bathing, the exit site should be kept dry. Since VAD patients are susceptible to infections, they should avoid situations that could place them at an increased risk (contact with sick individuals, poor hygiene and living conditions, and so on) and notify their healthcare team immediately with any signs or symptoms suspicious for infection, along with routine assessment of nutritional status. In addition, driveline exit sites should be documented with photographs at each outpatient follow-up visit. If the patient has any concern regarding exit site or driveline management, they can call the clinic and are often able to send a representative photo to the outpatient VAD coordinator for review (Table 49.14).

Table 49.14 Percutaneous driveline exit site care

Step	Procedure	Example
1	1. Remove jewelry (e.g., rings, watches, etc.) 2. Wash hands with soap and water 3. Perform hand hygiene	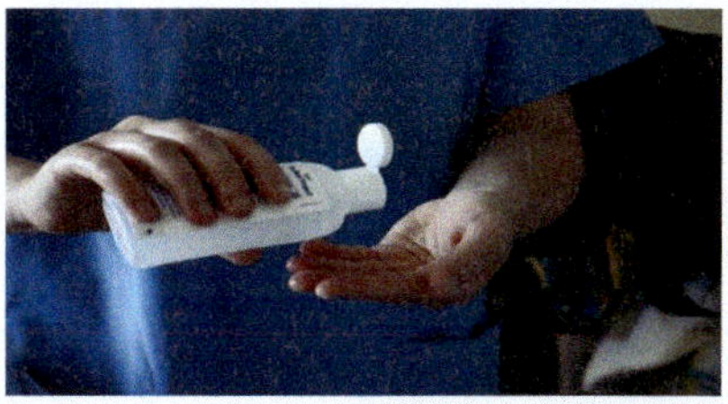
2	1. Clean the tray table with surface disinfection 2. Prepare sterile wound dressing pack 3. Prepare sterile materials (gauze 7 × 5 cm, with slit), a special gel support dressing (8 × 10 cm*), and a driveline fixer 4. Add antiseptic wound solution on the gauze *this may vary between countries	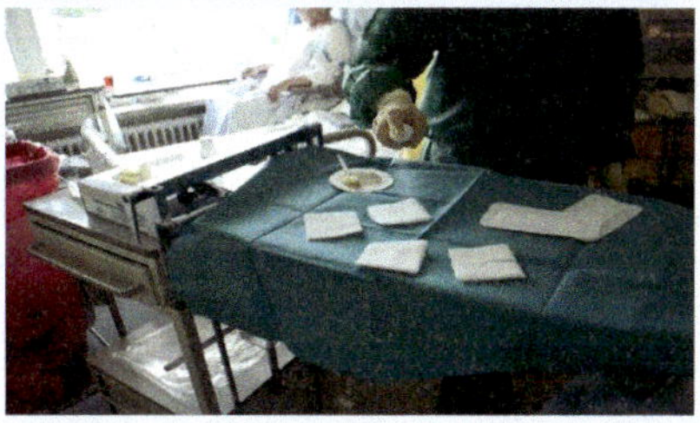
3	1. Don disposable gloves 2. Remove old dressing 3. Inspect exit site carefully for redness, swelling, pain, discharge, or odor 4. Remove and discard disposable gloves	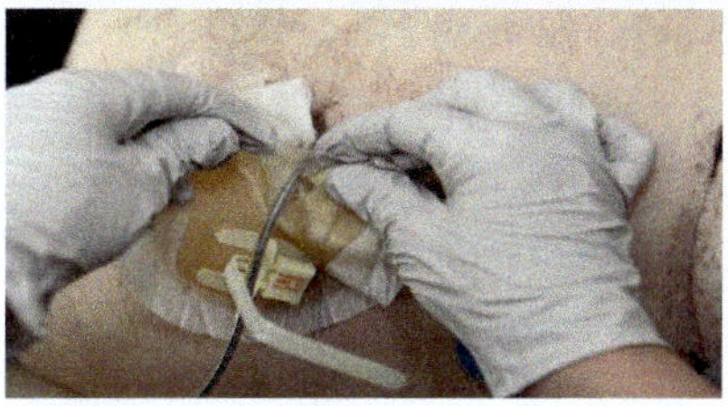
4	1. Perform hand hygiene 2. Don sterile gloves 3. Clean the exit site with gauze stroking from inside to outside 4. Let antiseptic dry	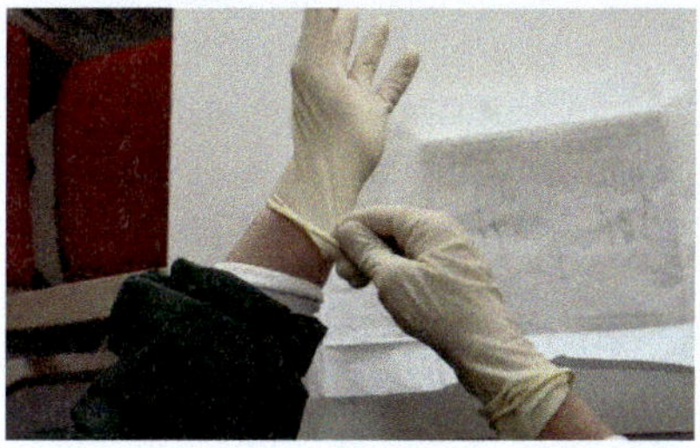
5	1. Clean the driveline with gauze by wiping from the exit site along the cable 2. Fix driveline by completely covering with slit gauze 3. Apply the special gel support dressing	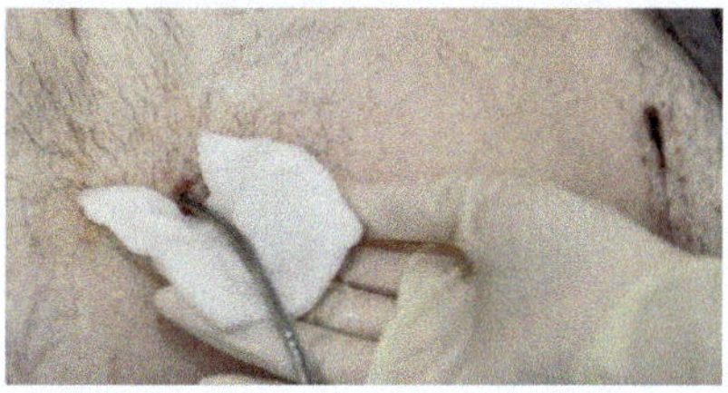
6	1. Put on the driveline fixer 2. Tighten fixer around driveline 3. Perform position control 4. Remove sterile gloves and perform hand hygiene	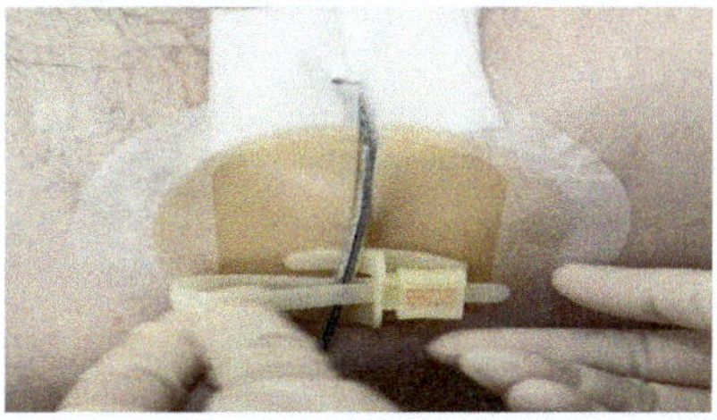

49.10 Treatment of PDL Infection

The majority of infections occur at the driveline exit site, beginning with a disruption or trauma to the barrier between the skin and driveline and sometimes spreading deeper. Once infections develop, they can be difficult to eradicate [52, 53] because VAD patients are subject to continuous hospital treatments and risk contamination with nosocomial resistance organisms [54–56].

When infection of the driveline site is suspected, prompt culture and Gram stain of the discharge from the exit site, along with blood cultures, should be obtained prior to the initiation of broad-spectrum antibiotic. The use of antibiotics in the outpatient setting should be judiciously guided by infection experts and the surgical team by phone consultation with each case subsequently discussed at MDT meetings to guide changes and choices of appropriate antibiotics or antifungals when needed in the same way as for inpatient management. In the case of superficial driveline infection, it is possible to treat this cohort on an outpatient basis using oral antibiotics. Treatment of superficial infections should include also aggressive wound care by increasing the frequency of dressing changes and reviewing dressing change protocols to ensure compliance and close monitoring. The PDL-ES and dressing should be kept clean and should be immobilized to prevent disruption of the area surrounding the driveline itself. For moderate infections, additional treatment may involve local debridement and weekly clinic visits. If the patient has signs of systemic infection such as fever or leukocytosis, inpatient treatment should be considered. If the infection appears to be deep, surgical drainage and incision of driveline site with driveline revision may be required to remove necrotic tissue and allow for faster wound healing. Several reports have demonstrated success with repositioning of the driveline when the infection is isolated to the exit site [57]. The surgical incision and debridement should always be done in the operating room under sterile conditions. After surgical debridement, negative-pressure wound therapy (NPWT, vacuum therapy) can be used to accelerate wound healing. NPWT is a therapeutic technique using a continuous vacuum dressing to promote wound healing and has been successfully applied in select driveline infection cases as an adjuvant to antibiotic therapy; however, the efficacy of this method remains to be tested in larger patient cohorts [58, 60]. Additional methods are to reject infected tissue and cover the driveline with well-perfused tissue such as rectus muscle or to use antimicrobial beads [61] and novel therapies such as Mepilex™ or Aquacel® dressing changes. If all of these fail, another measure to combat prolonged infection is to move the driveline into the peritoneal space, wherein a completely new exit site is created and the driveline covered with omentum.

In the case of recurrent driveline infections, long-term intravenous or oral antibiotics may be necessary to suppress and prevent recurrence of infection. Close consultation with infection experts is required to guide suppression therapy and treatment durations. While device exchange can be performed for severe cases, recurrences are common [53, 62]. However, for those patients who refused or may be unable to undergo pump exchange surgery, the only option may be wide debridement of the driveline and the use of local antibiotic beads and NPWT. These patients should also be placed on chronic suppressive antibiotic therapy. For patients stratified to destination therapy, the treatment options can be limited and may require lifelong continuous suppressive antibiotic therapy. Changing strategy and escalating patients to urgent heart transplant status may be a good option in VAD patients who have chronic infection.

49.10.1 Pump-Pocket Treatment

The initial treatment of a pump-pocket infection (PPI) is similar to those with a PDLI. Imaging typically demonstrates the presence of fluid surrounding the device when PPIs occur. Therefore, surgical drainage in combination with IV antibiotics is essential for the management of PPI [63]. If IV antibiotics and percutaneous or surgical drainage are unsuccessful and the patient continues to exhibit signs and symptoms of ongoing infection, a device pocket revision may be necessary. In this case, the infectious tissue should be debrided and three to five samples sent for Gram stain, KOH and Calcofluor white stain, bacterial and fungal culture, and broad-range PCR. The pump pocket and the surrounding tissue should be lavaged several times with saline. NPWT-assisted closure of a pocket wound may assist with wound healing after surgical incision and drainage and should be considered [58, 64]. The presence of Gram-negative bacteria or yeast can also require more invasive management and complete revision of the driveline tract or an exchange [65]. As an alternative therapy with less systemic side effects, the use of antibiotic-impregnated beads applied locally to the pump pocket should be considered in select cases [63]. After either percutaneous or surgical incision or drainage, aggressive wound care is critical to successful treatment of an infected VAD pocket. Patients should undergo sterile daily dressing changes and monitoring for signs of continued infection. Severe cases of pump-pocket or mediastinal infections with tissue defects may benefit from use of muscle or omental transposition flaps, although these procedures are associated with a high mortality [66, 67]. If all of these fail, another measure to combat pump-pocket infection is to exchange the full pump particularly in the presence of VAD-associated infective endocarditis [58, 59]. While there is no data to support any specific approach to therapy of VAD-associated infective endocarditis, clinical decision making for device exchange or explantation is generally based on the patient's overall status including, but not limited to, presence of sepsis, end-organ dysfunction, progressive cachexia, and/or septic emboli.

49.10.2 Pump and/or Cannula Treatment

In the case of pump and/or cannula infection, device replacement should be performed because this type of infection portends a poor prognosis. The principle of early rather than late replacement is to be preferred. If VAD replacement is not an option, then aggressive IV antibiotic therapy should be pursued and continued for a prolonged period of time. Many patients with persistent pump or cannula infection will ultimately require lifelong oral suppressive therapy. An infection expert should always be consulted to guide chronic antibiotic therapy. Selected VAD patients with chronic pump and/or cannula infection should be considered for urgent cardiac transplant listing. VAD patients with chronic infections can be successfully transplanted with subsequent eradication of their infection.

References

1. Kirklin James K et al (2015) Seventh INTERMACS annual report: 15,000 patients and counting. J Heart Lung Transplant 34(12):1495–1504
2. Hannan MM, Husain S, Mattner F, Danziger-Isakov L, Drew RJ, Corey GR, Schueler S, Holman WL, Lawler LP, Gordon SM, Mahon NG, Herre JM, Gould K, Montoya JG, Padera RF, Kormos RL, Conte JV, Mooney ML, International Society for Heart and Lung Transplantation (2011) Working formulation for the standardization of definitions of infections in patients using ventricular assist devices. J Heart Lung Transplant 30(4):375–384
3. Monkowski DH, Axelrod P, Fekete T, Hollander T, Furukawa S, Samuel R (2007) Infections associated with ventricular assist devices: epidemiology and effect on prognosis after transplantation. Transpl Infect Dis 9:114–120
4. Holman WL, Rayburn BK, McGiffin DC et al (2003) Infection in ventricular assist devices: prevention and treatment. Ann Thorac Surg 75:S48–S57
5. Baddour LM, Bettmann MA, Bolger AF et al (2003) Nonvalvular cardiovascular device-related infections. Circulation 108:2015–2031
6. Dembitsky WP, Tector AJ, Park S et al (2004) Left ventricular assist device performance with long-term circulatory support: lessons from the REMATCH trial. Ann Thorac Surg 78:2123–2129 (discussion 2129-30)
7. Matthews PC, Berendt AR, McNally MA, Byren I (2009) Diagnosis and management of prosthetic joint infection. BMJ 338:b1773
8. Li JS, Sexton DJ, Mick N et al (2000) Proposed modifications to the Duke criteria for the diagnosis of infective endocarditis. Clin Infect Dis 30:633–638
9. Sohail MR, Uslan DZ, Khan AH et al (2007) Management and outcome of permanent pacemaker and implantable cardioverter-defibrillator infections. J Am Coll Cardiol 49:1851–1859
10. Solomkin JS, Mazuski JE, Bradley JS et al (2010) Diagnosis and management of complicated intra-abdominal infection in adults and children: guidelines by the surgical infection society and the infectious diseases society of America. Clin Infect Dis 50:133–164
11. Mermel LA, Allon M, Bouza E et al (2009) Clinical practice guidelines for the diagnosis and management of intravascular catheter-related infection: 2009 update by the infectious diseases society of America. Clin Infect Dis 49:1–45
12. Stevens DL, Bisno AL, Chambers HF et al (2005) Practice guidelines for the diagnosis and management of skin and soft-tissue infections. Clin Infect Dis 41:1373–1406
13. Centres for Disease Control and Prevention. CDC/NHSN surveillance definition of healthcare-associated infection and criteria for specific types of infections in the acute care setting. http://www.cdc.gov/nhsn/PDFs/pscManual/17pscNosInfDef_current.pdf.
14. Zierer A, Melby SJ, Voeller RK et al (2007) Late-onset driveline infections: the Achilles' heel of prolonged left ventricular assist device support. Ann Thorac Surg 84:515–520

15. Restrepo CS, Martinez S, Lemos DF et al (2009) Imaging appearances of the sternum and sternoclavicular joints. Radiographics 29:839–859
16. Dell'Aquila AM et al (2016) Ann Thorac Surg 101(1):87–94
17. Poston RS, Husain S, Sorce D et al (2003) LVAD bloodstream infections: therapeutic rationale for transplantation after LVAD infection. J Heart Lung Transplant 22:914–921
18. Hill JA, Mokadam NA, Rakita RM (2014) Intracranial mycotic aneurysm associated with left ventricular assist device infection. Ann Thorac Surg 98(3):1088–1089
19. Coakley G, Mathews C, Field M et al (2006) BSR & BHPR, BOA, RCGP and BSAC guidelines for management of the hot swollen joint in adults. Rheumatology (Oxford) 45:1039–1041
20. Moran E, Byren I, Atkins BL (2010) The diagnosis and management of prosthetic joint infections. J Antimicrob Chemother 65(Suppl 3):iii45–iii54
21. Muller M, Morawietz L, Hasart O, Strube P, Perka C, Tohtz S (2008) Diagnosis of periprosthetic infection following total hip arthroplasty—evaluation of the diagnostic values of pre- and intraoperative parameters and the associated strategy to preoperatively select patients with a high probability of joint infection. J Orthop Surg Res 3:31
22. Klug D, Lacroix D, Savoye C et al (1997) Systemic infection related to endocarditis on pacemaker leads: clinical presentation and management. Circulation 95:2098–2107
23. Schuhmann MU, Ostrowski KR, Draper EJ et al (2005) The value of C-reactive protein in the management of shunt infections. J Neurosurg 103(3 suppl):223–230
24. Elliott TS, Foweraker J, Gould FK, Perry JD, Sandoe JA (2004) Guidelines for the antibiotic treatment of endocarditis in adults: report of the working party of the British society for antimicrobial chemotherapy. J Antimicrob Chemother 54:971–981
25. Carr CM, Jacob J, Park SJ, Karon BL, Williamson EE, Araoz PA (2010) CT of left ventricular assist devices. Radiographics 30:429–444
26. Roman CD, Habibian MR, Martin WH (2005) Identification of an infected left ventricular assist device after cardiac transplant by indium-111 WBC scintigraphy. Clin Nucl Med 30:16–17
27. Hannan MM, O'Sullivan KE, Higgins AM et al (2015) The combined impact of surgical team education and chlorhexidine 2% alcohol on the reduction of surgical site infection following cardiac surgery. Surg Infect (Larchmt) 16(6):799–805
28. Bratzler DW, Dellinger EP, Olsen KM et al (2013) Clinical practice guidelines for antimicrobial prophylaxis in surgery. Am J Health-Syst Pharm 70:195–283.29
29. Edwards FE, Engelman RM, Houck P et al (2006) The society of thoracic surgeons practice guideline series: antibiotic prophylaxis in cardiac surgery, part I: duration. Ann Thorac Surg 81:397–404.31
30. http://www.cdc.gov/nhsn/PDFs/pscManual/17psc NosInfDef_current.pdf
31. Husain S et al (2016) The 2015 international society for heart and lung transplantation guidelines for the management of fungal infections in mechanical circulatory support and cardiothoracic organ transplant recipients: executive summary. J Heart Lung Transplant 35(3):261–282
32. http://www.cdc.gov/nhsn/PDFs/pscManual/9pscSSI current.pdf
33. Uriel N, Naka Y, Colombo PC et al (2011) Improved diabetic control in advanced heart failure patients treated with left ventricular assist devices. Eur J Heart Fail 13(2):195–199
34. Raymond AL, Kfoury AG, Bishop CJ et al (2010) Obesity and left ventricular assist device driveline exit site infection. ASAIO J 56(1):57–60
35. Dang NC, Topkara VK, Kim BT, Lee BJ, Remoli R, Naka Y (2005) Nutritional status in patients on left ventricular assist device support. J Thorac Cardiovasc Surg 130(5):e3–e4
36. Fleissner F, Avsar M, Malehsa D, Strueber M, Haverich A, Schmitto JD (2013) Reduction of driveline infections through doubled driveline tunnelling of left ventricular assist devices. Artif Organs 37:102–107
37. Aaronson KD, Slaughter MS, McGee E et al (2010) Evaluation of the HeartWare® HVAD left ventricular assist device system for the treatment of advanced heart failure: results of the ADVANCE bridge to transplant trial. Circulation 122:2215–2226 (Abstract)
38. Topkara VK, Kondareddy S, Malik F et al (2010) Infectious complications in patients with left ventricular assist device: etiology and outcomes in the continuous-flow era. Ann Thorac Surg 90(4):1270–1277
39. Slaughter MS, Rogers JG, Milano CA et al (2009) Advanced heart failure treated with continuous-flow left ventricular assist device. N Engl J Med 361(23):2241–2251
40. Williams MR, Oz MC (2001) Indications and patient selection for mechanical ventricular assistance. Ann Thorac Surg 71(3 Suppl):S86–S91
41. Schaffer JM, Allen JG, Weiss ES et al (2009) Evaluation of risk indices in continuous-flow left ventricular assist device patients. Ann Thorac Surg 88(6):1889–1896
42. Rojas SV, Avsar M, Uribarri A, Hanke JS, Haverich A, Schmitto JD (2015) A new era of ventricular assist device surgery: less invasive procedures. Minerva Chir 70(1):63–68
43. Schmitto JD, Molitoris U, Haverich A, Strueber M (2012) Implantation of a centrifugal pump as a left ventricular assist device through a novel, minimized approach: upper hemisternotomy combined with anterolateral thoracotomy. J Thorac Cardiovasc Surg 143(2):511–513
44. Hanke JS, Rojas SV, Avsar M, Haverich A, Schmitto JD (2015) Minimally-invasive LVAD implantation: state of the art. Curr Cardiol Rev 11(3):246–251
45. Schibilsky D, Benk C, Haller C et al (2012) Double tunnel technique for the LVAD driveline: improved management regarding driveline infections. J Artif Organs 15(1):44–48
46. Chinn R, Dembitsky W, Eaton L, Chillcott S, Stahovich M, Rasmusson B, Pagani F (2005) Multicenter experience: Prevention and management of left ventricular assist device infections. ASAIO J 51(4):461–470 ISSN: 1058-2916

47. Slaughter MS, Pagani FD, Rogers JG, Miller LW, Sun B, Russell SD, Starling RC, Chen L, Boyle AJ, Chillcott S, Adamson RM, Blood MS, Camacho MT, Idrissi KA, Petty M, Sobieski M, Wright S, Myers TJ, Farrar DJ (2010) HeartMate II clinical investigators. (2010) clinical management of continuous-flow left ventricular assist devices in advanced heart failure. J Heart Lung Transplant 29(Suppl 4):S1–S39 ISSN: 1053-2498
48. Singh A, Russo MJ, Valeroso TB et al (2014) Modified HeartMate II driveline externalization technique significantly decreases incidence of infection and improves long-term survival. ASAIO J 60(6):613
49. Hieda M, Sata M, Seguchi O, Yanase M, Murata Y, Sato T, Sunami H, Nakajima S, Watanabe T, Hori Y et al (2014) Importance of early appropriate intervention including antibiotics and wound care for device-related infection in patients with left ventricular assist device. Transplant Proc 46:907–910
50. Feldman D, Pamboukian SV, Teuteberg JJ et al (2013) The 2013 international society for heart and lung transplantation guidelines for mechanical circulatory support: executive summary. J Heart Lung Transplant 32(2):157–187
51. Baronetto A, Centofanti P, Attisani M et al (2014) A simple device to secure ventricular assist device driveline and prevent exit-site infection. Interact Cardiovasc Thorac Surg 18(4):415–417
52. Sharma V, Deo SV, Stulak JM et al (2012) Driveline infections in left ventricular assist devices: implications for destination therapy. Ann Thorac Surg 94(5):1381–1386
53. Koval CE, Thuita L, Moazami N, Blackstone E (2014) Evolution and impact of drive-line infection in a large cohort of continuous-flow ventricular assist device recipients. J Heart Lung Transplant 33(11):1164–1172
54. Beiras-Fernandez A, Kur F, Kiefer S, Sodian R, Schmoeckel M, Weis M, Reichart B, Weis F (2009) Multidrug-resistant gram positive infections in patients with ventricular assist devices: the role of daptomycin. Transplant Proc 41(6):2589–2591
55. Leclercq R (2009) Epidemiological and resistance issues in multidrug-resistant staphylococci and enterococci. Clin Microbiol Infect 15(3):224–231
56. Howden BP (2005) Recognition and management of infections caused by vancomycin-intermediate *Staphylococcus aureus* (VISA) and heterogeneous VISA (hVISA). Intern Med J 35(Suppl 2):S136–S140
57. Walter V, Stock UA, Soriano-Romero M et al (2014) Eradication of a chronic wound and driveline infection after redo-LVAD implantation. J Cardiothorac Surg 9:63
58. Baradarian S, Stahovich M, Krause S, Adamson R, Dembitsky W (2006) Case series: clinical management of persistent mechanical assist device driveline drainage using vacuum-assisted closure therapy. ASAIO J 52(3):354–356
59. Garatti A, Giuseppe B, Russo CF, Marco O, Ettore V (2007) Drive-line exit-site infection in a patient with axial-flow pump support: successful management using vacuum-assisted therapy. J Heart Lung Transplant 26(9):956–959
60. Kawata M, Nishimura T, Hoshino Y, Kinoshita O, Hisagi M, Ando M, Morota T, Motomura N, Kyo S, Ono M (2011) Negative pressure wound therapy for left ventricular assist device-related mediastinitis: two case reports. J Artif Organs 14:159–162
61. Kretlow JD, Brown RH, Wolfswinkel EM et al (2014) Salvage of infected left ventricular assist device with antibiotic beads. Plast Reconstr Surg 133(1):28e–38e
62. Levy DT, Guo Y, Simkins J et al (2014) Left ventricular assist device exchange for persistent infection: a case series and review of the literature. Transpl Infect Dis 16(3):453–460
63. McKellar SH, Allred BD, Marks JD, Cowley CG, Classen DC, Gardner SC, Long JW (1999) Treatment of infected left ventricular assist device using antibiotic-impregnated beads. Ann Thorac Surg 67(2):554–555
64. Yuh DD, Albaugh M, Ullrich S, Conte JV (2005) Treatment of ventricular assist device driveline infection with vacuum-assisted closure system. Ann Thorac Surg 80:1493–1495
65. Tjan TD, Asfour B, Hammel D, Schmidt C, Scheld HH, Schmid C (2000) Wound complications after left ventricular assist device implantation. Ann Thorac Surg 70(2):538–541
66. Hutchinson OZ, Oz MC, Ascherman JA (2001) The use of muscle flaps to treat left ventricular assist device infections. Plast Reconstr Surg 107(2):364–373
67. Sajjadian A, Valerio IL, Acurturk O et al (2006) Omental transposition flap for salvage of ventricular assist devices. Plast Reconstr Surg 118(4):919–926

Acquired von Willebrand Syndrome

Anna L. Meyer and Ivan Netuka

© Springer International Publishing Switzerland 2017
A. Montalto et al. (eds.), *Mechanical Circulatory Support in End-Stage Heart Failure*,
DOI 10.1007/978-3-319-43383-7_50

The multicenter pilot trial for HeartMate II® (Thoratec, Pleasanton, CA) left ventricular assist systems in 2003 was noticeable, and the rate of bleeding complications was much higher than the rate of thromboembolic events [1]. Initial anticoagulation protocol was decreased; however patients still showed a dysfunction of the primary hemostasis thus showing very complex interactions irrespective of the level of anticoagulation only. Already back in 2005, the team of the Hannover Medical School diagnosed at the first time an acquired von Willebrand syndrome in a patient after continuous-flow left ventricular assist device (cfLVAD) implantation. The 23-year-old male patient was noticed with a nonstop bleeding from his earlobe after puncture for blood collection for blood sugar measurement. Subsequently, a lot of compelling data regarding the development of a von Willebrand syndrome after cfLVAD implantation have been published [2, 3].

50.1 Von Willebrand Factor

The von Willebrand factor (vWF) circulates in the blood as the largest soluble protein in the human body. VWF is a multimeric glycoprotein built from identical ≈250 kDa subunits into disulfide-linked multimers that may be >20,000 kDa [4], ◘ Fig. 50.1. The subunit contains among others binding sites for platelet glycoprotein receptors Ib and IIb/IIIa and collagen [5, 6]. Hereby, the vWF mediates platelet adhesion and aggregation at sites of vascular injury [7]. VWF also is a carrier protein for blood clotting factor VIII, and this interaction is required for normal factor VIII survival in the circulation [4]. So far, the role of the vWF is not completely explained in the regulation of angiogenesis [8].

VWF is synthetized in endothelial cells and megakaryocytes. After polymerization of monomers to gigantic linear multimers, these are packaged into

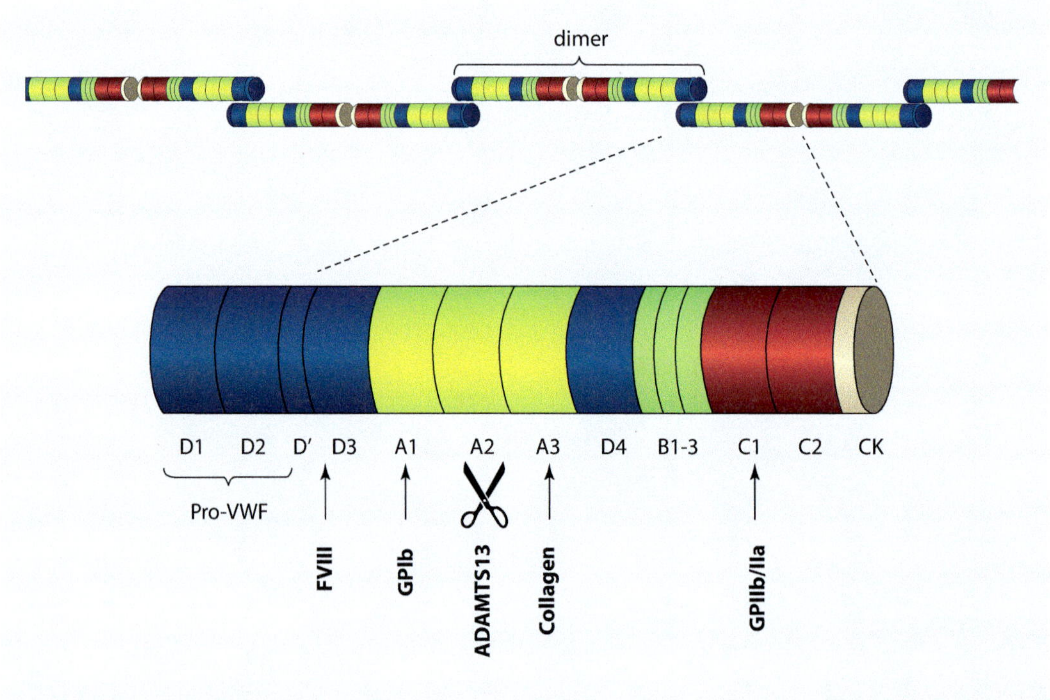

◘ **Fig. 50.1** Illustration of a von Willebrand factor with the subunits and specific functions (Reproduced with permission from De Meyer et al. [34])

secretory vesicles [5, 6]. Regulators of the secretion of the vWF are thrombin, histamine, epinephrine, and vasopressin [9].

50.2 Mechanism of AVWS Development

Under physiologic conditions, higher fluid shear stress elongates the vWF multimers from a globular state to an extended chain conformation, thereby exposing the cleavage site in the A2 domain to the metalloproteinase ADAMTS13 [10]. This causes a cleavage of high-molecular-weight multimers of vWF by this specific metalloprotease to shorter multimers [11]. This results in the presence of vWF multimers of different sizes that are characteristic of the circulating pool of vWF, ranging from a single up to 20 dimers (~10,000 kDa) [12].

However, in supraphysiologic shear stress, an excessive forced cleavage of the vWF by ADAMTS13 occurs. Originally, an interrelation between elevated shear stress and AVWS has been described in patients with severe aortic stenosis [13], referring to the clinical symptoms originally described as the Heyde's syndrome already in 1958 [14]. The same mechanism of action was further described in patients implanted with axial and centrifugal LVADs. The key feature of the acquired von Willebrand syndrome (AVWS) in patients with continuous-flow left ventricular assist devices (cfLVAD) is a lack of high-molecular-weight multimers (HMWM) of the vWF. Nevertheless, the reduction of HMWM is individual; therefore the percentage of remaining large multimers varies [2].

The larger multimers disappear significantly from the circulation by 2 h [15], ◘ Fig. 50.2. A recent publication documents in both in vitro and in vivo the vWF multimers variation even as early as within minutes of axial assist device operation [16]. The small vWF fragments have reduced hemostatic function [17]. Hereby, the primary hemostasis is disturbed [18]. The hemostatic potential of vWF multimers is governed by the multimer size [11]. These effects are explained

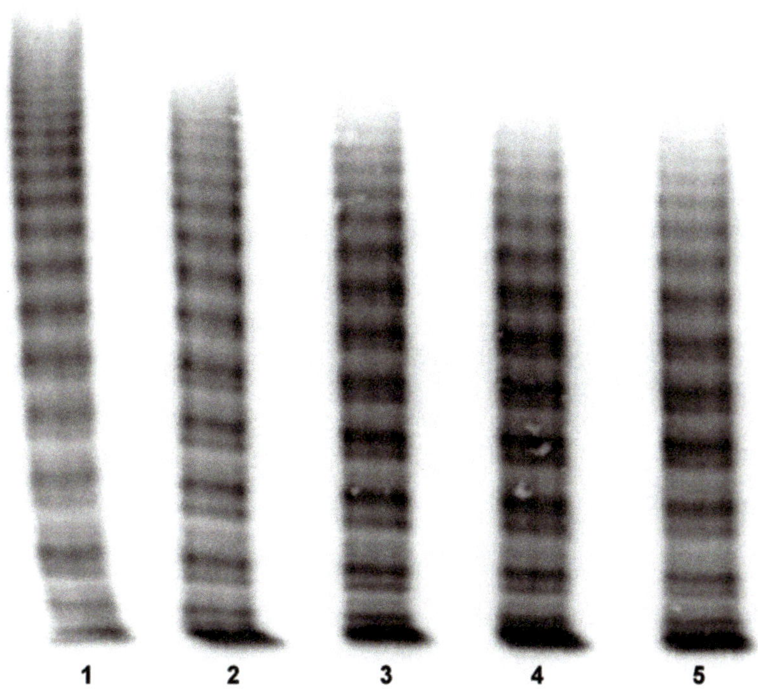

◘ **Fig. 50.2** Blood samples of a patient before **1** and after 2 h **2**, 6 h **3**, 12 h **4**, and 24 h **5** of LVAD implantation. After 2 h larger multimers disappear from the circulation **2**

by fewer binding sites of the smaller multimers and lower binding affinity between low vWF multimers and platelets, thus reducing both platelet adhesion and aggregation [19].

Patients exhibit increased bleeding from mucosa in the nasopharyngeal zone (epistaxis) and gastrointestinal tract (gastrointestinal bleeding) as well as prolonged bleeding after injury, during dental surgery, and prolonged menses and menorrhagia in women [11].

50.3 Diagnostic

A patient after cfLVAD implantation with an AVWS shows an abnormal platelet function test (PFA-100™). To diagnose an AVWS, the following tests are recommended: vWF antigen assays (vWF:Ag), vWF functional assays like vWF collagen-binding capacity (vWF:CB) and the functional ability of vWF to bind platelets (the ristocetin cofactor activity, vWF:RCo), and multimer analysis using electrophoretic separation. In AVWS a reduced vWF:RCo/vWF:Ag ratio of <0.6–0.7 indicates a selective loss or decrease in HMWM. A decrease in vWF:CB/vWF:Ag ratio may also indicate a loss or decrease in HMWM [20]. However, there is a general consensus to consider vWF multimer analysis as the gold standard for the detection of structural abnormalities in vWF indicating AVWS, since a decrease in HMWM may be the only way of detecting AVWS in patients with cardiovascular disorder who have normal vWF:RCo and vWF:CB and even normal vWF:RCo/vWF:Ag and vWF:CB/vWF:Ag ratios [3, 21].

50.4 Device-Type Association

In contrast to the first-generation volume-displacement assist devices [22], the acquired von Willebrand syndrome has been described in both axial and centrifugal long-term cfLVAD represented by the HeartMate II® and HVAD® (HeartWare® Ventricular Assist Device) with device-specific features [23]. Consequently, the same was confirmed with a use of continuous-flow pumps for short-term circulatory support in ECMO circuits or short-term cfLVAD as Impella® (Abiomed, Danvers, MA) or Levitronix® CentriMag® [24–26], and data shows a strong association with high prevalence of bleeding during the support and after transition to heart replacement therapy [24]. Preliminary analysis of HeartMate® III suggests also a certain reduction in HMWM; however degree and features of the device-specific phenomenon still need to be determined. Longitudinal analysis of HeartMate. 3 suggests lesser degree of HMWM degradation in contrast to HeartMate II; nonetheless potential implications need to be determined in larger clinical outcomes matched series [27].

50.5 Therapy

The coagulation disorder is reversible and thereby represents an indirect proof of the interplay between continuous-flow pumps and vWF. Patients after heart transplantation or LVAD explantation show reconstitution of its physiological pattern [28]. The vWF presence and function normalize during the first postoperative day after assist device explantation, thus supporting the observation of vWF turnover with a half-life of 12–20-h in vivo [29].

Current therapy still remains contentious. In a case report, the effect of human vWF/factor VIII concentrate was described [30]. In patients with aortic stenosis was described a reduced postoperative blood loss if desmopressin was administered during cardiac surgery (0.3 μg/kg in 100 mL of normal saline over 30 min) [31]. This therapeutic algorithm was adopted in some centers also for LVAD surgery.

Another approach is the inhibition of the metalloprotease ADAMTS13 which cleaves the vWF. In an in vitro study, the activity of ADAMTS13 could be reduced by the administration of doxycycline. Therefore, reduction of the smallest vWF degradation fragments was described. However, the dose was tenfold higher than the recommended daily allowance for antibiotic therapy [32].

A recent study also reported an up to 83±8% inhibition of the ADATMS13 activity with monoclonal antihuman anti-vWF antibodies that partially blocked vWF-ADAMTS13 interactions, but this is also an in vitro study and not certified for clinical use [33].

Ultimately, with current level of evidence, the only proven causal therapy of a vWF is the high rotational speed pump removal at a time of pump explantation, most commonly at a time of heart transplant.

References

1. Struber M, Sander K, Lahpor J, Ahn H, Litzler PY, Drakos SG, Musumeci F, Schlensak C, Friedrich I, Gustafsson R et al (2008) HeartMate II left ventricular assist device; early European experience. Eur J Cardiothorac Surg 34(2):289–294
2. Crow S, Chen D, Milano C, Thomas W, Joyce L, Piacentino V 3rd, Sharma R, Wu J, Arepally G, Bowles D et al (2010) Acquired von Willebrand syndrome in continuous-flow ventricular assist device recipients. Ann Thorac Surg 90(4):1263–1269 discussion 1269
3. Meyer AL, Malehsa D, Bara C, Budde U, Slaughter MS, Haverich A, Strueber M (2010) Acquired von Willebrand syndrome in patients with an axial flow left ventricular assist device. Circ Heart Fail 3(6):675–681
4. Sadler JE (1998) Biochemistry and genetics of von Willebrand factor. Annu Rev Biochem 67:395–424
5. Wagner DD, Fay PJ, Sporn LA, Sinha S, Lawrence SO, Marder VJ (1987) Divergent fates of von Willebrand factor and its propolypeptide (von Willebrand antigen II) after secretion from endothelial cells. Proc Natl Acad Sci U S A 84(7):1955–1959
6. Sadler JE (2009) Low von Willebrand factor: sometimes a risk factor and sometimes a disease. Hematology Am Soc Hematol Educ Program 106–112. doi:10.1182/asheducation-2009.1.106
7. Nichols WL, Rick ME, Ortel TL, Montgomery RR, Sadler JE, Yawn BP, James AH, Hultin MB, Manco-Johnson MJ, Weinstein M (2009) Clinical and laboratory diagnosis of von Willebrand disease: a synopsis of the 2008 NHLBI/NIH guidelines. Am J Hematol 84(6):366–370
8. Sami SS, Al-Araji SA, Ragunath K (2014) Review article: gastrointestinal angiodysplasia - pathogenesis, diagnosis and management. Aliment Pharmacol Ther 39(1):15–34
9. Rondaij MG, Bierings R, Kragt A, van Mourik JA, Voorberg J (2006) Dynamics and plasticity of Weibel-Palade bodies in endothelial cells. Arterioscler Thromb Vasc Biol 26(5):1002–1007
10. Siedlecki CA, Lestini BJ, Kottke-Marchant KK, Eppell SJ, Wilson DL, Marchant RE (1996) Shear-dependent changes in the three-dimensional structure of human von Willebrand factor. Blood 88(8):2939–2950
11. Stockschlaeder M, Schneppenheim R, Budde U (2014) Update on von Willebrand factor multimers: focus on high-molecular-weight multimers and their role in hemostasis. Blood Coagul Fibrinolysis 25(3):206–216
12. Tsai HM, Sussman II, Nagel RL (1994) Shear stress enhances the proteolysis of von Willebrand factor in normal plasma. Blood 83(8):2171–2179
13. Vincentelli A, Susen S, Le Tourneau T, Six I, Fabre O, Juthier F, Bauters A, Decoene C, Goudemand J, Prat A et al (2003) Acquired von Willebrand syndrome in aortic stenosis. N Engl J Med 349(4):343–349
14. Heyde E (1958) Gastrointestinal bleeding in aortic stenosis. N Engl J Med 259:196
15. Batlle J, Lopez-Fernandez MF, Lopez-Borrasca A, Lopez-Berges C, Dent JA, Berkowitz SD, Ruggeri ZM, Zimmerman TS (1987) Proteolytic degradation of von Willebrand factor after DDAVP administration in normal individuals. Blood 70(1):173–176
16. Van Belle E, Rauch A, Vincentelli A, Jeanpierre E, Legendre P, Juthier F, Hurt C, Banfi C, Rousse N, Godier A et al (2015) Von Willebrand factor as a biological sensor of blood flow to monitor percutaneous aortic valve interventions. Circ Res 116(7):1193–1201
17. Bartoli CR, Restle DJ, Zhang DM, Acker MA, Atluri P (2015) Pathologic von Willebrand factor degradation with a left ventricular assist device occurs via two distinct mechanisms: mechanical demolition and enzymatic cleavage. J Thorac Cardiovasc Surg 149(1):281–289
18. Chan CH, Pieper IL, Fleming S, Friedmann Y, Foster G, Hawkins K, Thornton CA, Kanamarlapudi V (2014) The effect of shear stress on the size, structure, and function of human von Willebrand factor. Artif Organs 38(9):741–750
19. Gralnick HR, Williams SB, Morisato DK (1981) Effect of multimeric structure of the factor VIII/von Willebrand factor protein on binding to platelets. Blood 58(2):387–397
20. Tiede A, Priesack J, Werwitzke S, Bohlmann K, Oortwijn B, Lenting P, Eisert R, Ganser A, Budde U (2008) Diagnostic workup of patients with acquired von Willebrand syndrome: a retrospective single-centre cohort study. J Thromb Haemost 6(4):569–576
21. Tiede A (2012) Diagnosis and treatment of acquired von Willebrand syndrome. Thromb Res 130(Suppl 2):S2–S6
22. Crow S, Milano C, Joyce L, Chen D, Arepally G, Bowles D, Thomas W, Ortiz NV (2010) Comparative analysis of von Willebrand factor profiles in pulsatile and continuous left ventricular assist device recipients. ASAIO J 56(5):441–445
23. Meyer AL, Malehsa D, Budde U, Bara C, Haverich A, Strueber M (2014) Acquired von Willebrand syndrome in patients with a centrifugal or axial continuous flow left ventricular assist device. JACC Heart Fail 2(2):141–145
24. Morrison KA, Jorde UP, Garan AR, Takayama H, Naka Y, Uriel N (2014) Acquired von Willebrand disease during CentriMag support is associated with high prevalence of bleeding during support and after transition to heart replacement therapy. ASAIO J 60(2):241–242
25. Kalbhenn J, Schmidt R, Nakamura L, Schelling J, Rosenfelder S, Zieger B (2015) Early diagnosis of acquired von Willebrand syndrome (AVWS) is elementary for clinical practice in patients treated with ECMO therapy. J Atheroscler Thromb 22(3):265–271

26. Davis ME, Haglund NA, Tricarico NM, Keebler ME, Maltais S (2014) Development of acquired von Willebrand syndrome during short-term micro axial pump support: implications for bleeding in a patient bridged to a long-term continuous-flow left ventricular assist device. ASAIO J 60(3):355–357
27. Netuka I, Kvasnička T, Kvasnička J, Hrachovinová I, Ivák P, Mareček F, Bílková J, Malíková I, Jančová M, Malý J et al (2016) Evaluation of von Willebrand factor with a fully magnetically levitated centrifugal continuous-flow left ventricular assist device in advanced heart failure. J Heart Lung Transplant 35(7):860–867
28. Uriel N, Pak SW, Jorde UP, Jude B, Susen S, Vincentelli A, Ennezat PV, Cappleman S, Naka Y, Mancini D (2010) Acquired von Willebrand syndrome after continuous-flow mechanical device support contributes to a high prevalence of bleeding during long-term support and at the time of transplantation. J Am Coll Cardiol 56(15): 1207–1213
29. Sadler JE (2003) Aortic stenosis, von Willebrand factor, and bleeding. N Engl J Med 349(4):323–325
30. Cushing M, Kawaguchi K, Friedman KD, Mark T (2012) Factor VIII/von Willebrand factor concentrate therapy for ventricular assist device-associated acquired von Willebrand disease. Transfusion 52(7):1535–1541
31. Steinlechner B, Zeidler P, Base E, Birkenberg B, Ankersmit HJ, Spannagl M, Quehenberger P, Hiesmayr M, Jilma B (2011) Patients with severe aortic valve stenosis and impaired platelet function benefit from preoperative desmopressin infusion. Ann Thorac Surg 91(5):1420–1426
32. Bartoli CR, Kang J, Restle DJ, Zhang DM, Shabahang C, Acker MA, Atluri P (2015) Inhibition of ADAMTS-13 by doxycycline reduces von Willebrand factor degradation during supraphysiological shear stress: therapeutic implications for left ventricular assist device-associated bleeding. JACC Heart Fail 3(11):860–869
33. Rauch A, Legendre P, Christophe OD, Goudemand J, van Belle E, Vincentelli A, Denis CV, Susen S, Lenting PJ (2014) Antibody-based prevention of von Willebrand factor degradation mediated by circulatory assist devices. Thromb Haemost 112(5): 1014–1023
34. De Meyer SF, Stoll G, Wagner DD, Kleinschnitz C (2012) von Willebrand factor: an emerging target in stroke therapy. Stroke 43(2):599–606

Concomitant Noncardiac Surgery During Mechanical Circulatory Support: Management of Therapy

Rachel A. Beaupré and Jeffrey A. Morgan

© Springer International Publishing Switzerland 2017
A. Montalto et al. (eds.), *Mechanical Circulatory Support in End-Stage Heart Failure*,
DOI 10.1007/978-3-319-43383-7_51

51.1 Introduction

As greater numbers of heart failure patients are given the option of mechanical circulatory support (MCS) as bridge-to-transplant therapy as well as destination therapy, physicians and practitioners across specialties will need to have working access to cursory knowledge of the physiology and anatomic placement of these cardiac devices. As this unique patient population experiences both enhanced length and quality of life, the incidence of patients on MCS who develop both acute and more slowly developing general surgical problems that require intervention will continue to rise. It is expected that over time this emphasis will shift from acute general surgical problems related to initial device placement to a greater proportion of outpatient and more traditional general surgical problems as both mechanical circulatory devices and care methods advance.

Thus it becomes necessary to establish protocols and models for inter-professional and inter-specialty communication and care systems to best and most comprehensively meet the needs of these patients. The general surgeon must possess a cursory knowledge of the pathophysiology, surgical placement of mechanical devices, and their unique operative challenges in order to adapt and formulate a therapeutic plan that addresses the need for innovation both to address intraoperative challenges and successfully accomplish the general surgical goals and minimize the instances of complications. The anesthesiologist must understand the cardiopulmonary pathophysiology and principles underlying the function of these devices in order to best develop an anesthetic care plan and prepare for effects of surgical manipulation and positioning and anticipate the unique needs of this patient population.

It is our hope that this chapter will serve as a guide to the unique general surgical issues faced by patients on mechanical circulatory support, strategies for patient management in the perioperative period, unique challenges posed by the patient on mechanical circulatory support, and the potential complications, outcomes, and effects of general surgical intervention in this growing patient population.

51.2 Preoperative Management

51.2.1 General Surgical Consultation for Patients with Mechanical Circulatory Support

General surgical issues that arise in the ventricular assist device (VAD) patient population can be broken down into early and late surgical issues. Early in the post-VAD implant period, most interventions consist of tracheostomy, wound infection, or thoracic procedures [1]. Most of the non-abdominal procedures are indicated for complications of VAD placement (thromboembolic or bleeding complications), whereas the need for abdominal intervention (other than GI bleeding) is often unrelated to VAD placement such as cholecystitis or appendicitis [2]. Therefore, understanding the time from implantation and the likely problems to be encountered is necessary for the consulting team as they initially approach the patient for assessment.

51.2.2 Selecting a Surgical Care Team

Coordinating care and choosing members of perioperative team and overall management strategy proves to be more challenging in this patient population over the more common general surgical patients. The potential for complications related not only to the general surgical procedure in and of itself but also the potential complications related to the device both from a surgical and intraoperative management perspective must be considered.

Several models of perioperative care have been utilized to provide support for patients undergoing noncardiac surgery. The necessity of having an LVAD technician present during the operation and the immediate availability of a cardiac surgeon should a complication or LVAD-related issue arise are essentials agreed upon across the literature. The presence of a specialized cardiac anesthesiologist or conducting the operation in a cardiac surgical suite has varied between described methods of care and appears to have no specific effects on overall patient outcomes [3–5].

It is the authors' opinion that admitting the patient to the heart failure unit staffed with nurses, clinicians, and other staff possessing expertise in the care of patients on mechanical circulatory support combined with the general surgical team overseeing the aspects specifically related to postoperative surgical management remains the best postoperative strategy for optimal patient recovery.

51.3 Anesthesia and Intraoperative Monitoring Considerations

The anesthesiologist, cardiac, or otherwise managing the patient on mechanical circulatory has a wide variety of monitoring options and techniques at their disposal that he or she must tailor to the individual needs of the patient and the specific nature of each noncardiac case.

The choice of vital monitoring formats has varied across the literature with physician preference, patient condition, and working experience with the LVAD patient population. In self-reported data, the routine use of invasive monitoring for noncardiac cases in LVAD patients was inversely associated with institutional volume and was reportedly used in up to 83% of the time for minor noncardiac surgical procedures in low-volume institutions (65% for high volume) and 50% reporting use of arterial catheters for blood pressure monitoring during endoscopic procedures [6]. However, since the VAD apparatus can provide data on cardiac output, it is possible to forgo invasive monitoring when appropriate for the individual. Ahmed et al. (2012) have shown in their series that it is possible to manage patients safely without routine central lines, Swan-Ganz catheters, and transesophageal echocardiography [7]. In a majority of cases, invasive arterial lines can be avoided for pressure monitoring provided pulsatility is preserved and external monitoring can be carried out [8]. This same principle applies to the use of pulse oximeter, which is sufficient for monitoring of oxygenation, though serial arterial blood gases can be used if there are concerns for its accuracy [1]. It is likely that in the absence of extensive comorbidities, the use of invasive monitoring is more closely associated with physician and staff familiarity with operatively managing patients on mechanical circulatory support and that incidence of its uses may decline as more widespread experiences with this patient population increase.

When initiating general anesthesia in this patient population, it is particularly important to take measures to ensure the peripheral effects of vasodilatory drugs, and mechanical ventilation does not interfere with proper VAD function. It is essential to maintain preload and support right ventricular function in the LVAD patient. Negative inotropic drugs should be used with caution, and the use of positive inotropes or selective pulmonary vasodilators may be employed if right ventricular dysfunction, signified by increasing central venous pressure in tandem with low cardiac output, is encountered [9, 10]. Routine use of prophylactic infusion of milrinone may be implemented to prevent dysfunction and guard against increases in the pulmonary vascular resistance according to physician preference [11]. Though conventional techniques are generally well tolerated and fluid requirements are not necessarily vastly different than the non-VAD patient in elective procedures, induction must proceed in a manner that supports the contractility of the right ventricle in the LVAD patient in order to maintain left-sided pump filling [10, 12, 13]. The possibility of preload reduction secondary to vasodilation combined with the negative effects of positive-pressure ventilation on venous return renders the need for adequate pre-procedural fluid optimization and appropriate tidal volume and PEEP settings essential to maintaining pump function as well as preserving pulsatility for external blood pressure monitoring [12–14]. In a similar manner, in axial-flow pump support reduction of increases in systemic vascular resistance and hypertension is advisable to guard against pump failure and poor perfusion [15]. These techniques can be used in combination or separately according to each patient's clinical scenario in order to best optimize intraoperative care and ensure the best possible patient outcome.

51.4 Operative Technique/Approach

Depending on the patient's particular surgical problem, type of device, and surgeon familiarity with conducting surgery in this unique patient population, the presence of mechanical circulatory support may or may not alter the surgical plan in regard to choosing the surgical approach, positioning, and other operative factors.

Secondary to the hemodynamics of LVAD devices, patient positioning can affect the filling pressures. The surgical and anesthesia teams should be well aware of the possibility for the development of position-dependent hypotension. Goldstein et al. (1995) note this complication with patients positioned in left lateral decubitus and remark that dobutamine therapy in an attempt to increase cardiac preload is counterproductive and worsened the development of hypotension; when fluid resuscitation was provided prior to induction, hemodynamic stability was achieved throughout the operative period in the subsequent cases eliminating the need for vasopressors or transfusion. As such, the patient's position and preoperative fluid balance must be taken into account in order to avoid intervention that can strain the heart and risk destabilizing pump mechanics.

Interestingly, despite the challenges that VADs pose for patient positioning, reported cases have shown that it is possible to safely conduct surgical procedures in the prone position. In one case, positioning was directed by the surgeon and perfusionist in order to avoid traction or excessive force on the driveline and other components and surgery proceeded uneventfully with the use of radial arterial line for pressure monitoring without the patient experiencing any hemodynamic instability [16]. Other cases, however, describe VAD patients experiencing decreases in right ventricular cardiac output due to the effects of positioning and low fluid status. It is thought that the compression of the RVOT by the outflow cannula led to the obstruction of flow in the first case, and both cases were remedied by patient response to fluid bolus [17]. Cases such as these demonstrate that with proper attention to detail and responsiveness to hemodynamic changes, VAD patients are able to tolerate a variety of positioning challenges.

When undertaking a laparoscopic approach, both the positioning of port sites in relation to the device and driveline and the potential consequences of pressurizing the abdomen must be taken into consideration. Insufflation may have significant effects on hemodynamic parameters such as cardiac preload. Second-generation LVADs are significantly dependent on preload, a cardiac parameter which may decrease with abdominal insufflation [14]. Insufflation should occur slowly with careful monitoring of the arterial blood pressure. Morgan et al. (2012) note that the typical positioning for laparoscopic procedures has the potential to exacerbate this aspect of pathophysiology by increasing upward pressure on the diaphragm and thereby decreasing venous return. In the series by Ahmed et al. (2012), patients undergoing laparoscopic procedures were insufflated to 10 mmHg and only increased to 12 mmHg in the event that better visualization was needed, no complications or adverse effects on cardiac function parameters at these pressures. Insufflation should commence slowly with caution and used in a manner that balances the optimization of surgical field of vision without destabilizing the patient's hemodynamic function.

When proceeding with a laparoscopic approach, in addition to ensuring careful insufflation, patient positioning, and cardiac parameter monitoring, one must also consider the appropriate placement of port sites. McKellar et al. (2012) describe this as the most common surgical modification and, in their series, most often necessitated by the need to avoid the device driveline, but also describe the need to place additional port sites in order to lyse prior surgical adhesions. For these reasons, the general or gynecologic surgeon unfamiliar with the LVAD patient may choose to pursue a traditional open approach as opposed to a laparoscopic one due to the uncertainty of LVAD positioning and potential for the said complications.

As technology progresses and greater proportion of patients with LVADs possess second- or even third-generation devices which have a smaller size of hardware implanted, it will become more feasible for laparoscopic procedures to be carried out more often and with less concern for interrupting hardware with more traditional port placement. Imaging technologies such as abdominal ultrasound may help guide the surgeon in choosing appropriate port site locations if concern for damaging or interrupting pump chambers and drivelines persists in the operating room [2–11]. Consultation with the cardiac surgeon responsible for implantation prior to surgery to discuss potential port sites may also be helpful [9]. Surgeons may choose to mark the abdomen in order to avoid the LVAD and driveline and avoid exposure of any of its components [18]. Successful laparoscopic Roux-en-Y in an LVAD patient without postoperative complications in order to help her become eligible for and receive heart transplantation has already been described in the literature [19] as well as in other patients with an implanted HeartMate II device [11] though certainly many more such examples are prevalent. Such laparoscopic bariatric surgery has also been undertaken complication-free in LVAD patients as an aid for ventricular recovery and eventual LVAD explantation [18]. Hoefnagel et al. (2012) comment that the positioning for gastric bypass in this manner may actually circumvent some of the aforementioned difficulties that laparoscopic surgery may pose in the VAD patient as the head-up positioning helps relieve pressure on the diaphragm. As such cases demonstrate its safety and feasibility, it is expected that the incidence of laparoscopic surgery in the LVAD-possessing patient will increase.

When conducting surgical planning for open abdominal operations, it is of utmost importance to consider surgical incision sites as well as working planes in relationship to the presence and positioning of both the pump pocket and the driveline course. It may become necessary to alter incision direction or placement in order to preserve and avoid any complications to these sites and precious equipment. For example, Garatti et al. (2009) remark that cholecystectomy and hepatic resection procedures can be performed through a right subcostal incision. However, McKellar et al. (2012) describe an instance of altering incision placement and/or direction for both an exploratory laparotomy and cholecystitis patient in order to avoid the drivelines. In abdominal procedures such as colectomy/ileostomy creations, it may be necessary to opt for a low transverse incision as opposed to a midline in order to avoid device components which can pose surgical difficulties and possibly lead to suboptimal ostomy placements [21]. Incision placement and surgical approach may vary widely depending on the present surgical need and anatomic placement of the device and driveline. The need for alterations in the choice of surgical incision site may be even more pronounced in patients with first-generation mechanical circulatory support devices to the nature of their larger size and thus larger device pockets and drivelines [15]. The noncardiac surgeon thus must plan not only the best surgical approach to access the underlying pathology but also consider alternations to preserve the integrity of the mechanical circulatory device.

The presence of the device and its pocket can present a specific challenge for left-sided surgical procedures. In order to gain access to the spleen, left kidney, or other structures on the left side, it may be necessary to pursue a lateral and/or lumbar approach to avoid disruption of the device pocket [20]. Alteration of incision placement may also be influenced by the presence of the VAD in association with other implantable devices such as defibrillators or previously placed surgical mesh [21]. Therefore, careful pre-surgical planning must be undertaken to optimize surgical exposure while maintaining the integrity and position of both the VAD device and any other devices that patients may possess.

51.5 Morbidity and Mortality in Comparison with LVAD Patients with No Concomitant Noncardiac Surgery

When considering the need for general surgery intervention in the LVAD patient, the importance of accurate prognostication and future outcomes that correspond with therapeutic goals before the advent of the general surgical intervention becomes vividly apparent in the need to accurately counsel patients on MCS as well as their families and support system.

51.6 Successful Bridge to Transplant

One important factor in the long care of this patient population is determining whether prior therapeutic goals, specifically bridge-to-transplant therapy goals, are attainable at even rates with the LVAD patient who requires no general surgical interventions.

Most studies indicate that patients undergoing noncardiac surgery are able to undergo a successful bridge-to-heart transplantation at the same rate as their peers.

Schmid et al. (2001), Garatti et al. (2009), and Stehlik et al. (2009) have reported successful forwarding to transplantation of 50%, 54.5%, and 72% of patients in their studies, rates which are concordant with the LVAD population who did not undergo any noncardiac surgical procedures. Interestingly, all procedures in the Schmid et al. (2001) study, excepting one, were conducted on an urgent or emergent basis.

Arnaoutakis et al. (2014) report that 30% of their study patients underwent orthotopic heart transplantation through the duration of their study, noting that acute care surgery patients were less likely than their counterparts to receive transplant; however, this difference was not significant in patients with a HeartMate II device. All three of the patients with a Novacor device who underwent noncardiac abdominal surgery in Eckhauser et al. (2006) reports eventually received heart transplantation.

In addition, it appears that even after encountering surgical complications did not implicate a worse long-term prognosis. In a study comparing the outcomes for patients with and without surgical complications, 63% of patients were forwarded to heart transplant as compared to 33% of their counterparts whose recovery was uneventful [20]. Thus, patients who have undergone general surgical intervention seem to have no further complications after the need arose for such intervention that would preclude them from progressing along the same therapeutic course as other VAD patients and are able to undergo heart transplantation at similar rates.

51.7 Perioperative Mortality

Data regarding the perioperative mortality of LVAD patients undergoing noncardiac surgical procedures indicates that such patients fair as well as their peers who have not undergone such procedures. Both Morgan et al. (2012) and Brown et al. (2009) report no significant difference in 1-year survival between these patient populations. Stehlik et al. (2009) conclude that the difference in survival for patients on the destination therapy pathway was no different from their peers who required no general surgical intervention, and at the time of the study, conclusion had been living an average of another year [22]. Patients had an operative mortality of 0% and 12% 30-day mortality. Taghavi et al. (2014) had low perioperative mortality of 6.2% [23]. An additional study demonstrated a 30-day mortality rate of 10%, the causes for which were cerebral hemorrhage and multiorgan failure unrelated to the noncardiac surgical procedures undertaken [17]. Ahmed et al. (2012) also demonstrated the safety of NCS in LVAD patients in their study which included patients on destination therapy. After surgery most patients are able to be extubated in the operating suite, and greater than 50% recover in the PACU as opposed to the ICU environment [4–6]. This reflects that the operative risk for patients with an LVAD device is not significantly high to preclude general surgical intervention.

Mortality and morbidity can vary significantly depending on patient status and comorbidities preoperatively. The need for certain surgical procedures is likely to correlate to the severity of the patient's condition and therefore reflects a different prognostic class compared to peers whose interventions are less likely to reflect poor preoperative condition. These differences become evident when examining the data comparing patients undergoing elective vs. emergent surgical intervention.

Whether the surgery was performed on an emergent basis contributes to patient mortality and quality of life. Arnaoutakis et al. (2014) remark that the need for tracheostomy was associated with higher 1-year mortality and thus a lower likelihood for receiving heart transplantation. This should come as no surprise as the need for tracheostomy is generally associated with poorer patient outcomes due to its reflection of the severity of patient condition in the overall general surgical population itself. Among HeartMate II patients receiving destination therapy, there was a 10% 30-day mortality; however, 50% of these procedures were emergent neurosurgical procedures for intracranial hemorrhage, and the other 50% consisted of emergent abdominal procedures; excluding these six patients, the average lifespan after noncardiac surgery was 448 days with over 54% of patients continuing to survive for greater than 2 years [8].

This is also dependent upon the given context in which the need for surgical intervention arose. Patients who required emergent intervention after VAD implant have worse outcomes than patients who were later admitted with a less immediate surgical need [2]. In addition, earlier need for intervention tends to reflect a poorer, less optimized preoperative patient condition.

When taking all patients into consideration, Arnaoutakis et al. (2014) show that cumulative survival for LVAD patients undergoing general surgical procedures was equivalent, thus leading to the conclusion that general surgery intervention is not a tool to be dismissed or disregarded simply due to the complexity of this patient population. Similarly, there was no difference in the time between LVAD placement and patient death between those undergoing NCS and those who had experienced no such need for intervention [2]. Schmid et al. (2001) found no difference in prognosis for the patients undergoing noncardiac operation nor in the patients experiencing postoperative complications.

51.8 Perioperative Management of Anticoagulation

Deciding on a management strategy for perioperative anticoagulation therapy requires considering all pertinent options to select a method that will best balance the risk of bleeding against the risk for potential thromboembolic device-related events.

As devices require the persistent use of anticoagulation to guard against thromboembolic complications, the decision of how to best proceed with the cessation, or reversal of, Coumadin and whether to bridge with heparin and/or continue with antiplatelet therapy.

Optimizing anticoagulation strategy is imperative in guarding against the event of surgical bleeding and essential to the goal of avoiding transfusion whenever possible and in the patient's best interest. In the case of need for emergent or urgent surgical intervention, the traditional approach of reversing warfarin's effects via the administration of vitamin K and FFP is tolerated in this patient population. Continuous-flow circulatory support devices are less likely to cause a thromboembolic event with short-term subtherapeutic INR levels due to the constant movement and circulation of blood through the device which limits the potential for stagnation and therefore clot formation. Stehlik et al. (2009) found that the risk for postoperative bleeding was no worse in the group of patients who had previously been anticoagulated and required either tapering and substitution with heparin or emergent reversal.

In contrast to the standard protocol for immediate anticoagulation reversal in the need for emergent or urgent surgical, a variety of management approaches have been used in the perioperative period for non-emergent or elective procedures.

In the case series reported by Morgan et al. (2012), no transfusions were required for procedures with aspirin as the sole anticoagulant on board or for patients whose warfarin was bridged with heparin therapy preoperatively with or without the use of aspirin. However, bleeding which required transfusion did occur in all patients who were on both warfarin and aspirin preoperatively. Chacon et al. (2014) attribute the low rate of transfusions (15%) to be due to the preoperative clinical optimization and fluid-management strategies. Transfusion was required in 90.9% of patients in the Garatti et al. (2009) study in the first 24 h postoperatively. In Brown et al. (2009) study, 48% of patients required transfusion. Among destination therapy patients, 38% of patients required transfusion in Bhat et al. (2013) patient series, 38% of whom were undergoing gastrointestinal procedures, and all transfusions were due to intraoperative blood loss. These differences reflect the preoperative INR values, whether full reversal of anticoagulation was possible prior to emergent surgery, and the generation of devices found in these patients. Patients with first-generation/pulsatile devices are more likely to require blood transfusion in the perioperative period as the hemodynamics do not allow for full reversal of anticoagulation due to the increased risk for thromboembolic complications as compared to the newer continuous-flow devices in which anticoagulation can be safely interrupted for short periods of time without causing significant risk for said complications.

51.9 Surgical Complications

Overall, the most common surgical complications encountered in noncardiac operations are intraoperative and postoperative bleeding and the need for transfusions. Stehlik et al. (2009) note that bleeding complications were more frequently encountered in abdominal procedures and postulate that the VAD weight and function leads to increased intra-abdominal pressure and motion in the surgically manipulated areas. McKellar et al. (2012) noted that these complications were more common in patients possessing first-generation VADs and that the decreased size of second-generation devices may have contributed to the decreased number of complications seen in this specific subset of LVAD patients.

In a series of 63 noncardiac surgeries in Heart Mate II patients, only one complication other than bleeding was encountered – three episodes of ventricular tachycardia were successfully reversed with external defibrillation during cranial hematoma evacuation [8]. Other complications to be avoided include the possibility for electrocautery interference with the VAD or other implanted devices which could trigger changes in output or cause arrhythmias [10, 11]. Proper grounding should be ensured to avoid such interference and arrhythmia.

The potential for postoperative surgical infections necessitates a strict adherence to protocols that preserve sterility of the operating environment and proper selection of antibiotic coverage. The most common surgical site infections in LVAD population are due to methicillin-resistant *Staphylococcus aureus* and *Pseudomonas aeruginosa* (Topkara). With proper coverage, infectious complications are similar to the risk of the general VAD population [2]. Therefore, preoperative antibiotic prophylaxis should be certain to cover for these organisms as well as other potential sources of nosocomial infectious agents to ensure patients are safeguarded from infectious agents.

51.10 Conclusion

The proliferation, availability, and advancements made in the area of mechanical circulatory support continue to increase the number of patients who are eligible for assist device placement. The enhancements made to patient quality of life and lengthened lifespan create clinical scenarios in which patients on support require not only acute but also later occurring general surgical presentations. Increased collaboration between both surgical and nonsurgical physicians and medical staff along with greater awareness of assist device physiology and anatomy, along with surgical and management strategies, becomes ever important in this evolving patient care environment. The anesthesiologists must be aware of the importance of hemodynamic monitoring, patient positioning, and a strong knowledge of troubleshooting interventional techniques for this patient population in a noncardiac procedure. The general surgical physicians and staff must take care in developing surgical strategies that maximize the success of operation while minimizing manipulation and sources of infection for the device, pump, and drivelines of the support system. They must also remain vigilant in guarding against unique post-surgical complications with additional awareness of anticoagulation strategies. Counseling patients will require expressing the potential effects of noncardiac surgical procedures on patient mortality, morbidity, potential for future cardiac transplantation, and any effect on long-term prognosis. This chapter has outlined these issues and provided a basis for such understanding, serving as a springboard into deepening individual physician knowledge of this particular subset of patients on mechanical circulatory support.

References

1. Slininger KA, Haddadin AS, Mangi AA (2013) Perioperative management of patients with left ventricular assist devices undergoing noncardiac surgery. J Cardiothorac Vasc Anesth 27(4):752–759. doi: 10.1053/j.jvca.2012.09.022. Epub 2013 Jan 17. Review. PubMed PMID: 23332965
2. Brown JB, Hallinan WM, Massey HT, Bankey PE, Cheng JD, Stassen NA, Sangosanya AT, Gestring ML (2009) Does the need for noncardiac surgery during ventricular assist device therapy impact clinical outcome? Surgery 146(4):627–633; discussion 633-4. doi: 10.1016/j.surg.2009.06.033. PubMed PMID: 19789021
3. Arnaoutakis GJ, Bittle GJ, Allen JG, Weiss ES, Alejo J, Baumgartner WA, Shah AS, Wolfgang CL, Efron DT, Conte JV (2014) General and acute care surgical procedures in patients with left ventricular assist devices. World J Surg 38(4):765–773. doi: 10.1007/s00268-013-2403-0. PubMed PMID: 24357244
4. Barbara DW, Wetzel DR, Pulido JN, Pershing BS, Park SJ, Stulak JM, Zietlow SP, Morris DS, Boilson BA, Mauermann WJ (2013) The perioperative management of patients with left ventricular assist devices undergoing noncardiac surgery. Mayo Clin Proc 88(7):674–682. doi: 10.1016/j.mayocp.2013.03.019. PubMed PMID: 23809318
5. Morgan JA, Paone G, Nemeh HW, Henry SE, Gerlach B, Williams CT, Lanfear DE, Tita C, Brewer RJ (2012) Noncardiac surgery in patients on long-term left ventricular assist device support. J Heart Lung Transplant 31(7):757–763. doi: 10.1016/j.healun.2012.02.023. Epub 2012 Mar 14. PubMed PMID: 22425233
6. Sheu R, Joshi B, High K, Thinh Pham D, Ferreira R, Cobey F (2015) Perioperative management of patients with left ventricular assist devices undergoing noncardiac procedures: a survey of current practices. J Cardiothorac Vasc Anesth 29(1):17–26. doi: 10.1053/j.jvca.2014.07.001. Epub 2014 Nov 11. PubMed PMID: 25440639

7. Ahmed M, Le H, Aranda JM Jr, Klodell CT et al (2012) Elective noncardiac surgery in patients with left ventricular assist devices. J Card Surg 27(5):639–642. doi: 10.1111/j.1540-8191.2012.01515.x. PubMed PMID: 22978844
8. Bhat G, Kumar S, Aggarwal A, Pauwaa S, Rossell G, Kurien S, Kumar A, Pappas PS, Tatooles A (2012) Experience with noncardiac surgery in destination therapy left ventricular assist devices patients. ASAIO J 58(4):396–401. doi: 10.1097/MAT.0b013e31825b8d36. PubMed PMID: 22713727
9. Kartha V, Gomez W, Wu B, Tremper K (2008) Laparoscopic cholecystectomy in a patient with an implantable left ventricular assist device. Br J Anaesth 100(5):652–655. doi: 10.1093/bja/aen052. Epub 2008 Mar 15. PubMed PMID: 18344554
10. Goldstein DJ, Mullis SL, Delphin ES, El-Amir N, Ashton RC Jr, Gardocki M, Jordan DA, Catanese KA, Levin HR, Rose EA et al (1995) Noncardiac surgery in long-term implantable left ventricular assist-device recipients. Ann Surg 222(2):203–207. PubMed PMID: 7639586; PubMed Central PMCID: PMC1234779
11. Hoefnagel AL, Pasternak R, Curle AE, Eaton MP (2012) Laparoscopic gastric bypass in a patient with an implanted left ventricular assist device. J Cardiothorac Vasc Anesth 26(5):880–882. doi: 10.1053/j.jvca.2011.02.012. Epub 2011 May 4. PubMed PMID: 21546270
12. Ficke DJ, Lee J, Chaney MA, Bas H, Vidal-Melo MF, Stone ME (2010) Case 6-2010: noncardiac surgery in patients with a left ventricular assist device. J Cardiothorac Vasc Anesth 24(6):1002–1009. doi: 10.1053/j.jvca.2010.09.005.PubMed PMID: 21109156
13. Votapka TV, Pennington DG, McBride LR, Kaminski DL, Andrus CH, Swartz MT (1994) Noncardiac operations in patients supported with mechanical circulatory support devices. J Am Coll Surg 179(3):318–320. PubMed PMID: 8069428
14. McKellar SH, Morris DS, Mauermann WJ, Park SJ, Zietlow SP (2012) Evolution of general surgical problems in patients with left ventricular assist devices.Surgery 2012;152(5):896–902. doi: 10.1016/j.surg.2012.03.005. Epub 2012 May 8. PubMed PMID: 22575878
15. Garatti A, Bruschi G, Colombo T, Russo C, Milazzo F, Catena E, Lanfranconi M, Vitali E (2009) Noncardiac surgical procedures in patient supported with long-term implantable left ventricular assist device. Am J Surg 197(6):710–714. doi: 10.1016/j.amjsurg.2008.05.009. Epub 2008 Oct 16. PubMed PMID: 18926514
16. Connors CW, Poltak JM, Christie AA (2012) Noncardiac surgery in the prone position in patients with ventricular assist devices. J Cardiothorac Vasc Anesth 26(1):e6–e7. doi: 10.1053/j.jvca.2011.09.023. Epub 2011 Nov 17. PubMed PMID: 22100212
17. Chacon MM, Hattrup EA, Shillcutt SK (2014) Perioperative management of two patients with left ventricular assist devices presenting for noncardiac surgery in the prone position. A Case Rep 2(6):70–73. doi:10.1213/XAA.0000000000000002. PubMed PMID: 25611544
18. Morrow EH, Pellegrini CA, Mokadam NA, Khandelwal S (2014) Laparoscopic gastric bypass during left ventricular assist device support and ventricular recovery. J Heart Lung Transplant 33(8):870–871. doi: 10.1016/j.healun.2014.05.017. Epub 2014 Jun 4. PubMed PMID: 25063533
19. DeNino WF, Peura JL, Toole JM (2013) Orthotopic heart transplantation after left ventricular assist device implantation and laparoscopic Roux-en-Y gastric bypass. J Heart Lung Transplant 32(3):377–378. doi: 10.1016/j.healun.2012.11.032. Epub 2013 Jan 2. PubMed PMID: 23290460
20. Schmid C, Wilhelm M, Dietl KH, Schmid C, Hammel D, Scheld HH et al (2001) Noncardiac surgery in patients with left ventricular assist devices. Surgery 129(4):440–444. PubMed PMID: 11283535
21. Eckhauser AE, Melvin WV, Sharp KW (2006) Management of general surgical problems in patients with left ventricular assist devices. Am Surg 72(2):158–161. PubMed PMID: 16536248
22. Stehlik J, Nelson DM, Kfoury AG, Reid BB, Clayson SE, Nelson KE, Christensen BJ, Renlund DG, Movsesian MA, Cowley CG, Smith HK, Rasmusson BY, Long JW (2009) Outcome of noncardiac surgery in patients with ventricular assist devices. Am J Cardiol 103(5):709–712. doi: 10.1016/j.amjcard.2008.11.021. Epub 2009 Jan 15. PubMed PMID: 19231338
23. Taghavi S, Beyer C, Vora H, Jayarajan SN, Toyoda Y, Dujon J, Sjoholm LO, Pathak A, Santora TA, Goldberg AJ, Rappold JF (2014) Noncardiac surgery in patients on mechanical circulatory support. ASAIO J 60(6):670–674. doi: 10.1097/MAT.0000000000000140. PubMed PMID: 25232769

Miniaturization and Future Technologies

Contents

Novel HeartMate Cardiac Assist Systems (Thoratec)

Edward J. Burke and Christopher Parker

© Springer International Publishing Switzerland 2017
A. Montalto et al. (eds.), *Mechanical Circulatory Support in End-Stage Heart Failure*,
DOI 10.1007/978-3-319-43383-7_52

52.1 Introduction

Recent advances in mechanical circulatory support technology have escalated the use of ventricular assist devices (VADs) for treating a broad range of patients with severe heart failure [1, 2]. Current devices range from small, percutaneously inserted pumps for short-term use to durable left ventricular assist devices (LVADs) that support patients for a few months to many years. Innovations in blood pump technology and today's sophisticated acute cardiac care are helping more patients to survive major cardiac events and to extend survival for those with advanced-stage chronic heart failure [3]. Future designs of mechanical support technology seek a better overall performance profile to achieve lower morbidity with enhanced survival. New HeartMate technologies (St. Jude Medical, Inc., St. Paul, MN) are designed to meet these goals and are currently being tested in worldwide clinical trials.

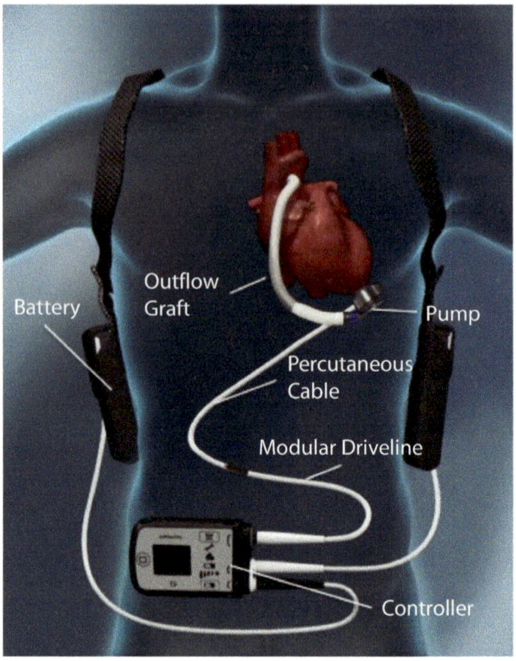

Fig. 52.1 The HeartMate III LVAS implanted and external components

52.2 HeartMate III Left Ventricular Assist System

The HeartMate III left ventricular assist system (LVAS) features a centrifugal flow pump that is designed to optimize hemocompatibility and reduce related adverse events. The miniaturized pump has a number of features to enhance surgical implantation and produce fewer effects on blood components [4, 5]. A fully magnetically levitated rotor (Full MagLev) with a wide blood flow gaps, a textured blood-contacting surfaces, and an artificial pulse are unique characteristics of the HeartMate III LVAS. These design features are intended to eliminate wear of the single moving component, reduce heat within the pump, lower shear stress on blood components, reduce thrombogenicity within the pump, and provide pulsatile flow for optimizing hemodynamics.

The implanted components of the HeartMate III system include the pump with 20 mm inflow cannula, a 14 mm sealed outflow graft with bend relief, and a modular percutaneous driveline. The electronics and software necessary to control the motor drive and levitation are integrated into the implanted motor. When implanted, the HeartMate III pump is positioned at the apex of the heart, with its integral inflow conduit inserted into the left ventricle (Fig. 52.1). The inflow conduit is secured in place with a low-profile, quick-connect apical cuff and titanium-locking ring. The outflow graft is anastomosed to the ascending aorta, and the percutaneous driveline is tunneled through the subcutaneous tissue of the abdomen to an exit site on either side of the abdomen. The external controller receives power from batteries or AC power and provides monitoring and control of the implanted pump. With the exception of the system controller, all external components are the same as for the HeartMate II LVAS.

The Full MagLev rotor eliminates the need for fluid or mechanical bearings, thereby avoiding wear of the single moving component. A single stator with back-iron poles, copper coils, and position sensors controls the rotation and levitation of the rotor. The radial position and rotational speed of the rotor are actively and independently controlled by measuring the position of a permanent magnet in the rotor and controlling the current in the drive and levitation coils. The attraction of the rotor's permanent magnets to the iron poles passively resists movement of the rotor in the axial direction. There are relatively large blood flow gaps between the rotor and the housing (Fig. 52.2). The gaps on the side of the rotor (radial) are approximately 0.5 mm; on the top and

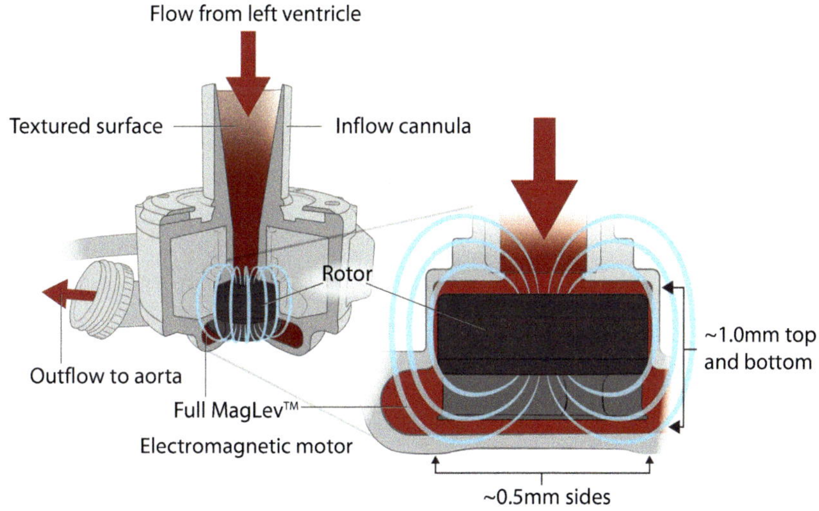

Fig. 52.2 Internal diagram of the HeartMate III showing the blood flow gaps and the magnetic fields

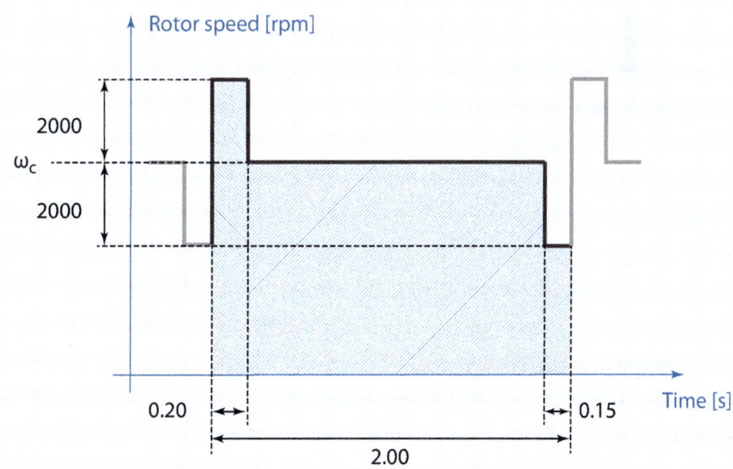

Fig. 52.3 A diagram showing the artificial pulse generated by the HeartMate III control

bottom (axial), the gap is 1.0 mm, which is 10–20 times greater than with a hydrodynamic bearing. Computational fluid dynamic analysis demonstrates well-organized flow fields across a wide range of flow (2–10 L/min), and surface shear forces are low compared to other types of pumps. An additional benefit of Full MagLev technology is that the large blood flow gaps are maintained regardless of rotor speed, even when not rotating. Therefore, it is possible to operate the pump at low speeds, which may be important for partial left ventricular assistance, right ventricular assistance, or weaning from support.

The pump is designed with large blood flow gaps to avoid stasis of blood and to reduce damage to blood components. The low hydraulic resistance in the gaps avoids stasis of blood in those regions. Low shear stresses reduce damage to blood components, which can minimize adverse events such as thromboembolism, hemolysis, and bleeding. Furthermore, since minor radial and axial divergence of the rotor is acceptable, levitation is maintained during patient physical activities, and an artificial pulse is facilitated. The artificial pulse is created as the rotor speed periodically decreases and increases from the set speed, permitting pressure and flow changes resulting from the LVAD (Fig. 52.3). The preset artificial pulse rate is 30 times per minute and is asynchronous with respect to the heart.

It has been established that a pulse during support with a continuous-flow LVAD is not necessary for adequate organ function and survival, but there are possible advantages for having some arterial pulsatility [6]. Changing flow within a rotary pump allows for a more complete washing of the blood-contacting surfaces for prevention of stasis. An artificial pulse may also help to avert adverse events, such as aortic insufficiency and bleeding from arteriovenous malformations.

In addition to reduction of shear and increased washing of the pump surfaces, enhanced hemocompatibility is also achieved by texturing internal pump surfaces, except for the rotor and rotor well. Surfaces textured with sintered titanium microspheres promote the adhesion of circulating cells and the development of a stable biological lining that reduces thromboembolic risk and the level of required anticoagulation therapy.

52.3 Clinical Experience

A multicenter clinical study evaluating the HeartMate III LVAS to meet the CE Mark requirements for clinical approval has been completed. CE Mark approval was granted in October of 2015. The trial involved 50 patients at ten centers in six countries and involved patients needing bridge-to-transplant support or support as destination therapy [7, 8]. The trial was designed to include "all-comers" with severe heart failure defined as New York Heart Association (NYHA) class IIIB or IV; ACC/AHA Stage D heart failure; ejection fraction <25%, cardiac index <2.2 l/min/m^2 without inotropes, or inotrope dependent on optimal medical management; or listed for heart transplant.

At the 6-month study end point, the performance goal of 88% survival was surpassed, with 92% of patients alive. Compared to the Seattle Heart Failure model, support with the HeartMate III reduced mortality risk by 66%. Two patients underwent successful heart transplant. There was a statistically significant improvement in NYHA class ($p < 0.0001$), quality of life ($p < 0.001$), and 6-minute walk distance ($p < 0.0001$). Adverse events included stroke and infection; however, there were no instances of device thrombosis or failure, and there was no hemolysis. In the USA, the 6-month results of a randomized multicenter study have recently been released. The Multicenter Study of MagLev Technology in Patients Undergoing Mechanical Circulatory Support Therapy with HeartMate III (MOMENTUM 3) has been conducted to compare clinical outcomes with the Full MagLev™ centrifugal flow HeartMate III LVAS versus the axial-flow HeartMate II LVAS in patients with advanced heart failure refractory to standard medical therapy. Patients were randomly assigned, in a 1:1 ratio, to receive the centrifugal-flow pump or the axial-flow pump. From September 2014 through October 2015, a total of 294 patients underwent randomization; 152 patients were assigned to the HeartMate III group and 142 to the HeartMate II group. One patient in the centrifugal-flow pump group and four in the axial-flow pump group did not undergo implantation in accordance with the protocol inclusion criteria. The remaining patients – 151 who underwent implantation of the centrifugal-flow pump and 138 who underwent implantation of the axial-flow pump – were included in the per-protocol population. The primary end point of event-free survival at 6 months was achieved in a higher percentage of patients in the centrifugal-flow pump group than in the axial-flow pump group (86.2% versus 76.8%). Study results demonstrated that non-inferiority was established of the HeartMate III LVAS as compared to the HeartMate II LVAS (absolute difference, 9.4 percentage points; 95% lower confidence boundary, −2.1; $P < 0.001$ for non-inferiority). The trial also specified a test for superiority, and it was demonstrated that at 6 months, the HeartMate III LVAS was superior to the HeartMate II LVAS (hazard ratio, 0.55; 95% confidence interval [CI], 0.32–0.95; two-tailed $P = 0.04$ for superiority). The rate of reoperation for pump malfunction was significantly lower in the HeartMate III group than in the HeartMate II. Only one patient (0.7%; 95% CI, 0 to 3.6) in the HeartMate III group underwent pump replacement (electrical malfunction), whereas 11 patients (7.7%, 95% CI, 3.9–13.4) in the HeartMate II group underwent either a device exchange (nine patients) or device removal with urgent transplantation (two patients) ($P = 0.002$) as a result of pump thrombosis. No significant differences between the two groups in the rates of death or disabling stroke resulted. The Kaplan-Meier estimate of the rate of actuarial event-free survival was significantly higher in the HeartMate III group (86%; 95% CI, 80–92) than in the HeartMate II (77%; 95% CI, 70–84; two-tailed $P =$

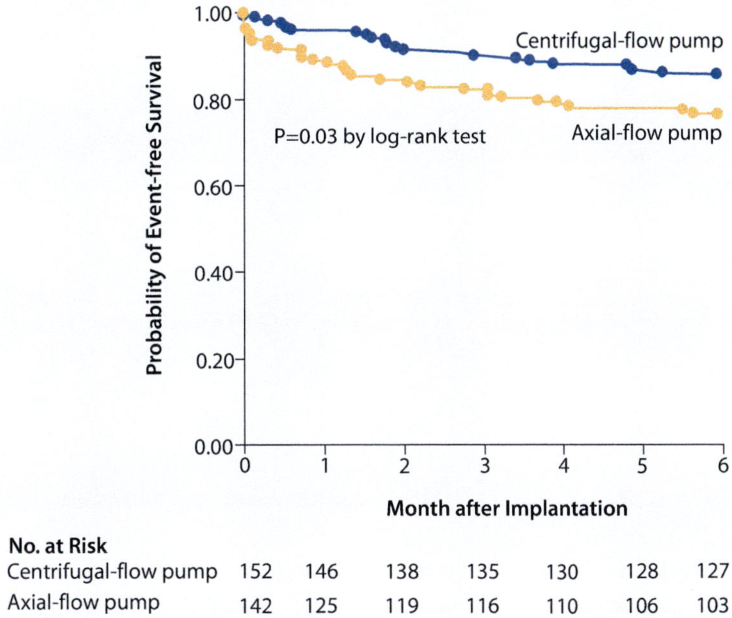

Fig. 52.4 Kaplan-Meier estimates of event-free survival in the intention-to-treat population (Reproduced with permission from Mehra et al. [9])

0.03 by the log-rank test) (Fig. 52.4). No patients in the centrifugal-flow pump group had suspected or confirmed pump thrombosis, whereas 14 patients (10.1%) in the axial-flow pump group suffered from 18 thrombotic events ($P < 0.001$). The data from the MOMENTUM 3 show that implantation of the fully magnetically levitated centrifugal continuous-flow pump HeartMate III was associated with a higher rate of survival-free of disabling stroke or survival-free of reoperation at 6 months after implantation compared to implantation of the continuous-flow pump HeartMate II among patients with advanced heart failure, irrespective of their eligibility for transplantation. The incremental benefits associated with the centrifugal-flow pump observed in this 6-month analysis were due to the absence of suspected or confirmed pump thrombosis leading to surgical pump exchange or urgent transplantation [9].

52.4 Percutaneous Heart Pump

The HeartMate Percutaneous Heart Pump (PHP) system (Fig. 52.5) is a catheter-based heart pump with control console designed to provide hemodynamic left ventricular support for many days to maintain adequate cardiac output. The key feature of the HeartMate PHP is its ability to be deployed percutaneously via a 14F arterial sheath and then expand to its full 24F dimension once in position across the aortic valve. This feature is made possible by a collapsible impeller and cannula mechanism, which is expanded upon deployment by the operator. The impeller pumps blood from the left ventricle, through the cannula, and into the ascending aorta. The HeartMate PHP is designed to provide average flow of 4–5 l/min. An external console provides device control and monitoring functions.

Potential clinical applications include cardiogenic shock following acute myocardial infarction, decompensated chronic heart failure, and acute cardiomyopathy/myocarditis. The HeartMate PHP may support patients during high-risk elective procedures, such as ventricular tachycardia (VT) ablation and high-risk percutaneous coronary intervention (HRPCI). It is ideally used to provide rapid hemodynamic stabilization of patients with compromised acute or acute-on-chronic ventricular deterioration. This will provide sufficient time for patient recovery or clinical decisions to be made regarding advanced surgical management, including options for bridging to long-term LVAD support. Figure 52.5 (middle) shows the HeartMate PHP in the sheath and partially and fully unsheathed. The sheathed PHP

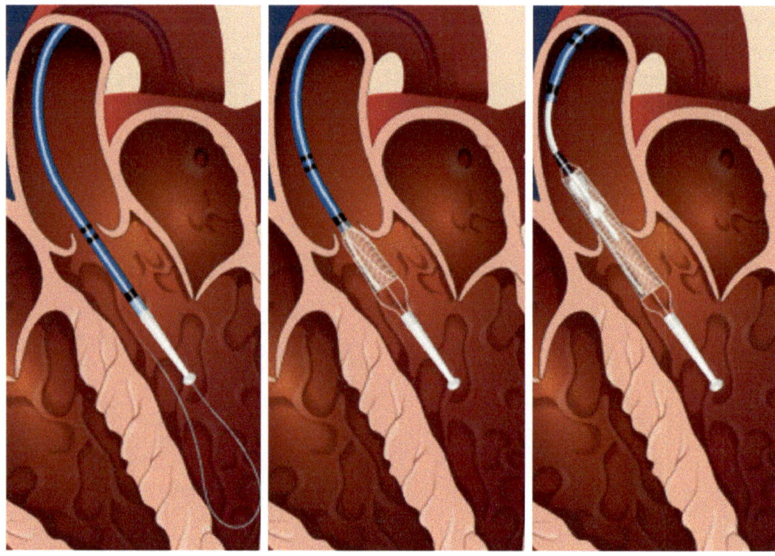

Fig. 52.5 The Heart Mate Percutaneous Heart Pump. The pump is introduced, via the femoral artery, across the aortic valve with the sheath fully withdrawn, allowing expansion of the elastomeric impeller and nitinol cannula

is inserted via the femoral artery and advanced across the aortic valve (left); then pullback of the sheath allows expansion of the device for operation (right). At the end of the support period, the cannula is re-sheathed, and the catheter pump is removed through the initial insertion site.

Recent European clinical experience with the HeartMate PHP includes the SHIELD I CE Mark study. Fifty high-risk patients were enrolled in a prospective, non-randomized, multicenter, open-label trial. The primary study performance end point was freedom from hemodynamic compromise during the PCI procedure, defined as mean arterial pressure (MAP) falling below 60 mmHg for more than 10 minutes during the PCI procedure and need for vasopressor/inotropic medication. The primary safety end point was a composite of major adverse events (MAEs), including: device-related cardiac death, new Q-wave myocardial infarction, surgical intervention due to device complications or malfunction, device-related access site complication requiring intervention or device-related limb ischemia, cerebrovascular accident, new or worsening aortic valve insufficiency, major bleeding complication (BARC $\geq$3), or severe hypotension. Secondary end points were efficacy of hemodynamic support and individual components of the major adverse event composite. Primary end points were evaluated post procedure or at hospital discharge. Patients were followed for 30 days post procedure.

Freedom from hemodynamic compromise following initiation of HeartMate PHP support during the PCI procedure was achieved in 98% of the patients. Five safety end point events occurred, including one access site complication requiring intervention, one cerebrovascular accident, one major bleeding complication, and two instances of new or worsening aortic insufficiency. No cardiac deaths, myocardial infarctions, or surgical interventions occurred. Hemodynamic stability was achieved in all patients, with a low incidence of adverse events. On the basis of results from the SHIELD I study, HeartMate PHP received CE Mark approval in July 2015 to support patients undergoing a high-risk PCI procedure. Further studies and formal clinical trials are planned to evaluate the HeartMate PHP system in high-risk PCI and other patient populations.

52.5 Other Considerations for Chronic Medical Circulatory Support

Along with advances in blood pump technology such as the HeartMate III, advances in patient-support equipment and clinical management of patients in the discharge setting are critical to advancing treatment with medical circulatory support (MCS) systems.

52.6 HeartMate Patient Peripherals

As the improvement in survival and outcomes on MCS therapy continue to improve [10], the focus on the patient-worn/patient-used hardware is increasingly important to enhance patient quality of life. Advances are underway via the miniaturization of external system controllers. Smaller and lighter controllers will allow patients to carry lighter hardware and allow it to adapt to the body habitus. Along with safety and reliability, emphasis is placed on smaller and lighter patient-worn controllers and batteries. Wearable accessories will facilitate patient comfort while providing secure and discreet accommodation of peripheral equipment.

52.7 Patient Management in the Discharge Setting

As the volume of chronic MCS patients increases and expectations of a high quality of life grow, the ability to monitor and support patents in the discharge setting is paramount. The use of established home monitoring systems in the cardiac rhythm management (CRM) therapy area is well established (Merlin.Net – SJM Corporation) [11]. The adaptation of such system to be applicable to future HeartMate patients will allow clinicians to better track and monitor patient status between clinic visits and potentially reduce adverse events.

References

1. Kirklin JK, Naftel DC, Pagani FD et al (2015) Seventh INTERMACS annual report: 15,000 patients and counting. J Heart Lung Transplant 34(12):1495–1504
2. Stretch R, Sauer CM, Yuh DD, Bonde P (2014) National trends in the utilization of short-term mechanical circulatory support: incidence, outcomes, and cost analysis. J Am Coll Cardiol 64(14):1407–1415
3. Long EF, Swain GW, Mangi AA (2014) Comparative survival and cost effectiveness of advanced therapies for end-stage heart failure. Circ Heart Fail 7(3): 470–478
4. Farrar DJ, Bourque K, Dague CP, Cotter CJ, Poirier VL (2007) Design features, developmental status, and experimental results with the HeartMate III centrifugal left ventricular assist system with a magnetically levitated rotor. ASAIO J 53(3):310–315
5. Bourque K, Cotter C, Dague C et al (2016). In Press Design rationale and pre-clinical evaluation of the HeartMate III left ventricular assist system for hemocompatibility. ASAIO J 62(4):375–383
6. Bourque K, Dague C, Farrar D et al (2006) In vivo assessment of a rotary left ventricular assist device-induced artificial pulse in the proximal and distal aorta. Artif Organs 30(8):638–642
7. Netuka I, Sood P, Pya Y et al (2015) Fully magnetically levitated left ventricular assist system for treating advanced HF: a multicenter study. J Am Coll Cardiol 66(23):2579–2589
8. Schmitto JD, Hanke JS, Rojas SV, Avsar M, Haverich A (2015) First implantation in man of a new magnetically levitated left ventricular assist device (HeartMate III). J Heart Lung Transplant 34(6):858–860
9. Mehra MR, Naka Y, Uriel N, Goldstein DJ, Cleveland JC Jr, Colombo PC, Walsh MN, Milano CA, Patel CB, Jorde UP, Pagani FD, Aaronson KD, Dean DA, McCants K, Itoh A, Ewald GA, Horstmanshof D, Long JW, Salerno C; for the MOMENTUM 3 Investigators* (2016) A fully magnetically levitated circulatory pump for advanced heart failure. N Engl J Med 376(5):440–450
10. Uriel N, Adatya S, Mehra MR (2015) Evolution in mechanical circulatory support: are we at the precipice of a disruptive innovation? J Am Coll Cardiol 66(23):2590–2593
11. Mittal S, Movsowitz C, Varma N (2014) The modern EP practice: EHR and remote monitoring. Cardiol Clin 32:239–252

HeartWare® HVAD® System

Daniel Tamez, Katherine Chorpenning, and Jeff A. LaRose

© Springer International Publishing Switzerland 2017
A. Montalto et al. (eds.), *Mechanical Circulatory Support in End-Stage Heart Failure*,
DOI 10.1007/978-3-319-43383-7_53

The HeartWare® HVAD® system is a miniature continuous-flow Ventricular Assist Device (VAD). The pump received Conformité Européenne (CE) Marking in 2009 [1–3] and US Food and Drug Administration (FDA) approval in 2012 [4, 5] for bridge to transplantation in patients with refractory heart failure (◘ Fig. 53.1). Currently, the HVAD system is one of the most extensively studied VADs available, having been implanted in approximately 2000 clinical trial patients to date and over 10,000 patients worldwide. The longest surviving patient has achieved over 8 years of device support.

Upon its introduction to the market in 2009, the HVAD system featured several important advantages over the contemporary competition. The device has an integrated inflow cannula that is inserted into the left ventricle apex and an outflow graft that is anastomosed to the arterial system. The integrated inflow cannula minimizes the pump footprint within the chest cavity and allows the pump body to be situated solely within the pericardial space, eliminating the need for a pump pocket (◘ Fig. 53.2) [6]. Pericardial placement is also advantageous in ensuring stable positioning that adapts to the ventricular and body habitus changes that occur post-implantation.

Additionally, despite its small size (160 g weight, 50 mL displacement volume), the HVAD pump allows for application in a broad patient

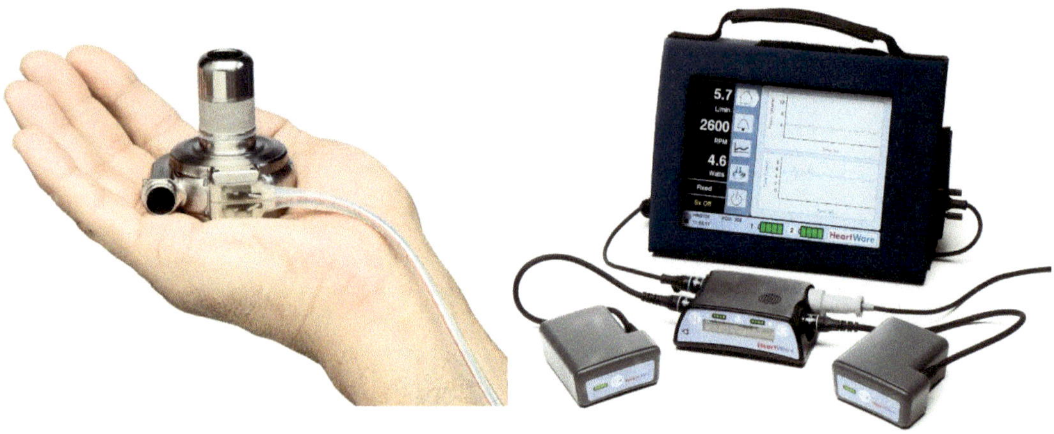

◘ **Fig. 53.1** The HeartWare HVAD system

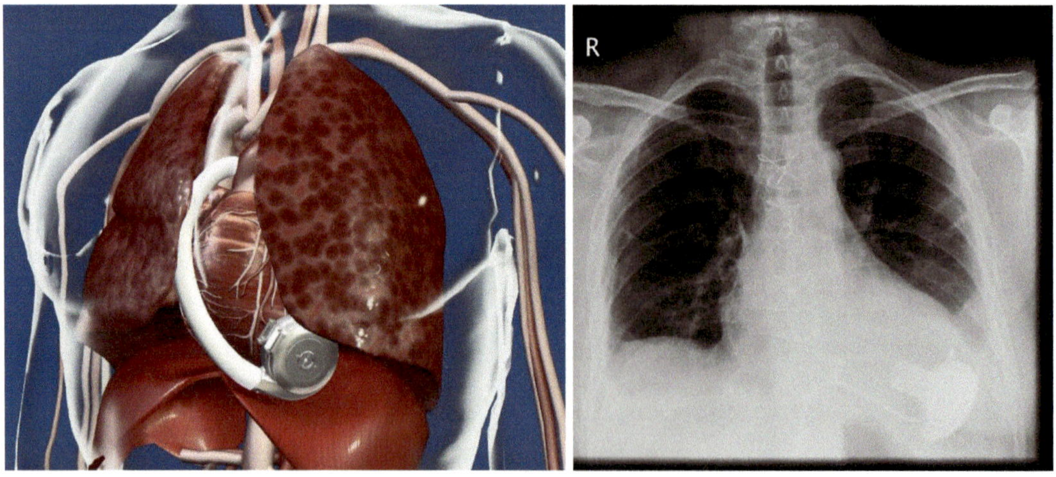

◘ **Fig. 53.2** The HeartWare HVAD pump implanted in the pericardial space

population without compromising clinical performance. Its design allows it to fit within small-framed patients yet is powerful enough to support large body habitus patients where circulatory demand may be higher. The key to developing a successful implantation technique was based on the standardization of the system's surgical tools. The simplistic design of the ventricle coring tool, sewing ring wrench, hex driver, and tunneler minimized user variability and allowed hospitals with varying levels of experience in the field of mechanical circulatory support (MCS) to achieve consistently excellent results.

The HVAD pump was also revolutionary in its application of magnetic suspension and hydrodynamic thrust bearing technology. Briefly, the pump consists of two redundant motor stators located within the upper and lower housing. Pump rotational speed ranges from 1800 RPM to 4000 RPM, and the device may generate up to 10 L/min of blood flow. It has one moving component – the impeller – which is passively suspended by magnets located within the pump centerpost. Hydrodynamic thrust bearings located on the four wide-channel impeller blades provide the necessary axial forces to balance the impeller's position within the pump housing. The success of the HVAD pump validates the concept that hydrodynamic thrust bearings may be used as an alternative to mechanical bearings to achieve a durable, "wearless" design. An impeller that is contact-free may theoretically operate for longer periods without the failures typically seen of its mechanical bearing counterparts [7].

As the field of MCS advanced, patient survival increased and ergonomics began to play a more prominent role in device design. Trends in pump miniaturization were similarly adopted for the peripheral equipment to enhance the patient's quality of life. The HVAD system controller is a wearable controller (13.4 × 10.5 × 5.1 cm) weighing 0.5 kg. This was the first MCS controller to have a display that provides real-time pump parameters (rotational speed, power consumption, and estimated VAD flow), alarm information, and troubleshooting messages to the patient. An intelligent interface between the controller and monitor allows users to view accurate pump flow estimation waveforms [8] with 50 Hz resolution. Clinicians are able to more effectively manage their patients by viewing both real-time waveforms as well as the historical trend information. Controller log files downloaded via the monitor provide insight to enhance patient management [9].

The HVAD pump introduced a novel design to the field of MCS and strongly influenced the growth of future technologies. HeartWare, Inc., has refined this first-generation technology and is currently developing a platform of miniaturized devices implantable by progressively less invasive surgery. The first of these devices is the MVAD Pump, which is 70% smaller than its predecessor (◘ Fig. 53.3). Many of the design aspects of the MVAD Pump were either derivations of or improvements in the HVAD pump. Some of these include the integrated inflow cannula, intrapericardial pump placement, gimbal sewing ring, and gel-impregnated outflow graft. The design, pump control algorithms, and alarm features of the MVAD Pump peripherals are the result of lessons learned from the HVAD controller, charger, power adapters, and batteries.

Reducing invasiveness of the implant procedure will allow access to patients at an earlier stage of their disease progression. The Longhorn® is in development for applications in elderly, full-support, and high-risk patients. It is an intraventricular axial-flow pump featuring an outflow cannula positioned across the aortic valve. The pump consists of a pedestal, a pump body motor assembly, and an outflow cannula with an internal vane diffuser. The motor assembly and impeller use same-core technologies developed with the MVAD Pump. The C-Pump® partial assist device (formerly known as the CircuLite® System) will support class III patients, and patients with heart failure with preserved ejection fraction, and may be implanted using a minimally invasive procedure.

HeartWare, Inc., has a strong miniature pump pipeline that began with the HVAD pump and which will continue with a family of smaller devices that leverage and enhance this original technology. It is the vision of HeartWare that availability of such miniaturized technology may help the MCS community to create a paradigm shift in the treatment of heart failure, further improving the adverse event profile and enhancing the patient quality of life.

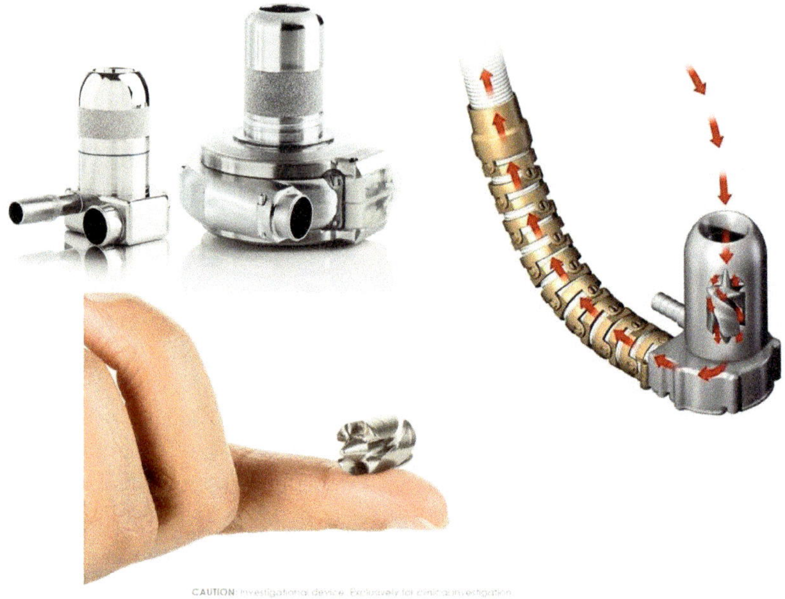

Fig. 53.3 The HeartWare MVAD pump

References

1. Wieselthaler GM, O'Driscoll G, Jansz P, Khaghani A, Strueber M (2010) Initial clinical experience with a novel left ventricular assist device with a magnetically levitated rotor in a multi-institutional trial. J Heart Lung Transplant. 29:1218–1225
2. Strueber M, O'Driscoll G, Jansz P et al (2011) Multicenter evaluation of an intrapericardial left ventricular assist system. J Am Coll Cardiol 57:1375–1382
3. Strueber M, Larbalestier R, Jansz P et al (2014) Results of a postmarket Registry to Evaluate the HeartWare® Left Ventricular Assist System (The ReVOLVE Registry). J Heart Lung Transpl 33:486–491
4. Aaronson KD, Slaughter MS, Miller LW et al (2012) Use of an intrapericardial, continuous flow, centrifugal pump in patients awaiting heart transplantation. Circulation 125:3191–3200
5. Slaughter MS, Pagani FD, McGee EC et al (2013) Use of the HeartWare® ventricular assist system for bridge to transplant: combined results of the ADVANCE and CAP trial. Journal of Heart and Lung Transplant 32:675–683
6. LaRose JA, Tamez D, Ashenuga M, Reyes C (2010) Design concepts and principle of operation of the HeartWare ventricular assist system. ASAIO Journal 56:285–289
7. Reyes C, Chorpenning K, LaRose JA, Gomez R, Tamez D (2014) Six-year in-vitro reliability results of the HeartWare HVAD pump. ASAIO Journal 60:541–544
8. Reyes C, Voskoboynikov N, Chorpenning K et al (2016) Accuracy of the HVAD pump flow estimation algorithm. ASAIO J 62:15–19
9. Chorpenning K, Brown MC, Voskoboynikov N, Reyes C, Dierlam AE, Tamez D (2014) HeartWare controller logs: a diagnostic tool and clinical management aid for the HVAD pump. ASAIO J (60):115–118

ReliantHeart: Forward Compatibility and TET

Antonio Loforte, Lucio Careddu, Emanuela Angeli, Luca Ragni, Gaetano Gargiulo, and Rodger G. Ford

© Springer International Publishing Switzerland 2017
A. Montalto et al. (eds.), *Mechanical Circulatory Support in End-Stage Heart Failure*,
DOI 10.1007/978-3-319-43383-7_54

54.1 Introduction

ReliantHeart (ReliantHeart Inc., Houston, TX, USA) HeartAssist5 (HA5) left ventricular assist device (LVAD) system is a miniaturized, implantable, second-generation axial-flow pump capable of long-term circulatory support in patients with end-stage heart failure. The device results to be the first continuous-flow LVAD ever implanted in human being. This compact axial-flow pump has been in development since 1988 named as MicroMed DeBakey [1] (MicroMed Cardiovascular Inc., Houston, TX, USA) whose design belongs to the second-generation pump category [2, 3].

54.2 History

In 1984 David Saucier, a NASA Johnson Space Center engineer, underwent a successful heart transplant under the care of Dr. George P. Noon and Dr. Michael E. DeBakey. It was during Mr. Saucier's clinical recovery that he had discussions with Drs. Noon and DeBakey in which they expressed their own desire to develop a long-term ventricular assist device.

The first formal meeting between the teams at Baylor College of Medicine and Johnson Space Center (JSC) occurred in 1988 when the Baylor team traveled to JSC to explore a cooperative effort to develop a new blood pump. At that time, the choice fell on a continuous-flow blood pump that would be able to achieve the desired small size and durability for human use. The design of the fuel injection pumps for the space shuttle was adopted and the continuous-flow pump developed. This pump was tested by Dr. Noon in animal experiments at Texas A&M University in College Station.

In 1995, after discussions with Dr. DeBakey's associates, Travis Baugh and Dallas Anderson founded the MicroMed Technology, LLC, with the intention of licensing and commercializing this technology from NASA. The focus of MicroMed was to (A) transform the ex vivo components into an implantable VAD, (B) demonstrate the long-term reliability of the pump, (C) develop all the external electronics and ancillary equipment, and (D) perform all necessary preclinical (in vitro and in vivo) testing and bring the technology to the patients who desperately need such a device.

After a decade of advance for optimized materials and manufacturing process for the human body for the conversion of the ex vivo pump into a long-term implantable pump, in November of 1998, the first implants of the DeBakey VAD were performed at the Deutsches Herzzentrum Berlin, Berlin Germany. Dr. Roland Hetzer and Dr. Matthias Loebe performed the implant with the assistance of Dr. DeBakey and Dr. Noon [4]. These landmark cases were the first ever of implantable rotary blood pumps to support long-term bridge to transplant patients. The lessons learned from these first two cases were invaluable in understanding continuous-flow devices and moving this new technology forward. The third and fourth patients were implanted at the Allgemeines Kranken Haus in Vienna, Austria, under the hands of Drs. Ernst Wolner and Georg Wieselthaler, again with assistance of Dr. DeBakey and Dr. Noon [5]. These two patients were the first to survive successful transplants after 74 and 115 days, respectively [6–8]. In 2001, the CE mark was obtained while the clinical trial of the DeBakey VAD in the USA was started in June 2000, at Methodist Hospital, Houston, with a patient implanted under the hands of Dr. Noon and of Dr. DeBakey.

One of the most compelling features of the DeBakey LVAD is the size. For this reason, Dr. Anthony Chang of Texas Children's Hospital approached Dr. DeBakey with the desire to make the DeBakey VAD available to the pediatric population that had no other options for mechanical circulatory support. With this new mission, MicroMed modified the adult version of the DeBakey VAD to provide a better anatomical fitting in the pediatric chest without modifying the pump's core components. As a result, MicroMed received a Humanitarian Device Exemption in 2004 for the DeBakey VAD Child, and the first patient implanted with this device was at Texas Children's Hospital in a 6-year-old girl.

54.3 Pump Characteristics

Since the first implants, a complete technical revision has been performed by time including changes in impeller geometry, inflow cannula, and front and rear gaps. The pump (◘ Table 54.1) is made up of titanium which surrounds the

Table 54.1 Comparison between most common LVADs (Courtesy by ReliantHeart Inc., TX, USA – ReliantHeart.com)

aVAD and HeartAssist5® vs. Other LVADs

COMPANY	Thoratec		HeartWare	ReliantHeart	
PRODUCT	HeartMate II	HeartMate III	HVAD	aVAD	HeartAssist5
WEIGHT (Grams)	292	220	145	84	92
PLACEMENT	Below Diaphragm	Pericardial Space	Pericardial Space	Pericardial Space	Pericardial Space
TYPE	Axial Flow	Centrifugal	Centrifugal	Axial Flow	Axial Flow
MEASURABLE PULSATILITY	Minimal [2]	Not Evaluated	Not Evaluated	Yes [2]	Yes [2]
PATTERNS OF PUMP CREATED THROMBUS	Reported [1] Stroke > 12% [4]	stroke rate of 12% 6 months of data [6]	stroke >28% [4]	Thrombus patterns Absent [1]	Thrombus patterns Absent [1] Stroke 0% [5]
HEMOLYSIS - Pfhgb vs. time at 5 liters/min	**16.67** [7]	**8.83** [7]		3.65 [7]	3.65 [7]
BEARING SYSTEM	**Ball in Cup**	**Active Magnetic Levitation**	**Active Magnetic Levitation**	Active Magnetic Stabilization & Directional Retention	Ball in Cup
TRUE FLOW MEASUREMENT				✓	✓
REMOTE MONITORING				✓	✓
PATIENT DIARY - INR TRACKER				✓	✓
Pump in or out of the Ventricle	OUT	OUT	OUT	**Intraventricular**	**OUT**
TET READY HA5 - Forward Compatibility to ***Liberty*** [3]				2018 [3]	2018 [3]
CE APPROVAL (Europe)	✓	✓	✓	Anticipated late 2016	✓
FDA TRANSPLANT ELIGIBLE (short)	✓	In Trial	✓	Trial early 2017	In Trial for Bridge to Transplant
FDA DESTINATION (long)	✓	In Trial	In Trial	Trial early 2017	

(1) Stony Brook Study, New York, December 1, 2013
(2) THI 2009 Report Frazier et, al.
(3) Forward compatibility – a design that gracefully accepts input designed for later versions of itself
(4) HeartWare Endurance 1 trial
(5) HeartAssist5 (rev6) EU commercial experience – no device related stroke
(6) Thoratec HeartMateIII, European Data on 50 patient study (doi: 10.1016/j.jacc.2015.09.083)...puslished December 15, 2015
(7) Hemolysis Testing – Average Plasma free Hemoglobin (Pfhgb) vs. time testing performed at 5 liters/min. ReliantHeart aVAD – final report from Texas Heart Institure August 21, 2015. Data on file. HMII and HMIII data from Bourque et. al. ASIO Journal, published ahead of print May, 18, 2016.

inducer-impeller, which is suspended by mechanical pivot bearings. The impeller operational range is 7500–12,500 rpm that is able to generate flows up to 6 l/min against a 100 mmHg pressure gradient. The principal technical features that diverge from most devices in the market is given by its dimensions of only 71 × 38 mm for a total weight of 92 g, and it consumes only 10 W of power. The device has a new long time battery support with quite 10 h of continuous functioning in battery mode. Moreover, the impeller inlet angle in the HA5 has been larger than its precursor, the MicroMed DeBakey VAD [2, 9]. This had led to a pump more responsive to changes in the pressure differential across the pump, due to changes in afterload, preload, or both.

The inlet cannula is also made of titanium and is inserted into the left ventricular apex. As mentioned previously, HA5 has optimized the design of the DeBakey-Noon LVAD especially in the impeller. Similarly to other axial LVADs, it has a flow straightener with three blades at inflow which also contribute to be a front bearing for the inducer-impeller with six blades and a flow diffuser with other six blades for the outlet, which function as rear bearing support for the impeller. The diffuser also helps to increase outflow pressure by directing the flow in the axial direction. Other main feature of the HA5 LVAD is the spinning direction of the impeller that is clockwise and differs from other devices available on the market. The wide stator was upgraded too with a new special arrangement of electromagnets. From the previous version with 5 magnets, the new version was upgraded with 8 magnets stator without changes in volume occupied. This also led a reduction in power consumption.

Numerical simulation and measurement of platelet activation rates in recirculation flow loops have showed that platelets are exposed to a lower stress accumulation and lower thrombus formation [10–13]. Early on during the development of what became MicroMed, Dr. Michael DeBakey directed the engineering team to design a pump that could drain a swimming pool full of water balloons without breaking a single balloon. Careful study of computational fluid dynamics and proprietary testing systems has allowed to refine the technology of the impeller, working with the flow straightener and diffuser, and draws blood more smoothly through the LVAD with the intended result of less damage to the blood's fragile components, including less platelet activation.

Moreover, this design study have made a device small enough to be implanted within the pericardium beside the heart and, unlike many LVADs today, implants above the diaphragm. An LVAD implanted in the abdomen can cause additional complications. Patients may feel prematurely full when they eat because an implant below the diaphragm can cause pressure on the stomach. Moreover, implantation of LVAD in the abdomen has a significantly larger blood path along nonhuman surfaces. The HA5 size can help to avoid many of the complications caused by nonhuman surface contact and by the stresses caused by cavitation as the blood flows through a larger device. In the second half of 2015, a new version of HA5 named first HA5 direct (HA5D) and then aVAD was released and entered clinical trials (◘ Table 54.1). This recent version differs from the standard HA5 for the taper inflow adaptor that allows the VAD to be inserted directly into the left apex (◘ Figs. 54.1 and 54.2). The aVAD has the same pump characteristics of HA5 allowing the same VAD performance and hemodynamics. The possibility of being inserted directly in the left apex allows the aVAD to be more similar to other pumps [2, 3] than standard HA5 allowing even a minimally invasive surgical implantation. Currently this novel device is still under investigation in trial centers in terms of FDA transplant eligible (short) and FDA destination (long) approval. Recently, on Tuesday, August 2, 2016, the company received CE mark approval for the aVAD usage (◘ Table 54.1).

In terms of outflow, the HA5 has a pre-embroidered Vascutek Gelweave (Terumo Cardiovascular System Corp., Ann Arbor, MI) vascular graft with another unique characteristic of an ultrasonic-flow probe placed around the outflow graft that provides real-time flow measurement, and data collected by the probe are continuously sent to the external controller. This graft together with all blood contacting surfaces are now Carmeda® BioActive (Carmeda AB, Sweden) biocompatible thus limiting the rate of thrombus formation which was commonly reported during the early experience with the device. The flow probe could accurately measure the flow inside the outflow graft, and this technology has been called "true flow." Also Frazier [14] and colleagues have demonstrated that HA5 is more "pulsatile" than other LVADs and previews MicroMed DeBakey VAD; in detail the HA5 could

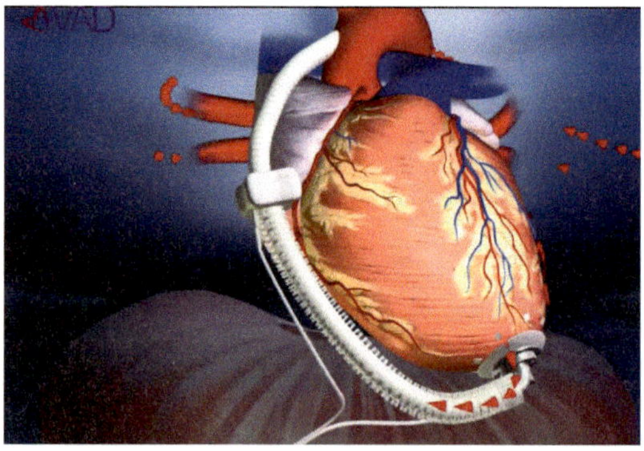

◘ **Fig. 54.1** aVAD (ReliantHeart Inc., TX) support system

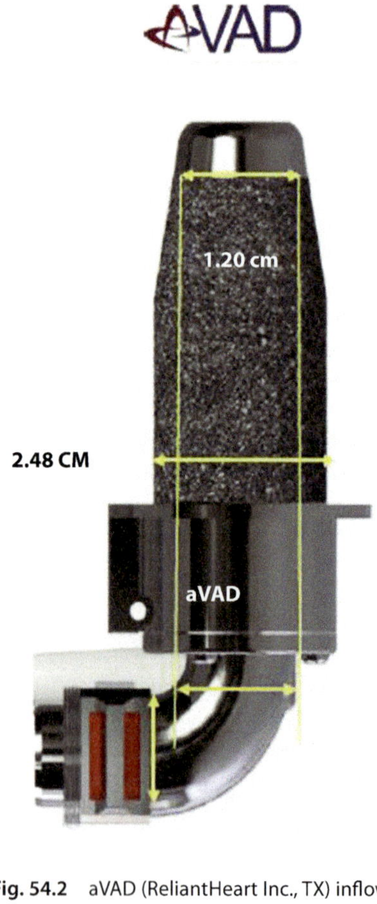

◘ **Fig. 54.2** aVAD (ReliantHeart Inc., TX) inflow cannula

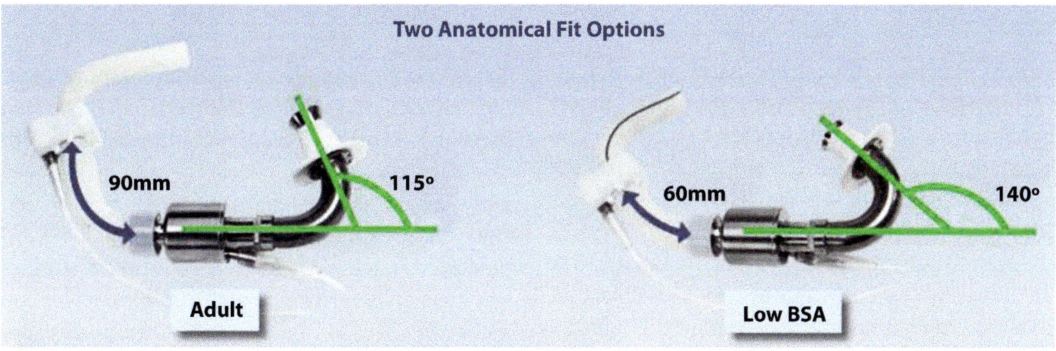

Fig. 54.3 Anatomical fit options according to inflow cannula angle of HeartAssist5 (HA5)

automatically adjust the pump flow rate on small changes in pump preload. The probe is connected with the device and could measure the aortic opening and mitral valve closure to ensure a more physiologic support for the left ventricle; this is a functional and capable option to better estimate and adapt the pump flow to the patient [14]. This information is useful when a patient is stable, but can prove vital if a patient is experiencing complications. This is an extremely reliable tool for the detection of cardiac arrhythmias such is atrial fibrillation in which is clearly viewable a modification in waveform and wave intervals.

Other LVADs rely on estimates by their software providings or they do not have flow data at all, which can leave the clinician flying blind whenever this information is the most needed. Flow measurement is unaffected by changes in blood or fibrin deposition, the ultrasonic flow probe has been proven highly accurate measuring real-time blood flow, and it is correctly positioned on the outflow graft to measure blood pumped from the HA5 as it moves into the aorta.

In addition to flow data, the HA5 tracks speed and electrical current usage by the pump motor, providing valuable information both about the volume of blood flow and its fluidity. All patients have specific characteristics which are continuously recorded by HA5; changes to this data can clearly indicate problems ranging from minor dehydration to more significant side effects.

Finally, all data are recorded by HA5 controller. The controller displays device main parameters such as pump flow (L/min), power consumption (watts), pump speed (rpm), and battery charge. The controller has a cellphone radio which automatically connects to vadlink.com. All data were constantly updated to the main server, and if Internet resource is absent, the data is stored in the controller and updated once network is available. Two rechargeable batteries serve as energy supply to the pump and the controller too. It is also used to connect the pump to the portable console, the HeartAttendant (HA). All data collected by the controller and the HA are stored in a remote sever at vadlink.com where the patients together with the physician could control remotely the all the information.

54.4 Indications for Implant

The pump comes in both adult and pediatric versions (Fig. 54.3), which differ in terms of inflow angle (140° for children and 115° for adults) and length of the outflow graft (60 mm for children and 90 mm for adults). The constant shortage of suitable donor hearts for transplantation has created the drive for more LVAD. For that reason, newer continuous-flow LVAD utilizing magnetic levitation technologies has proven to be more durable than previous-generation pulsatile-flow devices allowing them to be also used as a destination therapy [2, 15].

The development of HA5 in both adult and pediatric versions was approved as bridge to transplant (BTT) for the first time in 2010 and bridge to recovery and destination therapy (DT) in Europe, whereas FDA has approved the device only for humanitarian exemption from 2005 in children 5–16 years of age with end-stage heart failure and refractory to medical therapy while they are waitlisted for cardiac transplantation. The adult version is currently being tested in several centers across the USA as a BTT [16].

Current indication for LVAD implant from ESC is reported in the Guidelines of 2012 in which patients with severe heart failure (HF) with low LVEF (<25%) with frequent hospital admission for HF (>3), inotropic support, end-organ dysfunction due to low cardiac output and right-side deteriorating are candidate for LVAD implantation [17].

Anticoagulation management for patients with HA5 requires an INR value of 2.5–3.5 with a standard therapy with warfarin. From 2001 all devices are coated with Carmeda® BioActive and preliminary data report encouraging result on preventions of thromboembolic events; however, new data on this issue are still needed. HA5 together with Roche has incorporated in their remote database the INR information of the CoaguChek® device to improve safety of the device and monitoring of patients' therapy. Together with the anticoagulation therapy should be introduced an antiplatelet therapy; this has been proved to reduce risk of stroke and pump thrombosis [18]. In case of pediatric patients, this should be administered in the first 48–72 h from LVAD implant.

54.5 Surgical Technique

Traditionally, a complete median sternotomy is performed (■ Figs. 54.4, 54.5, 54.6, and 54.7). The skin incision is prolonged 5 cm below the xiphoid process. Central cardiopulmonary bypass is installed and the heart is arrested by usage of a cardioplegic solution. A pump holder ring is sewed with 8–12 U pledgeted stitches on the left ventricular apex. A star incision is performed with a surgical knife, and a coring device is utilized. The surgeon must pay attention during this procedure to ensure a full-thickness incision and detaching of the muscle in the apex to allow a perfect fit of the inflow cannula and the absence of chordae or myocardial trabeculae in front of the inflow cannula too.

Then the wire connector is tunnelized under the muscular fascia 3–5 cm above the iliac crest. The inflow cannula is then secured by sewing the inflow cannula ring to the previous apical fixation ring. The device is now tested and partial deairing is performed by filling the left ventricle. Finally, a connection between the embroidered graft and the ascending aorta is performed. This final suture could

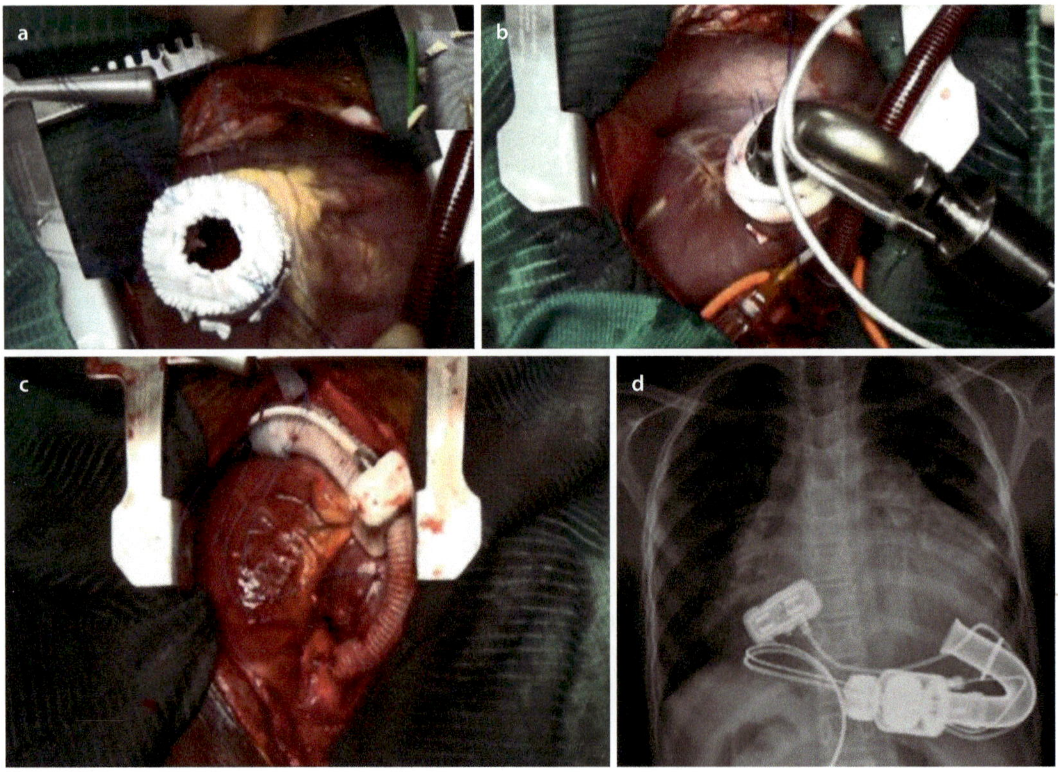

■ **Fig. 54.4** HeartAssist5 (HA5) surgical implantation in adolescents. Panel **a**, apical coring and sewing ring placement. Panel **b**, inflow cannula placement. Panel **c**, device in place. Panel **d**, X-chest ray postoperative view

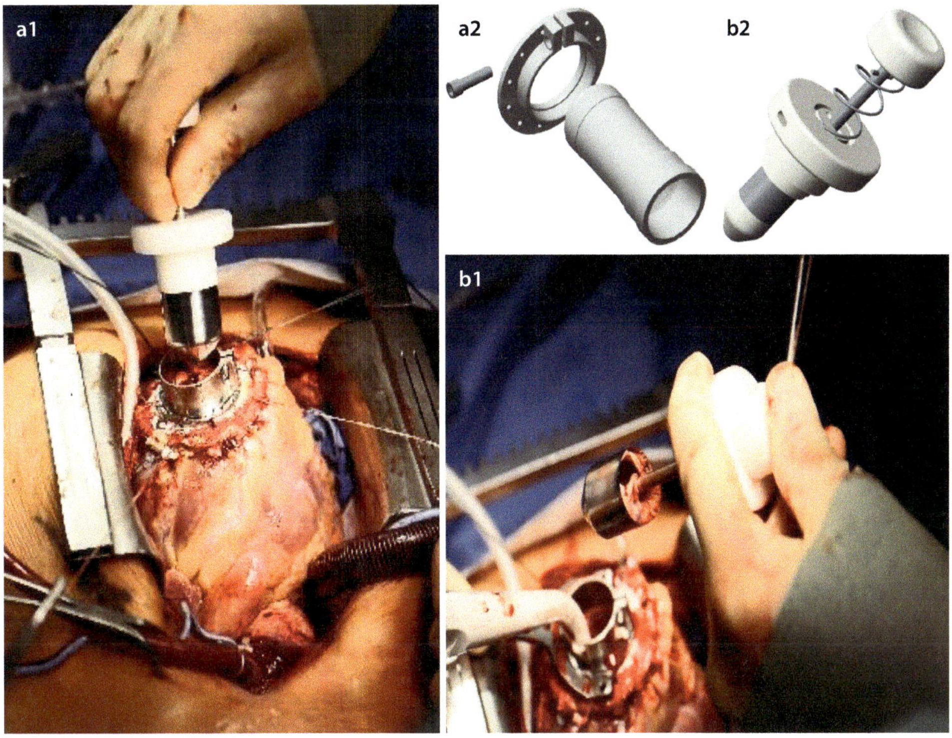

Fig. 54.5 aVAD (ReliantHeart Inc., TX) surgical implantation. Panels **a1**–**a2**, apical sewing ring and fast connect device placement. Panels **b1**–**b2**, apical coring by usage of aVAD core device

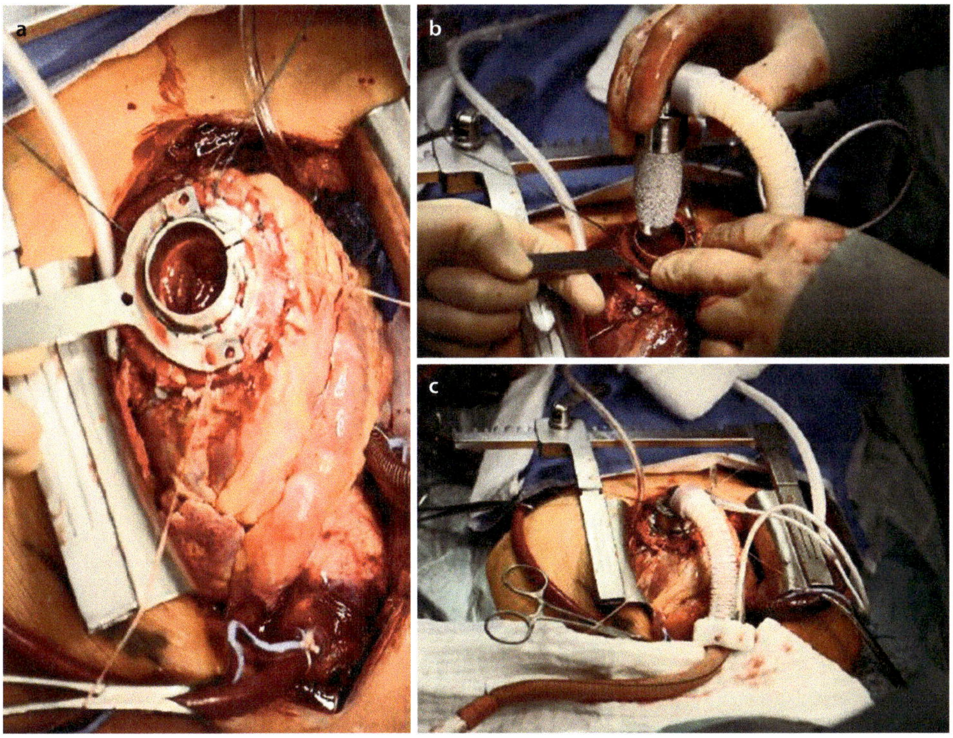

Fig. 54.6 aVAD (ReliantHeart Inc., TX) surgical implantation. Panel **a**, handle temporary fixation of apical sewing ring and fast connect device. Panel **b**, aVAD inflow cannula introduction. Panel **c**, left ventricular aVAD placement surgical view

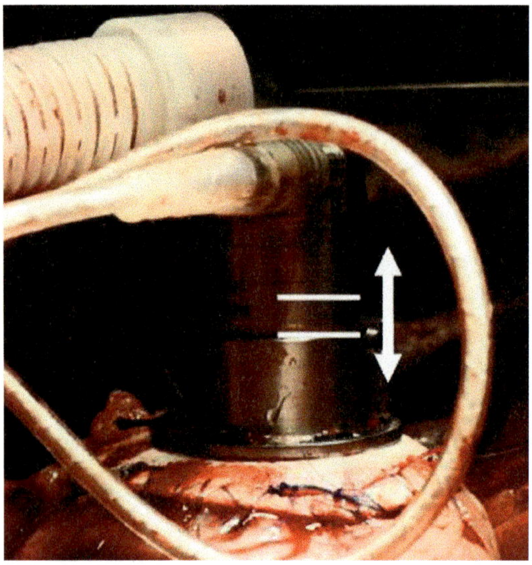

Fig. 54.7 Fast connect device adjustable depth (1 cm) for aVAD inflow cannula placement

be performed also on beating heart. After a careful deairing of the device and graft, the cardiopulmonary bypass can be stopped, and the chest can be closed (Figs. 54.4, 54.5, 54.6, and 54.7). This is the only surgical approach suitable in childhood patients. Other approaches (left thoracotomy or multiple mini-incisions) are not appropriate for the tiniest size of the thorax and might lead to a complex operation without benefits for the patient, and in some cases, this might only increase the number of perioperative complications. Nevertheless, in adult patients, the left thoracotomy (4th–5th intercostal space) allows the surgeon to a better view of the left apex, and the outflow graft can be anastomosed to the descending aorta. Another feasible choice for HA5 implant in adult patients is through multiple small incisions. A left mini-thoracotomy (4th–5th intercostal space) may be performed for left ventricle apex exposure. The outflow cannula anastomosis is instead performed through a right mini-thoracotomy or a J-shaped upper mini-sternotomy. In case of planned minimally invasive surgery, an CT angiography scan may be helpful to focus on preoperative anatomic features. Surely, in the near future, the novel aVAD (Figs. 54.1, 54.2, 54.5, 54.6, and 54.7) will get more facilities for minimally invasive surgical approaches.

We should not forget that both HA5 and aVAD have a disconnectable driveline which is easy to insert. Additionally, this offers the chance to remove the cable in case of driveline wound infection without need of full LVAD system replacement.

54.6 Remote Monitoring

Remote monitoring (RM) is an additional tool for ReliantHeart LVADs and enables monitoring of patients outside of conventional clinical settings (Fig. 54.8). RM in chronic disease, such as heart

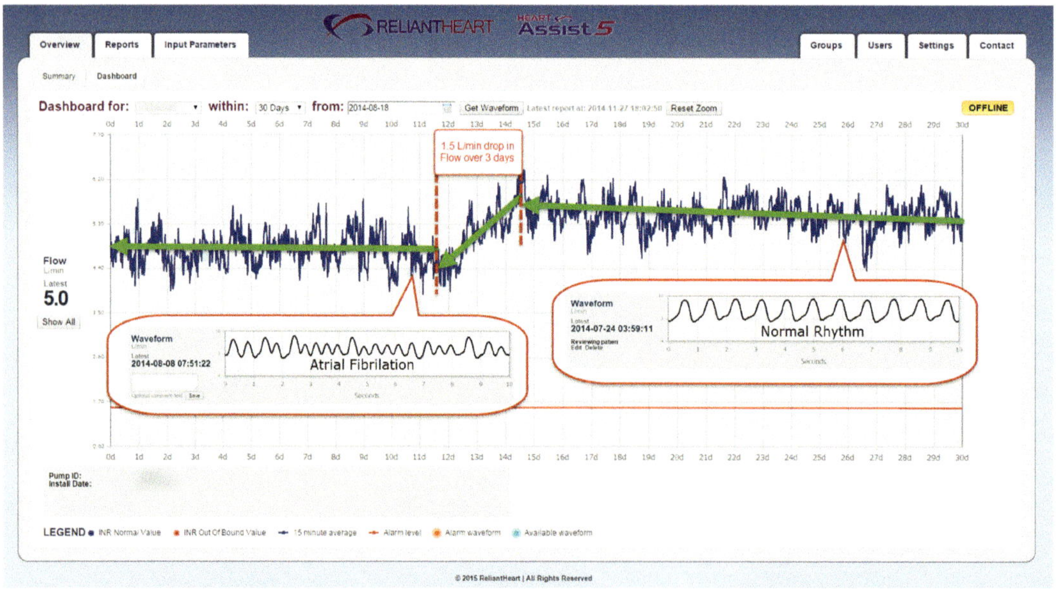

Fig. 54.8 Remote monitoring of hemodynamics and clinical status of patients while on aVAD support

failure, can significantly improve an individual's quality of life allowing the patients to maintain independence, prevent complications, and minimize personal costs. Nowadays, RM systems are integrated into pacemakers, ICD, loop recorders, etc. and have been commonly used for years with great benefits in such patients [19–22]. RM technology offers a safe, practical, and cost-effective alternative to the in-office follow-up visits especially in case Internet-based remote monitoring. Nevertheless, use of RM for left ventricular assist devices (LVADs) has become available only recently [4]; thus, no data is currently available in the literature.

Previous efforts to combine RM with ventricular assist devices have not been fully achieved [15]. Actually the HeartAssist5 LVAD is the unique LVAD with RM technology available in the market [2, 9, 23]. The HeartAttendant (HA) is the all-in-one portable console for the HA5 whose functions are (A) real-time blood flow data and (B) transmission of data via secure wireless Internet for remote home monitoring. The HA consists in a 17.5 × 13 cm touch screen monitor with an internal 9 V battery for the liquid crystal monitor, a memory card, and an Internet connection. It is connected to the LVAD with a two wire cables: one transferring instant pump flow data from the probe to the controller and the other transferring power from the controller to the pump motor.

With the HeartAssist Remote™ Monitoring System, HA5 patients feel more secure about their heart health while enjoying life at home or traveling.

All patients are requested to connect their controllers to the HA every day at least one time. At bedtime, patients connect their controller to their HA which then collects and stores data. This data can be viewed by physicians remotely helping to avoid unnecessary hospital admissions. In cases of concern, RM provides a head start, allowing for proactive response and possibly better results for the patient. This could lead to an effective deployment resulting in better use of the healthcare system's resources. Nowadays, the controller continuously records the pump parameters and transmits the data to the central registry through Internet connection with a GSM/3G radio cellphone embedded. The HeartAssist remote monitoring system consists of a secure remote central database (vadlink.com), which gathers the data obtained via the Internet. With this advanced RM system, all data is recorded and, if necessary, reviewed 24/7. The central database also sends email alerts to the authorized medical team whenever an alarm is received from a controller.

A fine-tuning of the pump could be performed by physicians in the ICU or ward and, after discharge from the hospital, in outpatient clinic during the clinical visits.

The major benefits of this advanced RM system include (A) improvement in clinical efficiency, (B) earlier patient intervention, (C) enhanced patient convenience, and (D) leveraged limited staff and healthcare resources.

Finally, patient privacy is guaranteed by a unique name and password and allows the patient's designated healthcare provider to access this data from their computer or device, including iPhone, Android, and Blackberry platforms (◘ Fig. 54.8).

54.7 Discussion

Since the introduction of LVADs, pulsatile volume-displacement devices have been successfully used as bridge to transplantation. However, adverse events such as infections, thromboembolic complications, and technical failures limited their use for long-term support. The recently introduced axial-flow devices (e.g., HA5) are much smaller and have a better long-term survival. They also show lower rate of both related complications and mechanical failures, which makes them suitable for extended time of bridge to transplantation or destination therapy. The experience with the predecessor of HeartAssist5, the DeBakey device, has been reported extensively in the past years [4, 5, 8, 16, 24]. Goldstein [16] and colleagues have reviewed 150 patients worldwide underwent the implant of the MicroMed DeBakey VAD as a bridge to transplantation between 1998 and 2002. From their review, 55% were either bridged to transplantation or recovery or are ongoing, and part of the patients have been followed in the outpatient clinic suggesting that bridging to transplantation can be approached with a low incidence of complication. Other subsequent reports have related the use of the HeartAssist5 LVAD has a valuable option for long-term support of patients awaiting heart transplantation.

Patients with these devices could achieve a good quality of life after discharge from the hospital. HA5 has also showed to be a reliable replacement option of other similar LVADs in case of pump complications in case of no immediate donor available [25].

In addition to routine clinical controls, RM results to be a useful and valuable tool in those who are discharged from the hospital after LVAD insertion thus providing to a continuous home monitoring of patients. All settings can be checked and optimized according to every single patient hemodynamics and characteristics for better fitting the difference in lifestyle.

We believe that RM is a useful technology improving patient care with an early detection and treatment of serious problems arising out of hospital. However, if a remote monitoring system allows automatic transmission of data from the device and may decrease the number of unnecessary ambulatory visits, still a question remains unresolved, whether the data are sufficient to accurately forecast the need for a clinical evaluation particularly in case of patients with chronic heart failure.

Medical, social, psychological, and economical benefits of RM in LVAD patients are still theoretical, and, despite all potential clinical benefits, RM should be taken as an add-on rather than a substitute from routine clinical patient follow-up.

54.8 Step into the Future: aVAD as a TAH and the Liberty (TET) System

A 90-day survival animal study at the Texas Heart Institute in Houston, TX, USA, has demonstrated that the novel aVAD-style total artificial heart is viable and dependable. Twenty animal implants over a period of 5 years have demonstrated that the aVAD is perhaps the foundation for the future total artificial heart (TAH) (◘ Fig. 54.9).

The aVAD Liberty system (◘ Fig. 54.10) will provide the platform for a totally implantable TAH. The common elements are energy transfer coils, sealed internal battery, tiny and efficient motor controller, power draw of just 5.5 watts combined for both the left- and right-side pumps, and accurate flow measurements that will confirm the generated pulsatility. The system can be implanted as a BVAD or a TAH and might be the key to produce a successful artificial heart in the near future.

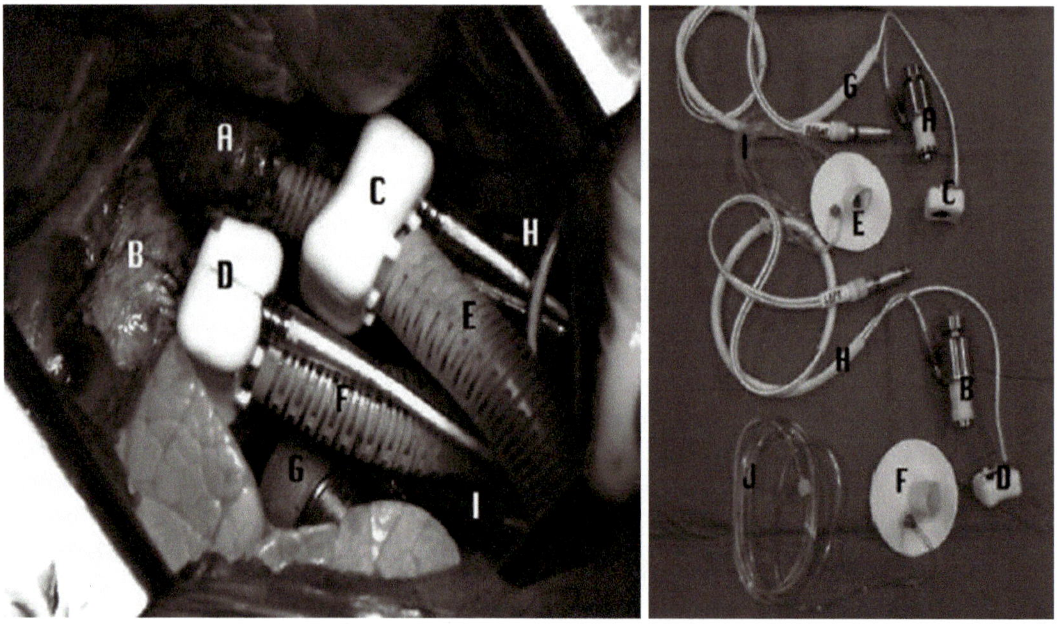

◘ **Fig. 54.9** Total artificial heart (TAH) setting by adoption of two aVAD rotary blood pumps

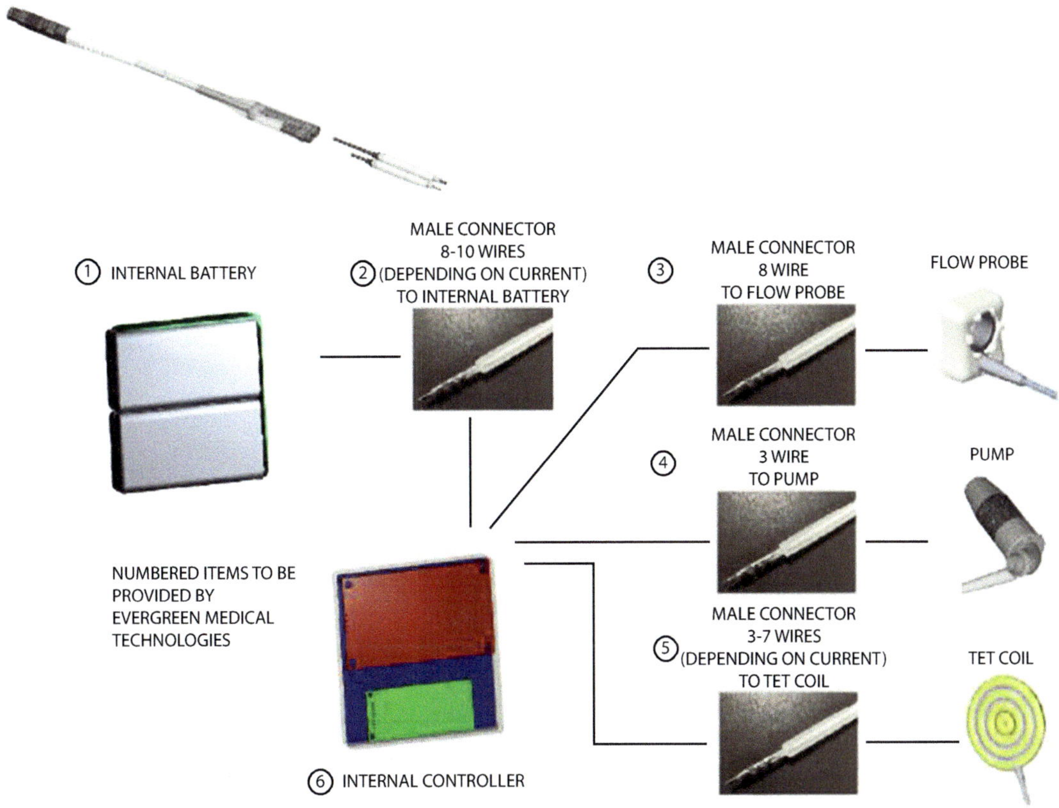

Fig. 54.10 The aVAD Liberty system setting

Acknowledgments Bologna University Hospital thanks Rodger G. Ford, CEO, Co-Founder, and Chairman of the Board of Directors of ReliantHeart Inc., TX, USA, for continuous discussions, information, and support.

Figures 54.1, 54.2, 54.3, 54.5, 54.6, 54.7, 54.8, 54.9, 54.10 and Table 54.1 are courtesy of ReliantHeart Inc., TX, USA (Relian Heart. com).

References

1. Noon GP, Loebe M (2010) Current status of the micromed debakey noon ventricular assist device. Tex Heart Inst J 37:652–653
2. Timms D (2011) A review of clinical ventricular assist devices. Med Eng Phys 33:1041–1047
3. Westaby S, Frazier OH, Beyersdorf F, Saito S, Siegenthaler MP, Pigott DW et al (2002) The jarvik 2000 heart. Clinical validation of the intraventricular position. Eur J Cardiothorac Surg 22:228–232
4. Noon GP, Morley DL, Irwin S, Abdelsayed SV, Benkowski RJ, Lynch BE (2001) Clinical experience with the micromed debakey ventricular assist device. Ann Thorac Surg 71:S133–S138 ; discussion S144-136
5. Wieselthaler GM, Schima H, Hiesmayr M, Pacher R, Laufer G, Noon GP et al (2000) First clinical experience with the debakey vad continuous-axial-flow pump for bridge to transplantation. Circulation 101:356–359
6. Wieselthaler GM, Schima H, Lassnigg A, Pacher R, Ovsenk T, Laufer G et al (1999) The debakey vad axial flow pump: First clinical experience with a new generation of implantable, nonpulsatile blood pumps for long-term support prior to transplantation. Wien Klin Wochenschr 111:629–635
7. Wilhelm MJ, Hammel D, Schmid C, Rhode A, Kaan T, Rothenburger M et al (2005) Long-term support of 9 patients with the debakey vad for more than 200 days. J Thorac Cardiovasc Surg 130:1122–1129
8. Wilhelm MJ, Hammel D, Schmid C, Stypmann J, Asfour B, Kemper D et al (2001) Clinical experience with nine patients supported by the continuous flow debakey vad. J Heart Lung Transplant 20:201
9. Thunberg CA, Gaitan BD, Arabia FA, Cole DJ, Grigore AM (2010) Ventricular assist devices today and tomorrow. J Cardiothorac Vasc Anesth 24:656–680

10. Chiu WC, Girdhar G, Xenos M, Alemu Y, Soares JS, Einav S et al (2014) Thromboresistance comparison of the heartmate ii ventricular assist device with the device thrombogenicity emulation- optimized heartassist 5 vad. J Biomech Eng 136:021014
11. Claiborne TE, Xenos M, Sheriff J, Chiu WC, Soares J, Alemu Y et al (2013) Toward optimization of a novel trileaflet polymeric prosthetic heart valve via device thrombogenicity emulation. ASAIO J 59:275–283
12. Bluestein D, Girdhar G, Einav S, Slepian MJ (2013) Device thrombogenicity emulation: a novel methodology for optimizing the thromboresistance of cardiovascular devices. J Biomech 46:338–344
13. Girdhar G, Xenos M, Alemu Y, Chiu WC, Lynch BE, Jesty J et al (2012) Device thrombogenicity emulation: a novel method for optimizing mechanical circulatory support device thromboresistance. PLoS One 7:e32463
14. Frazier OH, Khalil HA, Benkowski RJ, Cohn WE (2010) Optimization of axial-pump pressure sensitivity for a continuous-flow total artificial heart. J Heart Lung Transplant 29:687–691
15. Lahpor JR (2009) State of the art: implantable ventricular assist devices. Curr Opin Organ Transplant 14:554–559
16. Goldstein DJ (2003) Worldwide experience with the micromed debakey ventricular assist device as a bridge to transplantation. Circulation 108(Suppl 1):II272–II277
17. McMurray JJ, Adamopoulos S, Anker SD, Auricchio A, Bohm M, Dickstein K et al (2012) Esc guidelines for the diagnosis and treatment of acute and chronic heart failure 2012: the task force for the diagnosis and treatment of acute and chronic heart failure 2012 of the european society of cardiology. Developed in collaboration with the heart failure association (hfa) of the esc. Eur Heart J 33:1787–1847
18. Baumann Kreuziger LM (2015) Management of anticoagulation and antiplatelet therapy in patients with left ventricular assist devices. J Thromb Thrombolysis 39:337–344
19. Pektok E, Demirozu ZT, Arat N, Yildiz O, Oklu E, Eker D et al (2013) Remote monitoring of left ventricular assist device parameters after heartassist-5 implantation. Artif Organs 37:820–825
20. Pron G, Ieraci L, Kaulback K, Medical Advisory Secretariat HQO (2012) Internet-based device-assisted remote monitoring of cardiovascular implantable electronic devices: an evidence-based analysis. Ont Health Technol Assess Ser 12:1–86
21. Raatikainen MJ, Uusimaa P, van Ginneken MM, Janssen JP, Linnaluoto M (2008) Remote monitoring of implantable cardioverter defibrillator patients: a safe, time-saving, and cost-effective means for follow-up. Europace 10:1145–1151
22. Slotwiner D, Varma N, Akar JG, Annas G, Beardsall M, Fogel RI et al (2015) Hrs expert consensus statement on remote interrogation and monitoring for cardiovascular implantable electronic devices. Heart Rhythm 12:e69–100
23. Agarwal S, High KM (2012) Newer-generation ventricular assist devices. Best Pract Res Clin Anaesthesiol 26:117–130
24. Agati S, Bruschi G, Russo C, Colombo T, Lanfranconi M, Vitali E (2001) First successful italian clinical experience with debakey vad. J Heart Lung Transplant 20:914–917
25. Russo CF, Fratto PA, Milazzo F, Vitali E (2004) Successful replacement of malfunctioning tci heartmate lvad with debakey lvad as a bridge to heart transplantation. Interact Cardiovasc Thorac Surg 3:542–543

Early Experience with the CARMAT Bioprosthetic Artificial Heart

Piet Jansen, Christian Latrémouille, and Alain Carpentier

© Springer International Publishing Switzerland 2017
A. Montalto et al. (eds.), *Mechanical Circulatory Support in End-Stage Heart Failure*,
DOI 10.1007/978-3-319-43383-7_55

55.1 Introduction

Early development of mechanical circulatory support was aimed at replacing the native ventricles by a total artificial heart (TAH). However, progress was limited by the constraints of the then-available technologies and let to a shift toward implantable left ventricular assist devices (LVADs), supporting the left heart only. Over time, LVADs underwent a technological metamorphosis from valve-containing large devices placed in extra-thoracic pump pockets to valveless rotary flow devices that can be placed directly in the thoracic cavity using less-invasive surgical techniques [1]. These rotary flow devices contain narrow gaps and mechanical or hydrodynamic bearings and produce continuous flow in a high-shear environment. Despite the use of high levels of anticoagulation, pump thrombosis, acquired von Willebrand factor deficiency, and gastrointestinal bleeding have been observed with the use of these devices, indicating poor hemocompatibility [2, 3]. In addition, 10–40% patients with advanced left ventricular dysfunction treated by LVADs develop right ventricular dysfunction, resulting in complications related to right-sided congestion, such as renal failure and right heart failure [4].

The existing pneumatically driven TAH (SynCardia, Tucson, AZ) has synthetic blood-contacting surfaces and mechanical valves, requiring high levels of anticoagulation [5]. It uses external air compressors to activate the pumps, constraining patient's quality of life during mid- and long-term support.

The CARMAT total artificial heart (C-TAH) has been developed to address the issues of poor hemocompatibility and quality of life seen with the pneumatically driven TAH and external biventricular assist devices. It is intended to provide biventricular replacement therapy for patients with advanced heart failure.

55.2 Device Description and Functioning

The C-TAH is an electro-hydraulically driven single-unit device with the shape of a natural heart. The device has a polyetheretherketone (PEEK) body with a left and right ventricle. A double-layer hybrid membrane divides each ventricle into a blood compartment and an actuating liquid compartment. The blood-contacting layer of this membrane consists of bovine pericardial tissue chemically treated with glutaraldehyde [6]. The layer facing the actuating liquid side is made of polyurethane. The static surface of the blood compartment is covered with expanded polytetrafluoroethylene. The device is partially surrounded by a flexible polyurethane bag that serves as a reservoir and compliance chamber for the actuating liquid.

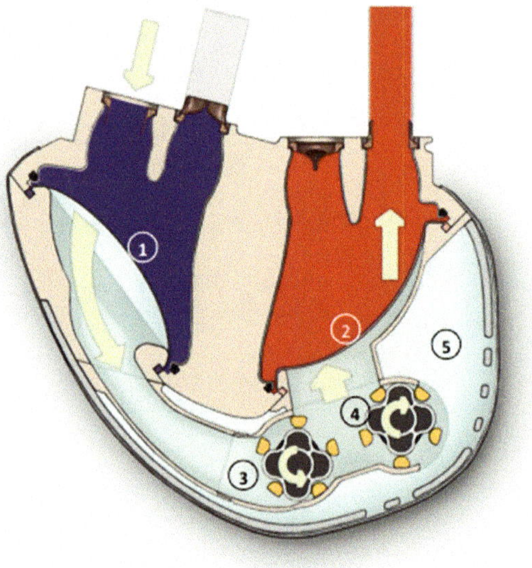

Fig. 55.1 Cross section of the CARMAT TAH. *1.* Right ventricle with membrane, *2.* left ventricle with membrane, *3.* main pump, *4.* auxiliary pump, *5.* silicon oil reservoir

Two volumetric side-by-side electrohydraulic pumps located in the liquid compartments of the prosthesis generate movement of the actuating liquid (Fig. 55.1). The principal pump shuttles the actuating liquid between the right and left ventricles, pulling and pushing the hybrid membranes. This results in a harmonious deployment of the hybrid membranes, with filling and emptying of the blood chambers in opposite phase. The auxiliary pump shuttles the actuating liquid between the left ventricle and the compliance chamber. With the auxiliary pump, it is possible to have a "cardiac cycle" with 2/3 diastole and 1/3 systole in standard conditions of 6 l/min flow. It is also possible to have different left and right stroke volumes, compensating for the bronchial circulation. The pumps always ensure full ejection of the blood cavities, to avoid stasis.

The beat rate ranges from 30 to 150 beats per minute, with a maximum stroke volume of

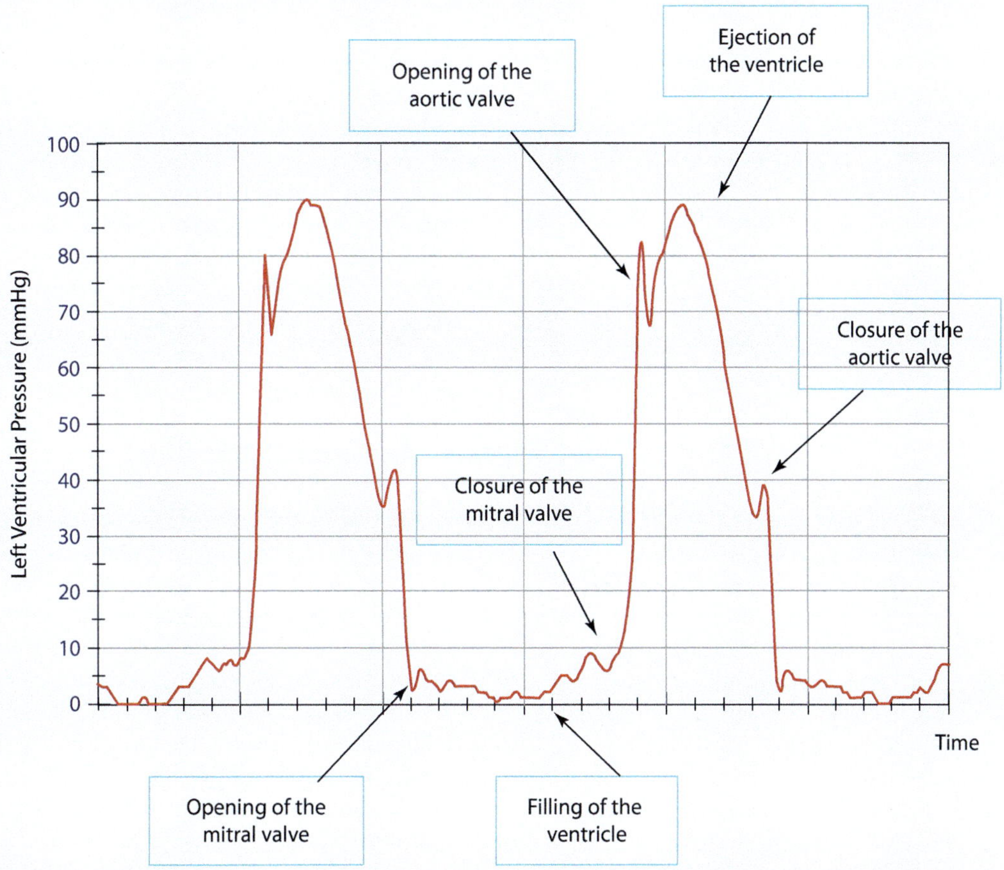

Fig. 55.2 *Left ventricular* pressure curve, obtained from the device pressure sensors and displayed on the hospital care console monitor. *Right ventricular* pressure curves are displayed in the same way

65 ml. Biological valves (M25 Carpentier-Edwards PERIMOUNT Plus 6900PT, Edwards Lifesciences, Irvine CA) at the inlet and outlet provide unidirectional pulsatile flow. The pumps do not generate pressure, but can operate within a pressure range from −10 to +250 mmHg on the left and right side.

The C-TAH is a self-containing system with the electronics that drive the pumps embedded inside the device. Pressure sensors are located in the actuating oil compartment of the left and right ventricle. They register ventricular pressures throughout the pumping cycle, providing instant information about filling and ejecting pressures. A third pressure sensor is located in the compliance chamber of the flexible polyurethane bag surrounding the prosthesis. This sensor provides information about pressure in the pericardial space and may be helpful in clinical detection of tamponade. Temperature sensors are embedded in the pressure sensors and monitor heat exchange in the ventricles and the pericardial space. An accelerometer located on the electronic board provides information about position changes of the prosthesis, used to correct/adjust the pressure measurements. Ultrasound transducers in each ventricle measure the position of the membrane.

The information gathered by the sensors and transducers is analyzed and processed by a microprocessor on the electronic board. This microprocessor communicates with another microprocessor that executes software whose algorithms control the activity of the motor pumps. Intraventricular pressure curves are displayed real time on the hospital care console monitor (Fig. 55.2).

A single percutaneous driveline of 8 mm in diameter delivers electrical current to power the prosthesis and provides information about its functioning. The driveline exits the skin at the lower left of the abdomen, where it is connected to an External Routing Module (ERM) maintained on the patient with a support belt. The ERM is connected to a controller, which is the interface between the prosthesis and the patient. The controller delivers power from two battery pockets providing approximately 4 h of untethered support. A small LED display on the controller provides information about battery status, device functioning, and alarms. The patient retains the controller and batteries in a carry bag.

55.3 Summary of Distinctive Features of the CARMAT TAH

- Bioprosthetic material in contact with blood
- No contact between blood and pumps
- Gradual deployment of stroke volume with minimal shear stress
- Pulsatile flow
- Self-containing system with on-board electronics and microprocessors
- Automatic response with variation in pump flow, according to the patient's needs
- Biventricular support
- Completely incorporated in the pericardial sac

55.4 Preclinical Testing

Device performance and durability of the C-TAH were tested in mock circulations and on durability bench tests. In vitro studies exposing the blood-contacting materials of the device to circulating fresh human blood verified the hemocompatibility of these materials [7]. Subsequent animal studies in a calf model were used to validate hemocompatibility and device performance in a physiological environment up to 10 days of support [8].

55.5 Anatomic Fit Studies

Standard two-dimensional thoracic computer tomography (CT) scans of potential candidates for C-TAH placement are analyzed preoperatively to ensure that the device fits in the thoracic cavity. From the 2D scans, a three-dimensional (3D) model of the thorax and its structures is created. The native heart is then replaced with a 3D model of the C-TAH. The inflow areas of the 3D model are placed at the right and left atrioventricular junctions and the outflow areas at the pulmonary artery and aorta. Based on these placements and the resulting position of the 3D model relative to the chest wall and diaphragm, the implanting surgeon determines whether the device fits (◘ Fig. 55.3).

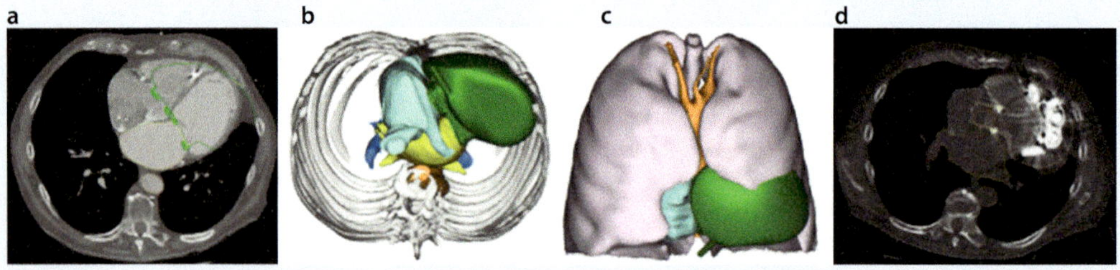

◘ **Fig. 55.3** Anatomic fit study. **a** 2D view of prosthesis contour (*green line*) relative to native heart. **b** 3D placement of the C-TAH, caudal view. **c** 3D placement of the C-TAH, frontal view. **d** 2D view of post-implant CT scan with prosthesis in place (*yellow line*, contour)

55.6 Implant Procedure

The bioprosthetic surfaces of the device, the atrial suture flanges, and the biological valves are preserved in glutaraldehyde. During the initial phase of the surgical procedure, these surfaces are carefully rinsed with heparin-containing saline according to a validated procedure.

The CARMAT TAH is implanted in orthotopic position. The pericardial space is accessed through a median sternotomy and a midline vertical incision of the pericardial sac. Cardiopulmonary bypass (CPB) is established with direct bicaval cannulation and an outflow cannula in the ascending aorta. After cross clamping, the native ventricles are excised up to the left and right atrioventricular junctions. The aorta and the pulmonary artery are transected just distally from the valve commissures. The diameter of the atrioventricular orifices is measured with sizing tools (30-35-40-45 mm). Bioprosthetic flanges with a circular central opening reinforced by a silicon ring are cut to size and sutured onto the mitral and tricuspid orifices. The silicone ring of each flange is connected to a single titanium interface device with two central openings. The C-TAH, with the inflow valves in place, is then clicked onto the interface device with the silicone rings ensuring hermetic sealing. Next, the aortic conduit (Dacron, 30 mm diameter) containing the outflow valve is sutured to the distal aorta. Finally, the pulmonary conduit (Dacron, 30 mm diameter) with outflow valve is sutured to the distal pulmonary artery. Both arterial suture lines are left open to facilitate deairing.

The percutaneous driveline leaves the C-TAH just ventral of the interface device and is tunneled to exit the skin at the lower right abdominal quadrant. The driveline is then connected via the ERM and an external cable to the controller and hospital care console. The C-TAH can now be switched on for deairing of the device's ventricles.

Deairing cannulas are inserted through the suture lines of the aortic and pulmonary conduits and connected to open syringes, in which CPB suction lines can be placed. After unsnaring the caval cannulae, the C-TAH is switched on with beat rate 10/min and stroke volume 30 ml to eject the remaining air through the deairing cannulas, with local CO_2 insufflation. The pump rate can be manually increased but high pressure on the suture lines should be avoided. When deairing is completed (eventually confirmed by echo), the aorta clamp is removed. Weaning of CPB is done with decreasing CPB flow while increasing the prosthesis output. Guided by the left atrial and central venous pressure, the clinician can set the pump rate, the left ventricular stroke volume, and the ratio between the right and left ventricular stroke volume. When the C-TAH has obtained full flow, CPB is stopped and protamine injected. Meticulous hemostasis is performed; the pericardium and sternum are closed, leaving drains in place.

55.7 Device Operation

In the early postoperative phase, the device settings can be switched from manual mode to automatic response mode. The automatic mode of the C-TAH is mimicking two physiological functions of the native heart: response to preload changes (Frank Starling law) and baroreceptor-like response.

The automatic response uses filling pressure targets for the right and left atrium that are set by the clinician. The membrane deployment in diastolic phase is controlled to achieve the preset filling pressure and maximizes stroke volume without suction of the atria. As a result, the C-TAH automatically adjusts its stroke volume, pump rate, and balance between left and right stroke volume. When the preload is increased (e.g., physical effort or hypervolemia), the prosthesis increases the flow to maintain the preset inlet pressures.

In case of low systemic arterial pressure (e.g., low vascular resistance, hypotension), the TAH automatically increases its pump rate to reach a minimum ejection pressure ensuring organ perfusion. Once the status is treated medically, the TAH will recover its normal functioning.

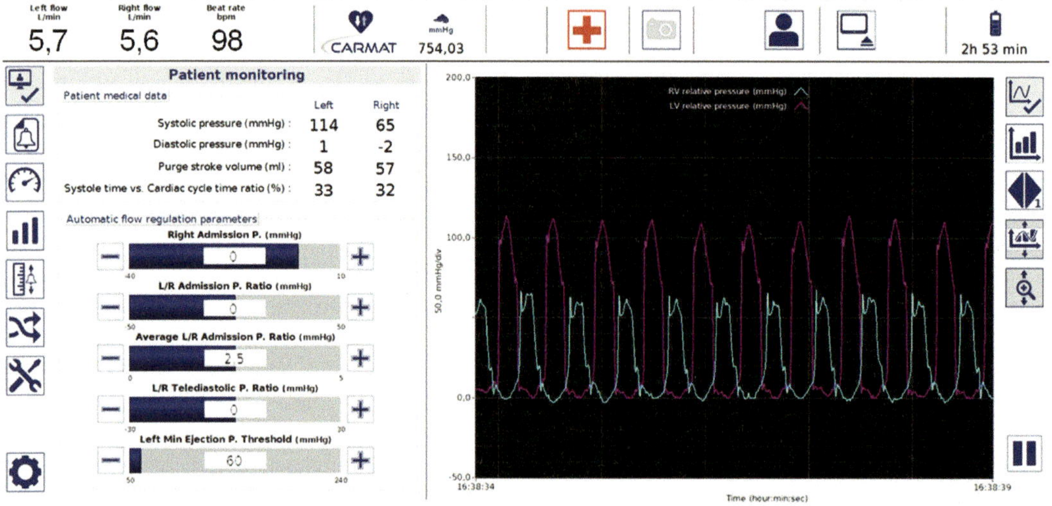

Fig. 55.4 Screenshot from the hospital care console monitor. *Left panel*: showing device parameters that can be adjusted by the clinician. *Right panel*: pressure curves from the left ventricle (*purple line*) and the right ventricle (*turquoise line*)

Figure 55.4 shows a screenshot of the hospital care console with the parameters of the automatic mode that can be adjusted by the clinician.

A Valsalva-response function is integrated in the automatic mode to prevent the prosthesis from increasing its blood flow in case of sudden intrathoracic pressure rise caused by coughing or defecation effort. If the right inlet pressure increases beyond 22 mmHg, the blood flow is maintained at the pressure level registered before sudden pressure rise. Once the right inlet pressure is below 18 mm Hg during five successive cycles, the prosthesis returns to its normal functioning.

55.8 Postoperative Management

Patients requiring TAH support often have concomitant renal insufficiency. The native ventricles are the main sources of B-type natriuretic peptide (BNP), which plays a critical role in renal perfusion. Their removal results in a depletion of BNP, increasing the risk of further deterioration of renal function in the postoperative phase. Supplementation of synthetic BNP, if available, may improve diuresis and renal function. In some cases temporary hemodialysis or hemofiltration is necessary to bridge a period of multiple weeks during which alternate sources of endogenous BNP secretion may restore the internal milieu [9].

In the postoperative phase, patients are extubated and mobilized as soon as possible and can start eating and drinking when intestinal peristaltic activity is confirmed. An educational program is initiated to prepare the patient and his personal caregiver in managing the external equipment.

55.8.1 Anticoagulation Guidelines

In the immediate postoperative phase, when thoracic drain production is minimal, intravenous unfractionated heparin is started (target anti-Xa activity 0.20 IU/mL). This is replaced by subcutaneous injection of low-molecular-weight heparin (e.g., tinzaparin) with a dose of 175 IU/kg/day when renal function is normalized. Oral antivitamin K is initiated when the D-dimer level is lower than 2000 ng/mL, typically 6–8 months after implantation. These guidelines are subject to modification according to clinical experience in the pivotal clinical study.

55.9 Clinical Experience

A first-in-man feasibility study of four patients was initiated in 2013 in France. The clinical teams participating in the study completed a training program that included multiple acute animal implants and device management sessions. The study population consisted of patients at high risk of death from end-stage biventricular failure and not eligible for transplant. A first step in the patient screening process was the assessment of anatomic compatibility by 3D virtual implantation of the C-TAH, as described above. Patient eligibility criteria are listed below:

55.9.1 Inclusion Criteria

- Age ≥18 years
- INTERMACS profile 1 or 2 [10]
- LVEF ≤30%
- Optimized medical treatment (European Society of Cardiology, American Heart Association recommendations)
- On intravenous inotropes ≥7 days
- BSA ≥1.7 m^2
- Anatomic compatibility verified by 3D modeling
- Signed informed consent

55.9.2 Exclusion Criteria

- Technical obstacle, high surgical risk
- Platelet count <150,000 cells per μL or INR ≥1.5 without anticoagulant therapy
- Hemorrhagic stroke <6 weeks
- Active uncontrolled bloodstream infection
- Hemodynamically significant peripheral vascular disease
- Malignant neoplasm with life expectancy <6 months
- On corticosteroid medication equivalent to prednisone 7.5 mg per day
- Irreversible cognitive dysfunction, psychosocial issues, and mental disorder that are likely to impair compliance

55.9.3 Clinical Cases

The first patient to receive the C-TAH was a 76-year-old male with severe biventricular failure based on nonischemic dilated cardiomyopathy. After an uneventful C-TAH implant procedure and a rapid initial recovery, he remained in the postoperative intensive care due to respiratory and renal failure, requiring hemofiltration. Bleeding complications prompted the clinicians to stop anticoagulation (heparin) at day 23. The patient was supported for 74 days when a device failure occurred and led to the patient's death. At autopsy, the blood-contacting cavities of the device were free from thrombus, and there was no thromboembolism in major organs, despite 51 days without anticoagulation [11].

The second case was a 68-year-old male with end-stage biventricular failure and not eligible for cardiac transplantation due to age. The surgical procedure and postoperative recovery were uneventful. After successful rehabilitation, the patient could be discharged from the hospital after 5 months. He spent 4 months at home, enjoying a reasonable quality of life. At 9-month support, he experienced a device failure resulting in death. The blood-contacting cavities of the device were free from thrombus, and there was no thromboembolism observed at autopsy.

The third patient was a cachectic 74-year-old male with severe biventricular failure based on nonischemic cardiomyopathy with an amyloid component and pulmonary hypertension. In the early postoperative phase, intermittent hemofiltration was needed to support renal recovery. Following a revalidation period at his referring hospital, the patient was discharged home at 5 months. Repeated re-hospitalizations for asthenia, cachexia, and renal insufficiency lead to the patient's death at 8 months.

The fourth case was a 58-year-old male supported by an extracorporeal life support system and on the high urgency list for transplant. While the surgical implant procedure was successful, the early postoperative phase was characterized by multiple re-interventions due to bleeding. The patient died after 20 days due to sepsis and multiorgan failure.

Detailed results of the feasibility study will be published in peer-reviewed journals. The preliminary clinical experience with the CARMAT TAH suggests that the development of total artificial hearts using bioprosthetic materials could represent an important contribution.

A European multicenter study was initiated in 2016. The objective of this pivotal study is to evaluate the clinical safety and performance of the C-TAH for the treatment of end-stage heart failure. The target study population consists of patients with end-stage heart failure, refractory to optimal medical management, requiring mechanical circulatory support but for whom LVAD is considered inefficient or contraindicated.

References

1. Kirklin JK, Naftel DC, Pagani FD, Kormos RL, Stevenson LW, Blume ED et al (2015) Seventh INTERMACS annual report: 15,000 patients and counting. J Heart Lung Transplant 34(12):1495–1504
2. Stulak JM, Lee D, Haft JW, Romano MA, Cowger JA, Park SJ et al (2014) Gastrointestinal bleeding and subsequent risk of thromboembolic events during support with a left ventricular assist device. J Heart Lung Transplant 33(1):60–64
3. Starling RC, Moazami N, Silvestry SC, Ewald G, Rogers JG, Milano CA et al (2014) Unexpected abrupt increase in left ventricular assist device thrombosis. N Engl J Med 370(1):33–40
4. Kormos RL (2014) The right heart failure dilemma in the era of left ventricular assist devices. J Heart Lung Transplant 33(2):134–135
5. Copeland JG, Copeland H, Gustafson M, Mineburg N, Covington D, Smith RG et al (2012) Experience with more than 100 total artificial heart implants. J Thorac Cardiovasc Surg 143(3):727–734
6. Carpentier A (2007) The surprising rise of nonthrombogenic valvular surgery. Nat Med 13(10):1165–1168
7. Jansen P, van Oeveren W, Capel A, Carpentier A (2012) In vitro haemocompatibility of a novel bioprosthetic total artificial heart. Eur J Cardiothorac Surg 41(6):e166–e172
8. Latremouille C, Duveau D, Cholley B, Zilberstein L, Belbis G, Boughenou M et al (2015) Animal studies with the Carmat bioprosthetic total artificial heart. Eur J Cardiothorac Surg 47:e172–e1e9
9. Quader MA, Goodreau AM, Shah KB, Katlaps G, Cooke R, Smallfield MC et al (2016) Renal function recovery with total artificial heart support. ASAIO J 62(1): 87–91
10. Stevenson L, Pagani F, Young JB, Jessup M, Miller L, Kormos R et al (2009) INTERMACS profiles of advanced heart failure: the current picture. J Heart Lung Transplant 2009(28):535–541
11. Carpentier A, Latrémouille C, Cholley B, Smadja DM, Roussel J-C, Boissier E et al (2015) First clinical use of a bioprosthetic total artificial heart: report of two cases. Lancet 386(10003):1556–1563

The ReinHeart Solution

Gero Tenderich, Sotirios Spiliopoulos, and Reiner Koerfer

© Springer International Publishing Switzerland 2017

A. Montalto et al. (eds.), *Mechanical Circulatory Support in End-Stage Heart Failure*,
DOI 10.1007/978-3-319-43383-7_56

The *ReinHeart* is an electrically driven TAH designed as an alternative to heart transplantation aiming to support patients for at least 5 years. The design requirements have been complete implantability, broad applicability, durability, and maintenance-free operation of the system [1].

56.1 System Components (Fig. 56.1)

56.1.1 Pump Unit (Fig. 56.2)

The pump unit consists of a *linear drive unit* and two *artificial ventricles* housing four mechanical valves and two polyurethane membranes. The linear drive unit consists of four coils on a bobbin and magnets. By variating the coil current, the bobbin can either be pulled into the magnetic field or pushed out of it. The resulting movement is guided by one central axis and ejects alternatively the left and right ventricle. A position sensing system detects the position of the bobbin along this central axis, and a temperature sensor reads the temperature of the drive unit. Inside the bobbin, durable springs provide the electrical connection to the coils.

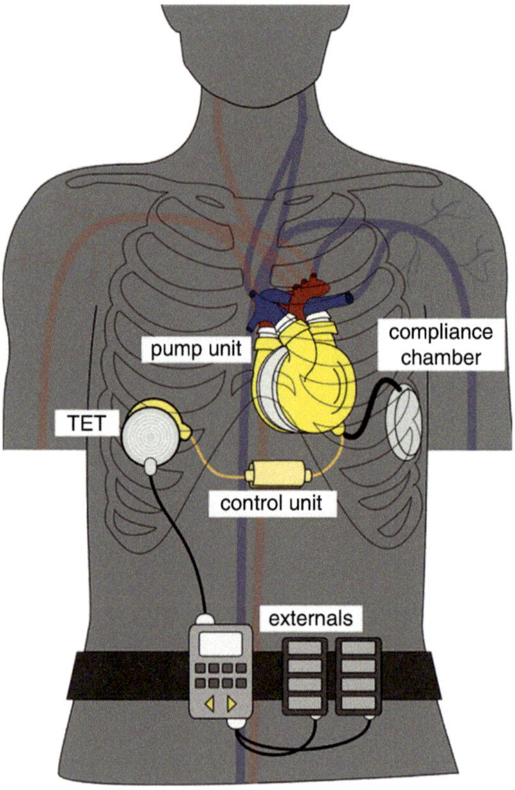

Fig. 56.1 System components

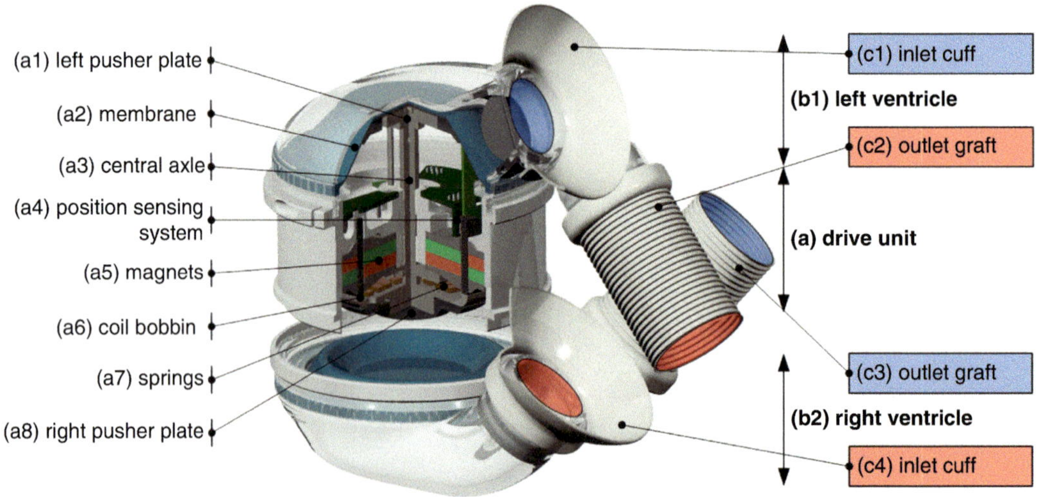

Fig. 56.2 Detailed view of the pump unit

Bobbin and springs are the only moving parts of the drive unit. This ensures low wear and high durability. A major characteristic of the system is that pusher plates are not fixed to the membranes, allowing a preload sensitive filling of the ventricles and thereby avoiding suction events. Ventricles provide a stroke volume of 60 ml. Depending on operational frequency and preload, the artificial ventricles can generate a pump flow of up to 7.5 l/min. Two inflow cuffs connect the pump unit to the left and the right atrium and two outflow grafts to the aorta and the main pulmonary artery. Four mechanical valves facilitate unidirectional blood flow. The pump currently weighs 850 g.

56.1.2 TET System

The TET system transmits electrical energy from an external to an internal coil. The subcutaneously implanted internal coil has a diameter of 70 mm. The external coil has an inner diameter of 70 mm and an outer diameter of 100 mm. Power from external batteries or other power supplies is converted to high-frequency AC voltage and then converted back to DC voltage by electronics included in the implantable controller. Power losses are remarkably low and local heating is minimal. The TET system is able to support the TAH up to a distance of 30 mm.

56.1.3 Implantable Controller

The implantable controller is a printed circuit board containing power and communication electronics as well as four battery cells and is connected by three microplugs to the pump unit, the compliance chamber, and the TET coil. It acquires data of the position sensing system and distributes current to the motor coils depending on the position of the coil bobbin and its pusher plates in the pump unit. Electronics are powered by the TET system or the implanted batteries. The batteries get charged by connecting the outer coil of the TET system and can support the device for about 45 min at full capacity.

56.1.4 Compliance Chamber

The compliance chamber is connected to the drive unit, and its operation is controlled by the implantable controller. It prevents suction events and regulates balance between left and right ventricular output by diminishing sharp pressure peaks in the drive unit. Furthermore an integrated pump adjusts air pressure and supports movement of the polyurethane membranes.

56.1.5 External User Interface

Intrinsic data of the TAH system is stored in an external user interface. It delivers operational data and enables adjustment of all clinically relevant parameters.

56.2 Current State of Development

Results from ongoing long-term, in vitro durability testing of the main components [2] suggest that safe patient support up to 5 years is feasible. Up to now, the connection springs between the bearing and the electrical coils as well as the membranes have been tested with accelerated frequency under physiological conditions for 440 and 250 million cycles. This corresponds to a calculated duration of operation of 7 and 4 years, respectively.

In order to minimize clot formation, fluid-structure interaction simulation and particle image velocimetry were used to analyze and optimize the motion pattern of the membranes, the flow distribution inside the pump, and consequently its washout performance, currently amounting 99.4% [3, 4]. A standard anticoagulation regime has still to be elaborated.

The TAH system is currently being tested in a subchorionic bovine model. Following typical excision of the native ventricles, inflow cuffs are sutured to the remnants of the left and the right atrium, and anastomosis of the outflow grafts with the aorta and the main pulmonary artery is performed. Finally, the pump unit is connected with the grafts, inserted into the thorax, and connected to the control unit and the compliance chamber.

References

1. Koerfer R, Spiliopoulos S, Finocchiaro T, Guersoy D, Tenderich G, Steinseifer U (2014) Steinseifer Paving the way for destination therapy of end-stage biventricular heart failure: the ReinHeart-total-artificial heart concept. Eur J Cardiothorac Surg 46(6):935–936
2. Pelletier B, Spiliopoulos S, Finocchiaro T, Graef F, Kuipers K, Laumen M, Guersoy D, Steinseifer U, Koerfer R, Tenderich G (2015) System overview of the fully implantable destination therapy – reinHeart -total artificial heart. Eur J Cardiothorac Surg 47(1):80–86
3. Sonntag SJ, Kaufmann TAS, Büsen MR, Laumen M, Linde T, Schmitz-Rode T, Steinseifer U (2013) Simulation of a pulsatile total artificial heart: development of a partitioned Fluid Structure Interaction model. J Fluids Struct 38:187–204
4. Sonntag SJ, Kaufmann TAS, Büsen MR, Laumen M, Gräf F, Linde T, Steinseifer U (2014) Numerical washout study of a pulsatile total artificial heart. Int J Artif Organs 37(3):241–252

Health-Economic Aspects

Content

Health-Economic Aspects of MCS Therapy

Robin Bostic and Mark S. Slaughter

© Springer International Publishing Switzerland 2017
A. Montalto et al. (eds.), *Mechanical Circulatory Support in End-Stage Heart Failure*,
DOI 10.1007/978-3-319-43383-7_57

57.1 Background of Mechanical Circulatory Support

The use of mechanical circulatory support (MCS) began in the 1960s. The first implantation of a ventricular assist device (VAD) as a bridge to recovery (BTR) occurred in 1966, and this was followed with a total artificial heart implant as a bridge to transplant (BTT) in 1969 [1, 2]. These events, along with the first human heart transplant in 1968 [3], began an era of intense research into treating advanced heart failure with various forms of cardiac replacement or assist. It was well recognized during this era that there was a need for MCS systems that could provide physiologic levels of support for extended durations. As the outcomes of heart transplant proved to be less than satisfactory in the early 1970s, research and development efforts on durable MCS escalated. Forms of MCS that evolved were basically total artificial hearts (TAHs) and ventricular assist devices (VADs), both of which were intended to provide lifetime support as alternatives to transplant.

In the early 1980s, effective immunosuppression therapy renewed heart transplant, which soon became the treatment of choice for end-stage heart failure. The issue of donor organ shortage became apparent as the number of patients dying on the wait list escalated. The BTT application offered the possibility of survival for the sickest patients waiting for a suitable donor, but there was also a need for a well-defined population of heart failure patients to study the effectiveness of VAD support. Clinical trials were initiated, with the TAH used as a permanent support system, and VADs were used for either temporary support as BTR or BTT.

Numerous VAD systems have been used for the BTT indication, but implantable left ventricular assist devices (LVADs) became the configuration that was most suitable for ambulatory support lasting for months. Portable pneumatic drivers were first used; then electric motors were integrated into the implantable pump. Clinical trials for the BTT indication were carried out in the USA and Europe during the 1990s, with ultimate market approval for this indication [4–6]. The majority of supported patients benefitted from improved organ function, better physical status, and longer survival. The positive outcomes were achieved during these trials, and with patients being supported for extended durations (years), the concept of lifetime support (DT) evolved. The Randomized Evaluation of Mechanical Assistance for the Treatment of Congestive Heart Failure (REMATCH) was carried out to evaluate LVAD support against optimal medical therapy in patients with end-stage heart failure [7, 8]. This trial demonstrated superior survival for LVAD-supported patients compared to those with continuing medical therapy [9].

By the early 2000s, the HeartMate XVE-LVAD (formerly Thermo Cardiosystems, Inc., and Thoratec Corporation, now St. Jude Medical Inc., St. Paul, MN) was approved for both BTT and DT, and the Thoratec paracorporeal VAD (PVAD) (formerly Thoratec Corporation, now St. Jude Medical Inc., St. Paul, MN) was approved for BTR and BTT. The preference for PVAD use was in patients needing biventricular support or who were too small for the XVE-LVAD, and for those needing long-term left ventricular support, the device of choice was the XVE-LVAD. Commercial use of the XVE-LVAD grew to numerous medical centers worldwide, with hundreds of patients being supported for extended durations. Nevertheless, the results of the REMATCH trial and the post-trial experience revealed that adverse events such as bleeding and infection were substantial, and the durability of the electric motor in the XVE-LVAD was very limited [10]. The morbidity, mortality, and cost of care from the adverse events were sizeable – the major stimulus for the development of smaller and more durable LVADs.

Small axial-flow pumps with a single moving component for enhanced durability were introduced clinically in 2000 and have been studied extensively since that time [11–13]. The adverse event profile of these devices, particularly their durability, is considerably improved over the prior generation of pulsatile devices. The HeartMate II LVAD (formerly Thoratec Corp., now St. Jude Medical Inc., St. Paul, MN) has completed clinical trials for BTT and DT, with FDA and CE mark approvals for these indications in 2008 and 2010, respectively [14–16]. The HeartMate II is the most widely used durable MCS device, with now more than 23,000 implants worldwide. Another device used for BTT is the HeartWare HVAD (HeartWare International, Inc., Framingham, MA), a centrifugal flow pump that has also been demonstrated to be durable for long-term support [17]. The survival rates for the BTT application for both the HeartMate II and the HVAD have reached 85% at

1-year end point, with no reports of device failure. However, pump thrombosis and gastrointestinal bleeding are adverse events seen in both devices, which are topics of much discussion and research today [18–20].

The most recent LVAD system to be introduced clinically is the HeartMate III (St. Jude Medical, Inc., St. Paul, MN) [21]. The HeartMate III is designed to have improved hemocompatibility with its full magnetically levitated rotor that has wide blood flow gaps for reduced shear stress on blood components. An artificial pulse and textured blood-contacting surfaces may also contribute to improved hemocompatibility. A clinical trial at 10 centers in Europe, Canada, Australia, and Kazakhstan enrolled 50 patients with the mixed indications of BTT and DT [22]. The trial completed in 2015 resulted in a 6-month survival rate of 92%, which exceeded the performance goal of 88%, and there were no instances of pump thrombosis, hemolysis, or need for pump exchange. CE mark approval was obtained in 2015 and a large multicenter clinical trial is underway in the USA.

57.1.1 Global Review of MCS Cost-Effectiveness

Support with a durable LVAD decreases morbidity and mortality for patients with end-stage heart failure. Supported patients may be discharged from the hospital and resume most activities with few physical limitations. Patients living at home with LVAD support has considerably less expense than when being hospitalized and receiving medical therapy. Clinical studies have shown that the potential benefits are quality-of-life improvement and functional status improvement (NYHA classification improved from NYHA class III or IV to class I or II for the majority of patients), and there are potential economic savings by reducing pharmacological treatments and decreased length of stay in intensive care unit and hospitalization duration [23, 24]. For these reasons, the American College of Cardiology, American Heart Association, and The European Society of Cardiology recommend the use of MCS for patients meeting criteria for severe heart failure while receiving optimal medical therapy [25, 26].

An analysis of costs associated with hospital discharge of patients who underwent LVAD support showed that this treatment provides effective and economical outpatient support and is associated with limited morbidity, with satisfactory quality of life [27]. In parallel with the REMATCH clinical study, Oz et al. [28] reported on cost and utilization data for 52 of the 68 REMATCH LVAD recipients. The mean cost to implant an LVAD was $210,187, including the cost of the device. This was comparable to other life-saving organ replacement procedures, such as liver transplant. They also commented on technologic and surgical improvements that were on the horizon and speculated on how these adjustments might influence the cost-effectiveness of the therapy. Many of these improvements have come to fruition in the "post-REMATCH" era, including refined patient selection and a newer, more robust, and reliable LVAD. Patient survival and quality of life are improving while costs of treatment are decreasing in the post-REMATCH era.

The cost of LVAD implantation, which excludes professional fees, was significantly lower for the post-REMATCH patients compared to the trial patients ($141,000 versus $210,000, $p < 0.001$) [34]. This was in part due to a shorter mean initial hospitalization for the post-REMATCH patients (31.6 days) compared with the general REMATCH cohort (43.5 days, $p = 0.01$) and with the late-REMATCH patients (45.0 days, $p = 0.01$). In the REMATCH study, an analysis of costs associated with end of life of end-stage heart failure patients receiving drug therapy was published [35]. The data of the 41 patients analyzed dealt with cost and resource utilization in 3-month intervals and focused on the last 2 years of life. The cost of medical management in the final 2 years of life was $159,302.90, with 52.0%, or $82,833.83, occurring in the final 6 months. REMATCH demonstrated a 2-year survival <10% in the medical management group. In another cost analysis of two large, very experienced centers, the cost of LVAD implant dropped significantly over time [36]. Outcomes with use of LVADs as DT have improved in the post-REMATCH era, including significantly lower hospital costs as well as trends toward better survival to hospital discharge and shorter average length of stay. During the HeartMate II DT clinical trial, costs were captured for all implanted devices, and when compared to the cost reported in the REMATCH trial, there was nearly 50%

reduction in cost for HeartMate II-implanted patients [36] (◘ Table 57.1).

Heart transplant without an LVAD bridge is the most cost-effective course, but the sickest patients often cannot continue waiting without circulatory support. BTT with transplant requires two major operations with considerable hospital time for both procedures, expectedly making this approach costly [29]. Studies have identified reimbursement for LVAD support as inadequate when compared to transplant; however, third-party payer reimbursement has improved along with better survival making BTT more cost-effective [30, 31]. In a more recent head-to-head cost comparison of heart transplant to LVAD support at 1 year, the average cost was approximately $40,000 high for LVAD support, but this difference was not statistically significant [32]. Comparison of LVAD support to heart transplant is problematic since patients undergoing LVAD implant for BTT are likely to be much sicker or are at higher risk of death than patients undergoing elective transplant. Furthermore, LVAD support in the sickest transplant candidates optimizes organ function and physical status lowering the risk of post-transplant complications. Cost-effective comparisons inherently give transplant an advantage [33].

In the Center for Medicare Medicaid Services, Medicare Provider Analysis and Review (MEDPAR) file contains data from claims for services provided to beneficiaries admitted to Medicare certified inpatient hospitals. MEDPAR 2013 hospital cost reported the volume, length of stay (days), and average cost for implanting an LVAD and heart transplantation (◘ Table 57.2). The hospital cost for implanting an LVAD, which includes the additional expense of the device and accessories, is becoming similar to heart transplantation cost.

The UK National Institute of Health Research, analyzing the clinical effectiveness and cost-effectiveness of LVADs as BTT, completed a systematic review and cost-effectiveness model [37]. The aims of this study were to determine the clinical effectiveness and cost-effectiveness of continuous-flow LVADs used for BTT versus medical therapy and BTT versus destination therapy. The systematic review included devices approved for BTT by the US Food and Drug Administration and Conformité Européenne (CE) approved – the two systems with results were the HeartMate II and the HVAD. Forty publications were identified to provide the outcome data, while cost-effectiveness data was gathered from implants performed at six institutions in the United Kingdom. There were no randomized controlled trials in the analysis. A semi-Markov model with multiple sensitivity analyses varying survival, utilities, and cost inputs to the model was used. The model outputs were incremental cost-effectiveness ratios (ICERs), cost-/quality-adjusted life-years (QALYs) gained and

◘ **Table 57.1** Comparison of REMATCH and HeartMate II DT costs

Implant Cost	REMATCH	HeartMate II DT Trial	*p*-Value
N	54	98	<0.01
Cost ($)	384,260 ± 340,456	193,812 ± 71,027	
Median ($)	245,445	186,156	

◘ **Table 57.2** Comparison of heart transplant and implantable assist device

MS-DRG 1 case mix	Case volume (N)	Average length of stay (days)	Average calculated cost ($)	Average organ acquisition cost ($)	Average total cost ($)
Heart transplant (ICD-9 Px 33.6 and 37.51)	648	32	116,265.71	28,406.14	144,673
Implantable heart assist (ICD-9 Px 37.52 and 37.66)	1259	34	196,595.26	Not applicable	196,026

cost/life-year gained (LYG). They reported that the 3-year, 10-year, and lifetime ICERs for BTT with an LVAD compared to medical management are higher than generally applied to willingness-to-pay thresholds. Nonetheless, at a lifetime time horizon, the ICERs approximate the threshold values used in end-of-life assessments. They had determined that LVADs for BTT yields ICERs of £122,730, £68,088, and £55,173, respectively, when compared with medical management.

At a lifetime horizon, using VADs as an alternative to transplant (ATT) rather than as a BTT was complex and had a reduced cost and reduced quality-adjusted life-years (QALYs). ATT when evaluated over a lifetime was £20,637 less costly than BTT for each QALY year. An important conclusion from this study was the need of published studies that include cost with survival, quality of life, functional capacity, and adverse event rates.

During the HeartMate II clinical trial, a Markov model was developed to assess cost-effectiveness of DT as compared to medical management [38]. Survival, hospitalization rates, quality of life, and cost data were analyzed for advanced heart failure patients treated with LVAD support or medical therapy. Clinical outcomes were obtained from the medical therapy arm of the REMATCH trial and from patients treated with an LVAD in the HeartMate II destination therapy clinical trial. The cost of heart failure admissions was estimated with Medicare prospective payments, and the cost of LVAD implantation was obtained from hospital claims during the clinical trial. Compared to patients treated with optimal medical therapy, continuous-flow LVAD patients had higher 5-year costs ($360,407 versus $62,856), QALYs (1.87 versus 0.37), and life-years (2.42 versus 0.64). The ICER of the continuous-flow device was $198,184 per QALY and $167,208 per life-year. This equates to a 75% reduction in ICER compared to the $802,700 per QALY for the pulsatile-flow device. The results were most sensitive to the cost of device implantation, long-term survival, cost per re-hospitalization, and utility associated with patients' functional status. This study concluded that cost-effectiveness of LVAD support was improving for patients treated for destination therapy with the newer continuous-flow LVAD. These results were attributed to better survival, lower costs of implantation, and better functional capacity of supported patients. Although the ICER/QALY was higher than the conventional $50,000, the high rate of cost reduction was very encouraging. The observed 75% reduction in QALY/year occurred during a time when LVAD implants were increasing substantially with the anticipation of further improvements. The findings and conclusions of this study were at a time when the use of continuous-flow LVADs was relatively early, and with clinical experience, efficiency and survival are likely.

57.2 Evolving Cost-Effectiveness: How It Is Changing

A number of cost-effectiveness studies have been performed with retrospective data on patients supported with the older generation of pulsatile LVADs [39–41]. These studies conclude that improvements in LVAD technology are necessary to improve cost-effectiveness, and continued reassessment is desired. Over the past decade, there has been a continual improvement in outcomes of durable continuous-flow LVAD support, with 6-month and 1-year survival rates for BTT near 94% and 85%, respectively [42]. This compares to the early results, which showed rates of 75% at 6 months and 68% at 1 year [43]. For sicker patients supported for DT, survival at 1 year has increased from 68 to 74%, and at 2 years, the increase was 58–61% [44]. These improvements are largely due to better timing of LVAD implant, preoperative optimization, postoperative management protocols, and refinements in the technology [45]. The overall rate of serious adverse events has steadily declined, which has a significant impact on hospitalization time, the number of interventions, and the total cost of care. Therefore, overall effectiveness of LVAD therapy is continuously evolving in a positive direction, but the longer survival time increases overall cost and offsets some of this gain [46, 47].

The evolution of LVAD therapy for advanced heart failure has been unique when compared to other devices and pharmacological therapy [48]. The change from pulsatile- to continuous-flow LVAD technology was relatively rapid as clinicians identified the benefits of the smaller and more durable devices. The "learning curve" associated with the application of the continuous-flow devices was relatively short, and outcomes have improved steadily over the 15 years since their inception [42]. In this same time

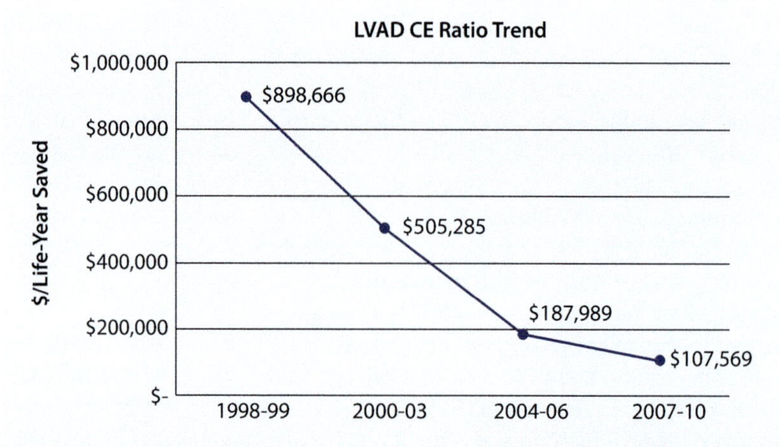

Fig. 57.1 LVAD CE ratio over time

frame, the ICER for pulsatile LVADs during the REMATCH trial was $602,361, which then decreased to $187,989 in the post-trial time and then to $107,569 with the use of the current continuous-flow devices (Fig. 57.1) [48]. This level of ICER nears the $100,000 mark of willingness to pay per life-year saved. This progress in cost-effectiveness is compelling, yet controlled unbiased data from clinical trials that guides policy decisions is needed. Furthermore, because LVAD technology is constantly evolving and patient care improves with experience, cost-effectiveness analysis also needs to be continuous and its methods developed.

Although LVAD support for both BTT and DT extends survival and the majority of patients experience improved quality of life, current cost-effectiveness studies indicate that further reduction in adverse events is necessary for this therapy to exceed cost-effectiveness thresholds [49–51]. Re-hospitalization and follow-up care for both BTT and DT indications are significant drivers for the high cost of LVAD support [52]. In particular, gastrointestinal bleeding (GIB) and infection are the leading causes for readmission, with the median cost of each readmission at approximately $7500 [53]. Unfortunately, GIB is very common with the current generation of continuous-flow LVADs, and it is currently unknown how to avoid this complication. Infection readmission is also common and is one of the more costly adverse events seen in the LVAD population. Less frequent, yet costly events occurring over the course of LVAD support are pump thrombosis requiring pump exchange and stroke. Methods for reducing device-related adverse events, particularly driveline infection, may prove to have a positive impact in reducing costs. Careful monitoring of outpatients and further development of shared-care resources may help to identify problems sooner, allowing for more effective diagnosis and treatment [54, 55].

57.2.1 Discussion

One of the past limitations for the use of LVADs was the requirement by protocol to implant these devices in the sickest patients whose chance of having a positive outcome was already limited. Since the commercialization of the continuous-flow LVAD, outcome measures have steadily improved while costs have remained fairly constant. Following clinical trials with the continuous-flow LVADs, there was a rapid expansion in the use of these devices worldwide. Indeed, some inexperienced centers had to pass through the "learning curve" before outcomes were at par with long-established centers where the clinical trials were conducted. Interestingly, centers without extensive experience in implanting LVADs can achieve excellent outcomes without high morbidity [56].

Early results from a HeartMate III clinical trial showed there were no instances of device exchange, pump thrombosis, or hemolysis [22]. With this reduction in adverse events, the HeartMate III may further reduce the cost of LVAD therapy. For patients who are ineligible for cardiac transplantation, this technology offers the clinician an increasingly cost-effective treatment option that prolongs survival and dramatically improves quality of life compared to traditional medical management. Progress made in device design and patient selection lowers cost and maximizes effectiveness of DT. With continued device-related improvements and clinical experience, LVAD implantation for DT will offer a cost-effective solution to heart failure patients ineligible for transplantation.

Published reports on LVAD therapy cost-effectiveness have come from the USA, United Kingdom, Italy, and Norway. Interpretation of the results in these studies must be done cautiously due to the considerable variability in the cost of delivering care and in the outcomes achieved. Larger controlled studies with well-defined methods are needed to better evaluate the cost-effectiveness of LVAD therapy. As LVAD technology improves and patient care experience progresses, better outcomes will be achieved at lower cost. Optimizing reimbursement requires a continuing assessment of this therapy.

57.3 Summary

Use of the LVAD for BTT and DT has evolved gradually, with results improving dramatically since these indications were first applied. Cost-effectiveness of LVAD therapy has progressed much, while further improvement is necessary to gain better acceptance from government agencies, third-party payers, and the general public. Clinical research must continue to further refine practices for reduced morbidity. Continued innovation by engineers should help to further refine device technology for optimizing biocompatibility and usability. Novel blood pump designs may offer improved biocompatibility, while clinicians must apply these devices in a cost-effective manner by selecting suitable candidates and employing standard practices.

References

1. Cooley DA, Liotta D, Hallman GL, Bloodwell RD, Leachman RD, Milam JD (1969) Orthotopic cardiac prosthesis for two-staged cardiac replacement. Am J Cardiol 24:723–730
2. DeBakey ME (1971) Left ventricular bypass pump for cardiac assistance. Clin Ex Am J Cardiol 27:3–11
3. Ratchford P (1968) Groote Schuur Hospital, Cape Town, The first human heart transplant operation. SA Nurs J 35:24–26
4. El-Banayosy A, Arusoglu L, Kizner L et al (2000) Novacor left ventricular assist system versus Heartmate vented electric left ventricular assist system as a long-term mechanical circulatory support device in bridging patients: a prospective study. J Thorac Cardiovasc Surg 119:581–587
5. Frazier OH, Rose EA, Oz MC et al (2001) Multicenter clinical evaluation of the HeartMate vented electric left ventricular assist system in patients awaiting heart transplantation. J Thorac Cardiovasc Surg 122:1186–1195
6. Farrar DJ, Lawson JH, Litwak P, Cederwall G (1990) Thoratec VAD system as a bridge to heart transplantation. J Heart Transplant 9:415–422; discussion 22–3
7. Rose EA, Moskowitz AJ, Packer M et al (1999) The REMATCH trial: rationale, design, and end points. Randomized evaluation of mechanical assistance for the treatment of congestive heart failure. Ann Thorac Surg 67:723–730
8. Rogers JG, Butler J, Lansman SL et al (2007) Chronic mechanical circulatory support for inotrope-dependent heart failure patients who are not transplant candidates: results of the INTrEPID Trial. J Am Coll Cardiol 50:741–747
9. Rose EA, Gelijns AC, Moskowitz AJ et al (2001) Long-term mechanical left ventricular assistance for end-stage heart failure. N Engl J Med 345:1435–1443
10. Long JW, Kfoury AG, Slaughter MS et al (2005) Long-term destination therapy with the HeartMate XVE left ventricular assist device: improved outcomes since the REMATCH study. Congest Heart Fail 11:133–138
11. Griffith BP, Kormos RL, Borovetz HS et al (2001) HeartMate II left ventricular assist system: from concept to first clinical use. Ann Thorac Surg 71:S116–20; discussion S4–6.
12. Frazier OH, Delgado RM 3rd, Kar B, Patel V, Gregoric ID, Myers TJ (2004) First clinical use of the redesigned HeartMate II left ventricular assist system in the United States: a case report. Tex Heart Inst J 31:157–159
13. Noon GP, Morley DL, Irwin S, Abdelsayed SV, Benkowski RJ, Lynch BE (2001) Clinical experience with the MicroMed DeBakey ventricular assist device. Ann Thorac Surg 71:S133–S138; discussion S44–6.
14. Struber M, Sander K, Lahpor J et al (2008) HeartMate II left ventricular assist device; early European experience. Eur J Cardiothorac Surg 34:289–294
15. Pagani FD, Miller LW, Russell SD et al (2009) Extended mechanical circulatory support with a continuous-flow rotary left ventricular assist device. J Am Coll Cardiol 54:312–321
16. Slaughter MS, Rogers JG, Milano CA et al (2009) Advanced heart failure treated with continuous-flow left ventricular assist device. N Engl J Med 361:2241–2251
17. Slaughter MS, Pagani FD, McGee EC et al (2013) HeartWare ventricular assist system for bridge to transplant: combined results of the bridge to transplant and continued access protocol trial. J Heart Lung Transplant 32:675–683
18. Stulak JM, Dunlay SM, Sharma S et al (2015) Treatment of device thrombus in the HeartWare HVAD: success and outcomes depend significantly on the initial treatment strategy. J Heart Lung Transplant 34:1535–1541

19. Stulak JM, Lee D, Haft JW et al (2014) Gastrointestinal bleeding and subsequent risk of thromboembolic events during support with a left ventricular assist device. J Heart Lung Transplant 33:60–64
20. Starling RC, Moazami N, Silvestry SC et al (2014) Unexpected abrupt increase in left ventricular assist device thrombosis. N Engl J Med 370:33–40
21. Schmitto JD, Hanke JS, Rojas SV, Avsar M, Haverich A (2015) First implantation in man of a new magnetically levitated left ventricular assist device (HeartMate III). J Heart Lung Transplant 34:858–860
22. Netuka I, Sood P, Pya Y et al (2015) Fully magnetically levitated left ventricular assist system for treating advanced HF: a multicenter study. J Am Coll Cardiol 66:2579–2589
23. Rogers JG, Aaronson KD, Boyle AJ et al (2010) Continuous flow left ventricular assist device improves functional capacity and quality of life of advanced heart failure patients. J Am Coll Cardiol 55:1826–1834
24. Starling RC (2010) Improved quantity and quality of life: a winning combination to treat advanced heart failure. J Am Coll Cardiol 55:1835–1836
25. Yancy CW, Jessup M, Bozkurt B et al (2013) 2013 ACCF/AHA guideline for the management of heart failure: a report of the American College of Cardiology Foundation/American Heart Association Task Force on Practice Guidelines. J Am Coll Cardiol 62(16):e147–e239
26. McMurray JJ, Adamopoulos S, Anker SD et al (2012) ESC guidelines for the diagnosis and treatment of acute and chronic heart failure 2012: the task force for the diagnosis and treatment of acute and chronic heart failure 2012 of the European Society of Cardiology. Developed in collaboration with the Heart Failure Association (HFA) of the ESC. Eur J Heart Fail 14:803–869
27. Morales DL, Catanese KA, Helman DN et al (2000) Six-year experience of caring for forty-four patients with a left ventricular assist device at home: safe, economical, necessary. J Thorac Cardiovasc Surg 119:251–259
28. Oz MC, Gelijns AC, Miller L et al. (2003) Left ventricular assist devices as permanent heart failure therapy: the price of progress. Ann Surg 238:577–583; discussion 83–5
29. Mishra V, Geiran O, Fiane AE et al (2010) Costs and reimbursement gaps after implementation of third-generation left ventricular assist devices. J Heart Lung Transplant 29:72–78
30. Digiorgi PL, Reel MS, Thornton B, Burton E, Naka Y, Oz MC (2005) Heart transplant and left ventricular assist device costs. J Heart Lung Transplant 24:200–204
31. Bostic RR (2005) Heart transplant and left ventricular assist device costs. J Heart Lung Transplant 24:1997–1998
32. Patel SR, Sileo A, Bello R, Gunda S, Nguyen J, Goldstein D (2015) Heart transplantation versus continuous-flow left ventricular assist device: comprehensive cost at 1 year. J Card Fail 21:160–166
33. Moreno SG, Novielli N, Cooper NJ (2012) Cost-effectiveness of the implantable HeartMate II left ventricular assist device for patients awaiting heart transplantation. J Heart Lung Transplant 31:450–458
34. Miller LW, Nelson KE, Bostic RR, Tong K, Slaughter MS, Long JW (2006) Hospital costs for left ventricular assist devices for destination therapy: lower costs for implantation in the post-REMATCH era. J Heart Lung Transplant 25:778–784
35. Russo MJ, Gelijns AC, Stevenson LW et al (2008) The cost of medical management in advanced heart failure during the final two years of life. J Card Fail 14:651–658
36. Slaughter MS, Bostic R, Tong K, Russo M, Rogers JG (2011) Temporal changes in hospital costs for left ventricular assist device implantation. J Card Surg 26:535–541
37. Sutcliffe P, Connock M, Pulikottil-Jacob R et al. (2013) Clinical effectiveness and cost-effectiveness of second- and third-generation left ventricular assist devices as either bridge to transplant or alternative to transplant for adults eligible for heart transplantation: systematic review and cost-effectiveness model. Health Technol Assess 17:1–499, v–vi
38. Rogers JG, Bostic RR, Tong KB, Adamson R, Russo M, Slaughter MS (2012) Cost-effectiveness analysis of continuous-flow left ventricular assist devices as destination therapy. Circ Heart Fail 5:10–16
39. Clegg AJ, Scott DA, Loveman E et al. (2005) The clinical and cost-effectiveness of left ventricular assist devices for end-stage heart failure: a systematic review and economic evaluation. Health Technol Assess 9:1–132, iii–iv
40. Sharples LD, Dyer M, Cafferty F et al (2006) Cost-effectiveness of ventricular assist device use in the United Kingdom: results from the evaluation of ventricular assist device programme in the UK (EVAD-UK). J Heart Lung Transplant 25:1336–1343
41. Rohde LE, Bertoldi EG, Goldraich L, Polanczyk CA (2013) Cost-effectiveness of heart failure therapies. Nat Rev Cardiol 10:338–354
42. Uriel N, Adatya S, Mehra MR (2015) Evolution in mechanical circulatory support: are we at the precipice of a disruptive innovation? J Am Coll Cardiol 66:2590–2593
43. Miller LW, Pagani FD, Russell SD et al (2007) Use of a continuous-flow device in patients awaiting heart transplantation. N Engl J Med 357:885–896
44. Jorde UP, Kushwaha SS, Tatooles AJ et al (2014) Results of the destination therapy post-food and drug administration approval study with a continuous flow left ventricular assist device: a prospective study using the INTERMACS registry (Interagency Registry for Mechanically Assisted Circulatory Support). J Am Coll Cardiol 63:1751–1757
45. Pagani FD (2016) Adverse event burden and mechanical circulatory support: looking toward the future. J Thorac Cardiovasc Surg 151:10–12
46. Pulikottil-Jacob R, Suri G, Connock M et al (2014) Comparative cost-effectiveness of the HeartWare versus HeartMate II left ventricular assist devices used in the United Kingdom National Health Service bridge-to-transplant program for patients with heart failure. J Heart Lung Transplant 33(4):350–358
47. Shah N, Agarwal V, Patel N et al (2016) National trends in utilization, mortality, complications, and cost of

care after left ventricular assist device implantation from 2005 to 2011. Ann Thorac Surg 101(4):1477–1484
48. Gelijns AC, Russo MJ, Hong KN, Brown LD, Ascheim DD, Moskowitz AJ (2013) Dynamics of device innovation: implications for assessing value. Int J Technol Assess Health Care 29:365–373
49. Long EF, Swain GW, Mangi AA (2014) Comparative survival and cost effectiveness of advanced therapies for end-stage heart failure. Circ Heart Fail 7(3):470–478
50. Patel SR, Sileo A, Bello R, Gunda S, Nguyen J, Goldstein D (2014) Heart transplantation vs continuous flow LVAD: comprehensive cost at one year. J Card Fail 21(2):160–166
51. Droogne W, Jacobs S, Van den Bossche K et al (2014) Cost of 1-year left ventricular assist device destination therapy in chronic heart failure: a comparison with heart transplantation. Acta Clin Belg 69:165–170
52. Neyt M, Van den Bruel A, Smit Y et al (2013) Cost-effectiveness of continuous-flow left ventricular assist devices. Int J Technol Assess Health Care 29: 254–260
53. Akhter SA, Badami A, Murray M et al (2015) Hospital readmissions after continuous-flow left ventricular assist device implantation: incidence, causes, and cost analysis. Ann Thorac Surg 100(3):884–889
54. Estep JD, Trachtenberg BH, Loza LP, Bruckner BA (2015) Continuous flow left ventricular assist devices: shared care goals of monitoring and treating patients. Methodist Debakey Cardiovasc J 11:33–44
55. Kiernan MS, Joseph SM, Katz JN et al (2015) Sharing the care of mechanical circulatory support: collaborative efforts of patients/caregivers, shared-care sites, and left ventricular assist device implanting centers. Circ Heart Fail 8:629–635
56. Katz MR, Dickinson MG, Raval NY et al (2015) Outcomes of patients implanted with a left ventricular assist device at nontransplant mechanical circulatory support centers. Am J Cardiol 115:1254–1259

Registries Perspectives

Content

The EUROMACS Registry of Patients Who Receive Mechanical Circulatory Support: Role and Perspectives

Theo M.M.H. de By, Evaristo Castedo, Thomas Krabatsch, Paul Mohacsi, Bart P. Meyns, Ivan Netuka, Jan Gummert, and On behalf of all EUROMACS members and contributors

© Springer International Publishing Switzerland 2017
A. Montalto et al. (eds.), *Mechanical Circulatory Support in End-Stage Heart Failure*,
DOI 10.1007/978-3-319-43383-7_58

58.1 Introduction

Considering the technological developments in mechanical circulatory support (MCS) for patients with end-stage heart failure, no clinician would doubt the need to register the events and data emerging from the application of this therapy.

Information about the events in individual patients, as well as the statistical evaluation of different groups of patients and the information about the functioning of devices over time, they can learn a lot about the safety of the applied therapy, freedom of adverse events, and survival. Such data lead to adaptation of clinical practice based on the registered outcomes and may result in new possibilities for improvement and/or in technical innovation. Physicians may use data for patient selection and the development of bespoke treatment strategies. Moreover, based on these data, the information to patients and their next of kin about the expected outcomes of MCS therapy may become more accurate.

The database offers individual hospitals a tool for benchmarking, while researchers may correlate data to gain science-based insights and define factors which influence patient care and outcomes.

The registry enables other stakeholders, such as the industry that produces the devices, to use data to initiate innovations and to measure the results of those.

58.2 Retrospective

As history shows, local registries, frequently developed by the treating physician(s) or their in-hospital ICT departments, became the source for professionals to demonstrate their local achievements.

Then, those who think big, and rightly so, develop initiatives to gather data on a larger geographical scale. While in the USA hospitals were obliged to provide data to INTERMACS, the Europeans created a voluntary registry, called EUROMACS, which connects with local and national databases. After an initiative of Prof. Roland Hetzer, in 2009, EUROMACS was founded as a nonprofit association which functions as a Committee of the European Association for Cardio-Thoracic Surgery. Forty-eight hospitals from 18 countries have now joined, and another 19 are taking steps to follow. The difference between EUROMACS and other registries is that EUROMACS provides data to professionals who wish to carry out clinical and/or scientific analyses. Further, data completeness checks by statisticians and on-site audits add to the quality of the data. The development of a near real-time dashboard will enable the participating sites to benchmark their outcomes by comparison with the anonymous data of the other hospitals.

For reasons of different regulatory environments and spans of control, an agreement with the IMACS Registry sees to the provision of data on a global level. Thus, we have connected the world of MCS from the ground up, from local to global, expecting that the clinical and scientific data will enable us to learn how to improve the care of patients with end-stage heart failure.

58.3 EUROMACS Organization

58.3.1 Structure

As a committee of the EACTS, EUROMACS is democratically structured. Members of the executive board, which have maximal five members, are elected by the members for a period of 3 years with a possibility to be re-elected for another 3 years. The extended board has a maximum of seven members and serves to reflect the diversity in nationalities of participants in the Registry. Extended board members are also chosen for a period of maximal 3 years, twice. While the executive board sees to the execution of the aims of the organization, the extended board approves the strategic planning, the annual report, and the financial report before it is sent to the members.

The executive board decided to appoint a managing director who manages the day-to-day business of the organization and facilitates the work of the board.

58.3.2 Providing Data to Clinicians and Scientists

The first aim of the EUROMACS Registry is to provide data to the community of clinicians and scientists.

1. On a regular basis (annual report)
2. Via the EUROMACS dashboard, after log-in
3. For scientific studies
4. Bespoke, e.g., for (national) statistics and for use on congresses

The first annual report was published in March 2015 [1]. The second report is expected in the spring of 2017.

Contributors of data, after they entered the EUROMACS Registry by means of their password, will immediately see the possibility to open a dashboard with statistics. These statistics not only provide general information about the number of cases in the registry, it also shows comparisons between the data from the hospital of the user with the entire EUROMACS database.

Further, any clinician or scientist can submit a study proposal to the EUROMACS committee and request anonymous data from the Registry. The applicant is asked to agree to use the data for the sole purpose of the study they were asked for. The data from EUROMACS were used for several studies and publications [2].

58.3.3 Collection of Data

A hospital that wishes to participate in the EUROMACS Registry is offered an agreement in which it accepts to provide pseudonymized baseline and follow-up data to the registry. A unique password allows the responsible physician and/or data manager to enter patient records and events. Three methods are at the disposal of the participants:

(a) Submitting the data patient per patient. This method is appropriate for hospitals which have a relatively low number of implants per year.
(b) Uploading from the local database. This method fits hospitals which historically have a local database in which they register the details of the treatment of MCS patients. The advantage is that uploading these data avoids double data entry.
(c) Regular data transfer from a national database, by means of a unique secure link, to EUROMACS.

The EUROMACS data set consists of several groups:

- Baseline data such as sex, age, primary diagnosis, laboratory data, and blood circulation data before MCS implantation. The number of mandatory data is limited to seven.
- Quality of life data (EQ. 5D).
- Perioperative data.
- Any event after the implantation. A distinction is made between major events and others, while routine follow-up is registered when the patient has come in for a checkup. The number of mandatory data is six.

The hospitals participating in the EUROMACS Registry have agreed to register events within 6 weeks after their occurrence. Every 6 months, as per June 30 and per December 31, they are asked to confirm that their data are up-to-date. The EUROMACS management offers them an overview of their patients and, if this would be the case, a breakdown of missing data. After completion and correction, the data are consolidated; from then on, they can be made available for analyses and studies.

58.3.4 Quality Control

Quality control, as referred to in the previous paragraph, consists of the statistical analysis of the data submitted by the participating centers. An overview of missing or inconsistent data is provided to the centers every 6 months. If data would be faulty, or missing, the centers are invited to correct the noncompliance.

On-site audits are a second instrument to guarantee that data collection and registration in the database reflects the reality in the participating clinics.

58.3.5 Global Cooperation

In 2013, EUROMACS and IMACS signed an agreement. The agreement sees to an annual anonymous data transfer from EUROMACS to IMACS. Whereas IMACS function is to gather data on MCS implants on a global level, EUROMACS focuses on information from hospitals in countries that are geographically, partly, or entirely on the European continent.

The first IMACS report was published in early 2016, in *The Journal for Heart and Lung Transplantation* [3].

58.3.6 Outcomes

◘ Figure 58.1 shows the result of all MCS implantations, registered in EUROMACS, in which the overall actuarial survival outcomes of 2850

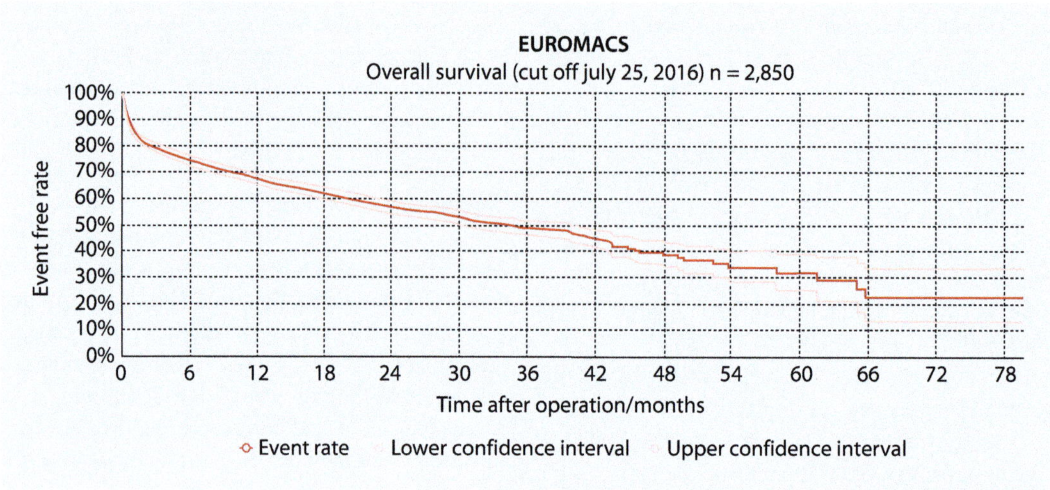

Fig. 58.1 Kaplan Myer analysis: overall survival of all MCS devices

Table 58.1 INTERMACS levels of 2172 VAD implantations

INTERMACS level	*n*	%
Critical cardiogenic shock	383	13.4
Progressive decline	879	30.8
Stable but inotrope dependent	697	24.5
Resting symptoms	509	17.8
Exertion intolerant	88	3.1
Exertion limited	37	1.3
Advanced NYHA class III	33	1.2
Unspecified	224	7.9
Total (%)	2850	100.0

NYHA New York Heart Association

primary implantations of all MCS implantations thru July 25, 2016.

The overall actuarial survival of 2850 patients receiving a primary implantation with a MCS device at 6 months, 1, 2, 3, and 4 years is respectively 73.7%, 66.5%, 56.2%, 48.4%, and 38.4%. Patients at risk are 488 (2 years), 178 (3 years), and 45 (4 years).

Table 58.1 provides a breakdown of the INTERMACS levels of the MCS patients in the EUROMACS registry.

The EUROMACS database shows that 55.3% of patients with MCS were in INTERMACS levels 2 and 3, whereas the seventh INTERMACS report showed a total of 55.7% of patients on these two levels [4].

Likewise, in comparison with the fifth INTERMACS report, wherein 19.7% of patients were in critical cardiogenic shock at the time of implantation, the EUROMACS database showed only 13.4% of patients in this category.

58.4 Perspective

Until the mid-2016, 48 hospitals from 18 countries contributed to the EUROMACS Registry. The registered implantations exceeded 2800, while the number of registered routine follow-up records and "events," such as transplantations, adverse events, pump exchange, and death, was more than 10,700. In the spring of 2016, a connection with the national MCS registry of Spain, Espamacs, could be established. Thus, participants in Espamacs have access to data on a European level. This access enables them to benchmark their results, as well as a possibility to retrieve data for scientific and/or clinical analyses.

As more individual hospitals and national databases such as the French, the Polish, and the Dutch join the Registry, it is expected that the number of registered implantations will be more than 4000 by 2017.

Starting in the summer of 2016, software to execute additional statistical analyses, such as frequency of follow-up, "near real-time" benchmarking of survival statistics, and freedom of adverse event comparisons will be introduced.

As part of the EACTS, the EUROMACS Registry will be able to benefit from the technology which is being developed within the framework of the EACTS QUIP project. This technology will open up new statistical pathways and interactive tools which enable, e.g., risk assessment, and create possibilities for participants to diversify their benchmarking according to patient morbidity, implant site, and size of the MCS program.

58.5 Conclusion

The EUROMACS database provides a multifunctional tool for cardio-thoracic surgeons, cardiologists, and other professionals who are engaged with providing care to patients with MCS. Registration in itself gives insight in the quantitative aspects of the therapy. While some hospitals use EUROMACS to keep track of their own implantations and follow-up, others have the objective to compare their outcomes with those of all participating centers. Likewise, national societies, such as the Spanish SECTCV, or the French SFCTCV, may use EUROMACS as a national database enabling measuring of the performance of all MCS programs in the country either individually or collectively. The link with EUROMACS and, on its turn, the links with the EACTS and IMACS enable all participants to use software and data with which they can benchmark themselves. The tools offered make it possible to identify strengths and weaknesses of the outcomes per hospital, or from a group of hospitals (if all those in that group agree), and to focus on improvements where necessary. It is expected that, over time, the available data will contribute to beneficial results for patients with MCS.

References

1. De By TMMH, Mohacsi P, Gummert J, Bushnaq H, Krabatsch T, Gustafsson F et al (2015) The European Registry for Patients with Mechanical Circulatory Support (EUROMACS): first annual report. Eur J Cardiothorac Surg. doi:10.1093/ejcts/ezv096
2. Bernhardt AM, De By TM, Reichenspurner H, Deuse T (2015) Isolated permanent right ventricular assist device implantation with the HeartWare continuous-flow ventricular assist device: first results from the European Registry for Patients with Mechanical Circulatory Support. Eur J Cardiothorac Surg 48(1):158–162. doi:10.1093/ejcts/ezu406
3. Kirklin JK, Cantor R, Mohacsi P, Gummert J, De By T, Hannan MM, Kormos RL, Schueler S, Lund LH, Nakatani T, Taylor R, Lannon J (2016) First annual IMACS report: a global ISHLT registry for mechanical circulatory support. J Heart Lung Transplant 35(4):407–412. http://dx.doi.org/10.1016/j.healun.2016.01.002
4. Kirklin JK, Naftel DC, Pagani FD, Kormos RL et al (2015) Seventh Intermacs annual report: 15,000 patients and counting. J Heart Lung Transplant 34:1495–1504

Service Part

© Springer International Publishing Switzerland 2017
A. Montalto et al. (eds.), *Mechanical Circulatory Support in End-Stage Heart Failure*,
DOI 10.1007/978-3-319-43383-7

Telemonitoring and Teleconsultation

The implant of a VAD is an economically costly answer for the treatment of advanced heart failure, which usually requires prolonged hospitalization and chronic drug treatments. Patients with an implantable VAD can be discharged and can be managed at home through an integrated hub-and-spoke model, requiring intensive cooperation between the reference center and peripheral structures. In this setting, a remote monitoring system using mobile telecommunication technology is crucial.

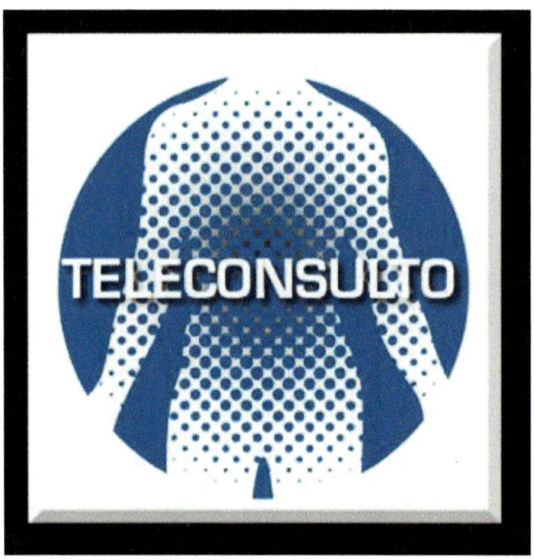

Fig. 1 Project logo

Our Institution has developed a Web application to offer 24 h healthcare and monitoring of outpatients with an implantable ventricular assist device (VAD) (Fig. 1).

The remote monitoring system allows an active control with the use of a tablet, which is provided to all patients at the time of their hospital discharge, through an innovative and functional interface, capable of exchanging clinical, laboratory, and instrumental data between the patient and a round-the-clock active consultation help center.

Specifically, a dedicated software application has been created for the detection and transmission of VAD-related health data and VAD monitoring. The application is a cross-platform one and can be downloaded on every PC, tablet, or smartphone and is easily accessible ("red heart" icon on the home page on the given tablet) (Fig. 2). This experimental telemonitoring and teleconsultation project is integrated with the creation of a dedicated website to collect real-time informations.

This system plays a two-way role: it makes possible for our institution to strictly follow the discharged patients and, on the other hand, allows patients and caregivers to easily and readily find an answer to any clinical problem.

Fig. 2 Program interface

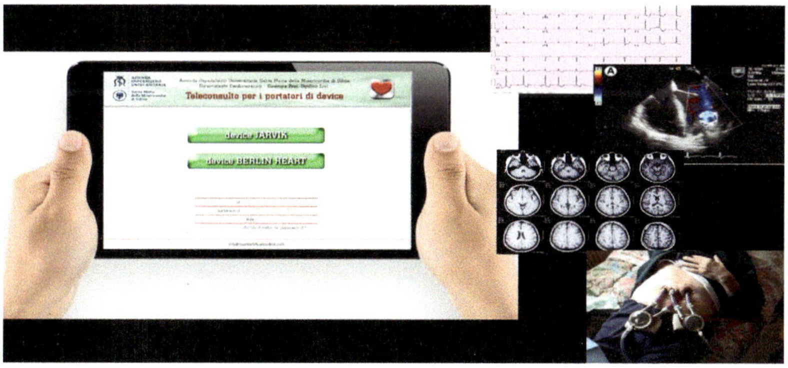

◘ Fig. 3 Possibility to send pictures and videoclips

In particular, the application consists of virtual modules which have to be filled in a simple and guided manner with a series of data regarding clinical status, anticoagulation, eventual problems, and so on. Also, it permits the uploading of high-definition pictures and video (e.g., clinical exams from other institutions, exit site of the device cable, etc.) allowing our center to follow these patients remotely. The system requires the use of passwords and usernames, in compliance with current privacy regulations (◘ Fig. 3).

The tablet is also equipped with an application that provides video chat and voice call services, through which patients and/or caregivers can reach our center (and vice versa) allowing the real-time sharing of the patient's problems, thus optimizing the opportunity of global management of the patient's problems. This system proved to be useful also as immediate support to less experienced clinicians who are facing emergency situations arising in such complex and particular patients.

The benefits of this monitoring are expressed in ensuring the non-hospital/home continuity of care of patients with VAD, with an early identification of problems related to them and thus in a more rapid activation for their resolution with a significant reduction in the patient's hospital accesses. Also there was a positive feedback by patients, who feel part of an integrated care pathway that revolves around their care and well-being, both from a clinical and social point of view. This application contains costs, by reducing the number of outpatients' examinations, unnecessary hospitalizations, and instrumental and laboratory tests, while making procedures more appropriate.

This heart remote assistance system improves the quality of life of patients by avoiding trips at risk of complications and problems for patients and families, while cutting down on overall costs.

The usefulness of this telemonitoring and teleconsultation system relies on a dedicated ambulatory, with a cardiac surgeon and a VAD coordinator guaranteeing round-the-clock availability. This setting is innovative in our national panorama.

All patients are requested to send instrumental, clinical, and physiological data twice a week. Individual interviews through the video chat are offered by our dedicated psychologist. Our VAD coordinator has the following tasks: daily telephone contacts with patients, monitoring the anticoagulation regimen, early identification of possible complications, and taking action to resolve them promptly if necessary. The cardiac surgeon doses the anticoagulation drug and is on call if needed. The "Teleconsulto" project started in November 2011, and since then, approximately 1.367 teleconsultations have been activated, with a solution found in 85% of cases within 45 min.

Our experience has shown us that this monitoring and management system delivers amazing results in terms of perceived safety, reduced anxiety, hospitalization rate, and clinical problem solving. Furthermore, it provided an overall improvement in the patients and the families' quality of life.